INFECTIOUS DISEASE EPIDEMIOLOGY

Oleksandr Hruzevskyi

ALLIED
HEALTH
PRESS

Infectious Disease Epidemiology

Author: **Oleksandr Hruzevskyi**

Allied Health Press
4164 Lakeshore Road
Burlington ON L7L 1A4
Canada
www.alliedhealthpress.com
Email: orders@arclereducation.com

ISBN: 978-1-77956-830-4

ABOUT THE AUTHOR

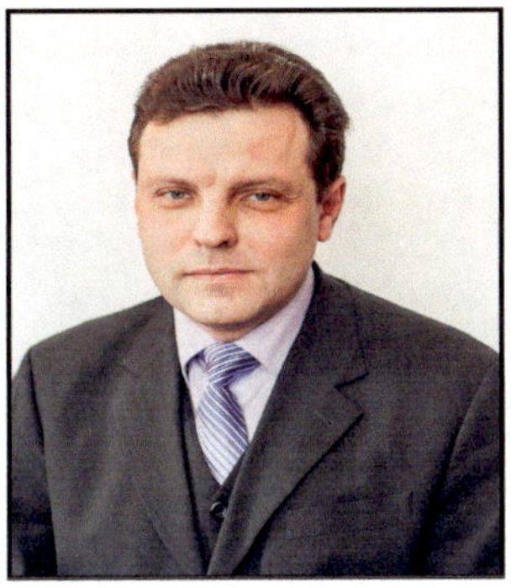

Oleksandr Hruzevskyi, MD, PhD, Doctor of Medicine, is a Professor at the Department of General and Clinical Epidemiology and Biosafety with a course on Microbiology and Virology at Odesa National Medical University. Dr. Hruzevskyi received his MD in 1996 (Diploma with Honors) from Odesa State Medical University, Ukraine, and subsequently defended his PhD (Candidate's Dissertation) in Microbiology in 2000 at the Research Institute of Microbiology and Immunology named after E.E. Metchnikoff (Kharkiv, Ukraine). In 2021, he was awarded the degree of Doctor of Medicine in Microbiology at the State Institution "Research Institute of Microbiology and Immunology named after E.E. Metchnikoff" of the National Academy of Sciences (Kharkiv, Ukraine), with certification as a Bacteriologist from the Kharkiv Academy of Postgraduate Studies. Dr. Hruzevskyi began his career as a sanitary worker at the Emergency Hospital in Mykolaiv, Ukraine, before working as a laboratory assistant at the Laboratory of Microbiology of the Odesa Institute of Clinical Biochemistry and Animal Sanitation. He completed his postgraduate studies at the Department of Microbiology, Virology and Immunology at Odesa State Medical University, where he later served as assistant professor, associate professor, acting head, and head of the department. Since 2022, he has been a professor at the Department of General and Clinical Epidemiology and Biosafety with a course on Microbiology and Virology at Odesa National Medical University.

His professional activities include teaching microbiology, virology, and immunology to students and postgraduates in Ukrainian, Russian, and English, developing and updating methodological materials, and conducting experimental scientific research and data analysis. Dr. Hruzevskyi is a member of the Trade Union of Health Professionals. His research interests focus on bacteriology, clinical microbiology, and the development of innovative diagnostic methods.

Brief Table of Contents

Detailed Table of Contents

CHAPTER 5

Surveillance and Monitoring of Infectious Diseases 145

CHAPTER 6

Infectious Disease Control Strategies 179

CHAPTER 12

Antimicrobial Resistance and Public Health 379

CHAPTER 13

Ethical Considerations in Infectious Disease Epidemiology 411

LIST OF FIGURES

PREFACE

Over the recent decades, the study of the mechanisms by which pathogens propagate across populations has become an urgent and rapidly evolving field of public health research. Understanding the patterns of infection dynamics, determinants of transmission, and their implications for individuals and populations is paramount to disease prevention and saving lives. This field combines information from biology, statistics, the social sciences, and policy analysis within an integrated framework for quantifying disease risk. Through the study of historical epidemics, combined with current surveillance data, researchers gain the ability to identify emerging threats and assess the efficacy of prevention efforts.

This corpus of research aims to answer key questions: What mechanisms and causes result in the occurrence of infection in a population? What environmental, behavioural, and biological factors influence the trajectory of an outbreak? What interventions result in the most significant benefits, and how can finite resources be allocated most effectively? These questions necessitate the employment of integrated methods—ranging from mathematical modelling and laboratory investigation to community-based research and health system analysis. Data generated not only inform public health policy but also enhance clinical practice, support global health initiatives, and inform international regulations aimed at protecting populations from both identified and emerging pathogens.

This book, *Infectious Disease Epidemiology*, aims to be a transparent, extensive, and cohesive description of the concepts, methods, and applications that characterise the discipline today. Consisting of contributions from a variety of distinguished researchers and practitioners, it integrates underlying theory with descriptive examples. To be read as a primary textbook by advanced students, a reference book for public health professionals, or a manual for multidisciplinary research groups, the book provides the depth and breadth necessary to meet the challenges posed by infectious agents in the 21st century.

Chapter 1 presents a perspective on the discipline of infectious disease epidemiology, from its origins in early observational studies to the current global networks that facilitate real-time surveillance of outbreaks. Chapter 2 covers the fundamental principles of epidemiology, including measures of disease prevalence, study designs, methods for reducing bias, and data analysis. In Chapter 3, readers will observe microbial pathogenesis and host response, considering the biological pathways by which pathogens invade, grow, and interact with immune systems. Chapter 4 discusses the mechanisms of infection transmission—that is, direct contact, airborne droplets, and vectors—and factors such as seasonality, population density, and human mobility that influence transmission patterns.

Building on this foundation, Chapter 5 discusses surveillance and monitoring systems, including sentinel networks, laboratory reporting, syndromic surveillance, and digital disease detection. Chapter 6 discusses the evaluation of control measures, focusing on the functions of case isolation, quarantine, mass drug administration, vector control, and non-pharmaceutical interventions (NPIs). Chapter 7 highlights new and re-emerging infections, and how globalisation, environmental change, and microbial evolution drive new threats and re-map the geography of disease.

Chapter 8 presents in-depth epidemiological profiles of prevalent infections, including respiratory viruses, foodborne pathogens, sexually transmitted diseases, and hospital-acquired pathogens, with case studies illustrating central principles in various settings. Chapter 9 covers vaccines and immunization programs, including design, delivery, coverage assessment, and how to overcome hesitancy. Chapter 10 situates infectious disease in the global health arena, covering international health regulations (IHR), cross-national cooperation, and the effect of socioeconomic inequality on disease burden.

Chapter 11 introduces risk assessment and mathematical modelling as methods for predicting outbreak evolution, assessing the effect of potential interventions, and guiding policy in conditions of uncertainty. Chapter 12 addresses antimicrobial resistance (AMR) and public health concerns, including resistance mechanisms, stewardship activities, and the therapeutic pipeline. Chapter 13 discusses ethical challenges, including balancing the rights of the individual with protection of communities, obtaining informed consent in investigation, and ensuring equity in resource allocation.

Chapter 14 discusses social and behavioural determinants such as the impact of cultural practices, risk perception, communication styles, and community involvement on disease control measures. Chapter 15 discusses health systems and their contributions to prevention, detection, and response, as well as infrastructure, workforce capacity, and integrated public health and clinical services.

This text is intended for graduate-level students in public health, medicine, veterinary medicine, and related fields; epidemiologists and biostatisticians seeking a general reference; clinicians and laboratory researchers interested in the population implications of infections; and policymakers and program managers responsible for designing and implementing control programs. Practitioners in government, nongovernmental, and international agencies will encounter relevant insights applicable to surveillance, outbreak control, and health system strengthening. Through the integration of theoretical frameworks and practical applications, this text provides readers with the knowledge and skills to tackle contemporary challenges and to create more effective defences against emerging threats.

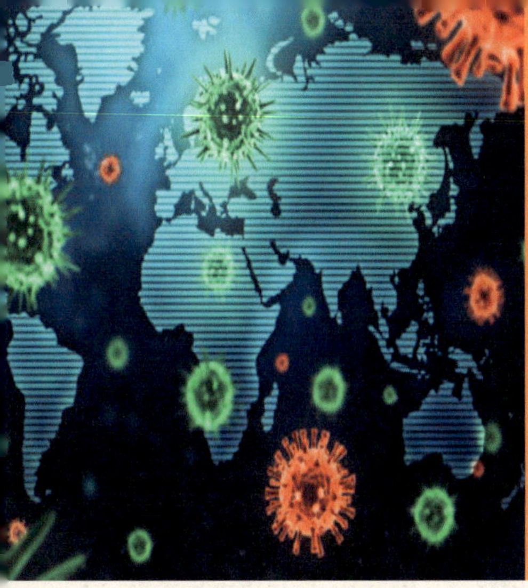

Chapter 1

INTRODUCTION TO INFECTIOUS DISEASE EPIDEMIOLOGY

Contents

Introduction

Infectious disease epidemiology is a fundamental field of epidemiology that involves the spread, determinants, and outcome of infectious diseases within populations in particular. Infectious disease epidemiology combines the biological and social sciences to explain how factors such as pathogen attributes, host attributes, and environmental factors contribute to disease transmission and progression. Understanding the dynamics of infectious diseases is crucial for designing effective public health interventions, surveillance, and response to outbreaks. By embracing a holistic approach symbolized by the epidemiological triad—agent, host, and environment—scientists are in a position to account for the complex interactions that lead to infectious disease emergence, transmission, and control (Iqbal, 2024). With changing public health conditions, the results emerging from infectious disease epidemiology are crucial to maintaining population health. One of the key aspects of infectious disease epidemiology is the ability to track multiple infectious diseases with distinct modes of transmission and population effects. For instance, infectious diseases such as tuberculosis or measles have unique epidemiological concerns, depending on their modes of transmission and their impact on public health in the past. The natural course of infections, that is, the progression from exposure to resolution or chronic disease, is required for the development of preventive and therapeutic strategies (Iqbal, 2024). Furthermore, recent worldwide health emergencies have highlighted the emergence of new diseases, which have encouraged more epidemiological research. Infectious disease epidemiology evolves as new knowledge and disease outbreaks emerge, thereby playing a crucial role in informing public health decisions. Digital tools have increased the ability of infectious disease epidemiology to gather and analyze data. It uses both organized and unorganized data from various sources to help track and respond to threats from infectious diseases as they happen. Remarkably, this was overhauled fundamentally during the COVID-19 pandemic, highlighting the intersection of technology and epidemiology in addressing new health challenges.

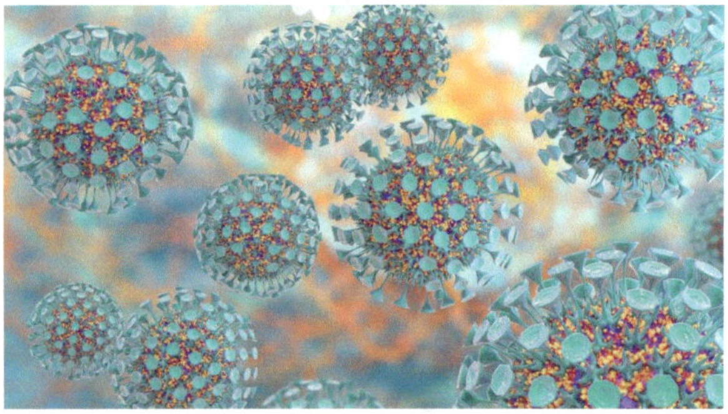

Figure 1.1. Infectious disease epidemiology.

Source: https://online.stanford.edu/sites/default/files/styles/figure_default/public/2020-08/Epidemiology-of-Infectious-Diseases_EPI231.jpg?itok=xkmJLZtE.

Incorporating digital data into mainstream epidemiological practice enhances the explanation of disease patterns, risk determinants, and population behavior and ultimately informs health policy and intervention planning. This thus signifies a new landscape of infectious disease epidemiology, enhanced by information technology, characterized by a resolve to address prevailing and emerging challenges adequately (Figure 1.1).

Explanation of Epidemiology

Epidemiology is a core field in public health that primarily focuses on the distribution and determinants of health-related states or events in defined populations. Epidemiology focuses on patterns of disease occurrence and their determinants, enabling policymakers to plan effective disease prevention and control strategies. Knowledge of how diseases are transmitted, who becomes infected, and why some groups become infected more easily than others enables epidemiologists to design interventions specific to a given context. The field encompasses several methodologies, utilising statistical analysis and data interpretation to draw conclusions about health trends over time. As the GBD, Injuries, and Risk Factors Study demonstrates, estimation of cause-specific mortality and morbidity is essential to identify the changing trends in health and disease in various regions, giving a distinct picture of public health trends and their inference on healthcare policy and resource allocation (Roth et al., 2018). The contribution of epidemiology extends beyond descriptive analyses, as it also involves identifying risk factors and implementing preventive interventions. Through the exploration of the complex determinants of health, such as environmental, behavioural, and genetic determinants, epidemiologists can design precise health interventions that address the aetiology of illnesses. Additionally, integration of epidemiological data with surveillance systems improves the capability of health agencies to respond effectively to new infectious diseases (EIDs). As noted in the European Society of Cardiology (ESC) guidelines, strict compliance to procedures and continuous screening, based on epidemiological research, is needed for effective healthcare policy (Adler et al., 2015). Ultimately, the integration of epidemiological information into public health practice enables communities to mitigate the impact of infectious diseases by promoting informed lifestyles, boosting vaccination rates, and enhancing overall health literacy. In addition, epidemiological data analysis encourages the appreciation of the intricate interplay between health and social factors. Sociodemographic factors like age, sex, socioeconomic status (SES), and geography have a significant impact on disease patterns and outcomes, underlining the need for an integrated strategy in epidemiological studies. Through such a framework, health inequities can be assessed well, and it helps design policies that address systemic inequalities and promote health equity. With data spanning many years, epidemiologists study trends that inform both local and global health policies, ultimately leading to lasting improvements in public health. Further, the reliance on continuous monitoring and evaluation of health trends serves to keep epidemiology as a dynamic science, adaptable to shifting society, healthcare services, and new infectious diseases (Roth et al., 2018). This way, epidemiology becomes central to public health because measures are based on evidence and address the details of disease transmission.

Importance of Studying Infectious Diseases

Infectious disease epidemiology is crucial for designing beneficial public health interventions and policies. With cross-country interactions increasing, so does the risk of pandemics and outbreaks, and thus, the study of infectious diseases becomes more relevant. Through analysing the dynamics of the transmission of the disease, the risk factors, and implications, epidemiologists can implement preventive interventions, allocate resources optimally, and safeguard vulnerable populations. Epidemiology models can estimate the spread of infectious diseases, so that early action can be taken against possible threats. Investigating these diseases benefits medical experts and helps policymakers understand the economic effects and health disparities between communities, leading to a more effective public health system. In addition, it is essential to study the connection between environmental factors and infectious diseases. For example, human microparasites are influenced by temperature and rainfall, but the details of these influences are still unclear. Experiments involving environmental variables in mathematical models can allow for improved modelling of disease transmission, for example, in schistosomiasis, in which there are several ecological stages which are part of the parasite lifecycle. With the integration of real-world environmental dynamics, researchers can design more targeted interventions for disease transmission control and improve health outcomes in diverse settings (Remais et al., 2010). Interdisciplinary approaches are essential for formulating comprehensive disease prevention and control strategies. Finally, infectious disease research extends beyond pressing public health concerns; it significantly advances knowledge of human behaviours and social patterns. For instance, virtual pandemics within Massively Multiplayer Online Games (MMOG) provide a helpful window of observation from which social interactions may be examined based on their effects on disease transmission. By applying epidemiological methods to these virtual worlds, game developers can learn about behaviour-influencing characteristics that have the potential to mirror genuine infectious disease patterns. This new method not only enhances the process of gaming but also the broader field of epidemiology by concluding contagion and intervention behaviors (Boman et al., 2007). This interdisciplinary approach works to highlight the importance of investigating infectious diseases, to bring attention to the influence of human behavior on the outcome, and to inform effective disease control interventions (Figure 1.2).

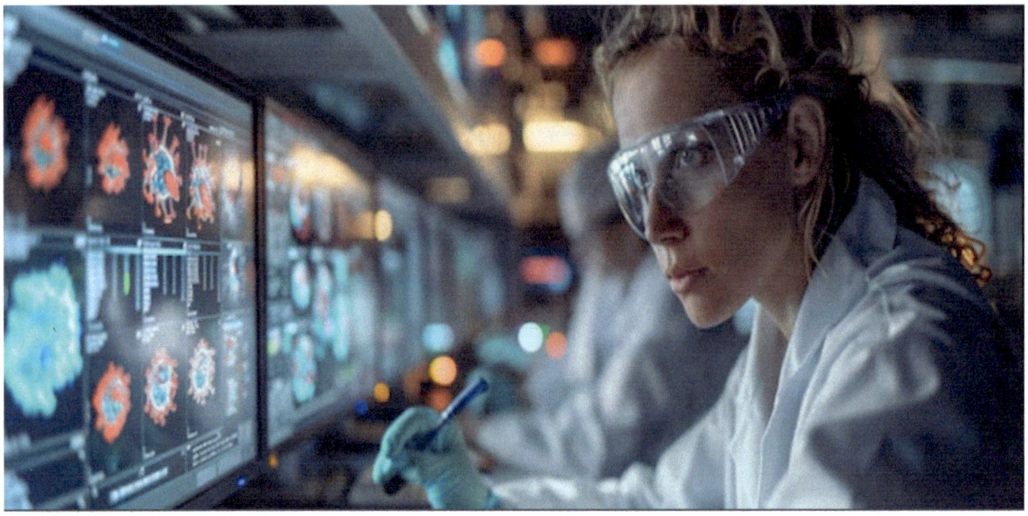

Figure 1.2. Studying infectious diseases.

Source: https://img.freepik.com/premium-photo/infectious-disease-specialist-studying-pathogens-wallpaper_987764-12241.jpg.

Key Terms and Concepts in Infectious Disease Epidemiology

Infectious disease epidemiology encompasses a collection of key terms and ideas that one needs to understand to grasp how infections become transmitted and controlled in populations. A key concept is distinguishing between incidence and prevalence, as both provide valuable details about how a disease spreads. Incidence refers to the number of new cases that develop within a specific time span, whereas prevalence is the total number of cases, both new and old, found in a population at any given time. Public health administrators need it to ascertain the effects of interventions and optimize resource allocation. Besides, the risk factor theory—behavioural, environmental, and biological—allows epidemiologists to identify at-risk groups for infection, thus guiding specific prevention strategies and health policies to curb the spread of disease. Transmission dynamics of pathogens is another significant term utilised in infectious disease epidemiology, in which one investigates how the diseases are transmitted from individual to individual or through vectors and the environment. Pathogen virulence, host immunity, and population density also affect the dynamics of transmission. Some pathogens can reproduce rapidly, making them more likely to infect susceptible individuals. Asymptomatic carriers can spread infections without knowing it, which makes it much harder to control outbreaks. Predictive modelling in these situations helps explain possible outbreaks and guides public health actions. When epidemiologists know these principles, they can design ways to prevent infectious diseases from spreading and lessen their effect on society. Finally, antimicrobial resistance (AMR) poses a significant challenge to the epidemiology of contagious diseases, representing a substantial threat to modern medicine. AMR refers to microorganisms developing resistance to medication and drugs that once cured them, leading to more cases of disease and death from infections that were previously treatable. There is a lot of information about the extent of AMR worldwide and recent reports show that in 2019, hundreds of thousands of people died due to bacterial resistance. Understanding AMR through epidemiology is essential for developing effective strategies and actions against the public health threat it poses. Solving this problem involves a multisectoral effort to improve information gathering, optimize antibiotic use, and promote research into new therapies. In addition, recognizing the connection between access to healthcare and AMR can inform just health interventions among various populations, especially in low-resource settings (Figure 1.3).

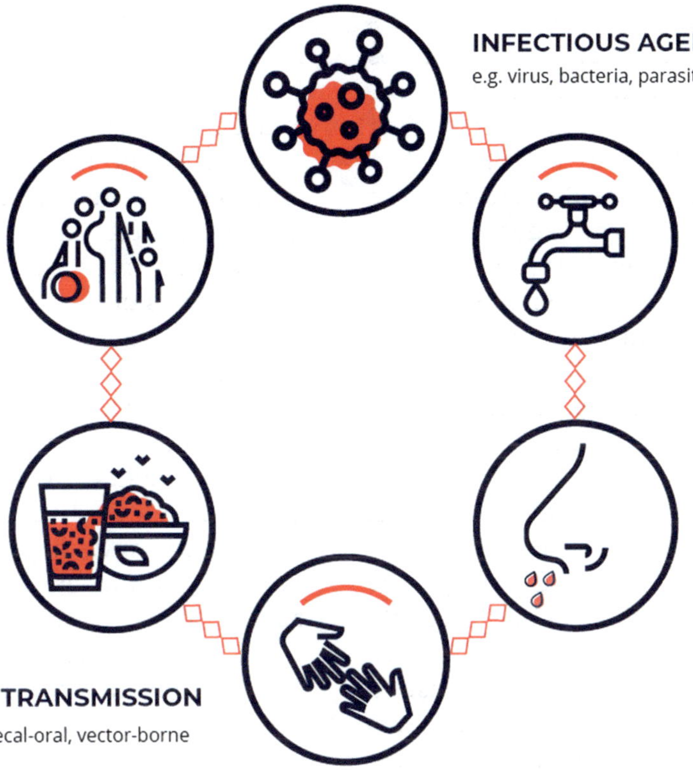

Figure 1.3. Key terms and concepts in infectious disease epidemiology.

Source: https://epidemics.ifrc.org/sites/default/files/inline-images/ECRM%20diagram%20v.3.png.

1.1. Historical Context

The background of infectious disease epidemiology reveals a lot about how public health has responded to epidemics. In the early days, epidemiology primarily involved observing how diseases spread, and the methods used were relatively basic. Epidemiology was greatly influenced by the cholera outbreaks in the 19th century, especially the one in London's Broad Street, which showed the value of collecting and studying data. John Snow's pioneering effort, which entailed case mapping and the identification of sources of contaminated water, defined the principles of epidemiological research. The pioneering study emphasised the need to study the social determinants of health because it accounted for issues such as population density as well as sanitation. These historical milestones laid the foundation for how society tackles public health issues today, including both biological and environmental determinants of infectious diseases. As infectious diseases continued to change, so did the paradigms used by epidemiologists to counteract them. Disease ecology came into being, reflecting an increased awareness of how human activities, environmental dynamics, and sociopolitical conditions converge to shape disease transmission. For example, in the history of HIV/AIDS in the late 20th century, the convergence of social stigma, limited access to healthcare, and socio-economic inequalities contributed substantially to the epidemic's course. This convergence is apparent in cities such as San Francisco, where efforts like the Getting to Zero campaign sought to tackle not just viral load declines but also structural causes. Yet, as Zaragoza et al. (2019) consider, these public health interventions often ignore determinants such as housing stability, which has a significant impact on health outcomes and remains a factor of disparity in the continuum of infectious disease epidemiology. The incorporation of historical context into infectious disease epidemiology sheds light on the necessity of multidisciplinary intervention that involves not only biological determinants but also social determinants. Modern public health efforts emphasise that effective disease prevention and control are contingent upon cooperation among multiple sectors, such as healthcare, urban planning, and community groups. For instance, San Francisco's experience with HIV interventions provides a key teachable moment: even with ground-breaking public health efforts, addressing root causes like housing and socio-economic status is still necessary for substantial health impact. According to Zaragoza et al. (2019), the interaction of class, race, and HIV health outcomes illustrates the general epidemiological principle that a rich past enriches present plans. A thorough look at these variables enables an improved response to infectious conditions, consequently improving public health outcomes among various populations.

1.1.1. Major Historical Pandemics and Their Impact

Historically large pandemics have effects that last longer than the health crisis, and they also impact societies and economies significantly. For instance, the Black Death that devastated Europe during the 14th century killed an estimated one-third of the continent's population. This crippling pandemic not only displaced economies but also introduced a series of social transformations, including the attenuation of feudalism and a reconfiguration of labour relations, with the resulting shortage of labour giving leverage to surviving labourers to negotiate for better wages and conditions of employment. Similarly, the 1918 pandemic of influenza forced governments to implement quarantine strategies and public health practices, emphasising the absolute need for planned interventions for the management of infectious diseases. These examples from the past emphasize learning about the social impact of pandemics as an inseparable part of infectious disease epidemiology, proving that the effects of such events can extend over generations. Analyzing pandemics from an epidemiological point of view illustrates that quantifiable definitions have a pivotal role in assessing their global impact. The absence of a standard definition of a pandemic results in difficulty in addressing such health crises, since the need for a more sophisticated definition that considers the reach of extensive dissemination and high morbidity and mortality has been called for. This precision is necessary because it enables public health authorities to target interventions and deploy resources effectively during an outbreak. Drawing from the heterogeneous past pandemics, say smallpox and cholera, one can hypothesize that the periodicity and scale of such events necessitate pre-emptive and well-coordinated public health intervention. Understanding the epidemiological characteristics of such pandemics assists in creating a reasonable plan for future preparedness, underscoring the need for robust surveillance systems and intersectoral convergence in public health (Dias, 2024). The examples of HIV/AIDS and the SARS-CoV-2 pandemic show how infectious diseases can change and affect human society in many ways. HIV/AIDS, which started in the late 20th century, was a significant public health issue and drew attention to the social stigma faced by people with the disease. Because of this shift in social opinion, policies and financial strategies were updated, which significantly changed the global health scene. COVID-19 has highlighted the existence of gaps in health systems, yet scientific progress and community involvement have made significant contributions. Both the historical and contemporary view of pandemics implies a need for sustainable interventions that not only suppress disease but also improve health equity and resilience in the affected populations (Brinks et al., 2024) (Figure 1.4).

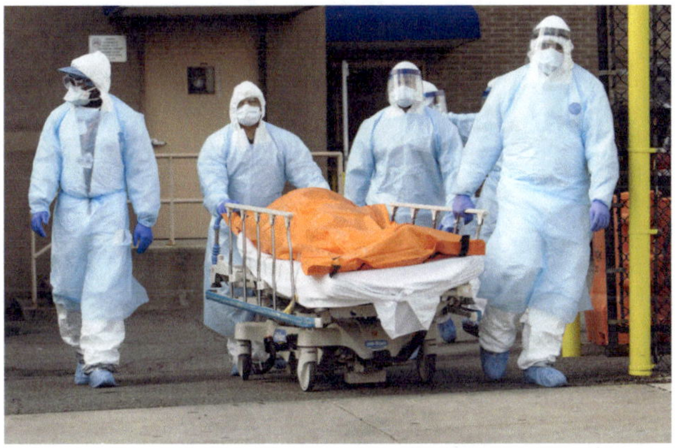

Figure 1.4. Major historical pandemics and their impact thc immediate public health.

Source: https://cdn.cnn.com/cnn/interactive/2020/health/covid19-pandemic-video-timeline/media/images/s_99007D8DF55266B31916FA69A21D93A5294AE6247684BF16E893FBB3B710C388_1587731433686_GettyImages-1208964807.jpg.

1.1.2. Development of Epidemiological Methods

The development of epidemiologic techniques has had a dominant part in the advancement of the knowledge of infectious diseases and in the molding of public health interventions. Early in its development, epidemiology relied on descriptive studies that dealt with describing the distribution of disease in populations. The field has, however, evolved to incorporate more sophisticated analytic approaches, including cohort and case-control studies, which have enabled scientists to examine risk factors and causation more effectively. Epidemiology has been transformed by using statistics, which makes it possible to analyze detailed data and observe trends in diseases. Because EIDs are on the rise, it is now more important than ever to develop reliable methods in epidemiology. Technology in epidemiology has made it possible to watch for and analyze infectious diseases in real time. Data visualization tools and Geographic Information Systems (GIS) are now part of the mapping of disease outbreaks, and it becomes simple for epidemiologists to pick easy targets and track the progress of infection. Furthermore, advances in technology for data collection through mobile health applications and wearable devices increase the granularity of data that can be processed. This technological alignment is particularly beneficial in analyzing the dynamics of disease transmission, as highlighted in recent studies of viral and bacterial diseases in Saudi Arabia, where researchers made use of massive surveillance datasets to provide insights on the epidemiology of infectious diseases common in the country (Aleyumlu et al., 2024; Alhumaid et al., 2024). The continuous development of such tools ensures that public health practitioners are well-equipped to address new challenges. Besides, advancement in epidemiological methods has highlighted the increased importance of multi-disciplinary research in tackling infectious diseases. Collaboration among interdisciplinary fields of microbiology, sociology, and environmental science has enriched a better pool of epidemiological research through diverse input and expertise. The interdisciplinary associations have been instrumental in resolving the complexities of infectious disease transmission dynamics and socio-behavioural determinants of disease transmission. The COVID-19 pandemic is a classic example of this shift, with the interface between epidemiology and behavioural science helping to navigate successful public health messaging and intervention. Through a full-spectrum approach that includes, but is not limited to, biological determinants, as well as social structures and behaviours, epidemiology can provide insights that inform effective public health policy and practice (Figure 1.5).

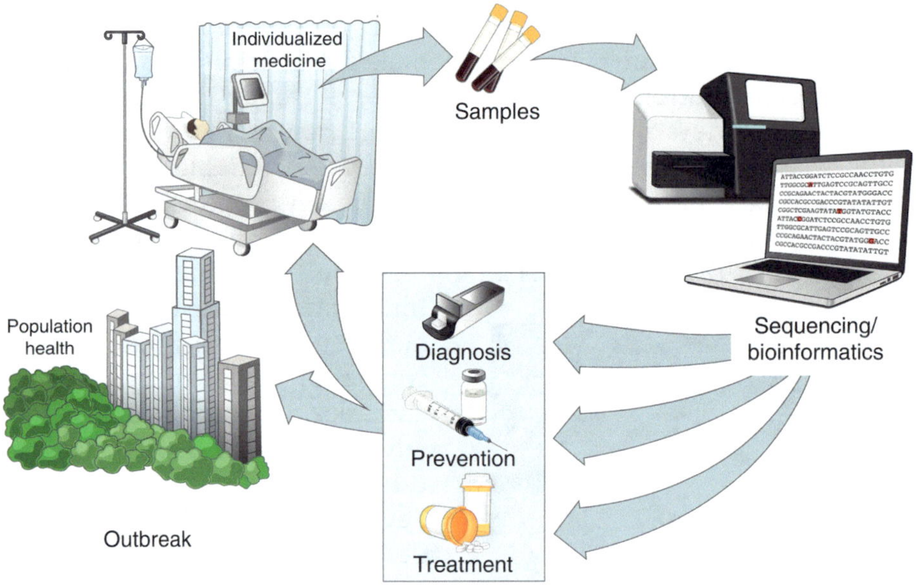

Figure 1.5. Development of epidemiological methods.

Source: https://media.springernature.com/full/springer-static/image/art%3A10.1038%2Fs41591-019-0345-2/MediaObjects/41591_2019_345_Fig1_HTML.png.

1.1.3. Contributions of Key Figures in the Field

Many important people in infectious disease epidemiology have helped to form the discipline and its techniques. For example, Edward Jenner's work on the smallpox vaccine in the late 18th century set the basis for vaccination, which has been improving ever since. Jenners' painstaking observation and experimentation shed light on the link between cowpox exposure and immunity to smallpox, thus establishing the foundation for immunisation practices that have resulted in this disease's global elimination. His efforts not only addressed pressing public health issues but also motivated future generations of epidemiologists to investigate the interaction between pathogens and human health, ultimately influencing vaccination practices worldwide. Therefore, Jenner's legacy continues to play an essential part in interpreting the historical context of infectious disease epidemiology and the ongoing battle against infectious diseases. John Snow is another central personality, commonly referred to as one of the fathers of modern epidemiology. In the mid-1800s, Snow used scientific inquiry to study the cholera epidemics affecting London, which significantly changed the field. Snow proved that environmental factors play a key role in infectious diseases by mapping cholera cases and identifying the sources of contaminated water. John Snow's work culminated in the removal of the pump handle from Broad Street, which halted the outbreak and demonstrated the importance of gathering and analysing vital data in public health. Snow's approach placed a premium on evidence-based interventions, a notion that remains at the heart of epidemiological research to this day. He contributed to understanding how infectious diseases spread and also highlighted the role of epidemiologists in advising on public health policies and actions to prevent outbreaks. Today, Priscilla Wald and other theorists have enriched infectious disease epidemiology by considering how culture and society influence the study of disease. Wald's work explores the intersection of scientific discourse, media portrayals, and cultural narratives of diseases like HIV/AIDS. She argues that the epidemic narrative plays a role by showing society's fears and attracting communities, which shape how people react to epidemics. Wald points out that using a combination of cultural, social, and political aspects in epidemiology helps explain how people perceive different health emergencies. Through her studies, Wald emphasises that knowing infectious diseases demands more than statistical data, since the story around disease has far-reaching effects on health policy and community outreach, closing the distance between science and society (McKay, 2009; Hewa et al., 2018) (Figure 1.6).

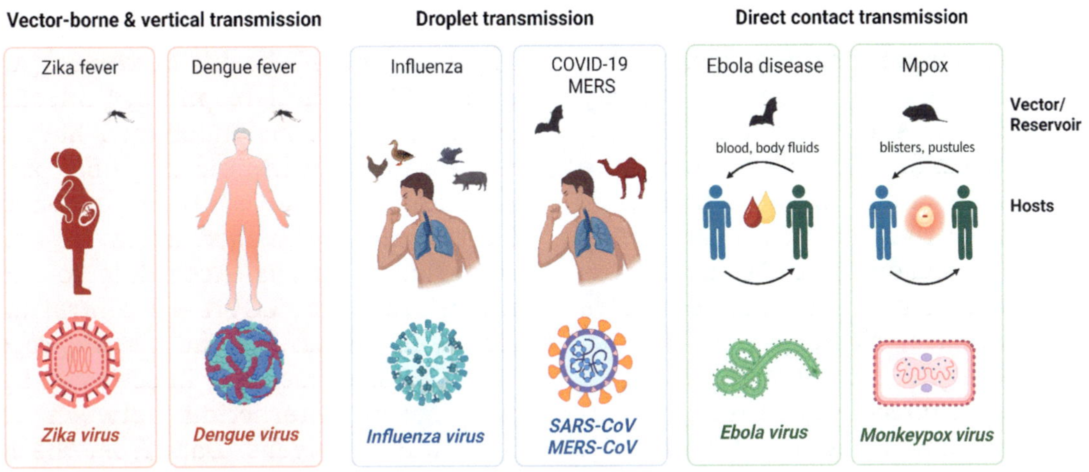

Figure 1.6. Contributions of key figures in the field.

Source: https://pub.mdpi-res.com/microorganisms/microorganisms-11-02618/article_deploy/html/images/microorganisms-11-02618-g001.png?1698128705.

1.2. Types of Infectious Diseases

Infectious diseases can be categorized into various groups according to their etiological agents, transmission modes, and clinical presentations. Generally, diseases are categorized into bacterial, viral, fungal, and parasitic infections. Each of these categories includes a wide variety of pathogens with distinct features and behaviors. For instance, bacterial diseases, such as tuberculosis and strep throat, are caused by single-celled microorganisms, while viral diseases, such as influenza and HIV, result from much smaller organisms that require host cells to replicate. In addition to their biological nature, both infectious disease types present distinct public health challenges, which determine the epidemiological methods for preventing and controlling them. One of the prominent categories is sexually transmitted diseases (STIs), and they encompass illnesses like genital herpes and human immunodeficiency virus (HIV). Genital herpes is of particular importance, caused by herpes simplex virus types 1 and 2 (HSV-1 and HSV-2) and characterized by being very prevalent; there are about 18.6 million Americans currently infected with HSV-2 alone. Despite continued research and the setting up of workshops like the CDC/NIAID Joint Workshop on Genital Herpes, the diagnosis and treatment of this disease are problematic. No cure or vaccine currently exists, highlighting the need for improved preventive interventions and treatments (Connolly et al., 2024). Understanding the details of these STIs helps develop better public health measures. In addition to STIs, the field of infectious diseases has expanded due to the availability of medical and administrative databases containing vital epidemiological data. There is now a large amount of medical information in the databases, which helps estimate the rates of infectious diseases. Yet, reliance on retrospective data is bedevilled by methodological issues, including the guarantees of targeting algorithm integrity employed for analysis. A scoping review identified 19 validation studies and nine capture-recapture studies on 20 infectious diseases in French medico-administrative databases, reporting potential flaws in data quality and completeness (Tassi et al., 2023). It is essential to resolve these methodological challenges to improve future epidemiological studies and, thus, gain better insights into infectious disease dynamics in clinical and community settings (Figure 1.7).

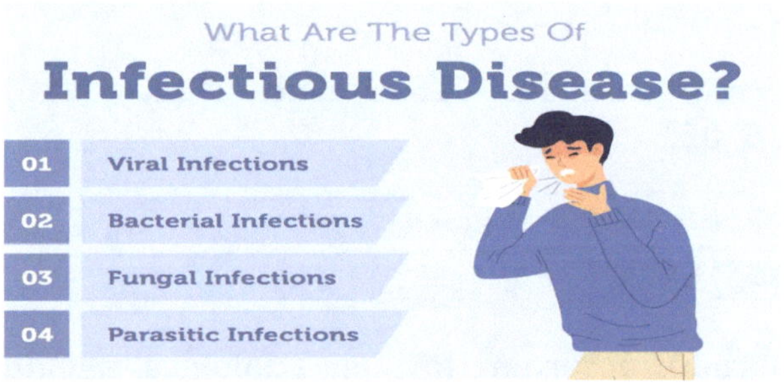

Figure 1.7. Types of infectious diseases.

Source: https://assets.lybrate.com/imgs/tic/enadp/what-are-the-types-of-infectious-disease.webp.

1.2.1. Bacterial Infections

Many people around the world are affected by bacterial infections, which have a significant influence on both disease and death rates. Many bacterial infections are common, but brucellosis, tuberculosis, and salmonellosis are particularly notable and often occur. Some populations, such as Saudi Arabia, show that closely observing these infections helps guide public health interventions. It was found that men are more likely to get brucellosis and tuberculosis, which means that epidemiological studies and public health plans should consider demographics. With knowledge of the epidemiological patterns of these bacterial infections, healthcare providers can identify more efficient prevention measures to limit their influence among susceptible communities, thereby improving public health outcomes (Alhumaid et al., 2024). Viral respiratory infections and secondary bacterial infections have become more critical during recent global pandemics. An example is the COVID-19 pandemic, which led to a significant increase in the number of bacterial infections. According to the study, the relaxation of COVID-19 control measures led to an increase in the prevalence of post-viral invasive bacterial infections, suggesting an ongoing interaction between bacterial and viral pathogens. Data from the National COVID Cohort Collaborative illustrated that kids had increased complication rates following certain bacterial infections, including iGAS and pneumonia, after viral respiratory epidemics. This relationship signifies that an increase in monitoring bacterial infections in the wake of viral pandemics is critical to identify vulnerable groups and take necessary measures to prevent worsened outcomes (Martin et al., 2024). In light of advances in infectious disease epidemiology, it is crucial to understand the epidemiological trends of bacterial infections in detail. Ongoing research is needed to develop active surveillance models that incorporate factors such as travel history, hospitalization, and demographics. As these factors are incorporated into surveillance systems, public health officials can strengthen the resilience of their data, allowing them to make more informed decisions regarding the management of bacterial infections. Furthermore, emerging research will also need to quantify the mortality impact of different bacterial pathogens to determine which infections pose the most significant threats. Collectively, such studies can allow for a better-informed public health response and, in turn, reduce the burden of bacterial infections on global health (Alhumaid et al., 2024) (Figure 1.8).

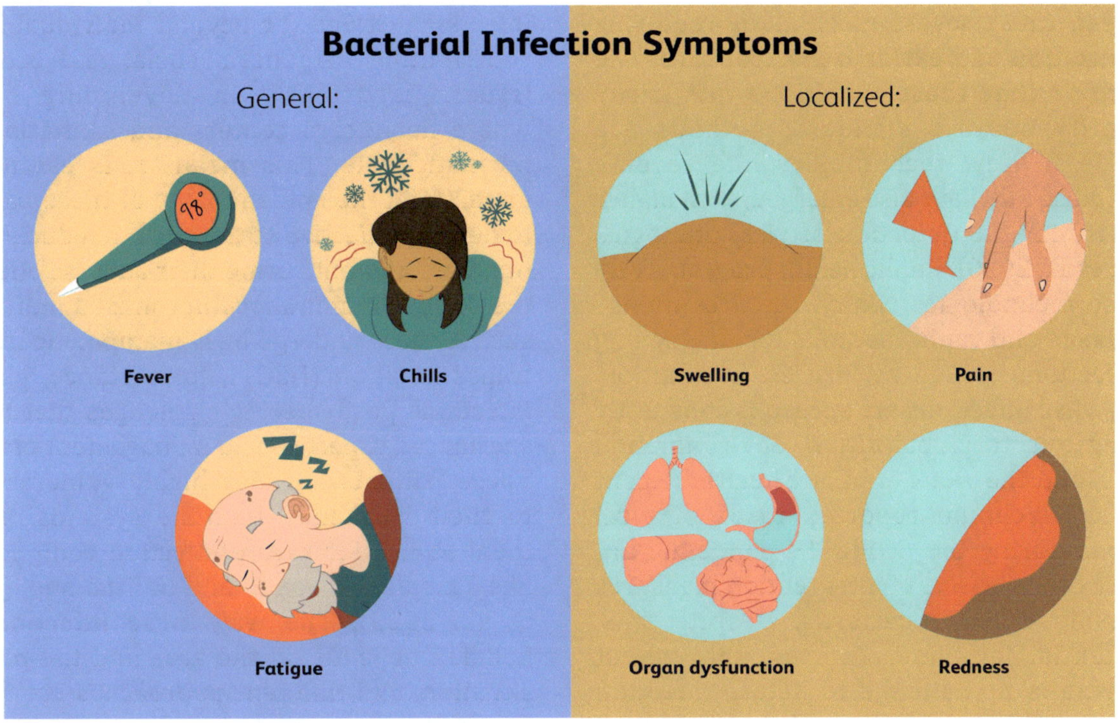

Figure 1.8. Bacterial infections remain a pervasive threat to public health.

Source: https://www.verywellhealth.com/thmb/ZTU2ZRdkJjNqzFp_opBrLWuJiLo=/6000x4000/filters:no_upscale():max_bytes(150000):strip_icc()/what-is-a-bacterial-infection-7705652_final-2f1b8b2429b2495c8333b584512d3afa.jpg.

1.2.2. Viral Infections

Viral diseases pose a significant challenge to global public health due to their diverse etiology and transmission patterns. Epidemiologists require knowledge of the viral pathogens when conducting research into patterns of infections within populations. An understanding of the pattern of occurrence and prevalence of infections such as hepatitis B and C, dengue fever, and influenza can be critical in understanding public health interventions. New research indicates that certain populations are more likely to have susceptibility demographics, notably men being more vulnerable to such infections (Aleyiydi et al., 2024). This can influence specific health interventions by highlighting the need to monitor viral infections to provide an effective public health reaction. Careful tracking of these infections not only prevents outbreaks but also underscores the importance of vaccination and protective practices in preventing the transmission of viral diseases. Beyond that, the situation with viral infections extends beyond routine, run-of-the-mill cases to encompass life-threatening neurological complications that require a different approach in diagnosis and treatment. Viral infections within the central nervous system (CNS) remain among the most up-to-date issues in virology and infectious disease epidemiology. These involve the cytomegalovirus, Epstein-Barr virus, and Japanese encephalitis virus, which can cause severe morbidities requiring hospitalization and extreme medical care. The problem is that these infections are tricky to identify because standard methods are not enough. New technologies like reverse transcriptase PCR have also emerged, with higher sensitivity for the detection of viral etiologies (Tiwari et al., 2020). Public health programs rely on these technologies, which require intense surveillance and rapid methods for diagnosing CNS infections caused by viruses. In addition, the way viral infections are spread is constantly changing due to globalization, environmental changes, and the work of public health. Recent trends of declining reported cases of viral infections during the COVID-19 pandemic are evidence of the effects of intervention measures in altering disease patterns. Despite this, the potential for underreporting throughout lockdowns is a challenge to actual infection rates and subsequent outbreaks (Aleyiydi et al., 2024). It is crucial to understand these trends in order to predict similar epidemics in the future. While they collect and study information, epidemiologists should plan for possible future threats from viruses, so that proper responses are ready for public health. In general, what we learn from viral infections helps inform epidemiology and reminds us that we should continue to investigate and update health policies.

1.2.3. Parasitic Infections

Parasitic infections are a significant part of infectious disease epidemiology, and they have profound public health importance, particularly in the tropics and subtropics. Among these infections, those caused by the *Adenophorean* nematodes have evoked interest due to their complex life cycles and unpredictable presentations. As emphasised in recent reviews, such parasitic infections, like trichuriasis and capillariasis, result from humans acting as final hosts by ingesting infected food or raw meat (Intirach et al., 2024). The implications of these infections extend far beyond individual health, contributing to general social and economic issues, particularly in developing nations where healthcare centers and sanitation may be inadequate. This means it is essential to understand the epidemiology of these parasites to develop effective strategies for reducing their numbers and mitigating their adverse effects on the public. In immunocompromised individuals, such as those undergoing hematopoietic stem cell transplantation (HSCT), for instance, parasitic infections pose specific challenges that require specialised expertise and management practices. These patients are also highly vulnerable due to their weakened immune systems, putting them at risk for severe infection complications like *Toxoplasma gondii* and *Giardia* spp. (Haque et al., 2023). The way these infections are handled depends on the area and the patient's situation, and different approaches are needed for diagnosis and treatment. Furthermore, health professionals are required to consider factors of risk, such as patients' exposure history and the immunosuppressive effect of their treatment regimen, to ensure timely interventions. It is crucial in this model to continually monitor and research to ensure the proper treatment plans for HSCT recipients and achieve better patient outcomes. Prevention and control of parasitic infections must be an integrated strategy combining public health measures, education, and improved sanitary habits. Proper preventive measures, such as health education based on proper food preparation and hygiene, can significantly reduce the prevalence rates of parasitic disease transmission (Intirach et al., 2024). Sanitary water supply and waste disposal community-level interventions are of great relevance in preventing environmental factors of the parasite lifecycle. Innovative investigations and public health actions to contain infectious agents, along with ongoing monitoring, play an important role in efficiently managing parasitic infections. Therefore, a combination of education, improved sanitation, and ethical healthcare systems is the solution to preclude the burdens caused by parasitic infections in vulnerable populations and in society at large (Figure 1.9).

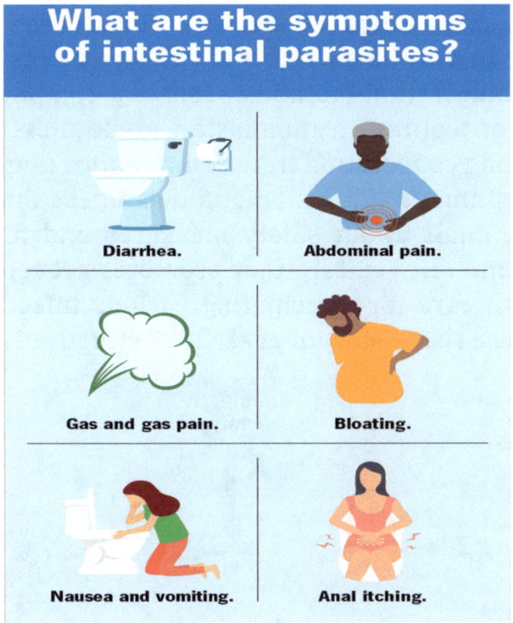

Figure 1.9. Parasitic infections represent a significant aspect of infectious disease epidemiology.

Source: https://my.clevelandclinic.org/-/scassets/images/org/health/articles/intestinal-parasites.jpg.

1.3. Transmission Dynamics

Understanding the transmission dynamics is essential to managing infectious diseases. Transmission dynamics refer to the routes by which a pathogen propagates through and among people and populations, and are based on intricate host behaviour, environmental, and agent features interactions. Mathematical modelling is beneficial because it allows public health practitioners to predict possible outbreaks and test the success of different intervention methods. These results, based on such models, are a key milestone in developing health policies and interventions targeted at controlling disease prevalence in the population as a whole (Haq et al., 2024).

Social causes are fundamental in shaping the way diseases spread. SES, the ability to get healthcare and social networking, are key factors in how likely someone is to get an infection and how they can access treatment. Recently, mathematical models have begun to incorporate these factors and illustrate the connections between them and health outcomes. It is essential to identify these disparities as a point of departure for formulating comprehensive strategies that take into account the specific vulnerabilities of various population segments. Hence, for example, models that were formed demonstrated that despite low-level contact between heterogeneous populations, they would generate extreme fluctuations in disease prevalence and disease spread (Surasinghe et al., 2024). Furthermore, the incorporation of novel measures, including structural causal influence (SCI), provides improved insight into how various populations conceptualise infectious disease transmission. By using SCI, researchers can quantify the relative susceptibility of a population's subgroups and determine how their differential exposure and healthcare access drive aggregate transmission patterns. It helps public health experts identify individuals at a higher risk of illness and develop strategies to prevent the spread of disease. Here, learning about the interaction between social determinants and health patterns is not merely book learning; it is a valuable process for formulating effective public health policy that can evolve to fit the dynamics of infectious disease epidemiology (Surasinghe et al., 2024).

1.3.1. Modes of Transmission

It is imperative to understand how infectious diseases are transmitted when creating public health strategies. Modalities of transmission are generally split into direct and indirect, and direct transmission means person-to-person contact using respiratory droplets or body fluids. Infection may be spread indirectly through vectors, objects, or the environment, which can occur when people come into contact with infected surfaces or are bitten by infected animals. It is crucial for deciding how to respond during an outbreak. For instance, the Mpox outbreak has spoken volumes on the complexity of the transmission dynamics and the importance of realising that zoonotic infections can shift to human hosts, new epidemiological challenges for public health systems, which require heightened surveillance and adaptive measures to cut down the risk profiles associated with multiple modes of transmission (Martini et al., 2023). The epidemiology of infectious diseases has witnessed an evolving understanding of specific pathogens, most notably regarding modes of transmission. Airborne infections, for example, are characterized by the capacity of pathogens to linger in the air for extended periods and spread disseminated outbreaks even between individuals who are distant from each other. This airborne characteristic has been a significant factor in determining the development of epidemics among populations. According to recent studies, the incidence of airborne diseases was the highest among all infections, suggesting that control measures should target airborne pathogens first to effectively break the transmission process (Samoylov et al., 2023). Besides, the comprehension of those transmission routes facilitates the assessment of the efficacy of interventions, highlighting the value of both vaccination and behavior changes to reduce the potential for airborne epidemics. Investigations into the modes of infection of most infectious diseases also shed light on the public health issues inherent in social activities and environmental determinants. Recent classification changes to Mpox, for instance, recognize a shift in perception regarding the transmission of the virus, particularly its initial association with men who have sex with men. With evolving attitudes to methods of transmission, approaches towards public communication and education to reduce stigma and observance of health procedures also have to grow. Strategic and culturally sensitive communication methods become a component of controlling transmission dynamics and eliciting cooperation from communities towards containment. Education and awareness inform individuals about safety measures and foster a community culture that promotes preventive health care for anticipating various infectious disease risks (Martini et al., 2023) (Figure 1.10).

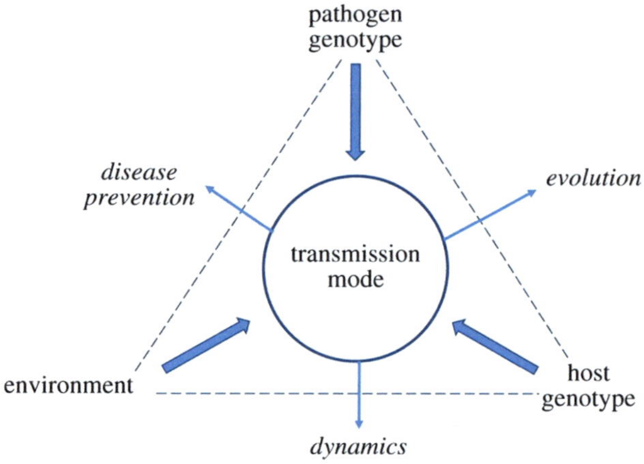

Figure 1.10. Modes of transmission.

Source: https://royalsocietypublishing.org/cms/asset/b8cd55e2-1464-4f6e-bc1d-400d3b567311/rstb20160087f02.jpg

1.3.2. Factors Influencing Transmission

The development of infectious diseases is influenced by a combination of factors, ranging from environmental to biological and sociocultural determinants. Climatic, urbanization, and geographical factors form the core of environmental influences in determining the presence and actions of the pathogens and their vectors. For instance, certain diseases are more prevalent in temperate climates, where pathogens such as mosquitoes thrive, thereby increasing the likelihood of transmission. In addition, human activities that modify the environment, such as urbanization and deforestation, can potentially alter disease dynamics because they can bring human populations closer to animals, which may be harboring zoonotic pathogens. We must pay attention to these environmental factors when designing effective disease prevention and control plans, as climate change is likely to continue affecting diseases globally, requiring adjustments in public health approaches. Most of the spread of infectious diseases occurs due to biological factors.

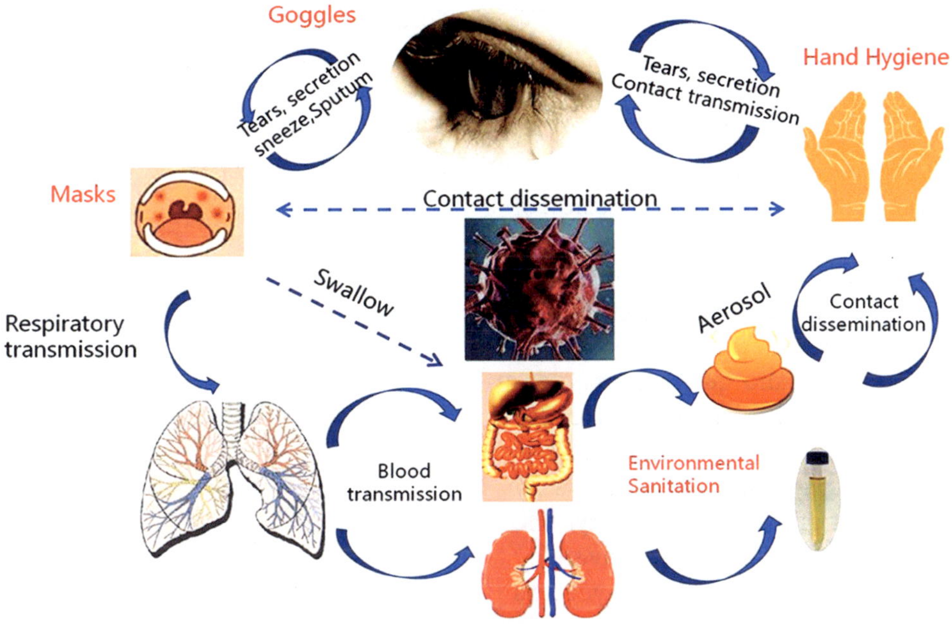

Figure 1.11. Factors influencing transmission.

Source: https://www.frontiersin.org/files/Articles/547355/fcell-08-00618-HTML/image_m/fcell-08-00618-g004.jpg.

A variety of viral strains among pathogens allows them to spread and cause more harm, making it difficult to manage them. For instance, studies on the Crimean-Congo Hemorrhagic Fever (CCHF) virus illustrate the various transmission dynamics and local prevalence caused by genetic mutations. With an estimated mortality rate of approximately 30%, trends in the transmission of CCHFV indicate that certain groups, such as livestock handlers and slaughterhouse workers, are at higher exposure due to close contact with infected animals and also ticks (Srivastava et al., 2024). The way infectious diseases are spread—through vectors, the air, or direct contact—also affects their rate of spread, which means it is essential to use interventions suited to the specific biological factors. Unequal access to healthcare, education, and wealth among individuals also plays a significant role in the spread of infectious diseases. There are not enough resources for disease treatment and prevention in these regions, which makes poor people there more likely to get infectious diseases. This has been demonstrated by the high rate of COVID-19 transmission, where social determinants like housing and healthcare had a significant impact on spread and rates of morbidity (Foxman et al., 2022). In addition, cultural practices, such as burial rituals involving physical contact with the deceased, can enhance disease spread. Thus, resolving these socioeconomic determinants is not only crucial for acute containment but also for long-term strategies aimed at reducing the aggregate infectious disease burden through improved public health infrastructure and community engagement (Figure 1.11).

1.3.3. Role of Vectors in Infectious Disease Spread

The contribution of vectors to the transmission of infectious diseases is an essential consideration in epidemiology. Vectors are normally living organisms, such as mosquitoes, ticks, and sandflies, that can transfer disease-causing organisms from one host to another. These vectors enable the transmission of a range of diseases like malaria, dengue fever, and Lyme disease, which disproportionately affect populations by factors of environment and socio-economy. The population dynamics of vectors are driven by ecological forces and the actions of both vectors and their hosts, so differential equations provide an essential technique for modeling disease transmission. Using compartmental models, such as the SIR model, scientists consider how vectors behave within ecosystems and how interventions could alter these dynamics to decrease disease transmission. Knowledge of the ecological functions of such vectors will aid in formulating targeted control measures to mitigate their impact on public health (Vinodhini et al., 2025). Vectors can also be defined based on their impact on epidemiological trends of infectious diseases. For example, their ability to carry and transmit more than one pathogen makes disease spread more complex. Some of these vectors, including Aedes mosquitoes, have the capacity to transmit viruses such as Zika, chikungunya, and dengue simultaneously, which exacerbates the problems for public health officials. Such poly-microbial transmission not only enhances disease incidence but can also result in co-infections that complicate diagnosis and treatment. The vectors' contribution to the maintenance of such cycles of pathogens highlights the need to comprehend their ecology, behavior, and interface with environmental components. Through the use of sophisticated modeling methods and ecological research, epidemiologists can more accurately forecast outbreaks and design successful intervention protocols focused on interrupting the transmission routes enabled by such vectors (Lobello et al., 2025).

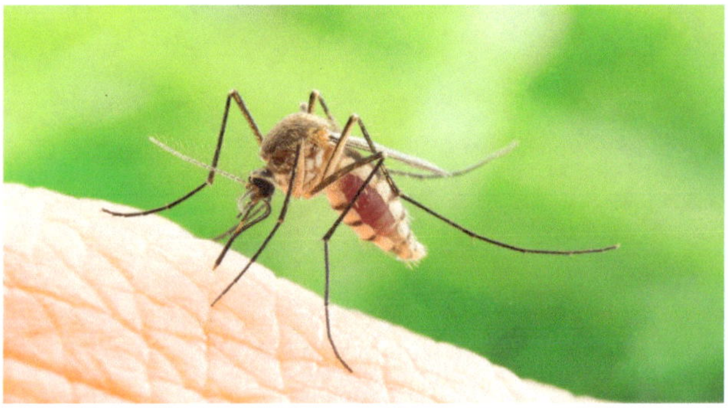

Figure 1.12. Role of vectors in infectious disease spread.

Source: https://s7g10.scene7.com/is/image/biomerieux/Aedes%20aegypti%20Mosquito.?qlt=85&wid=480&ts=1674036282490&dpr=on,2.625.

Furthermore, discoveries regarding vector biology, including microbiota, present promising avenues for developing novel methods to control infectious diseases. Recent research suggests that the microbiota of the skin of animals such as vultures plays a vital role in resisting pathogens and can be utilised to devise strategies for vector control. The complex interaction between vectors and their microbial flora provides a more informed understanding of how pathogens are maintained or abated within environmental conditions. Understanding such interactions allows scientists to discover intervention targets that may limit the vector's ability to spread disease. This holistic strategy not only improves our understanding of infectious disease ecology but also brings to the fore the urgent necessity of converging ecological and epidemiological methods in addressing the transmission of vector-borne diseases (Vinodhini et al., 2025) (Figure 1.12).

1.4. Surveillance and Data Collection

The epidemiological setting of infectious diseases relies heavily on effective surveillance and data gathering measures to inform public health interventions. Systematic observation of associated events to the state of health is performed by epidemiologists, allowing for a detailed examination of disease patterns among populations.

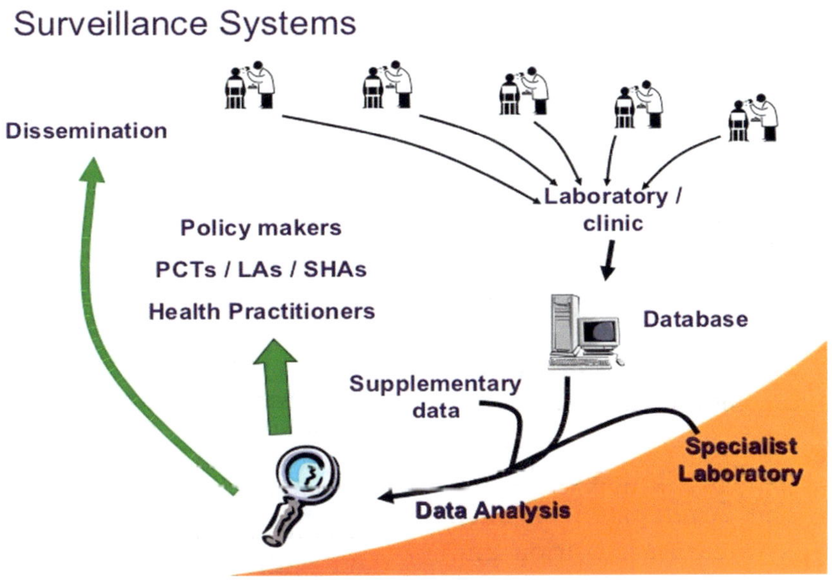

Figure 1.13. Surveillance and data collection.

Source: https://image.slidesharecdn.com/20100427alexkeenanintrotoepidemiology1-110725054744-phpapp01/95/introduction-to-epidemiology-and-surveillance-7-728.jpg?cb=1311574996.

The frequency, distribution, and determinants of disease are incorporated into such an exacting approach to produce critical information that facilitates timely interventions. When strong surveillance systems are in place, health authorities can detect outbreaks early and utilise resources effectively. What is learned from these surveillance activities is used to plan policies that help control and limit the spread of infectious diseases among people. The way surveillance and public health outcomes are linked shows how using data in epidemiology can benefit people's health. The COVID-19 pandemic has highlighted weaknesses and limitations in existing surveillance mechanisms, particularly in countries like Kazakhstan. The variability in the dynamics of disease throughout the pandemic has made it difficult to evaluate other infectious diseases, such as influenza. The decline in reported influenza cases created gaps in data collection, which hindered the evaluation of vaccine effectiveness and the planning of vaccination campaigns. Quoted in the review of Kazakhstan's health infrastructure, these gaps emphasize the importance of strong and dynamic surveillance systems capable of weathering such public health crises. Moreover, the review highlights the importance of public awareness of disease prevention and vaccination, underscoring the value of effective data collection in bridging the knowledge gap between the public and health authorities. Refining inefficiencies and knowledge gaps in surveillance systems is essential for strengthening epidemiological outputs. As with Kazakhstan, membership in international networks, such as the Global Influenza Hospital Surveillance Network (GIHSN), can enhance a country's surveillance capabilities, but grassroots-level activities should accompany this. Tailoring surveillance measures to the specific epidemiological characteristics of each region facilitates more accurate disease monitoring. Moreover, international collaboration is required, especially in monitoring zoonotic diseases that could lead to new outbreaks. The development of such systems with improved data acquisition and analysis will not only enhance the productivity of vaccine delivery but also better guide public health policy. These efforts will eventually result in more effective control of infectious diseases at the national and global levels, supporting the central role of surveillance in epidemiology (Figure 1.13).

1.4.1. Methods of Disease Surveillance

Knowing about disease surveillance is essential for the success of infectious disease epidemiology. Disease surveillance involves collecting, examining, and analysing health data to inform public health decisions. Through disease surveillanceit is possible to detect outbreaks, track changes in diseases, and assess the effectiveness of control efforts. Surveillance can be conducted in two ways: passively, where doctors report cases, or actively, which involves directly requesting information from healthcare centres and communities. These intensive data collection mechanisms enhance the overall quality of health information, which is essential for a timely response to emerging health threats. Furthermore, the use of sophisticated modelling techniques in disease surveillance can enhance the comprehension of disease dynamics within populations. For example, the quantitative estimation of contact rates enables researchers to develop models of disease transmission that predict potential interactions between human and animal populations. An example of such an application is simulating the transmission of rabies across wild and domestic dog interfaces, an application with direct implications for disease spread and interventions for disease control in northern Australia. These models provide vital insights into how diseases can spread, thereby guiding policymakers in designing evidence-based, targeted surveillance and intervention strategies to mitigate risks from zoonotic diseases that impact both humans and animals (Ward et al., 2024). Epidemiological data gathered through surveillance systems are a key element in guiding public health intervention as well as enforcing public health laws. Surveillance data, for instance, have been employed in Saudi Arabia to demonstrate trends in bacterial infectious disease over the last few years. By using statistical methods, scientists can calculate the most prevalent infections, such as brucellosis and tuberculosis, and characterise their demographic impacts. Such data not only aid in prioritising public health campaigns but also inform the distribution of resources to effective interventions. The data collected provides support for ongoing additions to disease surveillance infrastructures, potentially including variables like self-reported travel history and hospitalization ratios, in an effort to create a more advanced picture of the infectious disease climate and more effective inform public health strategies (Alhumaid et al., 2024) (Figure 1.14).

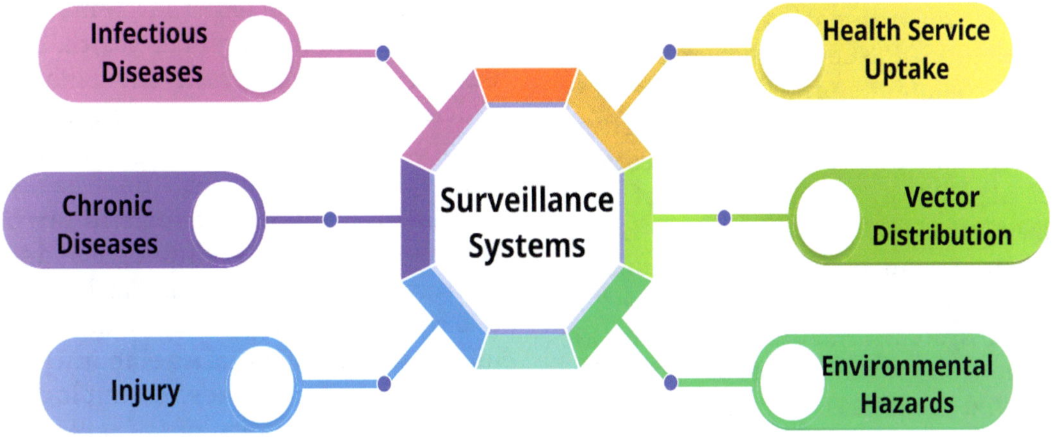

Figure 1.14. Methods of disease surveillance.

Source: https://publichealthprepared.org/wp-content/uploads/2022/09/Evaluating-Surv-System-Image-2.png.

1.4.2. Importance of Data Accuracy and Reliability

Reliability and accuracy of the data are critical in infectious disease epidemiology. Data accuracy forms the basis for effective public health decision-making and policy formulation. Inaccurate data may lead to ineffective public health interventions that can, in turn, exacerbate the epidemiology of infectious diseases. In epidemic settings, such as during outbreaks, accurate collection of data enables epidemiologists to track transmission patterns, identify high-risk groups, and implement targeted interventions. Poor data quality compromises critical analyses, which can damage the response to an infectious disease outbreak. Besides, good data fosters public trust in health authorities. As seen in the ongoing COVID-19 debate, accurate information has been crucial in shaping public attitudes and following health directives. For this reason, ensuring data accuracy is the most critical part of setting up and using effective epidemiological surveillance and response plans. If data is reliable in the methodology, public health interventions become more effective, especially during pandemics. Such approaches as serological surveys, case reports, and syndromic surveillance help to better understand the trends of diseases. The mixing of artificial intelligence (AI) technologies, as seen in the controversy over ChatGPT and its capabilities, is a testament to the potential for enriching data credibility through improved analytics. They can gather and display a vast amount of epidemiological data, which reveals previously unknown information. AI tools are used to monitor data in real-time and forecast results, thereby avoiding human errors in collecting and understanding data. Still, the accuracy of AI conclusions depends on the quality of the data it processes. The failure to take adequate measures to ensure data authenticity can lead to AI-based conclusions that mislead healthcare interventions, resulting in undesirable effects. The model of data validity and reliability must therefore be sufficiently robust to facilitate AI application in epidemiology (Alhur, 2024). In addition to facilitating short-term public health interventions, precise data are crucial in long-term studies and policy-making related to infectious disease epidemiology.

Historical data are crucial in analyzing disease trends, the efficacy of vaccines, and intervention effects over time. For instance, methodical collation of data regarding viral characteristics, as in the case of SARS-CoV-2 research during the COVID-19 pandemic, enables researchers to make substantive inferences regarding viral dynamics and public health implications (Bar-On et al., 2020). The advantage of such a historical approach is that it guides future research agendas and policy interventions by identifying probable areas of weakness within existing health systems. In addition, systematic data collection supports the global scientific community and facilitates cooperation in the struggle against infectious diseases worldwide. By doing this, putting effort into making data as precise and trustworthy as possible is not only a matter of response to public health emergencies in the current moment but also an investment in guaranteeing public health for future generations (Figure 1.15).

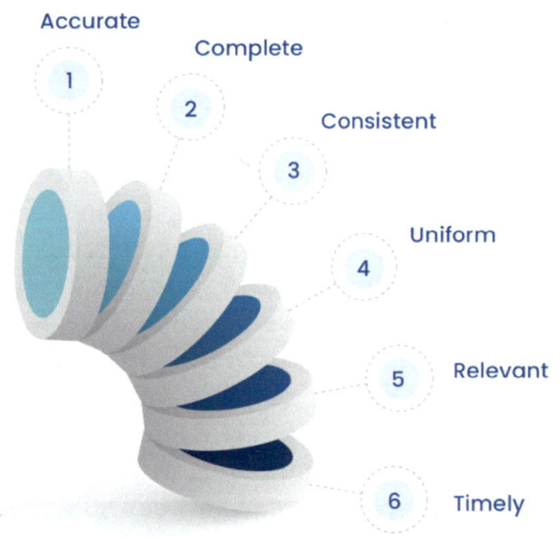

Figure 1.15. Importance of data accuracy and reliability.

Source: https://assets-global.website-files.com/62e17765d63bf58b55b9c94e/64b14f3415f803899cca3b37_Reliable-data.jpg.

1.4.3. Use of Technology in Surveillance

Infectious diseases that emerge pose a significant threat to global health. Due to these dangers, technology in surveillance is now crucial for disease monitoring and managing outbreaks. Because of AI, big data analytics, and GIS, epidemiologists can now easily monitor disease trends and anticipate future outbreaks. Because of these technologies, data can be captured and analyzed instantly, which makes it easier to identify areas with many diseases and possible hotspots. As elaborated in current studies, combining these technologies not only enhances the validity of surveillance data but also enables public health officials to implement timely interventions, thereby mitigating the impact of infectious diseases in populations (Zaman et al., 2025). Additionally, AI is helping to predict the spread of diseases and inform public health decisions. Employing sophisticated algorithms and machine learning (ML) techniques, researchers can develop dynamic models that simulate various cases of outbreaks. The models, such as the Susceptible-Infectious-Recovered (SIR) models, forecast transmission patterns and evaluate the effectiveness of control measures. Additionally, AI-powered surveillance systems heighten the capacity to trace and track contacts, which are all vital during public health responses to infectious diseases. Through an intense evaluation of these technologies, it is found that they have immense potential to aid in accurate decision-making and resource deployment in public health responses (Gawande et al., 2025). Despite the promising future of technology for surveillance applications, moral concerns and data privacy must be taken into account. The widespread use of digital health tools and AI raises concerns about data ownership, informed consent, and the potential misuse of sensitive information. As surveillancetechnologies increase in ubiquity in public health, there must be clear systems and guidelines of accountability to ensure compliance with ethical norms. Furthermore, equitable access to the technologies must be realised to prevent further exacerbation of existing health inequalities. Ultimately, a mutually harmonious balance that harnesses the strength of technological advancement while safeguarding citizens' rights and promoting inclusion will be essential to strengthening the international response to infectious disease outbreaks (Zaman et al., 2025) (Figure 1.16).

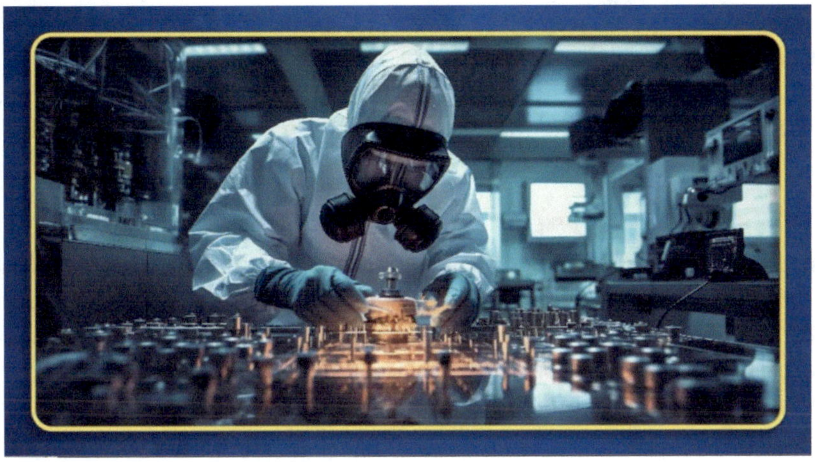

Figure 1.16. Use of technology in surveillance.

Source: https://www.pw.live/exams/wp-content/uploads/2024/04/Infectious-Disease-Surveillance-and-Control-01-jpg.webp.

1.5. Outbreak Investigation

Outbreak investigation is a scientific procedure for identifying the aetiology of infectious diseases and instituting effective public health interventions. In an outbreak situation, epidemiologists implement procedures such as case finding, outbreak mapping, and environmental surveys to determine the causes of disease transmission. The scrub typhus research in Nepal, particularly following the 2015 earthquake, is a testament to the importance of meticulous outbreak investigation protocols. Following this natural disaster, there was also an increase in scrub typhus infections, prompting the health authorities to collect epidemiological data from not only patients but also rodents and mites in the affected regions. The latter provided valuable information on the prevailing transmission ecology of the causative pathogen, *Orientia tsutsugamushi*. The remarks explain that studying the epidemiology of an outbreak helps explain its importance for public health. To investigate an outbreak, various methods may be employed, including laboratory tests and field research. After the earthquake in Nepal, teams quickly gathered samples from victims by using syndromic surveillance. Samples from blood, stool, and the throat, as well as tests on food and drinking water, are used to find any potential pathogens. The study enabled the discovery of Salmonella and influenza viruses, which played a crucial role in explaining the disease pattern following the disaster. By combining clinical and environmental information, epidemiologists can better understand the spread of infections, which enables them to develop effective public health measures that reduce the risk of new infections. Therefore, investigating all aspects of an outbreak is crucial for effective handling and preparation for epidemics. Last but not least, conclusions and implications from outbreak investigations inform public health policy and programming. Outbreak analyses of scrub typhus in Nepal have shown that the outcome not only directed to improve surveillance and early detection systems but also highlighted the necessity for educating the populace concerning preventive measures. The case fatality rate due to scrub typhus decreased significantly from 2015 to 2017, reflecting the effectiveness of public health actions based on prior studies. Furthermore, the inability to detect traceable pathogens in the environmental samples obtained from the post-earthquake survey revealed several key gaps that require addressing in future preparedness. With the continuous enhancement of methodological approaches in outbreak investigation and with early data sharing facilitated by it, public health experts can enhance response readiness to manage future infectious disease outbreaks, ultimately safeguarding population health.

1.5.1. Steps in Investigating an Outbreak

An outbreak investigation follows a specific process to determine the source, how the disease spreads, and what measures should be taken to stop it. The very first step is to confirm an outbreak, which requires finding cases that are higher than expected in a particular area or group of people. In addition, this step involves coordination with local health officials and proper reporting of epidemiologic information. Amidst emerging health threats, timely and efficient distribution of information, as identified in Yang et al. (2020), is critical to establishing a thorough understanding of the scope and direction of the outbreaks to support effective intervention measures.

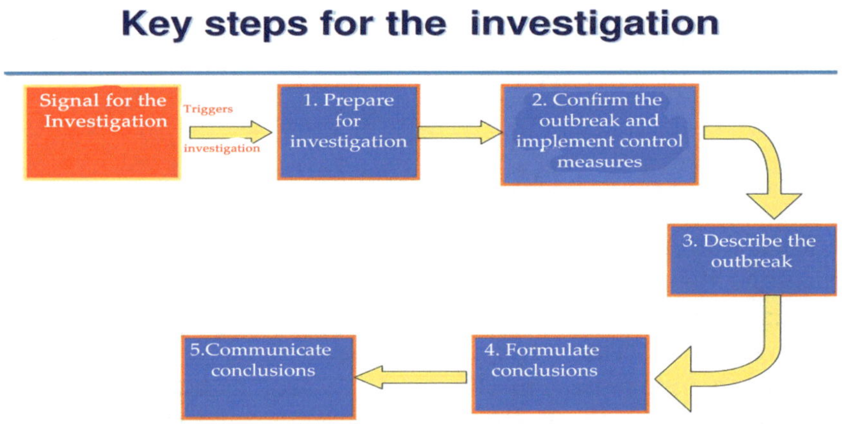

Figure 1.17. Steps in investigating an outbreak.

Source: https://image3.slideserve.com/5561486/key-steps-for-the-investigation-l.jpg.

After confirming an outbreak, the subsequent measure centres on defining the infected population and acquiring comprehensive information on the cases. Such involves gathering demographic information, clinical presentations, and comorbidities of infected individuals, as witnessed in studies exploring the incidence of underlying illnesses among patients with COVID-19, discussed in Yang et al. (2020). Such information not only accounts for the epidemiological profile of the outbreak but also helps identify probable risk factors responsible for the severe presentation of the disease. By this process of classification, researchers can map patterns of transmission and evaluate vulnerabilities within the community and eventually influence the response strategy customised to the needs of the affected population. The final phases of an outbreak investigation involve applying control measures based on the findings obtained through the previous steps and measuring their efficacy over a specified period. Vaccination campaigns, public health advisory notices, and upgraded sanitation procedures may be included in this phase, for which ongoing checks are necessary to validate effectiveness towards containing the outbreak. Additionally, the exchange of information and data gathered in the investigation is crucial in informing public health policy and enabling readiness for future epidemics, as noted in Wu et al. (2020). The combination of these efforts enables health agencies to establish a stronger framework for epidemiological practice, highlighting the importance of integrated response approaches and proactive interventions in infectious disease control (Figure 1.17).

1.5.2. Case Definition and Identification

The control and tracking of infectious diseases largely depend on correctly defining and finding each case. A case is usually characterised by clinical features, links with epidemiology, and laboratory tests that allow us to tell cases apart from non-cases. Such definitions are applicable for public health system standardisation, guidance of decision-makers in disease surveillance, outbreak investigation, and intervention planning. Strict case definition mechanisms ensure that epidemiologists can track routes of transmission and assess disease spread across groups. The data generated depends on the accuracy of case definitions, which must change over time as new evidence emerges and new infectious agents or strains become available. Quality infectious disease case identification calls for robust surveillance systems. These tools are the backbone for public health response through early case detection and reporting of infectious disease outbreaks. The availability of advanced methods, such as the Bayesian spatio-temporal model, enhances surveillance by enabling the forecasting of high-risk areas and providing evidence-based, targeted interventions. A fascinating aspect of new epidemiological methods is that they account for spatial and temporal trends, enabling resource planning and preventive interventions. The ability to analyze disease patterns and dynamics, for instance, with exceedance probability metrics, leads to greater specificity and sensitivity in outbreak detection and, ultimately, more effective control measures (Kim et al., 2024a). Understanding the dynamics of the domestic-wildlife interface is crucial for gathering information on the transmission of diseases with public health implications. For instance, the association between free-ranging domestic dogs and wild dogs in northern Australia presents a complex case study in infectious disease ecology. The dynamics between such populations, for instance, free-ranging domestic canines living in bushland and food-source-based wild canine activity, unveil the multifaceted nature of disease dissemination across the two groups. Epidemiologists utilise this knowledge to refine their models for disease transmission, enabling them to identify potential outbreaks and inform preventive measures. Merging epidemiological and ecological data highlights a pressing need for interdisciplinarity to fully address the challenge that infectious diseases pose at this interface (Ward et al., 2024).

1.5.3. Control Measures and Interventions

Control interventions and measures of infectious disease control are essential in preventing outbreaks and protecting public health. Early diagnosis, isolation of the patient, and strict infection control practices are the cornerstones of an effective public health response. Due to the uncertainties associated with most infectious diseases, interventions must be tailored to consider demographic and environmental factors to ensure that their impacts are successful. For instance, in dense populations, carrying out mass vaccination campaigns and awareness generation can significantly slow down transmission rates. These interventions are of particular importance in disease control for which there are no treatment options, emphasizing the importance of an active approach to epidemiological practice (Rahman, 2024). Public health guidelines based on systematic research are indispensable in ensuring that control measures reach the most vulnerable populations. As shown through disease studies, like the study on Mpox, young adults and specific segments in society, like men, have had higher rates of infection and so will be assisted by targeted control strategies (Rahman, 2024). Including education and public participation in control strategies will foster an educated public that is able to help public compliance and healthier practices. The application of training among healthcare practitioners on infection management and control can also enhance the effectiveness of these interventions by providing assurance that workers are well-trained to handle infectious cases effectively. The challenges created by EIDs, such as cutaneous leishmaniasis (CL), also highlight the need for adaptable and responsive control measures. Socioeconomic status and ever-changing environmental factors are among the variables that can influence disease epidemiology, necessitating ongoing research and investment in public health infrastructure. In the event of unexpected outbreaks or pandemic cases, existing healthcare systems may face increased pressure, potentially impacting other disease management efforts. Therefore, an elastic system with surveillance, rapid response coordination, and enhanced sanitary services becomes essential in mitigating the impacts of infectious diseases. An integrated strategy ensures that health systems are robust and well-equipped to address both present and emerging infectious challenges effectively (Figure 1.18).

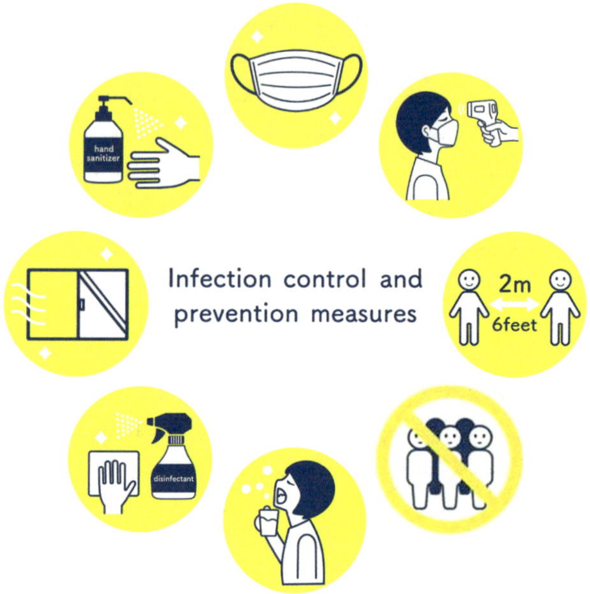

Figure 1.18. Control measures and interventions.

Source: https://engiomed.ae/wp-content/uploads/2022/04/IPC.jpg.

1.6. Public Health Implications

The environment and the distribution of resources in society have a significant impact on public health in infectious disease epidemiology. When public health receives less attention and funding, it may be unable to assist high-risk groups in a timely manner, which can exacerbate health disparities between groups. Public health institutions are being pushed harder to fix these inequalities, even though they must work through complex social and political situations. As Velasco et al. (2018) point out, the challenge is balancing the short-term calls for disease prevention with the need for long-term infrastructural development. Thus, successful approaches must include both immediate control of outbreaks and the creation of policies to support increased equity in health interventions. This two-pronged approach is crucial in mitigating the impact of infectious diseases across diverse populations. In addition, advances in digital tools in epidemiology portend significant changes in the practice of public health. The advent of so-called digital epidemiology is a sign of creative adjustment to the fast flow of information and the sophistication of new disease transmission. New sources of health data offer never-before-seen possibilities for rapid and effective action against outbreaks. Still, this movement also raises ethical concerns over data privacy and the abuse of personal health information. As highlighted in Velasco et al. (2018), interdisciplinary collaborations are beneficial for public health responses but must be approached with care to address the ethical considerations involved. Therefore, while digital approaches have a promising future, they must be incorporated judiciously to achieve effectiveness without eroding public confidence. An epidemiologic foundation of principles is essential in responding to the modern-day public health challenges. Fundamental elements, including causal associations, disease natural history, and screening protocol assessment, form the basis of evidence-based decision-making. Students in the field should not only understand the process of conducting epidemiologic studies but also critically evaluate the intervention for health effects and its implications on society. The broad curriculum in Chapter equips upcoming public health practitioners with the know-how to investigate the root causes contributing to the spread of disease, thereby informing prevention. Building this groundwork is critical to successfully addressing public health issues grounded in infectious disease processes so that practitioners can effectively contribute to population health gains (Figure 1.19).

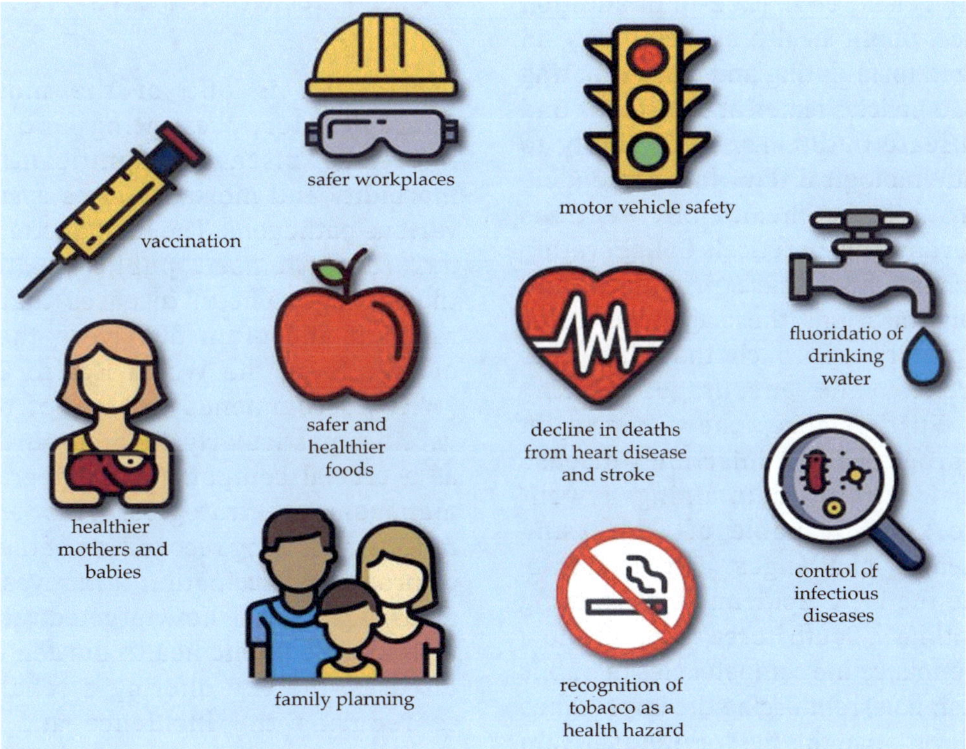

Figure 1.19. Public health implications.

Source: https://www.queensu.ca/gazette/sites/default/files/assets/alumnireview/articles/Public%20Health%20icons%20880x587%201.jpg.

1.6.1. Role of Public Health Agencies

The role of public health agencies in managing infectious diseases is foundational to the discipline of epidemiology. These agencies serve as the vanguard against health threats by implementing surveillance systems that monitor disease patterns within communities. By systematically collecting and analysing data on the incidence and prevalence of infectious diseases, public health entities can discern trends that may indicate outbreaks or emerging health crises. This proactive approach enables the early identification of potential hazards, allowing for swift interventions to mitigate their impact. According to the principles of epidemiology, effective data utilisation and timely response are critical for reducing morbidity and mortality associated with infectious diseases, as highlighted by Fehaid et al. (2024). In addition to surveillance, public health agencies play an essential role in formulating and disseminating evidence-based policies aimed at controlling and preventing disease outbreaks. Their ability to translate epidemiological data into actionable strategies ensures that health interventions are both relevant and practical. Collaborating with researchers, healthcare providers, and community organisations, these agencies foster a multidisciplinary approach that enhances public awareness and encourages healthy behaviours. Furthermore, the integration of training programs for infectious disease practitioners is key to maintaining a well-prepared workforce capable of addressing emerging health challenges. For example, programs like the Field Epidemiology Training Program Frontline in South Korea exemplify how agencies can enhance the competencies of public health professionals, reinforcing the importance of ongoing education in this field, as noted in Kim et al. (2024b). Moreover, public health agencies play a crucial role in coordinating responses during health emergencies, guiding the collective action necessary to combat infectious disease outbreaks. Their established frameworks for crisis management ensure that essential resources are allocated efficiently and effectively, minimizing disruptions to healthcare systems. These agencies serve not only as information hubs but also as leaders in directing public health initiatives that employ best practices in response management. By prioritizing competencies such as epidemiologic methods and crisis response in training programs, public health agencies cultivate a workforce equipped to handle the complexities of disease outbreaks. Ultimately, the role of these agencies is critical in fostering community resilience, enhancing health outcomes, and safeguarding public health on a broader scale, thereby underscoring their indispensable contributions to preventing and controlling infectious diseases.

1.6.2. Vaccination and Prevention Strategies

Vaccination is one of the most effective strategies for preventing and controlling infectious diseases, significantly reducing morbidity and mortality rates associated with various pathogens. The introduction of vaccines has revolutionised public health, enabling the management of diseases that were once rampant and often deadly. In the context of dengue fever, the World Health Organisation (WHO) recommends the use of the TAK-003 vaccine, particularly in high-burden regions, as a crucial component of integrated disease management strategies. This endorsement reflects a growing recognition of the importance of proactive vaccination initiatives in endemic areas, highlighting how targeted vaccination can mitigate the public health burden of infectious diseases, thereby offering a reliable pathway to reducing the incidence and severity of outbreaks (Torres et al., 2024). Moreover, the case of herpes zoster illustrates the potential of vaccination in addressing diseases that affect specific demographic groups. The introduction of the recombinant zoster vaccine (RZV) has been shown to provide an impressive vaccine efficacy of 97.2%, indicating its effectiveness in preventing herpes zoster and its complications, such as post-herpetic neuralgia. This is particularly pertinent given that a significant portion of the adult population may be at risk for this reactivation of a latent virus. By promoting vaccination strategies that target high-risk individuals, healthcare providers can diminish the risk of complications and enhance overall patient outcomes. This proactive approach highlights the crucial role of vaccination as a preventive measure against the resurgence of diseases associated with prior infections, thereby enhancing public health resilience (Lim et al., 2024).

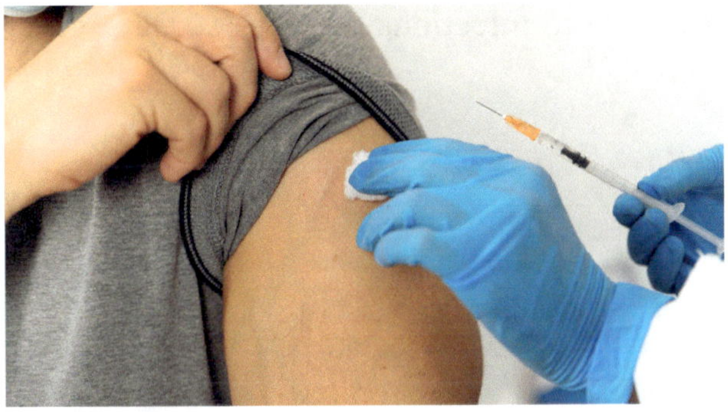

Figure 1.20. Vaccination and prevention strategies.

Source: https://www.cdc.gov/hepatitis-a/media/images/2024/04/hepatitis-a-prevention-control-thumbnail.jpg.

In conclusion, effective vaccination and prevention strategies are vital elements in the arsenal against infectious diseases, capable of altering their trajectory within populations. By focusing on widespread vaccine accessibility and public education, healthcare systems can improve immunization rates, reducing transmission and protecting vulnerable populations. Collaborative efforts involving health entities, social sectors, and scientific communities, as outlined in recommendations for dengue vaccination, exemplify the importance of an integrated approach to disease prevention. As seen with both the dengue and herpes zoster vaccines, successful implementation of vaccination programs hinges on a thorough understanding of epidemiological patterns and the specific needs of populations at risk. By synthesizing evidence-based practices with community involvement, we can enhance the effectiveness of vaccination campaigns and promote healthier societies (Lim et al., 2024; Torres et al., 2024) (Figure 1.20).

1.6.3. Global Health Initiatives and Collaborations

The global health landscape is becoming increasingly dominated by coalition-based efforts aimed at addressing infectious diseases through research, resource sharing, and capacity development. Efforts such as the Global Burden of Disease (BoD) study best illustrate this coalition response, where scientists and health bodies work together to measure the health effects of different diseases globally. The BoD strategy not only facilitates the generation of comparable data within regions but also identifies gaps that call for specific interventions. Through the adoption of a standardized approach, such collaborations attempt to simplify data collection and analysis, examining complex issues and informing stakeholders' decision-making. Finally, these collaborative efforts consolidate the system for measuring health outcomes, delivering vital information that guides public health strategies and resource distribution among countries, especially in those countries facing considerable disease burdens (Organized by Cost Action CA et al., 2020). Additionally, technological innovations further improve the prospects of global collaborations in health. Current technologies, such as GIS and remote sensing, enable epidemiologists to examine health data in a more refined manner, thereby refining efforts toward the elimination of infectious diseases like polio and malaria. For example, the use of GPS-enabled tracking during vaccination campaigns has been promising to maximize resource utilization and enhance coverage of hard-to-reach populations. Interdisciplinary collaboration between epidemiologists and digital health specialists creates new methods of responding to the continuously changing nature of disease dynamics. The integration of genomics and ML not only expedites insights into patterns of disease transmission but also facilitates the design of focused interventions, demonstrating the importance of interdisciplinary collaboration in promoting public health objectives. As new techniques keep arising, they have the potential to revolutionize the impact of global health programs (Eckhoff et al., 2015). Lastly, the success of global health partnerships depends on the willingness to bridge gaps in resources and methodology between nations. As some countries leverage sophisticated data analytics and holistic health systems, others struggle with traditional methods that hinder disease management. Efforts like the European BoD network have been instituted to counteract these imbalances by providing a collaborative platform for various international stakeholders. Through gap bridging of knowledge and capacities, these alliances facilitate nations to exchange best practices and strengthen their health systems. In addition, learning created through such collaborations not only assists in resolving existing disease burdens but also helps anticipate possible outbreaks of EIDs. Therefore, international global health efforts must continue to ensure an inclusive setting that upholds collaboration, knowledge sharing, and resource equity to maximize the international response to infectious diseases (Organized by Cost Action CA et al., 2020).

SUMMARY

The multidisciplinary character of infectious disease epidemiology makes a strong argument for the unification of public health functions. The development of epidemiological practices over time, including in institutions like the KTL/THL, provides evidence of how intentional organizational shifts can improve the efficiency of disease surveillance and response to outbreaks. In 40 years, KTL/THL had not only built a strong national surveillance infrastructure but had also modified its organization to give precedence to co-operation among microbiologists and epidemiologists. Such an integrative strategy is crucial in addressing the complexities of infectious disease control. It has shown that increased capability in producing and analyzing data can result in significant public health impact (Ruutu, 2024). With contagious diseases still on the frontline of global health threats, these lessons establish the critical need for continuous adaptation among public health institutions. The findings derived from the analysis of recent epidemiological data, exemplified by those in Saudi Arabia, further elucidate the complex dynamics of infectious disease occurrence. The monitoring observed significant trends in bacterial infections and accentuated the demographic differences that call for specific public health interventions. The observed decline in incidence during the COVID-19 pandemic underscores the interrelatedness of various infectious agents and the factors that influence disease transmission. Furthermore, emphasis on maximizing the specificity and sensitivity of disease reporting is critical in the identification of relevant health threats and prioritizing public health interventions (Alhumaid et al., 2024). These conclusions reinforce that a well-rounded knowledge of epidemiological trends is the basis for successful disease prevention and control programs. In conclusion, the significance of combining epidemiology with clinical microbiology and public health programs is immense. One such takeaway is the need for ongoing innovation in data collection and reporting systems to keep up with the changing dynamics of infectious diseases. Frameworks such as those of KTL/THL can serve as blueprints for implementation by other countries seeking to strengthen their epidemiological systems, particularly in areas where public health infrastructures are underdeveloped. Ongoing investment in research, surveillance, and stakeholder collaboration will ultimately enable countries to address the complexities relating to infectious diseases effectively. As we continue to evolve in our knowledge and utilization of infectious disease epidemiology, there is a need to prioritize flexibility and adaptability in public health policy to ensure that it can address existing, as well as future, health issues.

Infectious disease epidemiology provides key information on the dynamics of diseases that affect populations globally. The key area of focus is the classification of vector-borne diseases (VBDs), particularly those caused by parasites such as filariasis, leishmaniasis, and malaria. These diseases have common pathways of transmission and are serious threats to public health because of their prolonged morbidity and mortality. Knowledge of the epidemiology of these diseases is key in developing effective control measures. By promoting synergy among disease control programs and drawing lessons from comparative studies, researchers can reinforce strategies to curtail the incidence of these diseases, ultimately enhancing overall health outcomes for at-risk populations (Chaturvedi et al., 2025). Infectious disease epidemiology through this multidimensional strategy emphasizes a holistic approach when addressing complicated health issues. Another crucial area in infectious disease epidemiology is understanding the relationships at the wildlife-domestic interface. This interface plays a crucial role in determining the spread of zoonotic diseases from one animal population to another and occasionally to humans. Modelling the spread of disease is important in exploring these interfaces so that researchers can effectively visualise transmission dynamics. For example, the case study of rabies in northern Australia, which involves the wild dog-domestic dog ecosystem, demonstrates the intricacies of disease transmission. Key findings include the detection of free-roaming domestic dogs that often come into contact with wild populations, raising serious concerns about the spread of disease and control. This also highlights the importance of developing integrated strategies that consider both ecological and epidemiological insights, resulting in more effective surveillance and intervention measures (Ward et al., 2024). Some of the challenges persisting in infectious disease epidemiology involve the necessity for better data acquisition methods as well as coming up with strong models that consider numerous transmission dynamics. Reasonable estimates of contact rates between species are essential to develop dependable models of disease transmission, which can guide public health interventions. As the research on the facet of wildlife-domestic dog interactions influencing rabies transmission has shown, integrating full data on animal ecology and behavior can improve understanding considerably as well as mitigation initiatives. This emphasizes the need for interdisciplinary studies that bridge epidemiological and ecological gaps for the promotion of successful disease management. Ultimately, the integration of evidence from these diverse disciplines is likely to yield innovative solutions in infectious disease epidemiology and enhance global health security (Ward et al., 2024).

CLOSER LOOK

CENTRAL NERVOUS SYSTEM (CNS)

The central nervous system (CNS) is the core processing center of the human body, responsible for interpreting information, generating thoughts, and coordinating actions. It is composed of the brain and the spinal cord, two highly specialized structures protected by bone, membranes, and cerebrospinal fluid. Together, they form the command system that controls everything from movement and sensation to emotions, memory, and consciousness. The brain is the most complex organ in the body. It contains billions of neurons that communicate through electrical and chemical signals. These neurons form intricate networks that allow us to perceive the world and respond to it. Different regions of the brain handle different functions. For example, the cerebrum supports reasoning, language, decision-making, and voluntary movement. The cerebellum fine-tunes coordination and balance, allowing smooth, precise motions. The brainstem regulates essential automatic functions such as breathing, heart rate, and sleep cycles. Although these regions have distinct roles, they constantly communicate, ensuring that the brain functions as a unified whole.

Extending from the base of the brain is the **spinal cord**, a long bundle of nerve fibers that serves as the main pathway between the brain and the rest of the body. Sensory information from the skin, muscles, and organs travels up the spinal cord to reach the brain, where it is processed. Commands from the brain travel downward through the spinal cord to guide movement and control internal functions. The spinal cord also handles **reflexes**—quick, automatic responses that occur without involving the brain—to protect the body from harm.

The CNS is protected by several layers: the **skull** and **vertebrae**, which provide structural defense; the **meninges,** three protective membranes; and **cerebrospinal fluid**, which cushions the brain and helps maintain a stable environment. A deeper understanding of the CNS reveals how interconnected and delicate it is. Even small disruptions—injuries, infections, or degenerative diseases—can have major effects because the CNS coordinates so many vital functions. Despite its complexity, the CNS is remarkably adaptable, capable of learning and rewiring itself through a process known as **neuroplasticity**.

Overall, the central nervous system is the body's master control network, integrating information, shaping behavior, and enabling everything that makes us human.

REFERENCES

1. Abdulhakim, F., Alfehaid, S., Jazaa, S., Alharbi, S., Alkanfari, M. A. H., Almutairi, A. Z., Nasser, R., et al. (2024). Disease surveillance and public health: How epidemiology informs action. *Power System Technology*. https://www.semanticscholar.org/paper/fa74ec48fd18c3f1f9131239fb72f85c6f7dfa5e (accessed on 30th May 2025).
2. Adebola, O. A., Auta, H. S., Daniel, E. O., Emmanuel, et al. (2024). *Review of Global Burden of Disease Studies: Trends, Challenges, and Future Directions*. https://core.ac.uk/download/618286874.pdf (accessed on 30th May 2025).
3. Adler, Y., Charron, P., Imazio, M., Badano, L., Barón-Esquivias, G., Bogaert, J., Brucato, A., Gueret, P., Klingel, K., Lionis, C., Maisch, B., Mayosi, B., Pavie, A., Ristić, A. D., Tenas, M. S., Seferovic, P., Swedberg, K., Tomkowski, W., Achenbach, S., . . . Nesukay, E. (2015). 2015 ESC Guidelines for the diagnosis and management of pericardial diseases. *European Heart Journal, 36*(42), 2921–2964. https://doi.org/10.1093/eurheartj/ehv318Aleyiydi, M. S., Alshiban, N. M., Alajmi, A. M., Alosaimi, N. F., Alotaibi, M., Nassar, M. S., Alhumaid, N. K., et al. (2024). Epidemiology of viral infectious diseases reported in Saudi Arabia. *Infectious Diseases and Therapy, 13*, 1893–1905. https://www.semanticscholar.org/paper/e26ec01893069a935532dd6ed81b602e559280f6 (accessed on 30th May 2025).
4. Alhumaid, N. K., Alajmi, A. M., Alosaimi, N. F., Alotaibi, M., Almangour, T. A., Nassar, M., Memish, Z. A., et al. (2024). Epidemiology of reportable bacterial infectious diseases in Saudi Arabia. *Infectious Diseases and Therapy, 13*, 667–684. https://www.semanticscholar.org/paper/80889fccfb88b0b038f64bee778a60893cc8bd70 (accessed on 30th May 2025).
5. Alhur, A. (2024). Redefining healthcare with artificial intelligence (AI): The contributions of ChatGPT, Gemini, and Co-pilot. *Cureus*. https://doi.org/10.7759/cureus.57795.
6. Arthur, C., Banda, H., Chazya, R., Chijoka, et al. (2023). Epidemiological tools in focus: A comprehensive assessment of their role in addressing infectious disease challenges in Zambia. Journal for Research in Applied Sciences and Biotechnology. https://core.ac.uk/download/597862448.pdf (accessed on 30th May 2025).
7. Bar-On, Y. M., Flamholz, A. I., Phillips, R., & Milo, R. (2020). SARS-CoV-2 (COVID-19) by the numbers. *eLife, 9*. https://doi.org/10.7554/elife.57309.
8. Boman, M., & Johansson, S. J. (2007). *Modeling Epidemic Spread in Synthetic Populations – Virtual Plagues in Massively Multiplayer Online Games*. http://arxiv.org/abs/0705.4584 (accessed on 30th May 2025).
9. Brinks, R., & Hoyer, A. (2024). Approximation of the infection-age-structured SIR model by the conventional SIR model of infectious disease epidemiology. *Frontiers in Epidemiology, 4*. https://www.semanticscholar.org/paper/1047f62343d7a3b5b742c03357fece792b6d7792 (accessed on 30th May 2025).
10. Chaturvedi, R., & Sharma, A. (2025). Key facets for the elimination of vector-borne diseases: Filariasis, leishmaniasis, and malaria. *ACS Infectious Diseases*. https://www.semanticscholar.org/paper/6eda8858a1d6b721a2a67c6b3dc4fd9f8bba7d4a (accessed on 30th May 2025).
11. Connolly, K. L., Bachmann, L., Hiltke, T., Kersh, E. N., Newman, L. M., Wilson, L., Mena, L., et al. (2024). Summary of the Centers for Disease Control and Prevention/National Institute of Allergy and Infectious Diseases Joint Workshop on Genital Herpes: 3–4 November 2022.

Open Forum Infectious Diseases, 11(5), ofae230. https://www.semanticscholar.org/paper/5eec56195f3c1a8d19d853dabd16739eedae2c91 (accessed on 30th May 2025).

12. Dhimal, M., Dumre, S. P., Sharma, G. N., Khanal, P., Ranabhat, K., Shah, L., Lal, B., et al. (2021). An outbreak investigation of scrub typhus in Nepal: Confirmation of local transmission. *BMC Infectious Diseases, 21*. https://www.semanticscholar.org/paper/f34b3bf2357b5a651d2d5a2cd0a213f7791066c1 (accessed on 30th May 2025).
13. Dias, R. A. (2024). Towards a comprehensive definition of pandemics and strategies for prevention: A historical review and future perspectives. *Microorganisms, 12*. https://www.semanticscholar.org/paper/944819660a2e19eb025b92fdcda9d3cf02816a18 (accessed on 30th May 2025).
14. Eckhoff, P., & Tatem, A. (2015). Digital methods in epidemiology can transform disease control. *International Health, 7*, 77, 78. https://www.semanticscholar.org/paper/343fead12a016d8e5dca548159f56a5b2eece8f8 (accessed on 30th May 2025).
15. Foxman, B., & Mehta, S. (2022). Impact of technological developments on infectious disease epidemiology: Lessons from the first 100 years of the *American Journal of Epidemiology*. *American Journal of Epidemiology*. https://www.semanticscholar.org/paper/822dc26a68aa03678bd2a1349ef18b989a7da545 (accessed on 30th May 2025).
16. Fung, I. C. H. (2016). *PUBH 6533 – Epidemiology*. https://core.ac.uk/download/229147991.pdf (accessed on 30th May 2025).
17. Gawande, M., Zade, N., Kumar, P., Gundewar, S., Weerarathna, I. N., & Verma, P. (2025). The role of artificial intelligence in pandemic responses: From epidemiological modeling to vaccine development. *Molecular Biomedicine, 6*. https://www.semanticscholar.org/paper/611fd886ec9538f085ec154fff2e616a134144aa (accessed on 30th May 2025).
18. Geng, E., Hargreaves, J., Peterson, M., & Baral, S. (2019). Implementation research to advance the global HIV response: Introduction to the JAIDS supplement. *JAIDS Journal of Acquired Immune Deficiency Syndromes*. https://www.semanticscholar.org/paper/e37e88e74882b14eb9984ad1662867a7f6727330 (accessed on 30th May 2025).
19. Haque, E., Muhsen, I., Rasheed, W., Fakih, R., & Aljurf, M. (2023). Parasitic infections in hematopoietic stem cell transplant recipients. *Transplant Infectious Disease, 25*. https://www.semanticscholar.org/paper/f4a6cf13de908652ef05f16acc3fad6d9ffd79b0 (accessed on 30th May 2025).
20. Hewa, S., & Liu, B. (2018). Epidemiological transition and population health: Understanding social determinants of health in China. *Illness, Crisis & Loss, 26*, 223–246. https://www.semanticscholar.org/paper/23396a9d057b93391b02119548726528659b7e34 (accessed on 30th May 2025).
21. Hujatullah, M., Klivleyeva, N., Rabani, N. G., Glebova, T., Saken, K., & Bolatovna, K. A. (2024). Challenges in influenza control and surveillance in the Republic of Kazakhstan. *Journal for Research in Applied Sciences and Biotechnology*. https://www.semanticscholar.org/paper/56ded403892c38052cd3c8e175740481eb2ae87c (accessed on 30th May 2025).
22. Intirach, J., Shu, C., Lv, X., Gao, S., Sutthanont, N., Chen, T., & Lv, Z. (2024). Human parasitic infections of the class *Adenophorea*: Global epidemiology, pathogenesis, prevention and control. *Infectious Diseases of Poverty, 13*. https://www.semanticscholar.org/paper/749b2a1953a8a248a39a8b8e6d4b725f75d578be (accessed on 30th May 2025).

23. Iqbal, U. (2024). Book Review: Infectious disease epidemiology: History, transmission and prevention. *Herculean Research*. https://www.semanticscholar.org/paper/121a78e992146257eb7d1dd33aa3430fe65aa46e (accessed on 30th May 2025).

24. Johnson, D. E., Burtness, B., Leemans, C. R., Lui, V. W. Y., Bauman, J. E., & Grandis, J. R. (2020). Head and neck squamous cell carcinoma. *Nature Reviews Disease Primers, 6*. https://doi.org/10.1038/s41572-020-00224-3.

25. Kim, J., Lawson, A. B., Neelon, B., Korte, J. E., Eberth, J. M., & Chowell, G. (2024a). A novel Bayesian spatio-temporal surveillance metric to predict emerging infectious disease areas of high disease risk. *Statistics in Medicine, 43*, 5300–5315. https://www.semanticscholar.org/paper/d952982e454d5340f27eaca1fb3e640372867bc1 (accessed on 30th May 2025).

26. Kim, Y., Gwack, J., Kwon, Y., Cheong, M. J., & Lee, J. H. (2024b). Needs assessment for public health competency in infection prevention and control: Importance and performance analysis (IPA) of infectious disease response practitioners. *Journal of Korean Medical Science, 40*. https://www.semanticscholar.org/paper/96115965a74e58d31eade6d2ea34691f9c86fd86 (accessed on 30th May 2025).

27. Lim, D. Z. J., Tey, H., Salada, B. M. A., Oon, J., Seah, E. J. D., Chandran, N., & Pan, J. (2024). Herpes zoster and post-herpetic neuralgia—Diagnosis, treatment, and vaccination strategies. *Pathogens, 13*. https://www.semanticscholar.org/paper/d858848dd96414e74a4413aabd4d95f1e9183e9d (accessed on 30th May 2025).

28. Lobello, M., Bava, R., Castagna, F., Sotgiu, F. D., Berlinguer, F., & Tilocca, B. (2025). The role of vulture (*Accipitriformes*) cutaneous microbiota in infectious disease protection. *Microorganisms, 13*. https://www.semanticscholar.org/paper/186d62033d65e0420485fadc4a212d85e26ff298 (accessed on 30th May 2025).

29. Marahatta, S. (2015). Control of the outbreak of disease aftermath earthquake: An overview. *Nepal Journal of Epidemiology, 5*(2), 468, 469. https://www.semanticscholar.org/paper/a5c9117b3b7dac6788753e8a071119dc92b36a4b (accessed on 30th May 2025).

30. Martin, B., DeWitt, P. E., Russell, S., Haendel, M., Sanchez-Pinto, N., Albers, D. J., Jhaveri, R. R., et al. (2024). The recent increase in invasive bacterial infections: A report from the National COVID Cohort Collaborative. *The Pediatric Infectious Disease Journal, 44*, 217–227. https://www.semanticscholar.org/paper/ad41638630893f33ac7374d744ea2411b3800556 (accessed on 30th May 2025).

31. Martini, M., Behzadifar, M., Bragazzi, N., & Orsini, D. (2023). *Poc (Pox)*, a term for various infectious diseases in the history of public health and epidemiology: The dreaded smallpox, the almost unknown alastrim and the mpox. *Journal of Preventive Medicine and Hygiene, 64*, E209–E214. https://www.semanticscholar.org/paper/6ee62760c3b214e7c389df845d1f700fdde11e09 (accessed on 30th May 2025).

32. McKay, R. (2009). Priscilla Wald, contagious: Cultures, carriers, and the outbreak narrative, Durham, NC, and London, Duke University Press, 2008, pp. xi, 373, illus., £55.00 (hardback 978-0-8223-4128-4); £13.99 (paperback 978-0-8223-4153-6). *Medical History, 53*, 300–301. https://www.semanticscholar.org/paper/9d4958d15835fbb334d13c79104f1f68f0f5a4a3 (accessed on 30th May 2025).

33. Mesquita, S., Perfeito, L., Paolotti, D., & Gonçalves-Sá, J. (2023). *Digital Epidemiology After COVID-19: Impact and Prospects*. arXiv, abs/2312.04835. https://www.semanticscholar.org/

paper/387ea8d94a802aa3b82bf868cf5a9381f6d64d44 (accessed on 30th May 2025).

34. Murray, C. J. L., Ikuta, K. S., Sharara, F., Swetschinski, L. R., Robles, A. G., Gray, A. P., Han, C., et al. (2022). Global burden of bacterial antimicrobial resistance in 2019: A systematic analysis. *The Lancet, 399*, 629–655. https://doi.org/10.1016/s0140-6736(21)02724-0.

35. Organized by Cost Action CA, Milićević, M. Š., & Devleessch, B. (2020). 30.L. Workshop: European burden of disease network: Strengthening the collaboration. *European Journal of Public Health, 30*. https://www.semanticscholar.org/paper/4908d04d618513f98288e92fd451ce11fba02eff (accessed on 30th May 2025).

36. Rahman, M. M. (2024). Systematic review of the epidemiology, disease severity and preventive measures of mpox disease: A public health guideline for densely-populated countries. *F1000Research*. https://www.semanticscholar.org/paper/fd328435c8fe82919852b76c8134b62cee3ac63d (accessed on 30th May 2025).

37. Remais, J. (2010). *Modeling Environmentally-Mediated Infectious Diseases of Humans: Transmission Dynamics of Schistosomiasis in China*. https://core.ac.uk/download/323082019.pdf (accessed on 30th May 2025).

38. Roth, G. A., Abate, D., Abate, K. H., Abay, S. M., Abbafati, C., Abbasi, N., Abbastabar, H., et al. (2018). Global, regional, and national age-sex-specific mortality for 282 causes of death in 195 countries and territories, 1980–2017: A systematic analysis for the Global Burden of Disease Study 2017. *The Lancet, 392*, 1736–1788. https://doi.org/10.1016/s0140-6736(18)32203-7.

39. Ruutu, P. (2024). Building integrated epidemiology and National Microbiology Reference Laboratory (NRL) system for infectious disease control in Finland over 40 years. *Proceedings of the International Congress Public Health - Achievements and Challenges - Zbornik Radova*. https://www.semanticscholar.org/paper/ee5f0b950acd8aef48623d8ee2bc6512521e4b99 (accessed on 30th May 2025).

40. Samoylov, M. I., Borshchuk, E., & Pankov, A. S. (2023). Epidemiological characteristics of infectious disease statistics among the population of the Orenburg Region in 2013–2020. *ЗДОРОВЬЕ НАСЕЛЕНИЯ И СРЕДА ОБИТАНИЯ - ЗНиСО / Public Health and Life Environment*. https://www.semanticscholar.org/paper/55ab76a77442debd52722c0a1b6fdceb82a0857f (accessed on 30th May 2025).

41. Shakya, G., Marasini, B., Karki, K., Upadhaya, B., Acharya, J., Adhikari, S., Manjhi, R., et al. (2018). Outbreak investigation following the 2015 earthquake disaster in Nepal. *Journal of Nepal Health Research Council, 16*(1), 61–65. https://www.semanticscholar.org/paper/14d82a27fffe583206360e0cd1edb079cf58ec99 (accessed on 30th May 2025).

42. Shams, M., Rashidi, A., Mohamadi, J., Moradi, M., Pakzad, R., Naserifar, R., Abdi, J., et al. (2023). Real-time impact of COVID-19 pandemic on cutaneous leishmaniasis case finding and strategic planning, preventive interventions, control and epidemiology in a region with a high burden of cutaneous leishmaniasis and COVID-19: A cross-sectional descriptive study based on registry data in Ilam-Iran. *Health Science Reports, 6*. https://www.semanticscholar.org/paper/1ef9d3ba1afe6696f06fb3433abf4b11773de5d4 (accessed on 30th May 2025).

43. Srivastava, S., Kumar, S., Sharma, P. K., Rustagi, S., Mohanty, A., Donovan, S., Henao-Martínez, A., et al. (2024). Control strategies for emerging infectious diseases: Crimean-Congo hemorrhagic fever management. *Health Science Reports, 7*. https://www.semanticscholar.org/paper/0070505be9f28cb5bfef53d331b24da065a5ce2c (accessed on 30th May 2025).

44. Surasinghe, S., Manivannan, S., Scarpino, S., Crawford, L., & Ogbunugafor, C. B. (2024). Structural causal influence (SCI) captures the forces of social inequality in models of disease dynamics. https://www.semanticscholar.org/paper/c842d0a6de8f1de40c0799422a175b333b926625 (accessed on 30th May 2025).

45. Tassi, M. F., Le Meur, N., Stéfic, K., & Grammatico-Guillon, L. (2023). Performance of French medico-administrative databases in epidemiology of infectious diseases: A scoping review. *Frontiers in Public Health, 11.* https://www.semanticscholar.org/paper/0ab5c563d123204707a0c1361354066ae3bb3310 (accessed on 30th May 2025).

46. Tiwari, R. I., Bhullar, S., Chandak, N., Baheti, N., Daginawala, H., Singh, L., & Kashyap, R. (2020). Determination of etiology and epidemiology of viral central nervous system infections by quantitative real-time polymerase chain reaction in Central India population. *Neurology India, 68*, 1323–1330. https://www.semanticscholar.org/paper/5a776feba3962adb9e9eaf8c5c69ec03ac5c7a57 (accessed on 30th May 2025).

47. Torres, J. R., Brea-Del, C. J., Sáez-Llorens, X., Avila-Agüero, M. L., Coronell, W. R., Martinez-De, C. C., & Debbag, R. (2024). Regional molecular epidemiology of dengue and the potential optimization of its control through the use of vaccines: Report of the arbovirus committee of the Latin American Society of Pediatric Infectious Diseases, SLIPE. *Expert Review of Vaccines.* https://www.semanticscholar.org/paper/bffd9230f80f92f73eea18ffa8d9b599cc3d3339 (accessed on 30th May 2025).

48. Ul Haq, N., Tiwari, S. K., Porwal, P., & Ul Haq, I. (2024). Numerical models in the epidemiology of infectious diseases. *International Journal of Scientific Research in Science, Engineering and Technology*. https://www.semanticscholar.org/paper/652a610ee172fff09fd9dec84ee1785edba2c6eb (accessed on 30th May 2025).

49. Velasco, E. (2018). *Disease Detection, Epidemiology and Outbreak Response: The Digital Future of Public Health Practice.* https://core.ac.uk/download/199299749.pdf (accessed on 30th May 2025).

50. Vinodhini, R., Malini, M. T. N. M., Ramesh, P., Maragatham, R. S., Venkata, R. G., China, C., & Subba, R. (2025). Modeling infectious disease spread: Differential equations in population dynamics and epidemiology. *Communications on Applied Nonlinear Analysis.* https://www.semanticscholar.org/paper/a92a0b804bbaccc60074ff671d901bcb640f5717 (accessed on 30th May 2025).

51. Ward, M. P., & Brookes, V. (2024). An overview of the challenges and methods for defining the wildlife-disease interface in the context of disease spread modelling, including concepts of infectious diseases epidemiology. *Australian Zoologist.* https://www.semanticscholar.org/paper/1f864dda93a2b01a9de5602856bc305161c2f3af (accessed on 30th May 2025).

52. Wu, D., Wu, T., Liu, Q., & Yang, Z. (2020). The SARS-CoV-2 outbreak: What we know. *International Journal of Infectious Diseases, 94*, 44–48. https://doi.org/10.1016/j.ijid.2020.03.004.

53. Yang, J., Zheng, Y., Gou, X., Pu, K., Chen, Z., Guo, Q., Ji, R., et al. (2020). Prevalence of comorbidities and its effects in patients infected with SARS-CoV-2: A systematic review and meta-analysis. *International Journal of Infectious Diseases, 94*, 91–95. https://doi.org/10.1016/j.ijid.2020.03.017.

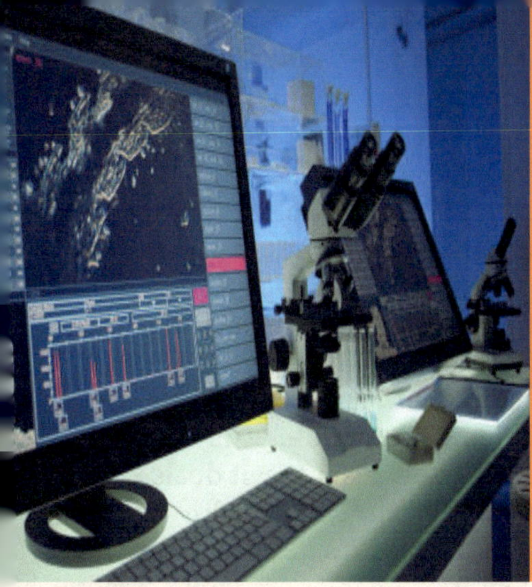

Chapter 2

PRINCIPLES OF EPIDEMIOLOGY

Contents

Introduction

Epidemiology is a cornerstone in public health, demonstrating the multifaceted relationship between health, disease, and populations. Through rigorous scientific investigation, epidemiologists examine the distribution and determinants of states or events of health in defined populations. Using a scientific approach, epidemiologists scrutinise diverse health phenomena, from infectious diseases to chronic illnesses, to determine patterns that guide interventions and policies. The relevance of incorporating population health principles into epidemiology is evident in the current trend toward value-based healthcare, which focuses on outcomes rather than just service provision. Appreciating epidemiological principles helps healthcare workers to cope effectively with this paradigm, ultimately enhancing health outcomes (an indispensable function in confronting the challenges that ensue from numerous social, economic, and Carmalt et al., 2018). By attending to both health determinants and health disparities, epidemiologists are engaged with environmental factors. Research methods should also be covered in an introduction to epidemiology because they are essential for testing hypotheses in health determinants. Cohort studies, case-control studies, and cross-sectional studies are beneficial for determining the causes and modes of disease transmission. Epidemiology is used in many areas of health to address existing problems, which makes it essential. This adaptability also encourages further responsibility at a population level, substantiating the fact that it is collective behavior that is imperative to disease prevention and health promotion (Cacrcp et al., 2023). As the profession evolves, it supports the fact that stakeholders must unite so that effective utilization of solutions towards addressing health problems is possible (Figure 2.2).

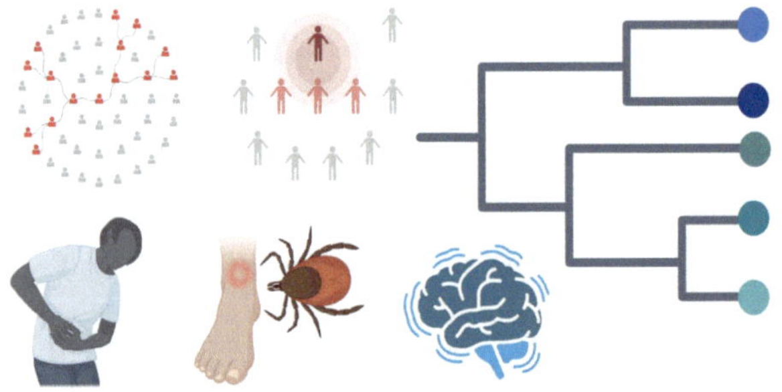

Figure 2.1. Epidemiology serves.

Source: https://microbenotes.com/wp-content/uploads/2024/09/Epidemiology.jpeg

Definition and Scope of Epidemiology

Epidemiology, when treated as a specific field of research, is more specifically concerned with the distribution and determinants of health-related states in defined populations. This summary highlights the discipline's focus on the transmission of diseases across various environments and populations. Most importantly, epidemiology is not merely interested in quantifying such events but also explores reasons and possible prevention. This interest is essential for the development of successful public health interventions and policies. By conducting a comprehensive evaluation of health patterns, epidemiologists can identify populations at risk and develop targeted interventions. This ties in with the ongoing need to adapt to complex health issues that arise in different sociocultural settings, leading to a healthier society through the process of informed decision-making and resource allocation. Epidemiology is not just the science of contagious diseases; it deals with chronic diseases, environmental health issues, and even social determinants of health. Having such a broad orientation enables epidemiologists to respond to various health issues by adapting their approaches and systems as needed. For example, to study interpersonal violence among athletes, epidemiologic techniques can be applied to identify cases, understand their patterns, and determine their causes. The 2024 International Olympic Committee's Consensus on Interpersonal Violence aims to integrate evidence and provide insight into the epidemiology of such acts, demonstrating the discipline's capacity to adapt and meet emerging public health challenges (Tuakli-Wosornu et al., 2024). As the discipline advances, it innovates through the incorporation of interdisciplinarity, which deepens its appreciation for complex health phenomena. In addition, the definition and scope of epidemiology are influenced by the need to be responsive to societal transformation and new health concerns. Of critical importance is the synthesis of data collection and analysis, which will inform local and international public health programs. For example, the definition of health statistics gives a basis for the identification of patterns and the development of hypotheses on causation and prevention. The versatility of epidemiology is evident in its application across various health domains, making it consistently relevant to modern world issues. The versatility also promotes an overarching responsibility across populations and highlights that group action is essential for promoting health and preventing disease (Cacrcp et al., 2023). As it continues to develop as a discipline, epidemiology realizes the importance of the coming together of stakeholders so that the effective implementation of solutions to complex health issues is possible (Figure 2.2).

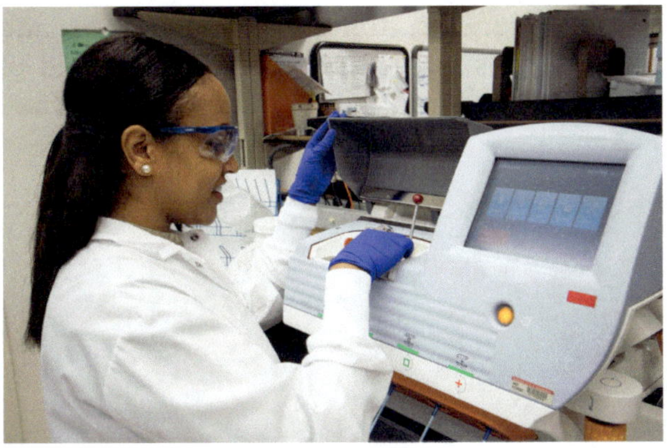

Figure 2.2. Scope of epidemiology as a distinct field of study.

Source: https://keystoneacademic-res.cloudinary.com/image/upload/element/13/134582_photo-1579154204845-5d7f8d4dc785.jpg.

Historical Development of the Field

Epidemiology's historical progression dates back to early civilizations, in which early theories of disease transmission were noted. Hippocrates, a Greek physician, is frequently regarded as being among the earliest epidemiologists because he understood the role of environmental factors as well as lifestyle factors in contributing to illness. He laid the foundation for understanding the cause-and-effect relationship between human populations and their environment. Throughout the centuries, the discipline underwent significant changes, especially in the 19th century when modern science began to develop. Trailblazers such as John Snow set new standards for conducting inquiries into the transmission of disease, particularly with his investigation of a cholera epidemic in London to a polluted water source. As a result of this episode, it became clear that epidemiology needed to focus on gathering and studying all the data, which was a key moment in the field's growth and the creation of its main principles. The recognition of public health as a profession in the 20th century facilitated the growth of epidemiology. At this time, several institutions and practices were established to monitor and improve the health of the population. Better vaccines and health campaigns led to a significant drop in infectious diseases, demonstrating the practical utility of epidemiology. Also, new ways of conducting studies like randomized controlled trials and cohort studies allowed researchers to draw clear conclusions about causes in public health. The use of statistics allowed researchers to measure both the risks and the outcomes seen in epidemiological data. As a result, the field gained recognition and was viewed as necessary, with main ideas emphasising the use of evidence to prevent and manage diseases. The COVID-19 pandemic has shown that epidemiology has a strong history, but also where it has not performed well in recent times. While governments rushed to deploy surveillance systems and control measures, it was quickly realized that many had inadequate infrastructures for successful disease monitoring and response. As identified by the recent literature, weak data systems and poor public health governance inhibited efforts to curb the virus transmission, exposing fundamental shortcomings in existing architectures (Morgan et al., 2021). Other countries, on the other hand, demonstrated examples of best epidemiological practice by rapidly marrying data and public health interventions. This contrast underscores the need for ongoing change in the discipline of epidemiology, emphasising the importance of enhanced coordination and integration of surveillance systems to leverage lessons learned from previous epidemics and inform subsequent public health policy (N/A, 2020).

Importance of Epidemiology in Public Health

Epidemiology is a foundation in public health that guides key strategies for the prevention of disease outbreaks and the improvement of population health. By studying the patterns, causes, and outcomes of health and disease conditions in specific groups, epidemiologists identify risk factors and provide evidence to support interventions that reduce them. For instance, monitoring the occurrence of foodborne illnesses affects public health policy decisions related to hygiene practices, food processing, and restaurant safety measures. Identification of *Escherichia coli* and other coliform bacteria as principal causes of foodborne illness is a classic case of the kind of vital information epidemiology provides, linking dirty conditions and eating contaminated food with health risks.

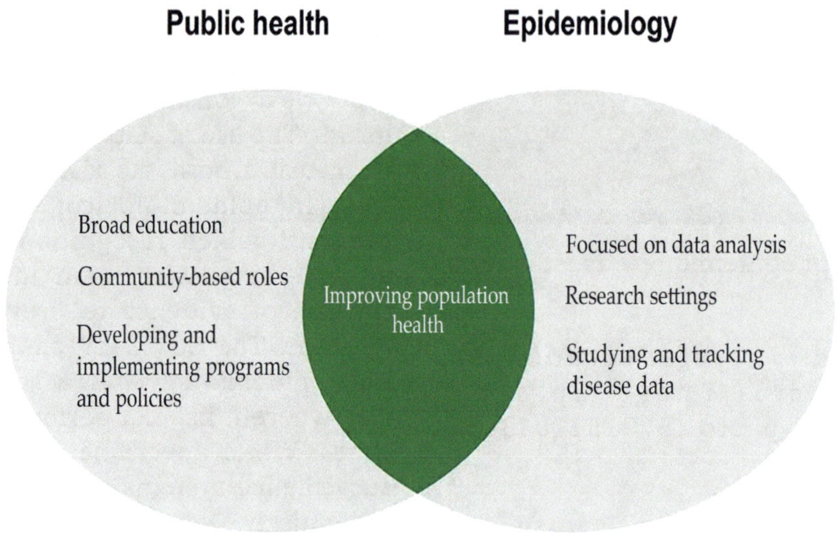

Figure 2.3. Epidemiology in public health.

Source: https://und.edu/blog/_files/images/core-differences-between-public-health-and-epidemiology-image.webp.

Efforts to contain these pathogens call for a concerted, global effort to ensure communities of adequate protection against foodborne diseases that endanger human health and economic stability. Ultimately, the contribution of epidemiology to public health is essential to designing effective prevention and health education programs (Dümen et al., 2019). In addition, the historical development of epidemiology has shown an increasing contribution to public health, particularly with advancements in laboratory technology. Significantly, however, the early contributions of public health giants such as Alexander Langmuir were predicated on the need for firm epidemiological practice over the sole dependence on laboratory results. This shift of paradigm underscored the role of field investigations and firm clinical case definitions in outbreak situations. As the discipline evolved, the incorporation of molecular epidemiology has transformed the ability of public health laboratories to identify disease-causing agents more accurately and better monitor infectious diseases. These developments have significantly enhanced the public health response to epidemics by amplifying the utility of epidemiological studies in informing laboratory practice and diagnostic capability. The ongoing evolution of epidemiological principles, therefore, remains to define the public health context and response to emerging health issues. Moreover, epidemiology is essential for more than disease avoidance because it helps us understand the social factors that affect health.

Epidemiological research studies how socioeconomic status, cultural beliefs, and environmental exposures affect the health of people in different populations. Through research, public health planners can identify the needs of at-risk groups and plan targeted interventions. An example of this is finding the disproportionate effect of a particular disease on poor populations that can be used to direct resources and health promotion efforts towards equity-based interventions. In addition, public health campaigns may be designed to educate such groups on preventing disease, thereby enhancing their resilience against public health threats. Therefore, epidemiology, apart from assisting in the control of disease, improves health equity, echoing the broader moral obligation of public health to advance the health of all. This vision as a whole highlights the central role of epidemiology in maximizing public health programs (Figure 2.3).

2.1. Key Concepts in Epidemiology

At the core of the epidemiology discipline is a number of central concepts that allow for the comprehension and study of health-related phenomena in populations. One of these concepts is the concept of disease distribution, which analyzes the nature of health events across various populations, including age, gender, and geographical location. Through such analysis using biostatistical methods, researchers can identify trends and causal factors in disease epidemiology.

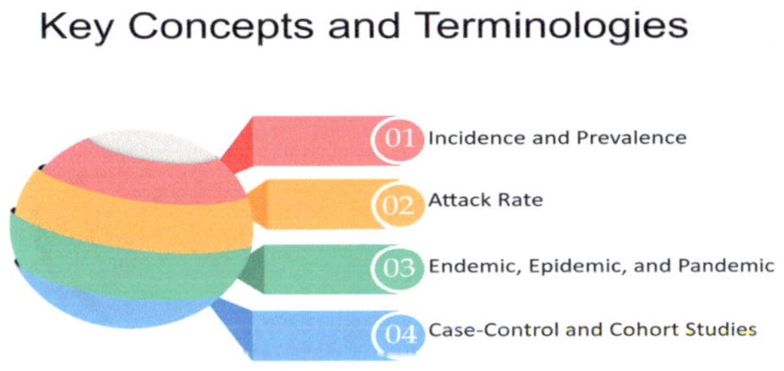

Figure 2.4. Key concepts in epidemiology.

Source: https://fastercapital.co/i/Survival-analysis-in-epidemiology--Unraveling-Disease-Dynamics--Key-Concepts-and-Terminologies.webp.

This practice allows public health practitioners to direct resources accordingly and conduct specific interventions. Moreover, identifying the social determinants of health is crucial, as conditions such as SES, education, and ecological determinants significantly affect health outcomes and disease vulnerability, reflecting the complexity of health issues in society. Another critical definition in epidemiology is that of causation, or the effort to establish an association between disease and risk factors. Epidemiologists apply mechanisms such as the Bradford Hill criteria to evaluate possible causal relationships, for example, the strength and consistency of associations. For instance, understanding how factors like smoking, nutrition, and physical exercise affect the incidence of chronic disease is crucial for informing public health policy. Furthermore, morbidity and mortality concepts enable the understanding of disease burden and facilitate the effective monitoring and evaluation of public health programs. By measuring the number of diseases and their prevalence, epidemiologists can design actions to prevent them, which leads to better population health. There has been a rise in the use of new technologies for training epidemiologists, especially by using virtual simulation. It has been seen that this approach helps improve teaching in epidemiology by providing a more engaging and interactive way for learners. Recent research has demonstrated that virtual simulations enhance learners' engagement with complex epidemiological principles and competencies, enabling them to learn about real-world public health scenarios. Spatio-temporal obstacles are removed by tools that enable learning, resulting in significant cost reduction and reducing risks in traditional learning environments. Nevertheless, problems such as initial foundation gaps and student discontent must be addressed to ensure the optimal use of virtual simulations in curricula. The implementation of such innovations results in a new era of public health professionals equipped with the necessary skills to deal with contemporary health issues across various populations (Li et al., 2024; Olowe et al., 2024) (Figure 2.4).

2.1.1. Disease Frequency and Measurement

Knowledge of disease frequency and measurement is central in epidemiology because these measures guide public health action and intervention. Disease frequency refers to the occurrence of health-related events in a given population over a specified time period. The event may be measured in different forms, such as incidence, which calculates new occurrences of a disease, and prevalence, which measures all events, new and old. Proper measurement of these frequencies is essential for the detection of trends, patterns, and future outbreaks. In addition, such information forms the basis for assessing health interventions and informing resource planning, especially during crises when timely and accurate information is critical. Scientists employ various approaches and tools to ensure that disease frequency measures are reliable. Using standard reporting guidelines is extremely important among them. Ontologies, which are used in nutritional epidemiology, help bring together and align different sets of data. For instance, ONE enables data to be linked by specifying research findings clearly and taxonomic relationships, for example, as illustrated in Ambayo et al. (2019). Through organizing data in a reasoned framework, such methods enable researchers to quantify disease frequency better, enhance study comparability, and ultimately qualify epidemiological studies better. In addition, the psychometric assessment of epidemiologic measurement instruments emphasizes the significance of validity and reliability in the accurate measurement of disease frequencies.

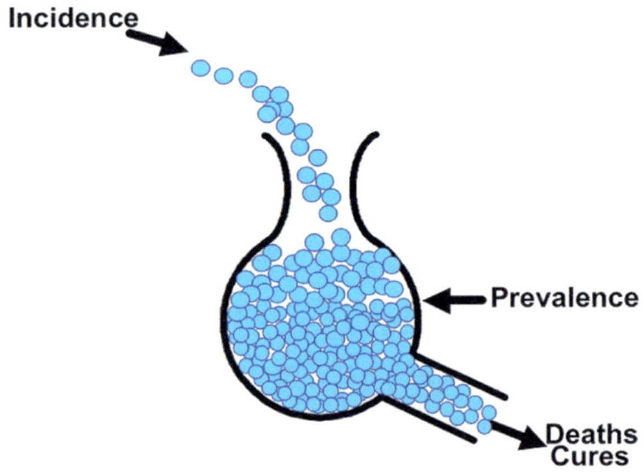

Figure 2.5. Disease frequency and measurement.

Source: https://upload.medbullets.com/topic/101004/images/incidence.jpg.

Current studies have identified the practical cross-cultural application of known tools, such as the Physical Activity Scale for the Elderly (PASE-I), for specific populations, highlighting the need for cultural adaptation and thorough testing of these devices (Berardi et al., 2018). Such a focus on evaluating the quality of measurement instruments helps ensure that data obtained from them is reliable, hence supporting the production of valid epidemiological findings. With the continued development of these tools by researchers, the future of epidemiological practice increasingly depends on sound measurement structures to grapple with the intricacies of disease frequency and its meaning for public health (Figure 2.5).

2.1.2. Risk Factors and Causation

Understanding the interdependence of causation and risk factors is core to the science of epidemiology. Risk factors, as exposures or characteristics raising the risk for disease occurrence, play a critical role in defining likely causative factors. An example, between gastric cancer (GC) and hypothyroidism, illustrates how chronic diseases influence the cancer susceptibility. The present research shows a high negative correlation of hypothyroidism with the risk of GC, indicating that hypothyroid patients will have a lower chance of having cancer of this type. These results are valuable for epidemiological preventative strategies since they underscore the importance of managing chronic diseases to decrease chances of cancer. This relationship illustrates how understanding risk factors influences our approach to disease prevention and highlights the importance of further research into the complex interactions within various populations (Zhang et al., 2024).

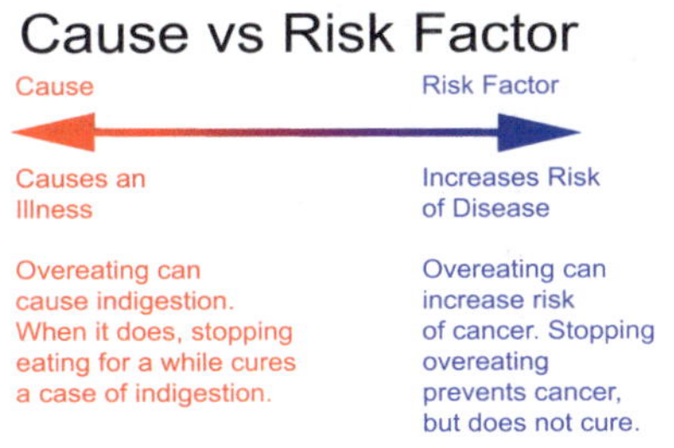

Figure 2.6. Risk factors and causation.

Source: https://healthicine.org/wordpress/wp-content/uploads/2018/09/RiskFactorvsCause-1024x740.jpg.

Besides chronic disease, specific subtypes of cancer also demonstrate different epidemiological patterns that are shaped by other risk factors. Gastric signet ring cell carcinoma (GSRC) is a case in point, with significant inconsistencies in incidence and mortality patterns according to demographic factors like age and sex. A comparison of trends using Surveillance, Epidemiology, and End Results (SEER) database data revealed a sharp rise in GSRC incidence from 1975 to 1998, followed by a decline in later years. These temporal patterns offer critical information regarding the risk factors involved in GSRC and highlight the significance of focused research further to establish our understanding of the causes of disease.

The prognostic factors obtained from these patterns also play a key role in building clinical models that can improve patient outcomes, showing how epidemiological investigation guides treatment approaches (Yu et al., 2024). It is crucial to recognise the differences in risk factors and causation to ensure an accurate public health intervention. Integrating evidence from different epidemiological studies allows researchers to construct a strong basis of knowledge regarding risk factors that lead to diseases. The discovery of mediators, including high cholesterol levels, in the relationship between hypothyroidism and GC, also helps to define the role of mediators through which risk factors affect diseases. Such information not only helps develop preventive strategies but also makes health communication more effective in terms of awareness generation among risk groups. In sum, an in-depth examination of risk factors and causation not only informs epidemiological research but also serves as a foundational element in the design and implementation of public health policies aimed at reducing the burden of diseases (Yu et al., 2024; Zhang et al., 2024) (Figure 2.6).

2.1.3. Epidemiological Transition

The theory of epidemiologic transition is central to explaining the change in patterns of disease and causes of morbidity with time as populations develop. First described by Abdel Omran in 1971, the model demonstrates a transition from high rates of fertility and mortality due to infectious diseases to low rates of mortality with non-communicable disease in developed countries. This change, in turn, reflects broader transformations in public health efforts, socioeconomic conditions, and advances in medical technology. More urbanization, improved sanitation, and enhanced healthcare systems led to the decline of infectious diseases, proving the importance of public health as a field of study in epidemiology.

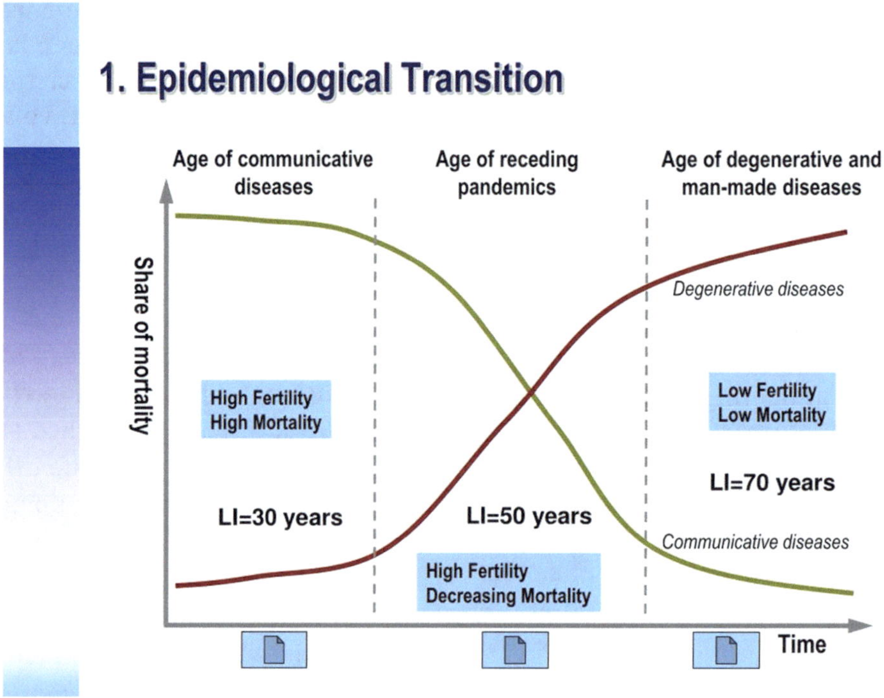

Figure 2.7. Epidemiological transition.

Source: https://image1.slideserve.com/2152309/1-epidemiological-transition1-l.jpg.

Moreover, as noted in the literature, wastewater-based epidemiology (WBE) has emerged as a crucial tool in this endeavour, providing key information on community health that informs public health decision-making and intervention planning (Girón-Guzmán et al., 2024). During the demographic and epidemiological transition, the main factors affecting health are the behaviors and environmental conditions of individuals. Especially since obesity, diabetes, and heart diseases are common, public health should focus on encouraging healthier ways of living. Epidemiological studies have found that things such as smoking, being inactive, and eating an unhealthy diet can significantly increase the risk of chronic diseases. An analysis of the health of retired contact sport participants reveals that, contrary to other suppositions, these athletes have superior risk profiles regarding dementia-related determinants compared to the general public (Department of Epidemiology et al., 2024). This finding suggests that there may be truncated understandings of present health, which emphasizes the complex determinants of health in various settings. Addressing the intricacies of the modern health trends, the addition of newer surveillance mechanisms is a requirement as we face the epidemiological transition dynamics. WBE is a good example of how classical frameworks were redefined to address newer health threats, such as pandemics and antibiotic resistance. Through the detection of viral loads and other traces of pathogens in community sewage, public health practitioners can tap into valuable information regarding epidemic trends and support timely interventions. Furthermore, the integration of health sectors, including the One Health initiative, underscores an inclusive approach recognizing the interrelatedness of animal, human, and environmental health. Such an integrated strategy is essential in the management of future health threats and the maintenance of public health gains in a period of high rate change and uncertainty (Girón-Guzmán et al., 2024) (Figure 2.7).

2.2. Study Designs in Epidemiology

The epidemiologic study designs are the basic structures used to examine the associations between exposures and health outcomes. Knowledge of these designs is critical for public health practitioners and researchers, as they determine how data are gathered, analyzed, and interpreted. Among the various designs available, RCTs, cohort studies, case-control studies, and self-controlled designs have distinct strengths and weaknesses that researchers must consider and navigate. RCTs are usually thought to be the gold standard because they tend to reduce bias and prove causation. Practicality and ethical considerations, though, may curtail their use in some contexts, and therefore, observational study designs have to be employed to reveal relationships between factors in everyday life. The complexities of each design underscore the need for methodological rigor to inform epidemiological research and guide the selection of appropriate study methodologies. Experimental studies are essential to epidemiology in that they offer the methodological backbone required to determine causal relations between exposures and health outcomes. Unlike observational studies that are susceptible to confounding variables, experimental studies allow scientists to manipulate independent variables and measure the effect on dependent variables under controlled conditions. This controlled manipulation promises to eliminate or reduce the typical biases that threaten observational data so that the internal validity of the results is optimized. An example is the way RCTs are a hallmark of experimental epidemiological research, ensuring comparability between the treated and control groups. Types of experimental design are necessary for drawing solid inferences about causality since they approximate hypothesis testing rigor in public health research. Experimental approaches in epidemiology are not without problems, however. One of the significant drawbacks is the ethical limitation of exposing individuals to potentially hazardous agents, making experiments difficult to conduct and implement. Second, the controlled conditions of the laboratory or field setting may not apply to real-world contexts, raising issues of external validity. This conceptual framework is especially relevant in measuring the validity of different types of studies, focusing on internal validity as well as possible extensions to external validity and general public health effect (Westreich, 2019). Within self-controlled study designs, the increasing acknowledgement of their methodological robustness facilitates subtle investigations of transient exposures and sudden health events. The case-crossover and self-controlled case-series study designs, for instance, facilitate investigators to adjust for time-invariant confounders, thereby enhancing capabilities for causal inference. A systematic review of self-controlled studies shows the expanding applicability of these study designs in epidemiological research (Cadarette et al., 2021). Standardization of language and shared paradigms for designing self-controlled studies not only allows researchers to communicate more effectively but also improves critical evaluation of results in published work. By distilling the conceptual basis of self-controlled designs, such activities ultimately enhance overall understanding of epidemiologic principles and spur the design of subsequent studies that adhere to optimal practices in research methodology (Figure 2.8).

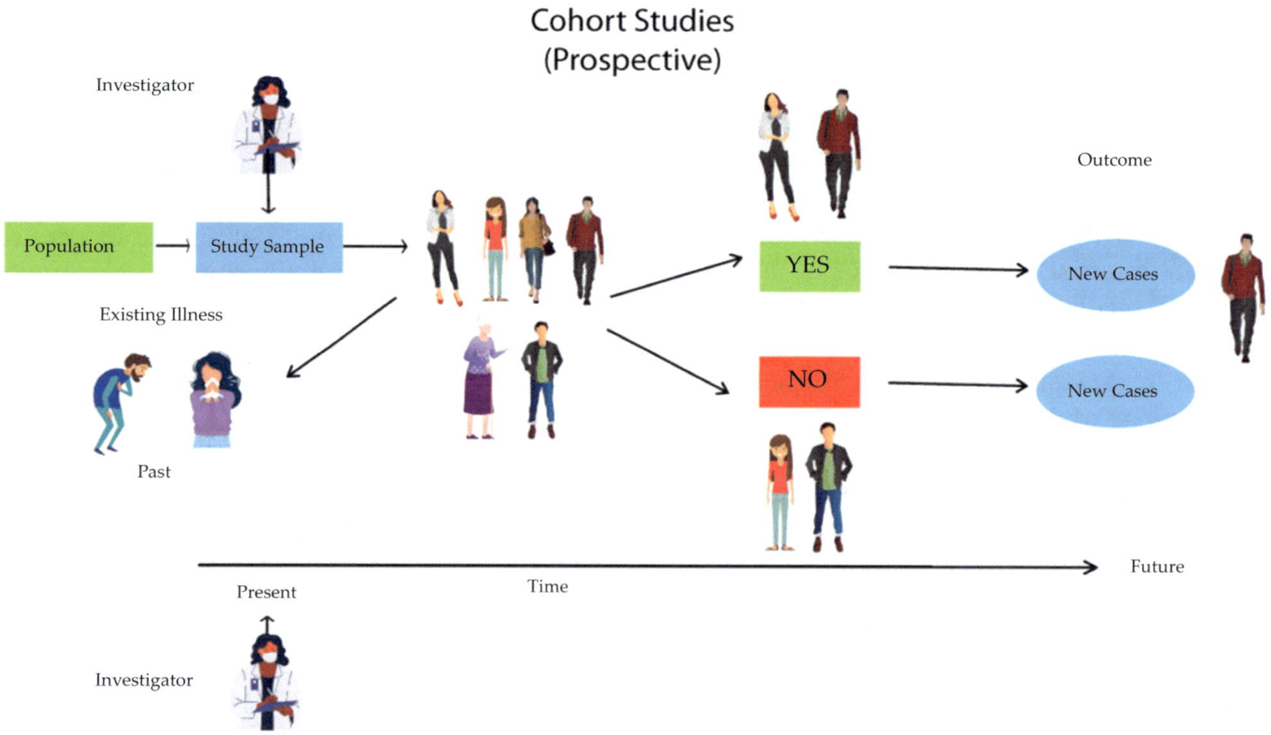

Figure 2.8. Study designs in epidemiology.

Source: https://pubrica.com/academy/wp-content/uploads/2021/04/Epidemiology-designs-1-1024x597.png.

2.2.1. Descriptive Studies

Descriptive studies play a crucial role within the discipline of epidemiology by providing a framework for understanding the occurrence of health-related events and illnesses within groups of individuals. Descriptive studies are defined by their emphasis on reporting occurrences of illnesses and health outcomes, along with recognizing patterns according to time, place, and person. For example, they can illuminate population characteristics such as age, sex, and socioeconomic status (SES) that can influence health trends. Researchers use information from patient records, surveys, and public health reports to form ideas about possible causes, which helps guide practical public health actions. Descriptive studies are useful because they help lay the groundwork for more advanced studies that aim to understand the underlying reasons behind a relationship. In several fields, including veterinary pathology, descriptive studies are crucial to increasing our comprehension of the dynamics of disease. Descriptive studies present an initial overview of disease prevalence and incidence, allowing researchers to identify regions with a heightened burden of disease. As observed in structured training workshops, such as those for OIE in partnership with CIRAD, the focus on developing descriptive epidemiology skills among health professionals highlights their importance. It is evident from these workshops how descriptive approaches can be integrated with practical practices, and the necessity of surveillance systems to monitor disease and evaluate methodologies for efficient intervention. Students tend to acquire enhanced abilities in case definition and sampling, and in the use of these methods for diseases like avian influenza, thereby demonstrating the beneficial cross-fertilization between theoretical and applied aspects of epidemiological education (Desvaux et al., 2007). In addition, the diligent planning of descriptive research includes awareness of their strengths and limitations, especially in observational studies. While they can show what is happening with health trends, descriptive studies do not prove that one thing causes another. This emphasizes the need for well-defined study rules and guidelines for who is included or excluded, which are necessary for reliable data collection. Researchers must address biases in observational methods, particularly selection bias, to ensure accurate results. Therefore, it is essential to conduct descriptive studies with attention to the proper techniques for validation and analysis. Through the grasp of these principles, investigators can substantially improve the quality of data derived, enabling descriptive studies to effectively inform subsequent research activities and public health interventions (Beck et al., 2018) (Figure 2.9).

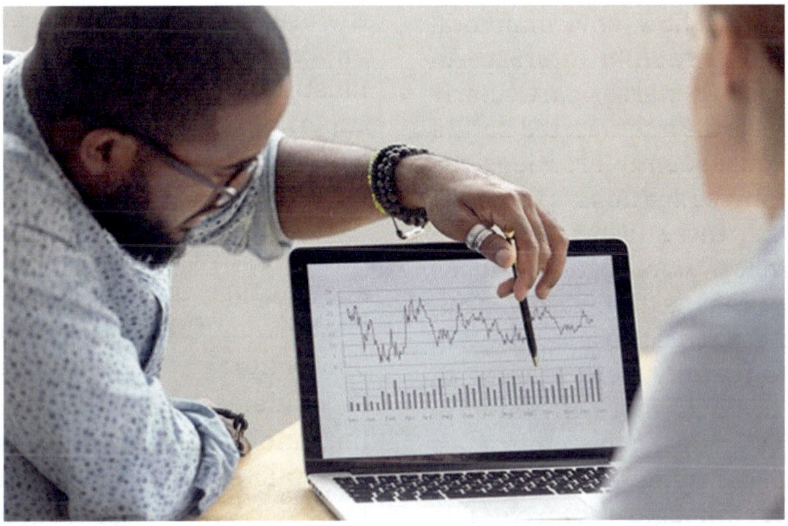

Figure 2.9. Descriptive studies.

Source: https://assets.everspringpartners.com/dims4/default/c8fce6c/2147483647/strip/true/crop/620x413+0+0/resize/620x413!/quality/90/?url=http%3A%2F%2Feverspring-brightspot.s3.us-east-1.amazonaws.com%2Fbf%2Fe4%2F0472f934481ebc7778c3f942f65c%2Fkent-epi-cvblog-descriptive-epi.jpg.

2.2.2. Analytical Studies

Analytical studies form the central element in epidemiological science, whose primary function is to unravel the association between exposure and health events. Both experimental and observational studies scrutinise causation, hence providing information critical in public health intervention. One of the most advantages of analytical research is that it can control for confounding variables, making it possible to isolate the effect of a given exposure on health outcomes. By applying tools like directed acyclic graphs (DAGs), complex relationships and biases that might otherwise affect outcomes are easier to depict. According to the literature, DAGs are effective instruments for detecting and minimising biases contained in observational data, validating the importance of methodological precision in epidemiological studies (Ellison et al., 2025). Scrutinizing these variables allows researchers to give the scientific community important information. Analytical studies are essential for more than testing hypotheses; they help find hidden biological reasons and affect clinical practices. Genetic and epigenetic factors are now being considered in epidemiology, illustrating how environmental factors and genetic susceptibility interact. An examination of epigenetic marks, particularly DNA methylation, reveals the multifaceted nature of phenotypes and consequently broadens the scope of analytical investigations (Jones et al., 2018). By studying these factors together, researchers can develop more detailed ideas about what causes diseases. As the field advances, the use of advanced statistical techniques will help epidemiologists identify new sources of bias, making their findings more meaningful and easier to interpret. Stressing the importance of well-designed analytic frameworks is key to the progress of epidemiologic research. The controversy surrounding DAGs' value and other conceptual tools underscores the importance of clear study design and reporting. Scientists must carefully control all variables relevant to their studies, including confounders, to ensure the validity of their analyses. It will remain challenging to precisely describe the complexity around these models as studies become increasingly methodologically advanced. Identifying these challenges paves the way towards future methodological innovation in study design and reporting practices. By fortifying the analytical research methodological foundation, epidemiologists can make better evidence and intervention contributions to public health, ultimately contributing to better health all over the world (Ellison et al., 2025).

2.2.3. Experimental Studies

Experimental research plays a vital role in epidemiology, as it provides the methodological framework necessary to establish causal associations between exposures and health outcomes. Unlike observational studies, which are susceptible to confounding variables, experimental studies enable researchers to manipulate independent variables and observe their effects on dependent variables under controlled conditions. By controlling the manipulation, researchers aim to reduce the usual biases in observations, which should improve the findings' internal validity. As an illustration, RCTs are a prominent feature of experimental studies in epidemiology, as they allow scientists to compare the effects on those treated with those in the control group.

They are essential for supporting conclusions about cause and effect because they are as rigorous as the testing done in public health epidemiology. Experimental methodologies in epidemiology, however, are not without limitations. One problem is that experiments may put people at risk, which makes it hard to design and perform them. Additionally, the controlled and simplified environment of the lab or field may not accurately reflect the true complexity of real-world situations, which can lead to issues with external validity. Hence, although experimental research yields pertinent information, in some cases, the information may not be easily transferable to population-level inferences. Experimental data must be critically evaluated to address these issues and gain a comprehensive understanding of the generalizability of the findings (Ellison et al., 2025). Further, investigators must exercise caution when interpreting this type of study since inferences based on idealized conditions might ignore important confounding variables typical of real-world clinical practice. In addition, recent advances in knowledge about frameworks like DAGs have enhanced the explanation of experimental research within epidemiology. DAGs provide a graphical representation of causal relationships, which makes it easier to explain how variables are involved across the research process. The methodological application makes it easier to have a clear framework for determining possible biases and causal pathways in experimental and observational research. The theoretical uses of DAGs can complement the examination of experimental data by giving information about unmeasured covariates and other difficulties involved in causal inference (Prueitt et al., 2024). Therefore, incorporating strategies such as DAGs into experimental study designs may provide new insights and contribute to better insight into various health outcomes associated with environmental exposures, enhancing the foundations of epidemiology as a science (Figure 2.10).

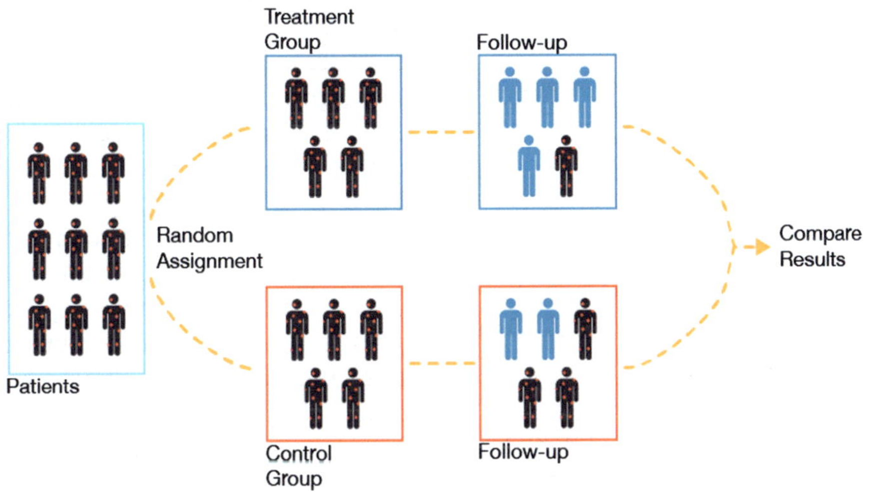

Figure 2.10. Experimental studies.

Source: https://betterthesis.dk/wp-content/uploads/2013/10/3.2.1-Figure-til-research-apporach2.png.

2.3. Epidemiological Measures

Epidemiological rates form the foundation of public health studies, providing a sound framework for understanding disease distribution and its determinants among populations. Incidence rates, prevalence rates, morbidity, and mortality rates are among the measures included, each of which provides significant information regarding the health condition of communities. Incidence rates indicate the rate at which new cases of a disease experience onset within a given time frame, and they provide insight into the dynamics of disease transmission. On the other hand, prevalence rates are concerned with the overall number of cases present in a population at a particular moment, which is of vital importance for resource planning and allocation in healthcare systems. Epidemiologists use these measures to detect risk factors linked to diseases and establish specific interventions to lower incidence and prevalence and improve public health strategies. Furthermore, the implementation of such epidemiological controls relies on reliable data sources and effective methods. For example, primary care electronic health records are being used more and more for epidemiology because they are so large in number and longitudinal in nature that they permit the examination of trends over time. However, they have pitfalls, such as misclassification and coding variability, which can lead to serious biases if not well-controlled. Technologies such as the "Data extraction for epidemiological research" (DExtER) tool are examples of data processing simplification efforts aimed at facilitating researchers to extract and organize health datasets for appropriate analysis efficiently. Through normalisation and standardisation of data inputs, DExtER improves the quality of epidemiological studies, which ultimately translates to more accurate public health surveillance and research results, crucial during and outside of health crises (Gokhale et al., 2020). The applicability of epidemiological measures has been specifically underscored in contemporary global health crises, including the COVID-19 pandemic. The rapid spread of the virus necessitated time-sensitive data to inform public health interventions and understand mental health outcomes across diverse populations. Surveys were used to determine the mental health status of targeted populations and reported high levels of anxiety and depression that worsened due to social isolation and health anxiety (Zhou et al., 2020). By using accurate epidemiological metrics, public health authorities can enhance their understanding of the psychosocial effects of pandemics and, in turn, develop more effective strategies for mental health care and community support programs. Thus, incorporating epidemiologic measures into public health models remains vital for mitigating infectious diseases and the mental health issues they cause, underscoring their pivotal role in epidemiology.

2.3.1. Incidence and Prevalence

Incidence and prevalence are both critical to the fundamental principles of epidemiology, as these measures help us understand disease dynamics within populations. Incidence is the number of new instances of a disease in a specified population over a specific period of time. It is an essential measure of the risk of contracting the disease and is critical for determining the effectiveness of preventive efforts. When public health workers follow incidence rates, trends can be detected, the effectiveness of interventions can be assessed, and resources can be allocated appropriately. Prevalence is a measure of all the cases, old and new, that exist at a particular moment. This distinction highlights the manner in which incidence can shed light on the chances of disease occurrence, while prevalence provides a snapshot of disease burden within a population (Manja et al., 2015). It is essential to notice differences in incidence and prevalence between populations when studying disease patterns. The way people are measured can be affected by where they live, their economic situation, and their demographics. In some cases, environmental factors or lifestyle choices can lead to certain diseases being more prevalent in specific areas. Still, the number of cases may be affected by healthcare access and cultural factors. Therefore, epidemiologists must consider these factors to accurately interpret data and design effective public health programs. Through the analysis of the incidence-prevalence relationship, scientists can also assess the effect of interventions over time and how changes in prevalence reflect the total impact of public health interventions on reducing rates of incidence (Bhopal, 2008). In public health practice, the incidence-prevalence relationship affects strategic planning and resource allocation. A high incidence would typically necessitate high-intervention efforts that are instant and directed towards prevention and disease control. In contrast, high prevalence might indicate periodic needs of care and management of chronic disease. For instance, during infectious disease outbreaks, a high incidence would prompt rapid public health responses in terms of vaccination drives as well as information campaigns. On the other hand, an increase in chronic disease prevalence, for example, diabetes, indicates the need for long-term management interventions, including patient education and health access enhancement. The comprehension of the dynamic interplay between these two terms not only improves epidemiological studies but also supports a better-informed public health intervention, leading toward an era of improved overall health in the population (Manja et al., 2015) (Figure 2.11).

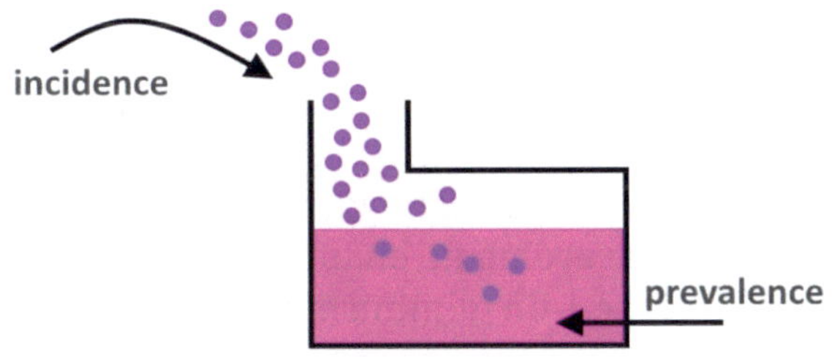

Figure 2.11. Incidence and prevalence.

Source: https://www.sltinfo.com/wp-content/uploads/2016/02/incidence-and-prevalence-1200x600-c-default.jpg

2.3.2. Mortality Rates

It is important to understand mortality rates in the study of epidemiology because they reflect very important information about the population's health status and the efficiency of healthcare systems. Mortality rates indicate the number of people in a population who die within a specified period, enabling public health officials to identify trends and implement suitable interventions. A review of death rates may point out that some groups, such as those who are older, of a different sex, or from a particular place, have higher death rates than others. These inequalities help find the areas with the greatest need for healthcare and also lead to research on the main reasons behind them. Trends in mortality can also push for public health actions to help prevent chronic diseases which have a significant impact on overall mortality rates. The study of individual diseases within mortality research is crucial for a comprehensive understanding of the epidemiological context. For instance, GSRC, a rare variant of GC, has shown variable mortality figures over time. A study using SEER data revealed that the rate of this cancer increased steeply through 1998 before dropping noticeably in later years (Yu et al., 2024). Patterns like these underscore the need for continuous monitoring and assessment of populations afflicted with specific diseases. Predictive models capable of predicting outcomes through well-documented risk factors are needed for improved management of such health disorders. This allows for more targeted intervention in the treatment, which eventually reduces death rates corresponding to only those diseases. Moreover, the integration of more sophisticated mathematical constructs into epidemiology enables us to understand the mortality rates in relation to infectious diseases more effectively. Applying fluid dynamics theories for modelling the spread of infections through space provides a fresh perspective in understanding how diseases spread across populations (Nnaji et al., 2024). The new approach depicts the dynamic processes of disease transmission as fluid densities of complicated equations. By doing this, epidemiologists can simulate various scenarios and identify the factors that contribute most strongly to mortality rates. The models' outcomes can be utilised to inform targeted public health interventions so as to allocate resources better, leading to a reduction in mortality rates. As epidemiologic modelling advances, it can transform how public health interventions are designed and implemented, and significantly impact the health of populations.

2.3.3. Morbidity Measures

Morbidity measures play a key role in epidemiology by showing the patterns of diseases and health conditions among people. Morbidity measures enable us to determine the prevalence of diseases and their frequency, allowing for comparisons between different groups and regions. Morbidity measures help public health officials assess the impact of diseases, inform decisions on health actions, and plan the allocation of resources. Most significantly, the distinction between incidence (new cases) and prevalence (existing cases) is significant because each yields different information regarding a population's health status. If the number of cases is high, it generally indicates a chronic health issue that requires management. Conversely, a high number of new cases typically signifies a recent outbreak or an exacerbating health situation. Understanding these factors is crucial for developing strategies that can lower disease rates and improve the health of everyone. Beyond prevalence and incidence, morbidity measures also comprise a range of metrics representing the burden of sickness on individuals and populations. Prevalent among these is the disability-adjusted life year (DALY), which combines years of life lost to premature death and years with disability. DALYs play a valuable role in comparing the total burden of health for different diseases, as they account for both morbidity and mortality, presenting a comprehensive picture of health loss in populations. It helps prioritize health issues for intervention and in measuring the effectiveness of health policy and programs. As epidemic trends shift, enacting such procedures can be an effective model to guide decision-making and policy formation in a way that optimizes the targeting of resources toward the most critical health problems confronting populations. The incorporation of morbidity measures into the precepts of epidemiology is not just about data gathering; it is about ethical and responsible public health practice. Valid morbidity measurements enable epidemiologists to recognize at-risk populations and direct interventions focused on diminishing disparities in health. Furthermore, the ethical implications of how these measures are utilised remain of utmost importance. For example, although software packages and analytical tools can assemble extensive health measures, interpretation and application thereof must be done with sensitivity to social, economic, and cultural contexts. Combatting biases and providing equal access to health resources requires the promise of transparency and community engagement in the epidemiological process, eventually encouraging a more equitable and efficient public health infrastructure (Afiaz et al., 2023; Hruz, 2023) (Figure 2.12).

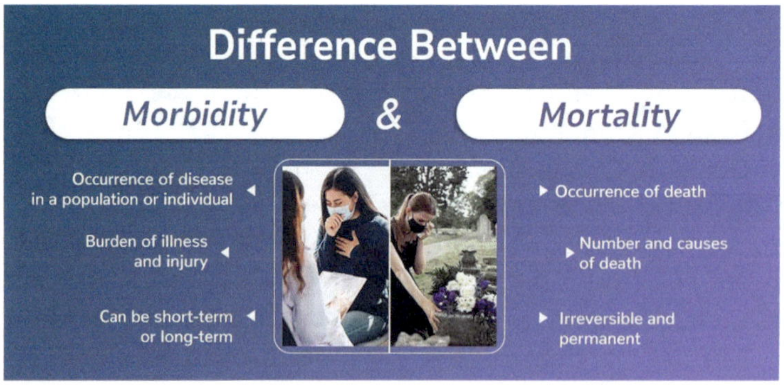

Figure 2.12. Morbidity measures are essential tools in epidemiology.

Source: https://media.geeksforgeeks.org/wp-content/uploads/20240409120405/Difference-Between-Morbidity-And-Mortality.webp.

2.4. Data Collection Methods

Effective methods for collecting data form the backbone of the discipline of epidemiology, for it is through these methods that researchers can collect, analyse, and interpret important health information. Quantitative techniques, including surveys and experiments, and qualitative methodologies, such as interviews and focus groups, cater to varied research objectives. Surveys are designed instruments offering comprehensive quantitative information, with which the researcher can establish trends, correlations, and causal factors. Conversely, qualitative techniques allow for more in-depth insight by recording individual histories and environmental circumstances that quantitative techniques may miss. The effectiveness of these techniques depends on their correspondence with the research purposes, the population being explored, and the precision of the epidemiological questions asked. As pointed out in field epidemiology training program (FETP) studies, the incorporation of sound data collection practices is essential for guiding public health actions effectively (Griffith et al., 2024).

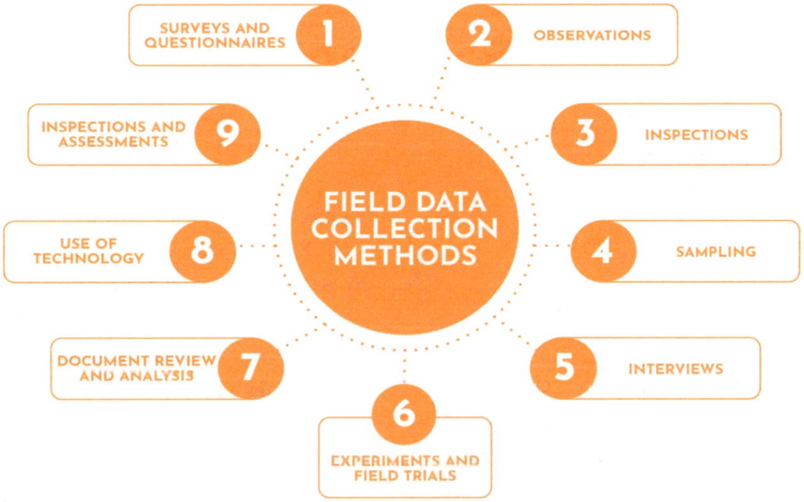

Figure 2.13. Data collection methods are fundamental to the field of epidemiology.

Source: https://irp.cdn-website.com/ed458e90/dms3rep/multi/field+data+colletion_methods.webp.

Data collection during epidemiological studies should also adhere to high standards of ethics, including ensuring participant confidentiality and obtaining informed consent. Ethical data collection practices enhance the validity of the research and foster community confidence in epidemiological evidence. For example, as the case of pediatric ocular injuries illustrates, collecting data from medical reports must adhere to ethical standards while protecting sensitive information that impacts vulnerable groups (Bamdad et al., 2024). This is especially crucial while working with disadvantaged groups or patients who experience stigmatization from specific health conditions. By embracing strict ethical procedures in combination with methodical data collection techniques, epidemiological studies can produce more precise, valid, and socially accountable results, ultimately advancing public health programs. Furthermore, the selection of the data collection method depends on the available resources as well as the nature of the targeted disease. In various epidemiological studies, researchers are increasingly adopting mixed-method strategies, which combine qualitative and quantitative data collection methods to gain a comprehensive understanding of health phenomena. For instance, the measurement of the prevalence of a disease could be complemented by following up with in-depth interviews to understand the experienced realities of the affected. This multi-component approach adds depth to the data gathered and allows for a more sophisticated analysis of patterns in epidemiology and determinants of health. Ultimately, the quality of data gathering efforts is integral to the validity of epidemiological research. It determines the interpretation and application of findings to public health practices, according to the training priorities for field epidemiologists (Griffith et al., 2024) (Figure 2.13).

2.4.1. Surveys and Questionnaires

Surveys and questionnaires are cardinal epidemiological tools, handy for collecting data on community perceptions of health, disease prevalence, and health behaviour. They enable the quantitative collection of information from various populations, allowing researchers to identify trends and make well-informed public health policy decisions. Surveys' design needs to be methodologically sound; they should include objective questions, valid response scales, and explicit instructions to ensure that the data collected truly represent the population's views and actions. For example, during the COVID-19 pandemic, surveys were used to measure community attitudes toward public health interventions and obtained valuable insights into common perceptions and concerns related to disease surveillance (LaJoie et al., 2022). This knowledge is critical to the development of successful health communication strategies and interventions. The effectiveness of surveys in epidemiological studies is further demonstrated by research that measures mental health outcomes during times of crisis, such as the COVID-19 pandemic. Researchers used online surveys to measure the psychological effects of social isolation and health anxiety in people from different demographics. In one piece of research, more than 2000 patients received a complete questionnaire, and among the findings were high levels of anxiety, depression, and insomnia in respondents (Zhou et al., 2020). The capacity to perform extensive surveys rapidly and cost-effectively, particularly over online media, attests to their adaptability and relevance in modern epidemiological work. This method enables researchers to obtain timely data, which is crucial in addressing public health crises and informing interventions that are responsive to the evolving needs of at-risk populations. Additionally, combining data received through surveys enhances the overall understanding of health issues in communities. To public health officials, this information aids in the identification of vulnerable populations and emerging health problems. By triangulating survey data with other epidemiological data sources, researchers can construct a more detailed picture of community health dynamics. Furthermore, the openness of the survey development process, including pilot testing and validation, lends strength to the credibility and reliability of the data obtained. As exemplified in wastewater-based epidemiological surveys, public perceptions based on surveys can inform community acceptance or opposition to new health monitoring approaches, helping policymakers in effective health regulation policy (LaJoie et al., 2022). Therefore, the intentional application of surveys and questionnaires plays a critical role in our understanding and application of epidemiology principles (Figure 2.14).

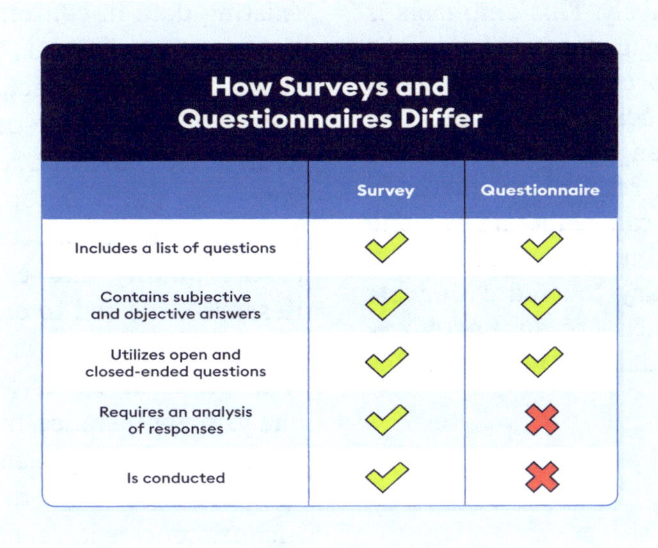

How Surveys and Questionnaires Differ

	Survey	Questionnaire
Includes a list of questions	✓	✓
Contains subjective and objective answers	✓	✓
Utilizes open and closed-ended questions	✓	✓
Requires an analysis of responses	✓	✗
Is conducted	✓	✗

Figure 2.14. Surveys and questionnaires.

Source: https://cdn.prod.website-files.com/63299e8be533faffbc123045/636ac7bd3d7b973f4b30e9e9_Surveys_and_Questionnaire_Differences.png.

2.4.2. Surveillance Systems

Surveillance systems are essential components of public health infrastructure, enabling early detection and response to potential health hazards. They form the basis for knowledge about the distribution and determinants of health-related states in populations. Efficient surveillance systems employ different methodologies for data collection, such as disease registries, health surveys, and laboratory reports. Data collection is necessary for detecting outbreaks, observing trends, and guiding public health interventions. In addition, the incorporation of advanced data analytics and technology increases the capability of these systems to anticipate and respond to health emergencies, thus enhancing public health outcomes. As explained in the investigation of public health practice, epidemiology plays a critical role in crafting effective interventions that respond to the prevailing epidemiological environment, as seen in the focus on adaptive methods of public health (Mwaura, 2024). During disease outbreaks, surveillance systems are an essential tool for outbreak investigation. They enable early detection of abnormal patterns that could be indicative of the onset of infectious diseases. Precise surveillance is essential for public health workers, who count on systematic methodologies to identify outbreaks from official and unofficial sources. Through verification of outbreaks and diagnoses, such systems assist investigators in collecting critical case information and performing descriptive epidemiology. As indicated in the principles of outbreak investigation, strong surveillance systems facilitate both the immediate response as well as a platform for continuous monitoring and risk communication to stakeholders (Iamsirithaworn et al., 2021). They play a central role in ensuring timely, effective, and appropriate intervention. Furthermore, the establishment and implementation of surveillance systems are crucial for promoting health equity and addressing disparities in healthcare access. Effective surveillance can shed light on gaps in public health services and identify at-risk populations with elevated risk of disease. By focusing on health equity, public health efforts can be structured to allocate resources and target interventions among vulnerable groups effectively. This emphasis is consistent with the strategic objectives of public health, which aim to improve health outcomes while considering the social determinants of health. Upcoming challenges, including EIDs and global health threats, require strengthened surveillance systems that can adapt and respond quickly. Therefore, continuous investment in such systems is necessary to create durable public health plans, which are supported by solid epidemiological evidence (Mwaura, 2024) (Figure 2.15).

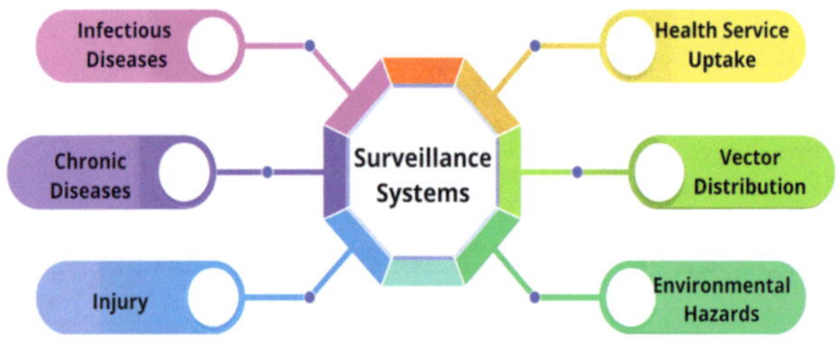

Figure 2.15. Surveillance systems are critical components of public health infrastructure.

Source: https://publichealthprepared.org/wp-content/uploads/2022/09/Evaluating-Surv-System-Image-1080x675.png.

2.4.3. Secondary Data Analysis

Secondary data analysis in the context of epidemiology is a valuable tool for combining existing data to inform decision-making in public health. Utilizing available datasets allows researchers to cost-effectively examine trends, detect health disparities, and assess intervention effects without the time and resource constraints of collecting original data.

This approach is especially beneficial where prompt action is required, as in public health crises. For example, research has shown that secondary electronic sources are highly effective in identifying pertinent studies related to interventions during health crises, demonstrating the significant value of existing data in contemporary epidemiological contexts (Levay et al., 2023). That reliance on secondary data reflects how important it is in supporting evidence-based practices in public health. Secondary data analysis has significant strengths, but it is not without its weaknesses. One major issue concerns the limitations related to the quality and extent of the data used. Researchers need to critically evaluate sources of secondary data to ascertain that they comply with the stringent criteria necessary for viable analysis. For instance, numerous epidemiological studies have emphasised how differences in data collection and definitions can introduce inconsistencies in results, negatively impacting the integrity of the analysis (Levay et al., 2023). In addition, the built-in biases in the raw data can also carry over through the analysis process. They can mislead researchers to incorrect conclusions if not adequately dealt with. These challenges necessitate a meticulous and informed approach to secondary data analysis, with a strong emphasis on methodological rigour. The use of secondary data analysis is most clearly realized in the examination of public health trends over time. Epidemiologists may utilize these data to identify trends, track the occurrence of disease outbreaks, and assess health policy effectiveness. Researchers may determine patterns by examining historical data and use these patterns to inform current health policies. For example, a retrospective study of pediatric surgical cases mirrored the working trends in a new unit, illustrating how past data can inform resource allocation and patient care decisions well (Aslam et al., 2023). This shows that secondary data analysis is not just about re-contextualizing available information; it is really about turning insights into usable public health policy. The convergence and analysis of secondary data, therefore, foster a deeper understanding of health dynamics, paving the way for improved health outcomes (Figure 2.16).

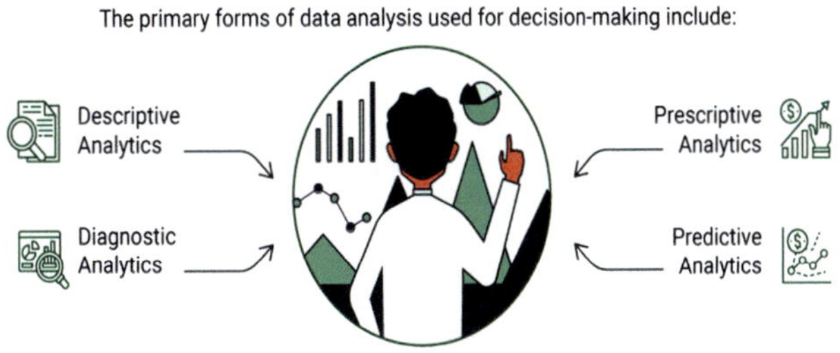

Figure 2.16. secondary data analysis serves as a critical tool public health decision-making.

Source: https://publichealth.tulane.edu/wp-content/uploads/sites/3/2022/08/blog-data-driven-decision-making-image-2-1024x540.jpeg.

2.5. Statistical Analysis in Epidemiology

In epidemiology, statistical analysis is one of the cornerstones that support many research studies aimed at defining patterns of health among populations. Through the use of sophisticated mathematical models and statistical measures, epidemiologists can recognize patterns between exposures and resultant health results and, thereby, influence public health policy. For example, biostatistical techniques enable researchers to evaluate the effect of different risk factors on the incidence and prevalence of disease, enabling one to forecast future health trends and modify interventions accordingly. As noted in Olowe et al. (2024), the foundational principles of biostatistics equip investigators with key competencies in probability theory and regression analysis, which are central to unravelling the complexities of health data in the context of a more interconnected global environment. Consequently, the inclusion of statistical methods in epidemiology promotes both scientific research and the efficiency of public health interventions. Furthermore, the use of advanced statistical methods has revolutionized the face of epidemiological research, especially in the situation of emerging health emergencies. In the case of the COVID-19 pandemic, for instance, public health professionals used statistical analysis to assess intervention approaches, track disease transmission, and analyze healthcare demands among populations. A good example cited in Tanese, Local Health Authority and Others (2023) is the use of District Operation Centers (DOCs) in Rome, where statistical surveys were used to gather information from healthcare workers. It was an evidence-based approach offering a foundation for knowledge on the effectiveness of innovative organizational approaches in addition to integrating primary care and public health systems more effectively. Through the implementation of stringent statistical analysis, these strategies not only addressed short-term healthcare needs but also ensured the resilience and flexibility of healthcare systems confronted with crises unparalleled in their history. In addition, the findings gleaned from statistical analysis extend beyond short-term health emergencies, influencing long-term epidemiological research and policy development. With the development of biostatistics, methodologies like big data analytics and machine learning (ML) are being used more to derive insights from vast datasets, allowing better comprehension of sophisticated determinants of health. These advances in methodology allow epidemiologists to carry out subtle analyses, especially in the management of chronic diseases and health inequities across various population segments. The continued focus on improving statistical methods, highlighted in Olowe et al. (2024), continues to be essential for assessing health interventions and guiding evidence-based public health policy.

Therefore, the significance of statistical analysis to epidemiology continues to be of great importance, providing researchers and practitioners with the ability to bridge the complex array of global health issues (Figure 2.17).

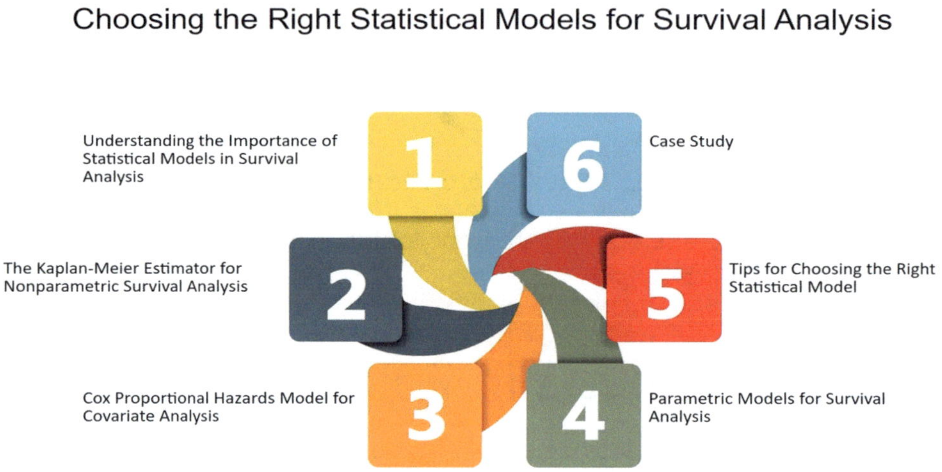

Figure 2.17. Statistical analysis in epidemiology.

Source: https://fastercapital.co/i/Survival-analysis-in-epidemiology--Unraveling-Disease-Dynamics--Choosing-the-Right-Statistical-Models-for-Survival-Analysis.webp.

2.5.1. Descriptive Statistics

Descriptive statistics is an integral part of epidemiology, as it gives various tools for summarizing and organizing data derived from population research. Using the measures of central tendency, that is, mean, median, and mode, scientists can communicate the average or typical values of health variables among various populations. Measures of dispersion, that is, range and standard deviation, also help in interpreting the variation in data sets. This statistical model enables epidemiologists to present sophisticated health data in a clear and easily digestible form, thereby enhancing the effectiveness of public health messages. By applying descriptive statistics effectively, professionals can consistently identify trends in disease prevalence, pinpoint areas requiring intervention, and allocate resources more efficiently, which is crucial in combating health disparities. In public health research, descriptive statistics also facilitate the visualization of data distributions by graphical means, including histograms or box plots. Beyond making large datasets easier to interpret, these visual aids reveal latent patterns that may not be as obvious through the analysis of numerical data alone. For example, identifying skewness in data can reveal disparities in health outcomes across demographic groups. Such information is invaluable for epidemiologists who seek to develop efficient public health interventions. Such practices are also rendered more critical by technological improvements that facilitate the efficient management of enormous volumes of health data, thereby enabling a more sophisticated understanding of population health trends across different phases of disease dynamics and intervention effectiveness. Additionally, the use of descriptive statistics in epidemiological research becomes critical while determining the influence of confounding variables in measuring causal relations. The given statistics provide a precise description of data properties and form the basis of more advanced inferential analysis, enabling researchers to examine possible correlations between exposure variables and health statuses. For instance, in Mendelian randomization studies, the appropriate deployment of descriptive statistics becomes essential to create a baseline against which causal conclusions could be inferred with less risk of biased results. This demonstrates the interaction between descriptive and inferential statistics, how strong descriptive analysis can add strength to epidemiological evidence. Therefore, the application of these statistical techniques, guided by epidemiological principles, underpins public health decision-making and policy development, ultimately leading to improved health outcomes on a larger scale (Skrivankova et al., 2021; Sallam, 2023) (Figure 2.18).

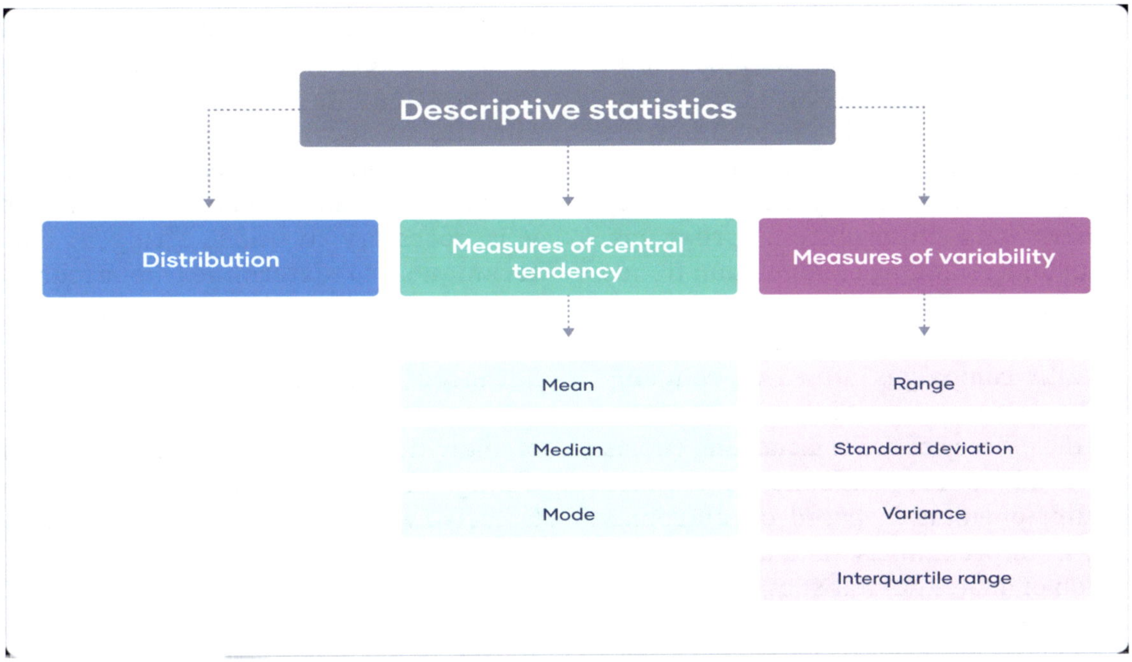

Figure 2.18. Descriptive statistics.

Source: https://www.scribbr.co.uk/wp-content/uploads/2023/01/Descriptive-statistics.webp.

2.5.2. Inferential Statistics

Inferential statistics are also crucial in epidemiology, as they enable predictions and inferences about population values based on sampled data. Such value is especially noted in relation to public health emergencies, like the COVID-19 pandemic. Inferential statistical analysis was used to assess the vast amounts of data collected on infection rates, duration of recovery, and the efficacy of different mitigation policies. The capacity to generalise results from a smaller group to a larger population enables epidemiologists to inform public health policy and resource allocation effectively. Further, by hypothesis testing and confidence intervals, inferential statistics create a system to evaluate the validity of assertions made about health outcomes so that evidence-based decision-making in the management of health crises such as COVID-19 can be supported (Latif et al., 2020). Inferential statistics' mechanics usually incorporate sophisticated modelling methods that estimate the relationships among several health-related factors. For example, in examining the impact of exercise on general health, epidemiologists can draw on compositional data analysis (CoDA) to consider how composite activities interact within a static 24-hour timeframe. With the help of CoDA, researchers can measure how time spent in different behaviours is associated with health outcomes, for example, body weight or cardiovascular health. This method emphasises the inherent interdependencies between activities of daily life and does not view them as distinct measurements. Therefore, inferential statistics not only quantify the associations but also explain the complex relationships in a holistic context that mirrors actual behavioural patterns (Dumuid et al., 2020). In addition, the use of inferential statistics is not just limited to data analysis; it critically shapes policy development and intervention programs. Through an understanding of population trends and the ability to draw sound conclusions from sample data, health officials can design targeted public health campaigns aimed at reducing health risks. Inferential statistics, for example, identified the efficacy of social distancing efforts during the COVID-19 pandemic as a cause for their implementation based on outcomes estimated from preliminary data analysis. The contribution of inferential statistics, therefore, is central to epidemiology because it bridges data-derived understandings with actionable public health interventions. This bridging highlights the imperative of using sound statistical techniques to ensure that public health measures are well-grounded and practical in protecting community health outcomes (Dumuid et al., 2020; Latif et al., 2020).

2.5.3. Interpretation of Epidemiological Data

Understanding patterns of disease and developing effective public health interventions require the interpretation of epidemiological data. One of the key features of this interpretation is the trend analysis over time, as observed in the examination of trends in HIV/AIDS epidemiology in the Philippines between 2010 and 2022. Using systematic collection and examination of longitudinal data, researchers established disconcerting gradients in the rise in HIV incidence, late diagnosis, and death rates in different geographic areas. This trend analysis presents key findings that call for focused community-level prevention efforts, especially among high-risk groups like migrant workers and commercial sex workers. Using the socioecological model, scientists can frame these observations within the broader context of social determinants, thereby informing interventions that are both pertinent and effective in alleviating the HIV/AIDS burden in the affected areas (Montegrico et al., 2024). When interpreting epidemiological information, it is necessary to utilise stringent analytical techniques to determine the accuracy and validity of outcomes. The discrete event simulation (DES) model represents one of these advanced techniques, permitting researchers to model disease progression through the use of individual traits and discrete events with timing. This model also differs significantly from conventional state-transition models in that it allows for a more subtle examination of diseases that could develop in multiple ways among individuals. For example, the use of DES in comparing the cost-effectiveness of screening protocols for diseases like abdominal aortic aneurysms illustrates its capability to account for time-dependent factors. This not only strengthens the evidence base for public health policy but also enables the interpretation of the impact of individual heterogeneity on disease outcomes, ultimately enhancing the quality of epidemiological studies and their applications (Wang et al., 2023). In addition, combining results across different analytical frameworks and longitudinal research extends the interpretation of epidemiological evidence by presenting a dimensional perspective of public health concerns. Through cross-matching trends realised from longitudinal data against models such as DES, public health practitioners can gain detailed insights that guide their strategic interventions. With ongoing observations of increasing trends in some diseases, there is a growing need to analyse data from a holistic perspective. This can develop creative prevention strategies and policy formulation guidelines for targeted groups, thus improving community health outcomes. Ultimately, a well-rounded interpretation of epidemiological data is crucial for addressing public health challenges effectively, ensuring that interventions are based on solid evidence and tailored to the community's needs (Wang et al., 2023; Montegrico et al., 2024) (Figure 2.19).

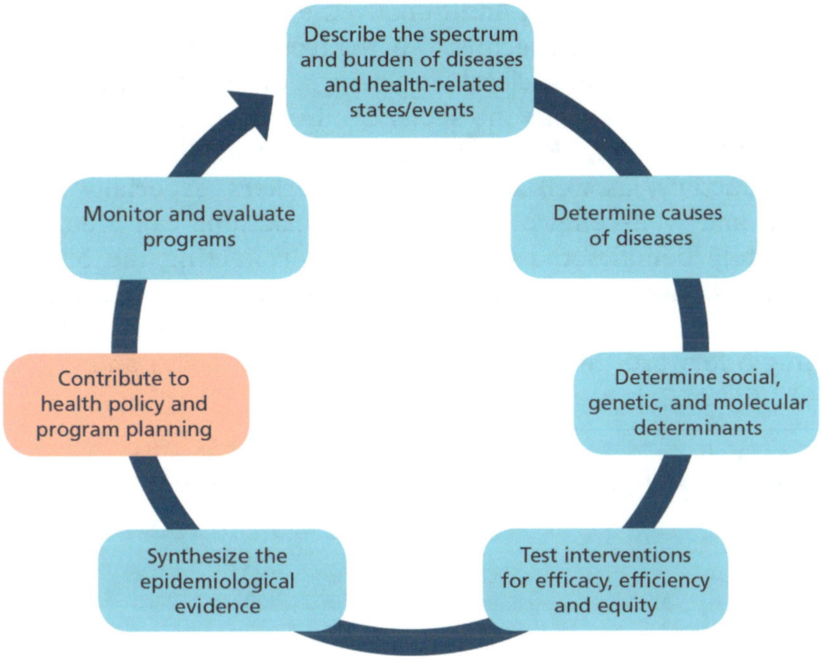

Figure 2.19. The interpretation of epidemiological data public health interventions.

Source: https://globalhealthdata.org/wp-content/uploads/2019/12/GHDMPP-Figure-18.1.jpg.

2.6. Applications of Epidemiology

The uses of epidemiology reach well beyond simply monitoring the occurrence and prevalence of illness; they actually shape public health policy and practice. By determining the causal association between exposures and health effects, epidemiologists can provide crucial evidence to guide interventions designed to reduce health risks. For instance, the epidemiological research on contagious diseases has facilitated the establishment of vaccination schemes that have dramatically reduced the occurrence of diseases like polio and measles. Additionally, epidemiological information guides health education campaigns, allowing communities to make enlightened decisions about their health habits. Thus, the incorporation of research evidence from epidemiology into public health programs helps to ensure that actions are based on scientific evidence that is the backbone of effective disease prevention and health promotion. Besides informing public health policy, epidemiology plays a vital role in resource allocation and healthcare planning. Through the identification of populations at increased risk and the identification of social determinants of health, policymakers can direct resources more purposefully. For example, the use of epidemiological approaches has helped to alleviate disparities in health outcomes between demographic groups. By being aware of those contextual determinants that contribute to these disparities, for example, SES or geography, health programs can be customized to address the specific needs of vulnerable populations. Along these lines, evidence obtained through epidemiological studies not only informs fund allocation but also underlies the development of targeted interventions intended to enhance overall health equity among populations. Additionally, the cross-disciplinary field of epidemiology has the capacity to influence numerous sectors, ranging from environmental health to occupational safety, thereby contributing to overall societal well-being. For instance, in the agricultural industry, improving labour productivity as well as the social conditions of workers has a close relationship with epidemiological understanding. Evidence shows that providing healthy working conditions leads to increased productivity as well as the SES of workers, especially in poultry farming. By prioritising the health and well-being of workers, organisations can create a more sustainable workforce that ultimately benefits the entire industry, reflecting the broader applications of epidemiological principles. The diverse use cases of epidemiology underscore its significance not only in solving urgent health issues, like investment policies in specific fields (Сметанин, 2024), but also in developing a forward-thinking paradigm to public health and personnel management (Zaporozhets, 2024) (Figure 2.20).

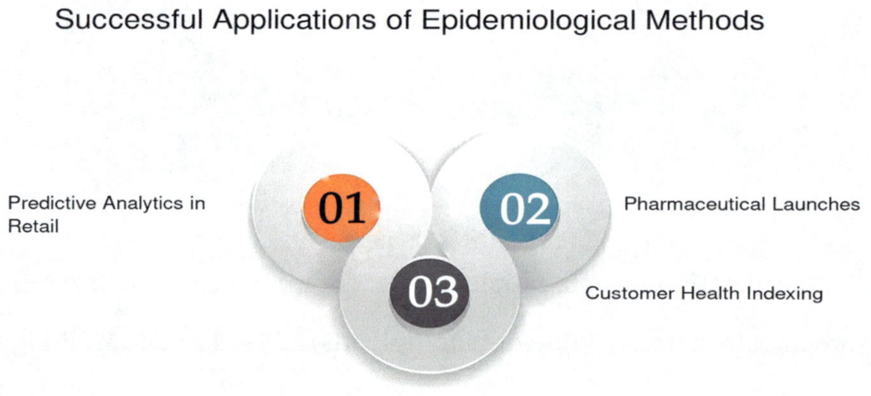

Figure 2.20. Applications of epidemiology.

Source: https://fastercapital.co/i/Medical-and-dental-public-health-and-epidemiology--Epidemiology-in-Business--Analyzing-Market-Trends-Like-an-Expert--Successful-Applications-of-Epidemiological-Methods.webp.

2.6.1. Disease Prevention and Control

Among public health, prevention and control of disease are pillars of epidemiological practice that target the reduction of incidence and morbidity of disease. Key strategies, such as vaccination, health education, and surveillance, form the basis of detecting and managing infectious pathogens. Vaccination interventions have proved very successful in controlling diseases such as polio and measles, emphasizing the significance of herd immunity. In addition, health education programs empower citizens with information on good hygiene practices, such as hand washing and sanitation, to help curb the transmission of infection. Surveillance mechanisms play a crucial role in observing disease patterns and responding in a timely manner to future outbreaks. Such forward-looking actions highlight the nature of epidemiology as a science devoted to knowledge and countermeasures against the risk of infectious diseases. As diseases themselves change over time, so too must response strategies evolve continuously, based on new patterns and evidence. A good example of this responsiveness is seen in the global response to the COVID-19 pandemic, where epidemiological principles have played a central role in informing public health guidance and interventions. Behavioral changes like wearing masks and social distancing are examples of how epidemiology intersects with social determinants of health. Public health workers have utilised contact tracing and testing to slow the transmission of the virus, providing valuable insights into its spread and the effects on vulnerable groups. Rapid case identification and isolation lighten the load on health systems and shield communities. In addition, disease control efforts are specifically designed to suit local conditions, maximizing their impact across various environments. Healthcare workers' role in the prevention and control of disease is of utmost importance, considering their exposure to possible sources of infection. The protection of healthcare workers through proper personal protective equipment (PPE) has become a vital aspect in consideration of recent pandemics. The experiences chronicled during the COVID-19 pandemic have brought into perspective the strict infection control measures in healthcare facilities. Through the adoption of extensive protective measures, hospitals can reduce the risk of transmission to both workers and patients. Disease control programs and guidelines that aim to protect healthcare workers are key elements of effective disease control programs. These procedures not only secure the safety of front-line individuals but also create public trust in the ability of healthcare systems to contain infectious risks (Ng et al., 2020; Su et al., 2020) (Figure 2.21).

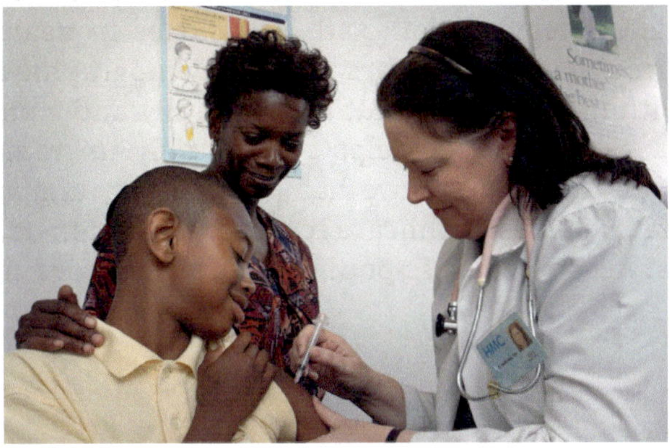

Figure 2.21. Disease prevention and control.

Source: https://cdn.britannica.com/82/192382-050-0DBDE346/nurse-vaccine-shoulder-muscle-injection-mother-boy.jpg.

2.6.2. Health Policy and Planning

Health planning and policy are central to the practice of epidemiology, determining the context under which public health programs are created and delivered. Policymakers need to understand the foundations of epidemiology to diagnose diseases that require attention and distribute resources effectively to address these issues. Through the use of epidemiological information, policymakers can identify at-risk populations, thereby making interventions not only evidence-supported but also informed by the intricacies of health determinants. The convergence of epidemiological concepts and policy-making results in more informed policies that can buffer against disease spread and improve population health outcomes. One of the central components in health policy development is concerned with the process of evidence assessment, which is essential for determining the impact of interventions.

Systematic reviews of the risk of bias in randomized trials are central to the process. Instruments like the Cochrane risk-of-bias tool are used to improve the reliability of the evidence base, enabling policymakers to determine which interventions work best at delivering better health outcomes. Otherwise, health policies could be based on hearsay rather than proven scientific principles. Integration of strong epidemiological knowledge into policy-making thus not only enhances transparency but also reinforces public confidence in health programs. Further, the use of the epidemiological tenets is not limited to the mere determination of health policies; it also affects the implementation of these policies in health service planning. Policy-makers have to navigate through several factors, such as demographic forces and social determinants of health, to come up with interventions that are culturally and contextually relevant. Knowledge of the epidemiological bases of diseases helps considerably in framing health promotion and prevention strategies. In addition, as literature has pointed out, understanding the links between risk factors and health states guides healthcare resource allocation decisions, thus ensuring maximization in the delivery of services to address population needs accordingly (Bhopal, 2016; Sterne et al., 2019) (Figure 2.22).

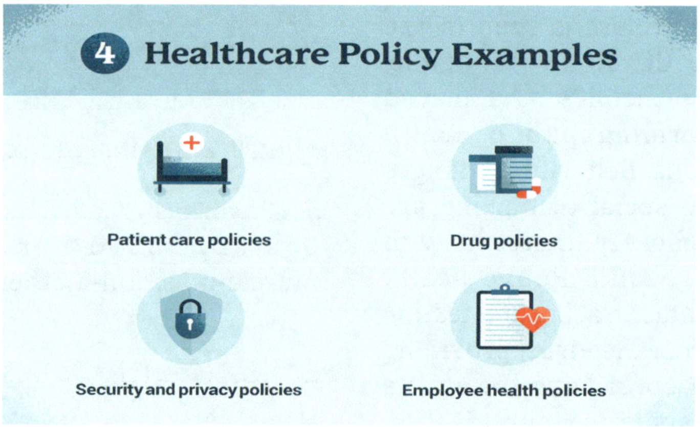

Figure 2.22. Health policy and planning.

Source: https://www.usa.edu/wp-content/uploads/2021/10/healthcare-policy-examples.png.

2.6.3. Global Health Initiatives

Global health programs are essential blueprints designed to address health issues that transcend national borders, upholding the principles of epidemiology. Such programs tend to emphasize infectious diseases, maternal well-being, and non-communicable diseases, promoting a multidimensional approach that combines country, NGO, and global organization efforts to support international cooperation. Through a multidimensional approach, involving policy change, community participation, and investment, global health programs aim to reduce health inequalities worldwide. For example, the growing number of HIV/AIDS cases has spurred many programs addressing education and access to care. These programs exemplify epidemiological approaches that promote evidence-based interventions responsive to the unique demographic and epidemiological demands of diverse populations, ultimately improving public health outcomes. Specific global health programs also illustrate how local programs can be derived from global recommendations. For instance, in Canada, a community-academic collaborative network has taken notable steps to look at the sexual and reproductive health and rights (SRHR) of women with HIV. They produced five important recommendations that promote the meaningful participation of affected groups, emphasizing the need to dismantle present power structures within health interventions. This model illustrates the extent to which global health programs can be adapted to local contexts while remaining aligned with overarching global standards. Combining principles of Equity, Diversity, and Inclusion, these programs increase awareness but also advocate participatory strategies that enable communities to own their health. This change towards community engagement is central to making sustainable improvements in health and ensuring interventions meet particular needs and conditions, as is the case with the initiative described in Osborne et al. (2025). Further, the global sepsis burden has necessitated focused efforts towards enhanced recognition, treatment, and prevention strategies. Sepsis is among the top causes of morbidity and mortality globally, and thus, there is a strong need for strong epidemiological evidence to direct public health interventions. Studies such as a recent one in Romania offer essential information concerning the epidemiology of serious infections, such as the most common pathogens, such as *Clostridium difficile*. These results are vital for establishing guidelines and interventions consistent with the concepts of epidemiology, which emphasize early detection and response to emerging health hazards. International health efforts targeting sepsis underscore the need for evidence-based strategies in informing healthcare responses, highlighting the imperative for vigilance and prompt action to address the consequences of this multifaceted disease on global health, as corroborated by the analysis in Grigorescu et al. (2025).

SUMMARY

In summarizing an examination of the Principles of Epidemiology, it is essential to emphasize the central role that epidemiologists play in helping to comprehend and counter public health hazards. Epidemiology serves as the foundation for successful public health measures by providing data-driven information on disease trends and health status. As indicated by the prevalence of conditions like prostate cancer, the second most common cancer in men globally, the importance of epidemiologic research cannot be emphasised enough (Rawla, 2019). Such findings enable directed screening programs and direct preventive actions, hence shaping healthcare practice and policy-making across populations. Finally, the conclusion made based on intensive epidemiologic research not only increases information but also translates into practicable strategies that protect public health and well-being. Furthermore, epidemiological principles are applicable beyond the reporting of statistics; they encompass a detailed examination of risk factors and social determinants of health that contribute to disease occurrence. The statistical research within the discipline reveals discrepancies in incidence rates, particularly across various demographics and geographic areas. For example, the significantly greater incidence of prostate cancer in African-American men underscores the importance of differential methods of screening and intervention (Rawla, 2019). This body of knowledge is essential for informing equal public health policy that aims to address and correct such disparities. By assisting with focused educational programs and health access enhancements, epidemiologists help shape a more equitable healthcare system, focusing on the needs of disadvantaged groups. Lastly, the professional ethical responsibilities of healthcare providers gain prominence in operationalising epidemiologic findings into clinical practice, as described by the guidelines of major health authorities. It is the duty of health practitioners to utilise epidemiological information wisely, making sound decisions based on both the overall results and specific patient conditions. Such practice is key to realising maximum health outcomes while minimising risks due to the misuse of data. Incorporating ethical considerations within epidemiological studies serves to reaffirm a patient-centered approach and the medical profession's shared responsibility for protecting public trust. Ultimately, principles of epidemiology provide a solid foundation for understanding health disparities, guiding preventive interventions, and ensuring that healthcare decisions align with the best principles of responsibility and ethical practice.

It is essential to understand the fundamental principles of epidemiology in developing effective public health strategies. The centre of epidemiology is the study of the distribution and determinants of health-related states or events. It emphasises that one should study the who, where, and when of the health outcomes to recognise patterns and likely risk factors. Additionally, the use of quantitative methods enables researchers to extract meaningful insights from health data, making evidence-based interventions possible. Fundamental concepts, including incidence and prevalence, serve as building blocks for measuring the frequency of disease in populations and making targeted public health interventions. Through incorporating these aspects, epidemiology aims not only to explain disease but also to reduce its impact through wise decision-making and resource allocation (Singhal et al., 2024). The other key principle of epidemiology is the recognition of the centrality of the population perspective in epidemiology. In contrast to clinical medicine, which tends to concentrate on the health of individuals, epidemiology aims to understand how diseases affect populations rather than single individuals. The population perspective is critical in the identification of social determinants of health, which may encompass SES, education, and healthcare access. By considering these larger contexts, epidemiologists are in a stronger position to design interventions that take into account systematic issues influencing health outcomes. Moreover, the value of teamwork from interdisciplinary fields enhances the validity of epidemiological studies; interdisciplinary collaboration fosters diverse perspectives that lead to more comprehensive solutions to public health problems (Fabre et al., 2023). The concept of prevention is the other pillar of epidemiology, informing efforts to decrease the occurrence and load of disease in populations. This forward-looking approach emphasises interventions like vaccination, education, and screening to identify diseases early and control risk factors well. In addition, epidemiological principles recommend the wise use of resources to achieve the most significant public health impact. For example, the application of focused health interventions can drastically reduce levels of disease transmission and increase the resilience of the community's health. By bringing research findings to public policy, the philosophy of prevention promotes a culture of health consciousness and stimulates active participation on the part of individuals and communities. Therefore, epidemiological principles provide the foundation for the comprehension and improvement of public health programs through a balanced approach towards disease prevention and control (Singhal et al., 2024).

CLOSER LOOK

REAL-WORLD CLINICAL PRACTICE:

Real-world clinical practice offers a uniquely authentic lens into how healthcare is delivered outside the controlled setting of randomized trials. While clinical trials remain the gold standard for determining efficacy and safety, they often operate under strict inclusion criteria, standardized protocols, and idealized follow-up schedules. In contrast, real-world practice reflects the complexity, variability, and imperfection of everyday medicine—factors that are increasingly recognized as essential for understanding how treatments perform in diverse patient populations. One of the central advantages of examining real-world clinical care is the ability to observe patient outcomes across a broad spectrum of demographics, comorbidities, and socioeconomic backgrounds. Real-world data (RWD), including electronic health records, insurance claims, pharmacy data, patient registries, and digital health tools, captures the experiences of individuals who may be excluded from traditional trials. This diversity allows clinicians and researchers to identify patterns of effectiveness, adherence challenges, and safety signals that might otherwise remain hidden.

Another important dimension of real-world practice is the role of clinical decision-making. Physicians must balance evidence-based guidelines with patient preferences, resource availability, and time constraints. These decisions, made in the flow of busy clinics and hospital wards, shape treatment trajectories that differ from the idealized pathways described in study protocols. Understanding these patterns helps illuminate why certain therapies succeed or fail when implemented broadly, and it highlights opportunities for guideline refinement, clinician education, and system-level support.

Real-world evaluation also reveals the impact of social determinants of health—factors such as housing stability, transportation access, and health literacy. These elements, often absent from clinical trial datasets, profoundly influence outcomes. By studying how they intersect with clinical care, health systems can design more equitable interventions, improve outreach strategies, and reduce gaps in treatment access. Moreover, the integration of real-world evidence (RWE) into regulatory and policy decision-making continues to grow. Regulators increasingly acknowledge that RWE can complement trial findings, inform post-market surveillance, and guide value-based care decisions. For clinicians, these insights support a more nuanced understanding of risks and benefits and enhance shared decision-making with patients.

In sum, taking a closer look at real-world clinical practice enriches our understanding of healthcare as it truly functions. It bridges the gap between controlled research and lived experience, ensuring that medical advances translate into meaningful, equitable improvements for all patients.

REFERENCES

1. Afiaz, A., Ivanov, A. A., Chamberlin, J., Hanauer, D., Savonen, C., Goldman, M., Morgan, M., et al. (2023). *Evaluation of Software Impact Designed for Biomedical Research: Are We Measuring What's Meaningful?* https://www.semanticscholar.org/paper/0393931546e45b591ab3438e5474b75c04a09d83 (accessed on 30th May 2025).
2. *Registries for Evaluating Patient Outcomes: A user's guide*. (2020). https://doi.org/10.23970/ahrqepcregistries4.
3. Ambayo, H., Bouwman, J., Bronselaer, A., De Baets, et al. (2019). An ontology to standardize research output of nutritional epidemiology: From paper-based standards to linked content. https://core.ac.uk/download/222452585.pdf (accessed on 30th May 2025).
4. Aslam, H., Jameel, M. K., Hameed, F., Butt, N. U. S., Ammar, M., Gondal, M. F., Abbasi, J., et al. (2023). Temporal trends and spectrum of pediatric surgical conditions operated in a tertiary care teaching hospital in Pakistan. *Proceedings*. https://www.semanticscholar.org/paper/73570a84fe34abd42a26e444ec0db37642681d0a (accessed on 30th May 2025).
5. Balaji, S., Manimegalai, R., & Nandhini, A. (2024). Enhancing cardiovascular disease prediction with EML-IoT integration. In *2024 International Conference on Smart Systems for Electrical, Electronics, Communication and Computer Engineering (ICSSEECC)*. https://www.semanticscholar.org/paper/ebbb317d2550caa5fa65c99c92b3c3b4b7e2f94a (accessed on 30th May 2025).
6. Bamdad, S., Shirvani, M., Shahriarirad, S., Tamaddon, M., & Attar, A. (2024). Epidemiology and characteristics of unintentional self-inflicted penetrating ocular injuries in children less than 6 years old. *BMC Ophthalmology, 24*. https://www.semanticscholar.org/paper/70489eb07dfb9dde5e0bfb9338de6af35fca641d (accessed on 30th May 2025).
7. Beck, A. P., Gröne, A., Caswell, J. L., Meyerholz, D. K., Dohoo, I. R., LaDouceur, E. E. B., Origgi, F. C., et al. (2018). *Observational Study Design in Veterinary Pathology, Part 1: Study Design*. https://core.ac.uk/download/160499856.pdf (accessed on 30th May 2025).
8. Berardi, A., Covotta, A., Gagliardi, M., Galeoto, et al. (2018). *Physical Activity Scale for the Elderly: Translation, Cultural Adaptation, and Validation of the Italian Version*. https://core.ac.uk/download/188824697.pdf (accessed on 30th May 2025).
9. Bhopal, R. (2008). *Concepts of Epidemiology: Integrating the Ideas, Theories, Principles and Methods of Epidemiology*. https://www.semanticscholar.org/paper/2e2216476a44207ef2b6eaa1940ed1661f79da4d (accessed on 30th May 2025).
10. Bhopal, R. (2016). *Concepts of Epidemiology*. Oxford University Press eBooks. https://doi.org/10.1093/med/9780198739685.001.0001.
11. CACRCP, T. Contents. (2023). *General Principles of Food Hygiene*. https://www.semanticscholar.org/paper/b8ec07028d330e3c3eeacf9e56973b451c4511e9 (accessed on 30th May 2025).
12. Cadarette, S. M., Maclure, M., Delaney, J. A., Whitaker, H., Hayes, K. N., Wang, S., Tadrous, M., et al. (2021). Control yourself: ISPE-endorsed guidance in the application of self-controlled study designs in pharmacoepidemiology. *Pharmacoepidemiology and Drug Safety, 30*, 671–684. https://doi.org/10.1002/pds.5227.
13. Carmalt, J. H., Caron, R. M., Hewitt, A. M., Hooker, et al. (2018). Teaching population health: Innovations in the integration of the healthcare and public health systems. https://core.ac.uk/download/286641618.pdf (accessed on 30th May 2025).

14. Department of Medical Epidemiology, Precision Breast, Faculty of Sport and, Department of Global Public, Institute for Molecular. (2024). Dementia risk factors in former contact sports participants: Prospective cohort study. *medRxiv*. https://www.semanticscholar.org/paper/cdaaf9f824998799d1a0d13148c861f6a8f27f1d (accessed on 30th May 2025).

15. Desvaux, S., & Molia, S. (2007). OIE training workshop on epidemiology, in particular of HPAI and TADs in the Philippines, in collaboration with CIRAD and Bureau of Animal Industry: Mission report, 29 January – 2 February 2007, Philippines. http://agritrop.cirad.fr/546445/1/document_546445.pdf (accessed on 30th May 2025).

16. Dümen, E., & Ekici, G. (2019). *Escherichia coli and Food Safety.* https://core.ac.uk/download/322441098.pdf (accessed on 30th May 2025).

17. Dumuid, D., Pedišić, Ž., Palarea-Albaladejo, J., Martín, F. J. A., Hron, K., & Olds, T. (2020). Compositional data analysis in time-use epidemiology: What, why, how. *International Journal of Environmental Research and Public Health, 17*, 2220. https://doi.org/10.3390/ijerph17072220.

18. Ellison, G. T. H., & Rhoma, H. (2025). Directed acyclic graphs as conceptual and analytical tools in applied and theoretical epidemiology: Advances, setbacks and future possibilities. *Mathematical Biosciences and Engineering*. https://www.semanticscholar.org/paper/e7db1888d82b7813ba7536bebd2dd5c5944bc5a3 (accessed on 30th May 2025).

19. Fabre, V., Davis, A., Diekema, D., Granwehr, B., Hayden, M., Lowe, C., Pfeiffer, C., et al. (2023). Principles of diagnostic stewardship: A practical guide from the Society for Healthcare Epidemiology of America Diagnostic Stewardship Task Force. *Infection Control & Hospital Epidemiology, 44*, 178–185. https://www.semanticscholar.org/paper/a4307808b8ecab2b64cdffbf212ede4c06eaf088 (accessed on 30th May 2025).

20. Girón-Guzmán, I., Sánchez, G., & Pérez-Cataluña, A. (2024). Tracking epidemic viruses in wastewaters. *Microbial Biotechnology, 17*. https://www.semanticscholar.org/paper/75b7668a1af065f800d6e69c06c89c02ed1c8c50 (accessed on 30th May 2025).

21. Gokhale, K., Chandan, J. S., Toulis, K. A., Gkoutos, G. V., Tiňo, P., & Nirantharakumar, K. (2020). Data extraction for epidemiological research (DExtER): A novel tool for automated clinical epidemiology studies. *European Journal of Epidemiology, 36*, 165–178. https://doi.org/10.1007/s10654-020-00677-6.

22. Griffith, M., Field, E., Huang, A. S., Shimada, T., Battsend, M., Housen, T., Pamphilon, B., et al. (2024). How do field epidemiologists learn? A protocol for a qualitative inquiry into learning in field epidemiology training programs. *BMJ Open, 14*. https://www.semanticscholar.org/paper/820e32b1058debb0a6bbab3eff328866d44c578d (accessed on 30th May 2025).

23. Grigorescu, A., Dumitrescu, F., Dorobanțu, Ș., Dragoș, A., Pîrvu, A., Roskanovic, M., on behalf of the FUSE study, et al. (2025). An epidemiological survey of sepsis in a tertiary academic hospital from Southwestern Romania. *Medicina, 61*. https://www.semanticscholar.org/paper/9ab36de167f621039885d43fce00e7341cd9f830 (accessed on 30th May 2025).

24. Hruz, P. (2023). A clarion call for high-quality research on gender dysphoric youth. *Acta Pediatrica, 112*. https://www.semanticscholar.org/paper/d101199f519ec66dd538b770511708666047a160 (accessed on 30th May 2025).

25. Iamsirithaworn, S., Thammawijaya, P., & Ungchusak, K. (2021). Principles of outbreak investigation. In *Oxford Textbook of Global Public Health*. https://www.semanticscholar.org/paper/c21cc615604e833e8eefb12fbb1746eaf653367b (accessed on 30th May 2025).

26. Jones, M. J., Moore, S., & Kobor, M. (2018). Principles and challenges of applying epigenetic epidemiology to psychology. *Annual Review of Psychology, 69*, 459–485. https://www.semanticscholar.org/paper/91a98eb6176924d0ff583534a36cad20f1bd67b7 (accessed on 30th May 2025).

27. LaJoie, A. S., Holm, R. H., Anderson, L. B., Ness, H. D., & Smith, T. (2022). Nationwide public perceptions regarding the acceptance of using wastewater for community health monitoring in the United States. *PLoS ONE, 17*, e0275075. https://doi.org/10.1371/journal.pone.0275075.

28. Latif, S., Usman, M., Manzoor, S., Iqbal, W., Qadir, J., Tyson, G., Castro, I., et al. (2020). Leveraging data science to combat COVID-19: A comprehensive review. *IEEE Transactions on Artificial Intelligence, 1*, 85–103. https://doi.org/10.1109/tai.2020.3020521.

29. Levay, P., & Craven, J. (2023). Systematic searching in a post-pandemic world: New directions for methods, technology, and people. *Evidence Based Library and Information Practice*. https://www.semanticscholar.org/paper/c5244136db386f6bd9763d71b0e01eca07956001 (accessed on 30th May 2025).

30. Li, W. Y., Li, H. Z., Zhan, S. Y., & Wang, S. F. (2024). Application of virtual simulation technology in epidemiology education: A systematic review. *Zhonghua Liu Xing Bing Xue za Zhi = Zhonghua Liuxingbingxue Zazhi, 45*(7), 1014–1023. https://www.semanticscholar.org/paper/e0ef30d3cce20fd443b55bda63d7930ca8f954a2 (accessed on 30th May 2025).

31. Manja, V., & Lakshminrusimha, S. (2015). Epidemiology and clinical research design, Part 2: Principles. *NeoReviews, 16*(2), e94–e108. https://www.semanticscholar.org/paper/2f31d84c69f86e2208093915c4ab34f25dd39dda (accessed on 30th May 2025).

32. Montegrico, J., Lee, J., & De Los Santos, J. A. A. (2024). A 13-year trend analysis of HIV epidemiology in the Philippines (2010 to 2022). *Journal of Community Health Nursing*. https://www.semanticscholar.org/paper/c17e00607fc67952fded37b589f001c2d7ead49c (accessed on 30th May 2025).

33. Morgan, O., Aguilera, X., Ammon, A., Amuasi, J., Fall, I. S., Frieden, T. R., Heymann, D., et al. (2021). Disease surveillance for the COVID-19 era: Time for bold changes. *The Lancet, 397*, 2317–2319. https://doi.org/10.1016/s0140-6736(21)01096-5.

34. Mwaura, F. M. (2024). The role of public health in promoting health standards. *Research Output Journal of Biological and Applied Science*. https://www.semanticscholar.org/paper/14befc27bb18967bb269e8a475dc85aa28e31769 (accessed on 30th May 2025).

35. N/A. (2025). *Laboratory Contributions to Public Health*. https://core.ac.uk/download/556244825.pdf (accessed on 30th May 2025).

36. Ng, K., Poon, B. H., Puar, T., Quah, J., Loh, W. J., Wong, Y. J., Tan, T. Y., et al. (2020). COVID-19 and the risk to health care workers: A case report. *Annals of Internal Medicine, 172*, 766, 767. https://doi.org/10.7326/l20-0175.

37. Nnaji, D. U., Kiogora, P. R., Onah, I. S., Mung'atu, J., & Aguegboh, N. S. (2024). Application of fluid dynamics in modeling the spatial spread of infectious diseases with low mortality rate: A study using MUSCL scheme. *Computational and Mathematical Biophysics*. https://www.semanticscholar.org/paper/d1ac94dd78deb2b8b50b7514dff0bc2ee7009872 (accessed on 30th May 2025).

38. Olowe, K. J., Edoh, N. L., Zouo, S. J. C., & Olamijuwon, J. (2024). Theoretical perspectives on biostatistics and its multifaceted applications in global health studies. *International Journal*

of Applied Research in Social Sciences. https://www.semanticscholar.org/paper/770c1b40594a4f13bfcdb002ef2e3c9b336feeb3 (accessed on 30th May 2025).

39. Osborne, Z., Habanyama, M., Cameron, B., De Pokomandy, A., Gagnier, B., King, E., Koebel, J., et al. (2025). Meaningful engagement as a cornerstone for implementing the key recommendations to advance the sexual and reproductive health and rights of women living with HIV across policy, practice, and research in Canada. *Journal of the International Association of Providers of AIDS Care, 24*. https://www.semanticscholar.org/paper/29e4acabf96bcfd1d03b2d5d98c6e0a889afd21d (accessed on 30th May 2025).
40. Priori, S. G., Blomström-Lundqvist, C., Mazzanti, A., Blom, N., Borggrefe, M., Camm, A. J., Elliott, P., et al. (2015). 2015 ESC guidelines for the management of patients with ventricular arrhythmias and the prevention of sudden cardiac death. *European Heart Journal, 36*, 2793–2867. https://doi.org/10.1093/eurheartj/ehv316.
41. Prueitt, R., Meakin, C. J., Drury, N. L., & Goodman, J. E. (2024). Evaluation of neural reflex activation as a potential mode of action for respiratory and cardiovascular effects of fine particulate matter. *Inhalation Toxicology, 36*, 125–144. https://www.semanticscholar.org/paper/68d18e734938c5f24cc2d06e55dccc99596c2c4c (accessed on 30th May 2025).
42. Rawla, P. (2019). Epidemiology of prostate cancer. *World Journal of Oncology, 10*, 63–89. https://doi.org/10.14740/wjon1191.
43. Richards, T. B., Croner, C. M., Rushton, G., Brown, C. K., & Fowler, L. (1999). Geographic information systems and public health: Mapping the future. *Public Health Reports, 114*(4), 359–373. https://www.semanticscholar.org/paper/cd15e878e17fb46435e8c76c0858e62d434c2a3e (accessed on 30th May 2025).
44. Sallam, M. (2023). ChatGPT utility in healthcare education, research, and practice: Systematic review on the promising perspectives and valid concerns. *Healthcare, 11*, 887. https://doi.org/10.3390/healthcare11060887 (accessed on 30th May 2025).
45. Singhal, T. S., Jain, J., Tejendra, A. R., Singh, A. J., Saad, J. D., Jain, M. K., Abdul-Zahra, A., Srivastava, A. P., et al. (2024). Eco-design of products and processes: A review on principles and tools for sustainable manufacturing. *E3S Web of Conferences*. https://www.semanticscholar.org/paper/09edee2b72e41355e9b66c899cef86b9e2291420 (accessed on 30th May 2025).
46. Skrivankova, V., Richmond, R. C., Woolf, B., Davies, N. M., Swanson, S. A., VanderWeele, T. J., Timpson, N. J., et al. (2021). Strengthening the reporting of observational studies in epidemiology using Mendelian randomization (STROBE-MR): Explanation and elaboration. *BMJ*. https://doi.org/10.1136/bmj.n2233.
47. Smetanin, V. N. (2024). *Some Aspects of HCAI Prevention in Medical Organizations*. https://doi.org/10.34660/inf.2020.81.58.013.
48. Sterne, J. A. C., Savović, J., Page, M. J., Elbers, R. G., Blencowe, N., Boutron, I., Cates, C. J., et al. (2019). RoB 2: A revised tool for assessing risk of bias in randomized trials. *BMJ*. https://doi.org/10.1136/bmj.l4898.
49. Su, H., Yang, M., Wan, C., Yi, L. X., Tang, F., Zhu, H. Y., Yi, F., et al. (2020). Renal histopathological analysis of 26 postmortem findings of patients with COVID-19 in China. *Kidney International, 98*, 219–227. https://doi.org/10.1016/j.kint.2020.04.003.

50. Tanese, M. A., Local Health Authority, & Others. (2023). Bridging public health and primary care in an Italian urban area: Lessons learnt from pandemic. *The European Journal of Public Health, 33.* https://www.semanticscholar.org/paper/c9b089292e3a3def19926b63b6ad2c020b9530af (accessed on 30th May 2025).

51. Thomas, L. B., Mastorides, S., Viswanadhan, N., Jakey, C. E., & Borkowski, A. (2021). Artificial intelligence: Review of current and future applications in medicine. *Federal Practitioner.* https://doi.org/10.12788/fp.0174.

52. Tuakli-Wosornu, Y., Burrows, K., Fasting, K., Hartill, M., Hodge, K., Kaufman, K., Kavanagh, E., et al. (2024). IOC consensus statement: Interpersonal violence and safeguarding in sport. *British Journal of Sports Medicine.* https://www.semanticscholar.org/paper/27d1b855fe1b396ab6a35fd75aed9b8469011309 (accessed on 30th May 2025).

53. Wang, J. M., Liu, Q., Gong, C., Zhang, M. L., Gao, P., Tang, X., & Hu, Y. (2023). Application of discrete event simulation model in analysis on cost-effectiveness of epidemiology screening. *Zhonghua liu Xing Bing Xue za Zhi = Zhonghua Liuxingbingxue Zazhi, 44*(3), 463–469. https://www.semanticscholar.org/paper/026766ae74ac6a1d5ea4484a1488322e1c0b330f (accessed on 30th May 2025).

54. Westreich, D. (2019). *Epidemiology by Design.* Oxford University Press eBooks. https://doi.org/10.1093/oso/9780190665760.001.0001 (accessed on 30th May 2025).

55. Yu, Z. H., Zhang, L. M., Dai, Z. Q., Zhang, M. N., & Zheng, S. M. (2024). Epidemiology and prognostic nomogram for locally advanced gastric signet ring cell carcinoma: A population-based study. *World Journal of Gastrointestinal Oncology, 16,* 2610–2630. https://www.semanticscholar.org/paper/a90040fb02650582c94ea7ec48b0ce184e2e9b55 (accessed on 30th May 2025).

56. Zaporozhets, V. V. (2024). *The Symbolism of Carols (From the "History of the Symbols of Slavic Mythology").* https://doi.org/10.34660/inf.2020.42.95.002.

57. Zhang, T., Qiao, J., Wang, Y., Zhou, Y., Hamoudi, H. J. A. S., Al Hendi, M. A. A., Wang, J. (2024). Causal link between hypothyroidism and gastric cancer risk: Insights gained through multivariable Mendelian randomization and mediation analysis. *Frontiers in Endocrinology, 15.* https://www.semanticscholar.org/paper/f1f718dc2067f5dcca5a2d0405740fde24922139 (accessed on 30th May 2025).

58. Zhou, J., Liu, L., Xue, P., Yang, X., & Tang, X. (2020). Mental health response to the COVID-19 outbreak in China. *American Journal of Psychiatry, 177,* 574, 575. https://doi.org/10.1176/appi.ajp.2020.20030304.

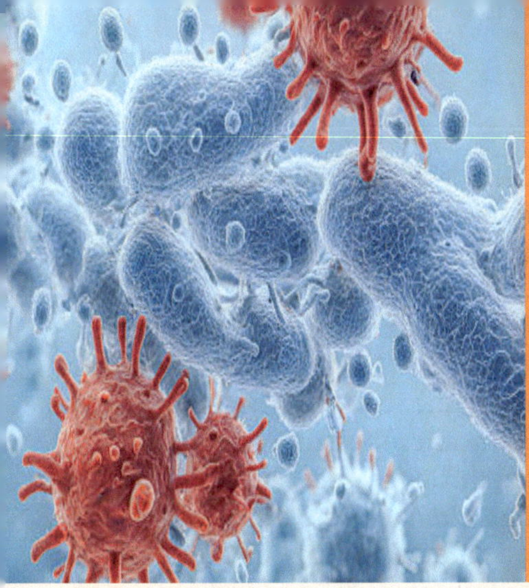

Chapter 3

MICROBIAL PATHOGENESIS AND HOST RESPONSE

Contents

Introduction

Understanding the connection between microbial pathogenesis and the host's response is a primary focus in biomedical research, particularly in elucidating disease development and treatment strategies. Because of their virulence factors, microbial pathogens can infect the body, avoid immune responses and damage important tissues. For example, research on periodontal disease has shown that infections involving Porphyromonas gingivalis bacteria can lead to significant bone loss and alterations in the immune system. This highlights the necessity of investigating not just individual pathogens, but also the collective behavior of microbial communities in their interaction with the host's immune system, particularly in localized infection models (Gao et al., 2020). Researchers hope to identify better ways to treat conditions that are made worse by microbial infections. The immune system helps make clear how microbes and the body's defenses interact. In many cases, chronic diseases are linked to immune system issues stemming from the persistent presence of microbes. For celiac disease, consuming gluten triggers the immune system to attack intestinal epithelial cells, resulting in damage due to abnormal T-cell responses. Such findings emphasize the multifactorial nature of these diseases, where genetic predisposition, environmental factors, and microbial dysbiosis converge to provoke adverse health outcomes (Cicerone et al., 2015). Learning about these interactions is crucial for figuring out the causes of inflammatory and autoimmune diseases, which in turn guides public health plans for managing them. It is necessary to employ multiple disciplines to investigate how microbes cause diseases and how the host responds to them. The method should use molecular biology, immunology, and microbiology to give a detailed view of how certain microbes impact the health and diseases of their hosts. Using advanced technologies such as high-throughput sequencing makes it possible for researchers to understand the microbes in a host and their effects on the immune system. Using a variety of techniques, scientists can gain a detailed understanding of the aspects of microbial infections. Ultimately, these efforts not only further our fundamental understanding of disease processes but also open avenues for innovative therapeutic interventions and preventative measures against pathologies associated with microbial infections and host responses (Figure 3.1).

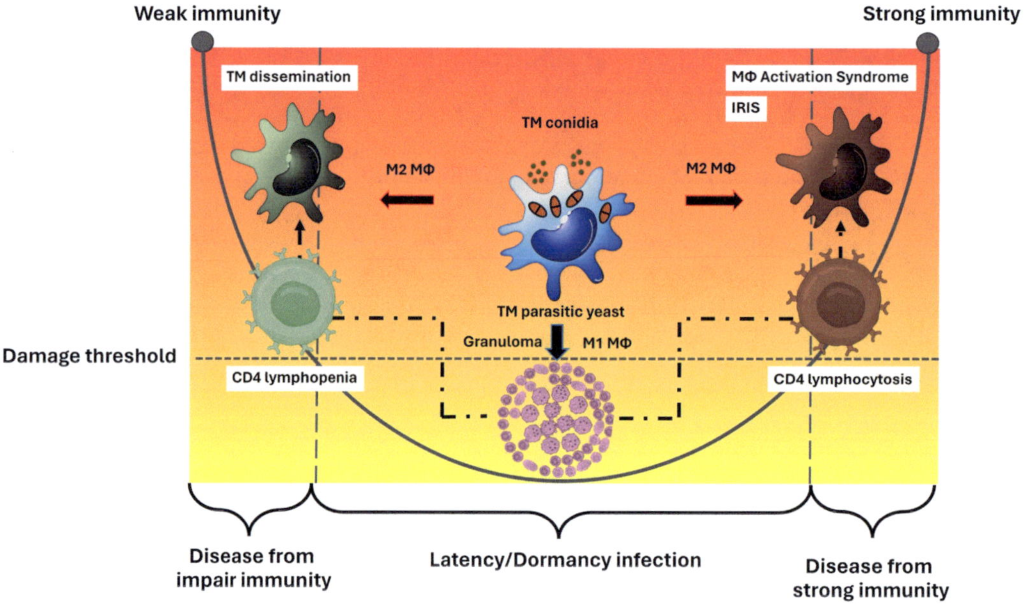

Figure 3.1. Microbial pathogenesis and host response.

Source: https://www.frontiersin.org/files/Articles/1448729/fimmu-15-1448729-HTML/image_m/fimmu-15-1448729-g002.jpg

Definition of Microbial Pathogenesis

Understanding how microbes cause disease is crucial for investigating their interactions with their hosts. Microbial pathogenesis mainly describes how microbes cause illness in a host body. It goes from the first colonization of the host's tissues to dodging the immune system and, finally, to the appearance of symptoms of the disease. The virulence factors of pathogens, for example, toxins, adhesion molecules, and enzymes, are essential in microbial pathogenesis. Additionally, the ability of microorganisms to survive in various environments often significantly affects their capacity to cause disease. Further research is showing that the health of the host, which depends on both genes and the environment, strongly affects the results of microbial infections. The relationship between microbial pathogenesis and the host immune response is particularly salient in understanding diseases such as inflammatory bowel diseases (IBD), which include both Ulcerative colitis and Crohn's disease. Researchers have found that an imbalance in the gut microbiome is crucial in causing IBD, highlighting the key role microbes play in maintaining intestinal health. Patients with IBD often show a decrease in beneficial bacteria capable of producing short-chain fatty acids (SCFAs), which have been linked to the regulation of immune responses within the gut. They help strengthen the gut barrier and also work on specific receptors to influence the immune system. Emerging evidence suggests that these microbial metabolites play a vital role in the host's ability to withstand pathogenic challenges, underlining the complexity of the host-microbe interaction in microbial pathogenesis (Venegas et al., 2019).

Moreover, the application of microbial biological control agents (MBCAs) provides an intriguing context for understanding microbial pathogenesis. MBCAs may play various roles with plants, which may make them more resistant to opportunistic plant pathogens. Such interactions typically require metabolic activities that are controlled and may occur through methods such as nutrient competition or the production of antimicrobial metabolites. Their usefulness depends on blocking pathogen growth as well as preparing the host to fight the disease. It is also necessary to understand how MBCAs function in disease management and to assess any potential risks they pose to people and the environment. Therefore, a comprehensive grasp of microbial pathogenesis is pivotal not only in clinical contexts but also in agricultural practices aiming to mitigate disease spread (Köhl et al., 2019) (Figure 3.2).

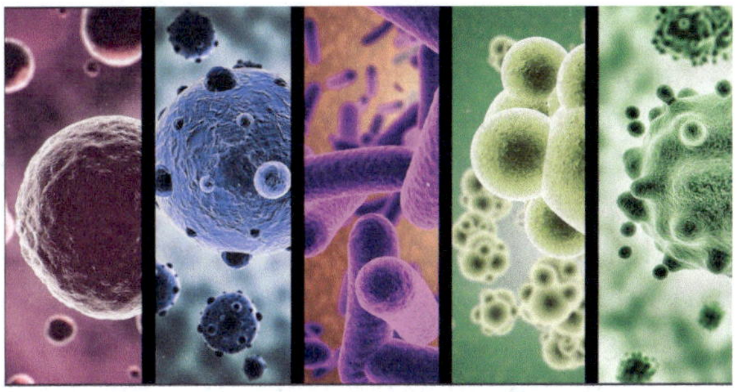

Figure 3.2. Microbial pathogenesis.

Source: https://static.wixstatic.com/media/4d76eb_ff9e3bc64d684864b0eb965c17262690~mv2.png/v1/fit/w_1000%2Ch_668%2Cal_c/file.png.

Importance of Studying Host Responses

Understanding host reactions to microbial infections is crucial in microbial pathogenesis, as it significantly influences whether an infection will succeed or fail. The relationship between pathogens and the immune system is complex and dynamic, continually evolving with each interaction. Examining these reactions can explain how hosts detect and manage microbial dangers, which is essential for designing helpful treatments. For example, discoveries about how the host immune system responds can be applied to making vaccines and new therapies, which help us better handle infections. Also, studying how some pathogens avoid these defenses can guide the search for new strategies to fight antibiotic resistance, which is now a significant issue in health care. Investigating the body's reactions to infection enhances our understanding of disease and is crucial for effective clinical treatment. Learning about the microbiota in the host gives a better understanding of the host's reaction. A variety of microbes that live in the gastrointestinal tract help maintain health by using homeostatic processes. The presence of eubiosis and dysbiosis in the microbiota can significantly impact the host's immune system and the likelihood of contracting an illness.

Examining the impact of microbial communities on the immune system may help us understand how imbalances in the microbiome contribute to IBD or obesity. Additionally, investigating the impact of these interactions on the host can lead to the development of new probiotic therapies aimed at restoring normal microbial levels and enhancing the immune system. Therefore, studying host responses in the context of microbiota composition is crucial for unraveling the complexities of health and disease in the face of microbial invasions, as highlighted in recent research on gastrointestinal microbial ecosystems (Cacciotti et al., 2016). Understanding how the host reacts to pathogens can help improve public health and food safety. As multidrug-resistant pathogens emerge, finding effective ways to combat them is crucial. For instance, research into ozone as a biocidal agent has demonstrated its potential in inactivating foodborne pathogens like *Campylobacter jejuni* and *Salmonella enteritidis*, emphasizing the need for innovative disinfection strategies in food processing (Anderson et al., 2003). Examining both the host's immune response and methods for destroying microbes enables us to develop more effective treatments for infections. With this research, food production becomes safer, and the public health guidelines are based on a detailed understanding of how microbes affect the body. For this reason, using this approach will improve our ability to prevent and control infectious diseases.

3.1. Mechanisms of Microbial Pathogenesis

There are many ways in which microbes invade and use their hosts, and these methods are not simple. The modulation of the host immune system is a crucial aspect, which can be achieved both through direct secretions from microbes and by the influence of the microbiota. For example, several commensal microorganisms are known to make substances that stop pathogens from infecting their host. A good example is the way *Tritrichomonas musculis* interacts with *Clostridioides difficile*: it helps protect the intestine by controlling neutrophil recruitment and interleukin-1 beta secretion which in turn strengthens the host's mucosal defense. Through these interactions, pathogens can manipulate their environment, escape immune detection, and, under the right conditions, thrive within the host, underlining the dynamic nature of host-pathogen interactions in microbial pathogenesis (Yang et al., 2024). Another vital way microbes cause disease is by altering the functions of host cells, primarily by affecting the production of interferons. When viruses or other pathogens invade a host, interferons are critical immune components that react. Recent studies have highlighted the significance of lambda interferons (IFN-λs) in combating periodontal pathogens and modulating immune responses. Unlike the other IFNs, IFN-λs play a different yet essential part, mainly by fighting viruses but less so against bacteria. They help the immune system fight off infections by impacting several inflammatory pathways and immune regulatory mechanisms, which also highlights how pathogens must avoid setting off too strong an immune response. This complexity in immune regulation illustrates how microbes can exploit specific host vulnerabilities to enhance their survival and pathogenicity (Ahmed, 2024). Additionally, the ability of pathogens to adapt to new situations can significantly impact the outcomes of infections, as is evident in many types of microbes. Pathogens have ways to avoid the immune system, such as changing their surface proteins, releasing substances that change the immune response, or forming a protective biofilm. The ability to change their surface antigens allows organisms, for example, *Neisseria gonorrhoeae*, to avoid being recognized by the immune system. They also protect microbes from the immune system of the host and from drugs meant to treat infections. They help bacteria take up nutrients and resist antibiotics, making infections more complicated to treat. Understanding these adaptive strategies not only elucidates the pathogenesis of various infectious agents but also underscores the challenges that healthcare professionals face when devising effective treatment protocols to combat infections caused by these resilient microbes (Figure 3.3).

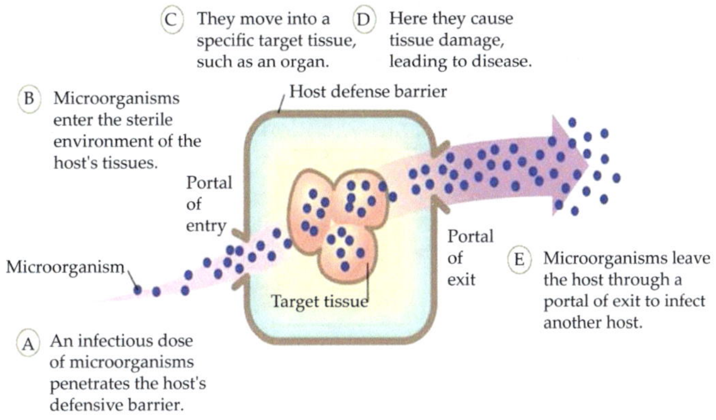

Figure 3.3. Mechanisms of microbial pathogenesis.

Source: https://slideplayer.com/14497280/90/images/slide_1.jpg.

3.1.1. Adherence and Colonization Strategies

It is essential for microbes to use strategies to stick to and colonize the host in order for infections to form. Bacterial or parasitic pathogens use different ways to stick to the host's tissues, which helps them avoid the host's immune responses. For example, Porphyromonas gingivalis and other oral bacteria have evolved to grow together in complex biofilms, which helps them remain in the mouth and disrupt the balance of microbes. If the balance of bacteria is disrupted, it can result in serious periodontal diseases. In periodontitis, the immune system fails to handle the infection effectively. The ability of these pathogens to assimilate and thrive on surfaces, coupled with their capacity to manipulate host immune reactions, highlights the intricate relationship between microbial adherence and host response mechanisms (Cui et al., 2025). Understanding these adherence strategies enables us to develop more effective methods for preventing and treating infections early on. Besides bacteria, intestinal parasites have been shown they interact with the host's microbiota, which affects their ability to adhere and settle. Helminths and protozoa reside in the gastrointestinal tract, where they interact with resident microbes to modulate their survival and pathogenesis. The gut microbiome has a dual role—it can help eliminate parasites and also create conditions that allow parasites to settle. When the types of microbes in the gut change, it can directly impact some protozoa's ability to stick to the intestinal lining and survive, which can change the course of the disease. Moreover, an altered microbial community can trigger immunological changes within the host, further affecting how well these parasites can establish themselves and interact with host defenses (Grondin et al., 2024). To effectively treat parasitic infections, we need to study how intestinal parasites interact with the microbiota. The knowledge of adherence and colonization strategies influences public health and the way infections are treated, not just the immediate situation of infection. Applying probiotics or specific antimicrobial therapies can help disrupt harmful microbes, thereby restoring balance and slowing down the progression of disease. In periodontal health, using methods that address how pathogens adhere to teeth may help individuals with gum disease recover more effectively. Additionally, approaches that alter the gut microbiota may be beneficial in treating intestinal parasitic infections and could impact the host's emotions and bodily functions. Ultimately, a comprehensive understanding of these strategies enables researchers and healthcare professionals to develop effective interventions that target not only pathogens but also the complex microbial ecosystems involved in host-pathogen interactions (Grondin et al., 2024; Cui et al., 2025) (Figure 3.4).

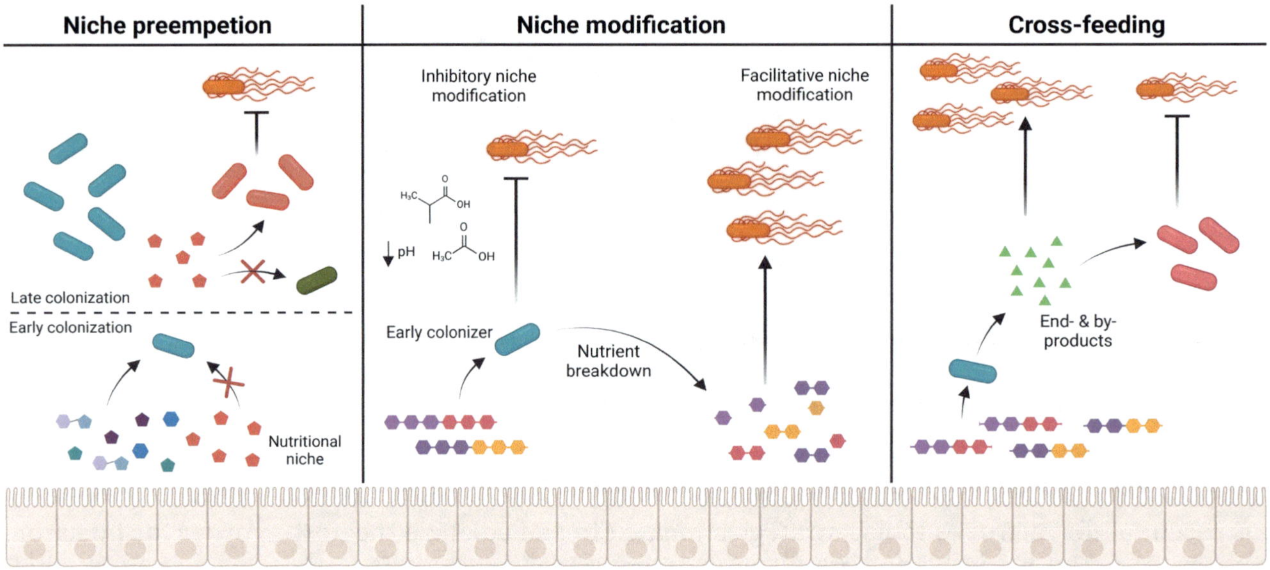

Figure 3.4. Adherence and colonization strategies.

Source: https://www.cell.com/cms/10.1016/j.chom.2024.05.002/asset/7a9c3eae-32fb-4b08-9253-da737af81c11/main.assets/gr2_lrg.jpg.

3.1.2. Invasion of Host Tissues

The invasion of host tissues by microbial pathogens represents a crucial step in the infection process, as it dictates the subsequent interactions between the pathogen and the host's immune system. There are many ways that microorganisms use to get past the epithelial barriers, which are the first barriers to infection. Bacteria such as *Staphylococcus aureus* have several virulence factors, such as adhesins and enzymes, that help them enter the body. After they are established, these pathogens can control host cell activities, which helps them live and multiply in the host's tissues. Understanding these mechanisms is crucial, as it enables researchers to identify potential therapeutic targets that aim to halt the invasion process before significant tissue damage occurs, thereby improving patient outcomes and expanding our knowledge of microbial pathogenesis (Masters et al., 2022). The infection known as osteomyelitis, which affects the bones, demonstrates how hard it is for bacteria to invade tissue. *Staphylococcus aureus* often leads to infections by forming biofilms and entering the osteocyte network, making it difficult for the immune system to deal with it. These bacteria are difficult to remove from the bone, which also demonstrates their significant influence on the host tissue's structure. Biofilms formed by microbes can cause infections to last a long time and the immune system may not notice them. Recent research emphasizes the importance of understanding these unique mechanisms of persistence, as it may lead to the development of novel interventions aimed at enhancing the host's ability to respond effectively against such resilient infections (Masters et al., 2022). Animal models have been beneficial in understanding how different pathogens invade host tissue. They help researchers study the various ways microbes and the host's immune system interact, which improves our knowledge of infection. Researchers have used ducks to demonstrate how responses to viral infections can alter the host's response, providing insight into tissue invasion. In addition, such models can explain how certain microbial factors control the immune response in the host, resulting in either infection or the host clearing the pathogen. By harnessing the knowledge gained from these experimental frameworks, researchers are better equipped to identify therapeutic targets and develop effective vaccines, ultimately paving the way for improved clinical approaches to managing infections (Figure 3.5).

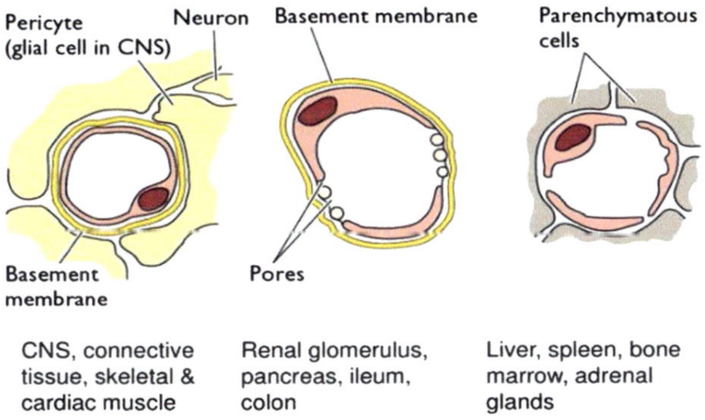

Figure 3.5. Invasion of host tissues.

Source: https://image3.slideserve.com/5730828/tissue-invasion-n.jpg.

3.1.3. Evasion of the Immune System

The numerous interactions between hosts and pathogens enable microbes to employ various strategies to evade the immune system. A significant way is for pathogens to change their surface antigens, which helps them hide from the immune system of the host. Because of antigenic variation, viruses and bacteria can survive in the host even after the immune system has fought them. For example, the influenza virus continually changes its hemagglutinin protein, which prevents people from fighting it with antibodies developed from previous infections or vaccinations. As a result, the immune system has to constantly deal with identifying and eliminating these pathogens, which causes the infection to keep coming back and highlights the pathogens' ability to escape being recognized by the immune system. Besides changing their antigens, pathogens may also use nutritional immunity evasion to get around the host's immune system. The host often stores essential micronutrients such as transition metal ions, to keep them away from invading microbes, which is called nutritional immunity. Because hosts attempt to block the entry of ions, pathogens have developed mechanisms to obtain the ions they need. For instance, certain bacteria deploy specialized metal acquisition systems, such as high-affinity transporters, to extract sequestered metals from host proteins competitively. This critical survival tactic enables pathogens to exploit the host's nutrient environment, thereby sustaining their growth and virulence while undermining the host's immune response, as recently reviewed findings (Diaz-Ochoa et al., 2014) elaborate. Furthermore, the intricacies of immune modulation are evidenced by some pathogens' ability to interfere directly with the host's signaling mechanisms. Viruses, in particular, have developed potent strategies to manipulate the host's immune system, including the interferon (IFN) response. When a virus infects, IFN from the innate immune system helps keep it from spreading, but many viruses have proteins that disrupt how IFN is produced and used. For instance, the African Swine Fever Virus (ASFV) appears to evade the IFN response, demonstrating the significant role of these viral proteins in enhancing pathogenicity. Studies have suggested that the K205R protein might influence IFN-mediated responses by hindering key signaling pathways, showing how virulence factors can subvert host defenses (Costa et al., 2011). Understanding these complex interactions is vital for developing effective therapeutic strategies against microbial infections (Figure 3.6).

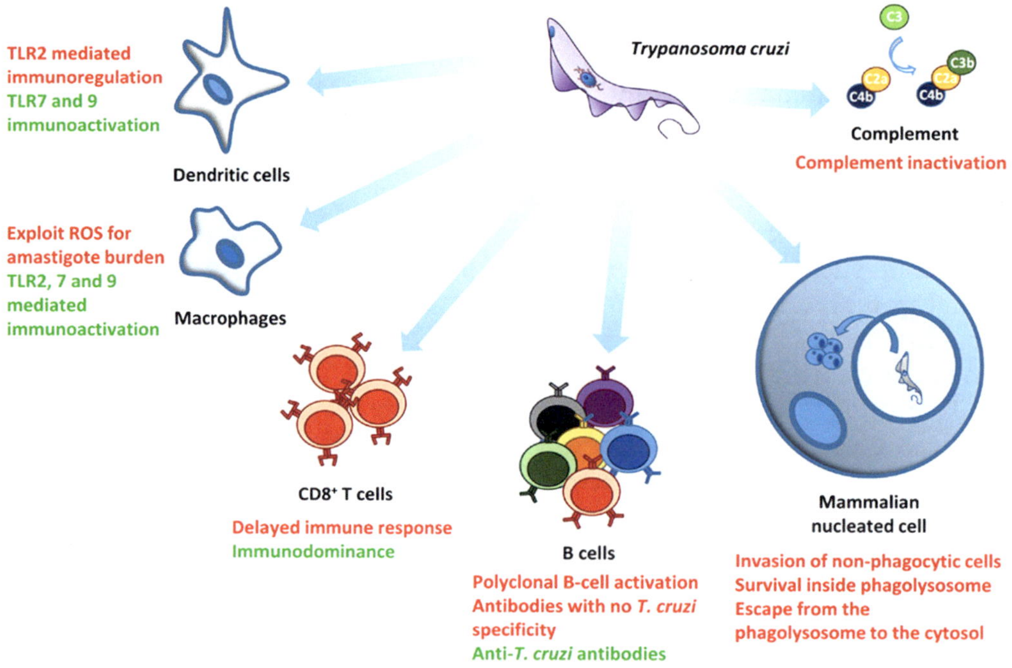

Figure 3.6. Evasion of the immune system.

Source: https://www.frontiersin.org/files/Articles/174016/fimmu-06-00659-HTML/image_m/fimmu-06-00659-g004.jpg.

3.2. Types of Microbial Pathogens

Bacteria, viruses, fungi, and parasites are the main types of microbial pathogens. All these groups have special traits, ways of infecting the host, and ways of interacting with the immune system. Bacterial pathogens can quickly increase in number inside the body, which can result in either local or systemic infections. They utilise various virulence factors, such as toxins and enzymes, to enter and harm the host's tissues. Unlike bacteria, viruses use the machinery of the host's cells to make more viruses, which can cause the cells to fail or die. Since bacterial and viral pathogens show a variety in how harmful they are, it becomes clear that microbial pathogenesis is not simple and that each type of pathogen has its own effects on the host. Fungal infections are different, since they cause immune responses that differ from those of bacteria. Unlike bacteria and viruses, fungi are eukaryotic, which makes them better able to evade detection by the immune system and also produce substances that alter how the immune system functions. Thermally dimorphic fungi, for example, *Talaromyces marneffei*, highlight the many facets of how fungi can cause diseases. The interaction between host immune responses and fungal virulence factors can either lead to adequate clearance of the pathogen or severe immunopathological outcomes, depending on the balance between response and pathogen aggressiveness. The intricate dynamics of host-fungal interactions underscore the need for targeted strategies in prevention and treatment, as highlighted in the current literature surrounding fungal infections and their management (Pruksaphon et al., 2024). Protozoa and helminths, which are parasites, also play a role in how microbes cause diseases. They have found ways to control the way their hosts respond, which enables them to live and multiply within the host. A lot of parasitic infections lead to chronic illnesses that can seriously affect a person's health. For example, certain parasites can change the proteins on their surface, which makes it hard for the immune system to notice them. Because of this, immune cells struggle to find and manage cancer, which makes treatment more difficult. The body's immune system may attack the parasites too aggressively, which can lead to tissue damage and exacerbate the disease. The dual nature of parasite-host interactions necessitates comprehensive research relationships and inform effective therapeutic approaches in combating parasitic diseases (Ahmed, 2024) (Figure 3.7).

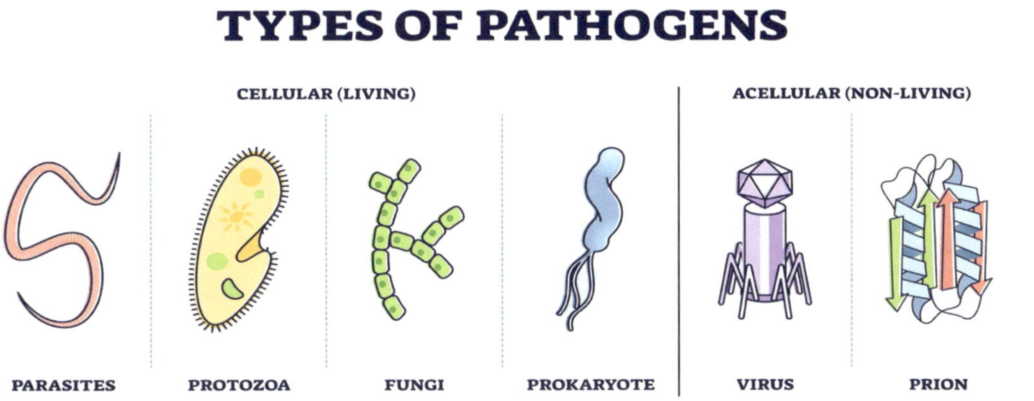

Figure 3.7. Types of microbial pathogens.

Source:

3.2.1. Bacterial Pathogens and Their Characteristics

Many types of bacteria invade hosts and cause diseases due to their unique traits. Several pathogenic bacteria possess virulence factors, including adhesins, toxins, and mechanisms that help them evade the immune system. As an example, adhesins help bacteria stick to host cells, which is a crucial initial step in establishing an infection. Exotoxins and endotoxins can also alter how cells function, leading to inflammation, which in turn helps bacteria multiply and remain in the body. Grasping these features is an essential step for figuring out the relationships between bacteria and humans, which may lead to new treatments for bacterial infections. In addition, the role of programmed cell death pathways, such as PANoptosis, in the development of microbial diseases has become increasingly important. PANoptosis combines apoptosis, pyroptosis, and necroptosis, facilitating the elimination of infected cells and triggering an inflammatory response. Because PANoptosis serves two purposes, it is clear that host defences against bacterial pathogens are complex; while it can stop infections, bacteria can sometimes turn it against the immune system. The exploration of PANoptosis offers insights into the host's cellular responses during infection and presents opportunities for the development of specialized therapies targeting these cellular processes (He et al., 2025). In addition to traditional virulence factors, bacterial extracellular vesicles (EVs) have emerged as crucial components in the pathogenesis of infections. They help bacteria communicate with the host cells, mostly among Gram-negative and Gram-positive pathogens. They carry pathogen-associated molecular patterns (PAMPs) that engage innate immune receptors, leading to cytokine production and initiating inflammatory responses. In any case, since bacterial EVs are complicated, they contribute to the way the immune system responds. Understanding the intricate interactions between bacterial EVs and the host immune system can enhance our knowledge of bacterial pathogenesis, paving the way for innovative diagnostic and therapeutic strategies, as well as promising developments in vaccine research (Peregrino et al., 2024) (Figure 3.8).

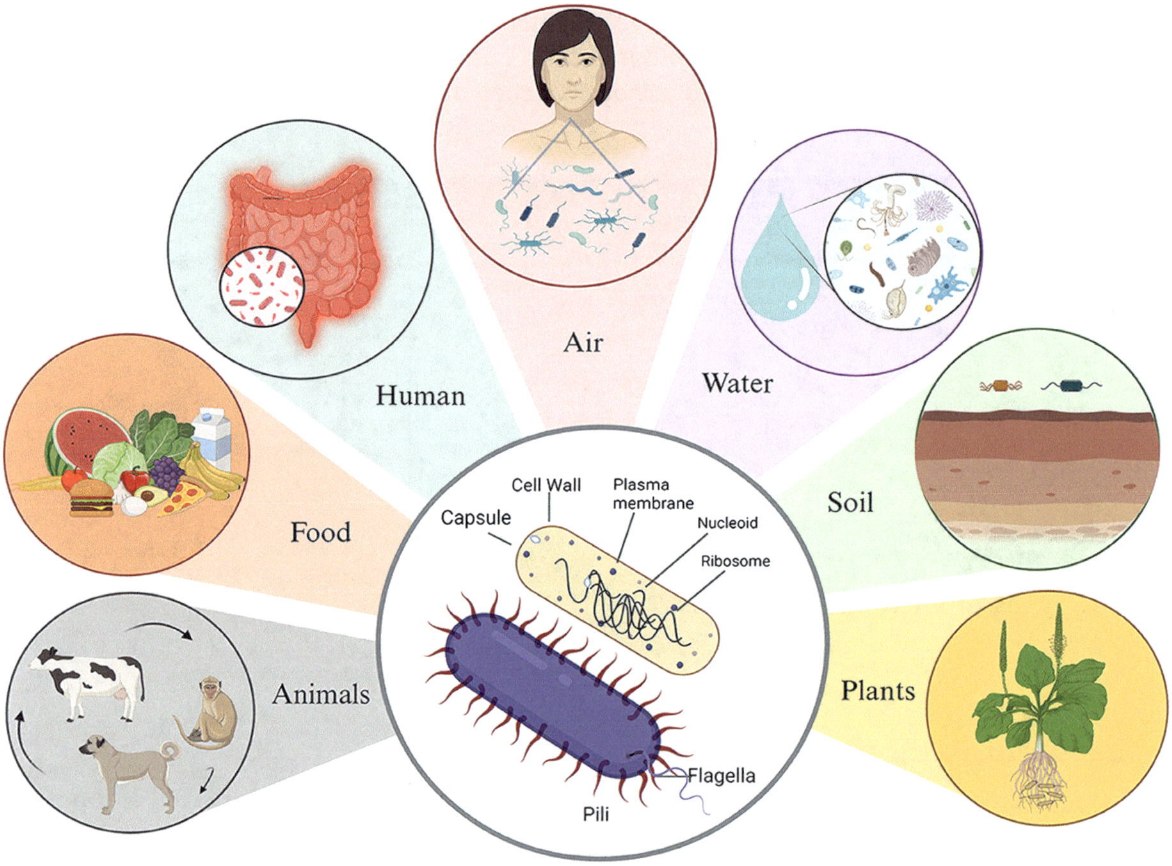

Figure 3.8. Bacterial pathogens and their characteristics.

Source: https://www.frontiersin.org/files/Articles/1370818/fmicb-15-1370818-HTML/image_m/fmicb-15-1370818-g001.jpg.

3.2.2. Viral Pathogens and Their Replication Strategies

Viral pathogens employ various ingenious methods to replicate within the cells they infect. While bacterial pathogens are made of complex cells, viruses only have simple genetic material covered by a protein coat. Because they are simple, viruses must use the host's own tools to reproduce. The first part of the core mechanism involves the attachment of the virus to the cell and its entry, followed by the uncoating of the viral genome. Inside the cell, the virus relies on the host's ribosomes and enzymes to make its proteins and reproduce its nucleic acids. The way viruses attack and the ways our cells defend against them are fundamental aspects of microbial pathogenesis, making it challenging to understand the host's response. Viruses use many different replication methods which allows them to adapt to other hosts and situations. HIV and similar viruses take their RNA genome and convert it into DNA once they enter the host, which then becomes part of the host's genome for continued survival. Unlike other viruses, influenza to recombine its genes when it infects the same cell, which significantly increases its ability to adapt. These methods make it harder for the host's immune system, which often leads to the host having a chronic infection or new strains of the virus appearing. Learning about the detailed mechanisms by which viruses reproduce is essential for virology and also guides research on antiviral drugs and vaccines, which are crucial for public health. How viral pathogens interact with the body's defenses shows that evolution is still happening. Viruses have developed several strategies to evade the immune system, including modifying their antigens and producing proteins that inhibit antiviral signals. At the same time, the host's immune system has adapted by developing new methods to identify and neutralize pathogens, illustrating an ongoing process of adaptation. For example, some viruses have been found to manipulate host cell signals, allowing them to replicate easily and prevent the body from responding with inflammation. Because of this, the process of viral infections is shaped, and it is also essential to understand how the virus and the host interact. As researchers delve deeper into these mechanisms, insights gained will be pivotal in designing innovative therapeutic approaches to combat viral diseases and improve health outcomes in affected populations (Figure 3.9).

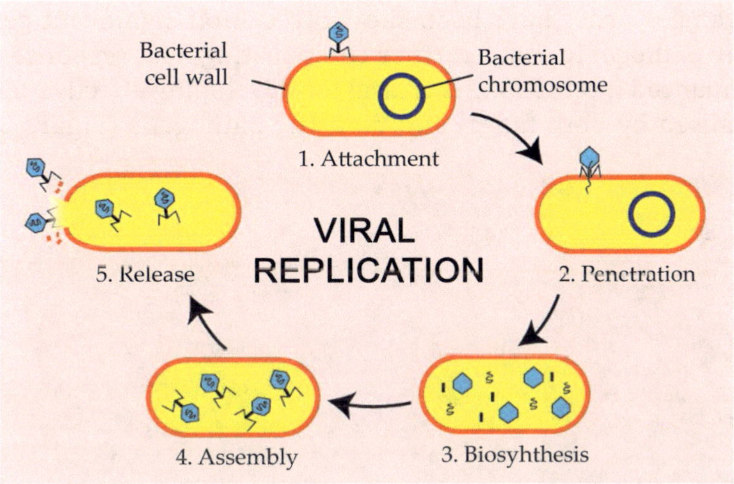

Figure 3.9. Viral pathogens and their replication strategies.

Source: https://encrypted-tbn0.gstatic.com/images?q=tbn:ANd9GcRbdqoe_j2kcnO3zfO_jglDu56V3ZPm4QHuhQ&s.

3.2.3. Fungal and Parasitic Pathogens

Many infectious diseases in humans are caused by fungal and parasitic pathogens, posing a significant threat to human health. Among fungi, the group called Onygenales (part of the Ascomycete order) contains several pathogens that can infect mammals, including *Histoplasma capsulatum* and *Coccidioides* spp. They can change their shape between yeast and filamentous forms, which helps them fit into the host and escape the immune system. Their ability to change their shape is essential for causing infections and allowing the disease to progress. Additionally, the rise of antifungal resistance exacerbates the challenges posed by fungal pathogens, necessitating the development of new treatments to combat infections effectively. It is essential to understand how these fungi evade host recognition to develop effective strategies for combating fungal diseases. Protozoa and helminths which are parasitic pathogens, also cause big problems for the immune system of the host. For example, some protozoan parasites, such as Plasmodium spp. and Trypanosoma spp., have complex life cycles and mechanisms to evade detection by the immune system, which enables them to survive and cause disease. They employ various methods, including altering their surface proteins and manipulating the immune system, to remain in the body and cause long-term infections. As a result of this persistence, many symptoms can appear, which can complicate both the diagnosis and the treatment. These parasites also cause inflammation in the body, which can lead to tissue damage and increase the illnesses linked to parasites. Studying how parasites interact with the immune system of their hosts helps find new treatments and improve ways to manage diseases. There is a complex and changing relationship between fungal and parasitic pathogens and the immune system of the host, which can lead to either protection or disease. The cytokine interleukin-17 (IL-17) exemplifies this dual role, as it is involved in the protection against various infections while also contributing to inflammation-related tissue damage. In the context of fungal infections, IL-17 plays a protective role by mediating the induction of proinflammatory molecules, which are essential for controlling pathogen growth (Das et al., 2017). When too much IL-17 is made, it can cause inflammation to become worse and damage tissues. Similarly, fungal pathogens like those of the Onygenales order have been shown to exhibit significant gene family expansions that may enhance their pathogenic traits, further complicating host responses (Taylor et al., 2015). Understanding these nuanced interactions is crucial for developing effective therapeutic approaches to manage diseases caused by both fungal and parasitic pathogens (Figure 3.10).

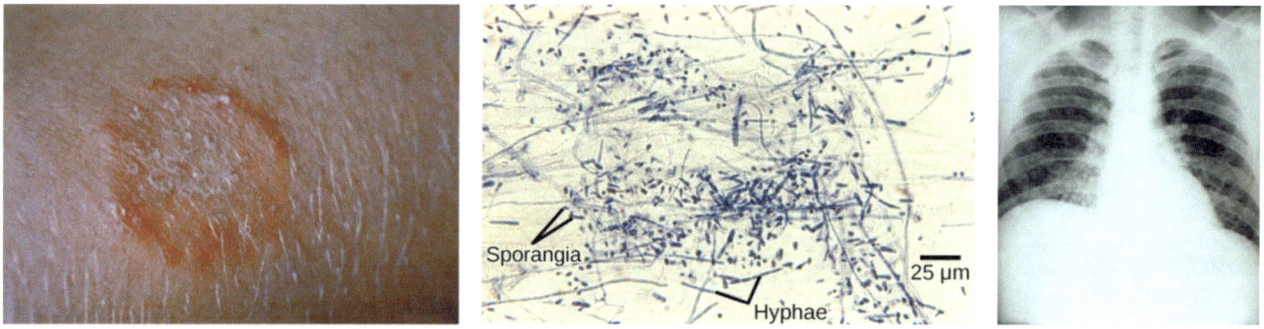

Figure 3.10. Fungal and parasitic pathogens.

Source: https://pressbooks-dev.oer.hawaii.edu/biology/wp-content/uploads/sites/26/2017/09/Figure_24_04_02abc.jpg.

3.3. Host Immune Response

It is essential to understand the host immune response to see how microbial pathogens function in the body. When pathogens invade, the immune system is the primary defense, using many different cells and molecules to respond to the infection. This defense involves both the innate immune response, which acts quickly but not specifically, and the adaptive immune response, which is specific and remembers threats. The two branches of immunity need to interact effectively, as a team effort can prevent pathogens from spreading and stop diseases from worsening. Yet, some microbial pathogens have adapted to exploit the body's weaknesses, resulting in a dynamic situation where the outcome of an infection depends on both the pathogen's virulence and the strength of the immune response. In specific cases, such as Clostridioides difficile infection (CDI), the host immune response is critically influenced by interactions with the gut microbiota. For example, *Tritrichomonas musculis* is a commensal organism that can affect the immune system, which means that not every interaction between microbes is harmful. Research suggests that T.mu prevents gut damage caused by CDI by inhibiting the accumulation of harmful neutrophils and promoting the differentiation of Th1 cells, which provide protection to the body. This complex relationship underscores the gut microbiome's role in shaping the host's immune system, as well as the impact of arginine-ornithine pathways on metabolism, which influences how pathogens affect the host and its immune system function. The findings emphasize that implementing microbiota-informed therapies may provide avenues for enhancing host defense mechanisms against specific pathogens (Yang et al., 2024). Additionally, the role of the host immune system becomes apparent when discussing the immunopathology of fungal infections. If the immune response is not strong enough, infections may persist, and if it is overly active, tissue damage can occur. The immune system of the host shows this balance by dealing with the virulence factors of *Talaromyces marneffei.* The damage response framework (DRF) aids in understanding how these interactions unfold, illustrating the intricacies involved in host defense and pathogen evasion strategies. In essence, the immune response must be finely tuned to eliminate threats without inadvertently causing harm to the host, which underscores the essential role of tailored therapeutic approaches in combating microbial pathogenesis effectively (Pruksaphon et al., 2024).

3.3.1. Innate Immune Response Mechanisms

The body relies on the innate immune response to defend against microbial pathogens, and it does this quickly and non-specifically. It consists of different cellular and molecular components that function together to detect and neutralise threats. A crucial aspect of the innate immune response is the presence of pattern recognition receptors (PRRs), which detect conserved microbial structures, or PAMPs, as well as damage-associated molecular patterns (DAMPs) released from injured or dying cells. When PRRs detect these molecular signatures, they launch signalling processes that start inflammation and attract immune cells to the infection area. So, the innate immune system provides quick protection and also helps initiate the adaptive immune system, which responds more precisely to future infections. Within the spectrum of innate immune cells, neutrophils, macrophages, and dendritic cells play pivotal roles in orchestrating host defence. Neutrophils are often the first responders to infection, exhibiting remarkable phagocytic activity and the ability to produce reactive oxygen species to eliminate microbes. Macrophages, while also being proficient phagocytes, engage in a more nuanced dialogue with their environment by secreting cytokines that modulate inflammation and facilitate tissue repair. Dendritic cells, in turn, are critical for linking the innate and adaptive immune responses; they process and present antigens to naïve T cells, thus facilitating a robust adaptive reaction. Together, they help the body respond to infections in various ways, which is why they are so crucial for maintaining the body's stability and health. Understanding how the innate immune system works in conjunction with microbial balance and the gut barrier is crucial for chronic inflammatory disorders, including IBD. Since IBD is thought to develop due to a combination of inherited factors, environmental influences, and immune system issues, the role of innate immune cells is crucial. As N/A (2024) discusses, these cells are crucial not only in initiating the inflammatory response but also in regulating interactions with the gut microbiome, which can be disrupted in IBD. Furthermore, the recognition of aberrant activation of PRRs, as noted in Adam et al. (2012), contributes to the understanding of both pathogen recognition and potential tissue injury in autoimmune diseases. Thus, exploring innate immune mechanisms not only expands our knowledge of microbial pathogenesis but also informs potential therapeutic strategies for disease management (Figure 3.11).

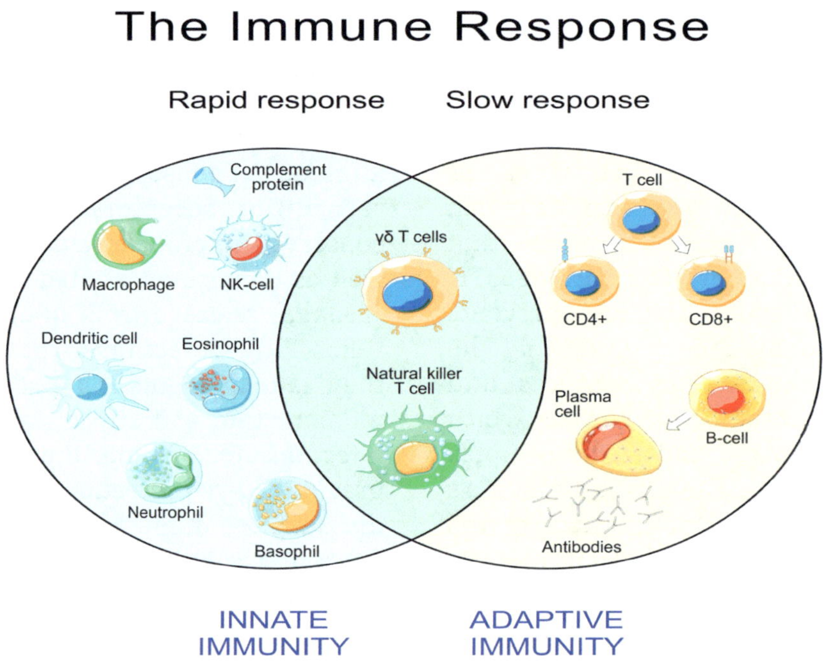

Figure 3.11. Innate immune response mechanisms.

Source: https://encrypted-tbn0.gstatic.com/images?q=tbn:ANd9GcRbdqoe_j2kcnO3zfO_jglDu56V3ZPm4QHuhQ&s.

3.3.2. Adaptive Immune Response Components

To fight microbial pathogens, the adaptive immune response utilizes a network of cells and mechanisms that are crucial. The central part of this response is lymphocytes, comprising B cells and T cells, each serving a distinct function in protecting the body. B cells are responsible for producing antibodies, which identify and eliminate pathogens. Once activated, B cells divide and become plasma cells, which produce a large number of antibodies tailored to the antigens in the body. By doing this, the immune system blocks pathogens and also tells other parts of the immune system to destroy them, which makes the response more effective. The engagement of B cells is particularly critical in the context of complex microbial infections, where antibody-mediated opsonization can significantly influence the pathogenicity of microbes within the host (Corriero et al., 2024). Additionally, T cells play a crucial role in adaptive immunity, distinguishing between various antigens and directing the immune system's responses. Cytotoxic T cells in the T cell group quickly eliminate infected cells, especially those containing pathogens. Otherwise, helper T cells, including Th1, Th2, and Th17, are essential for controlling the immune system. In this way, Th1 cells fight intracellular infections, and Th2 cells target infections that occur outside cells and allergens. The emergence of regulatory T cells (Treg) further underscores the complexity of T cell interactions, as they help maintain immune tolerance and prevent autoimmune diseases.

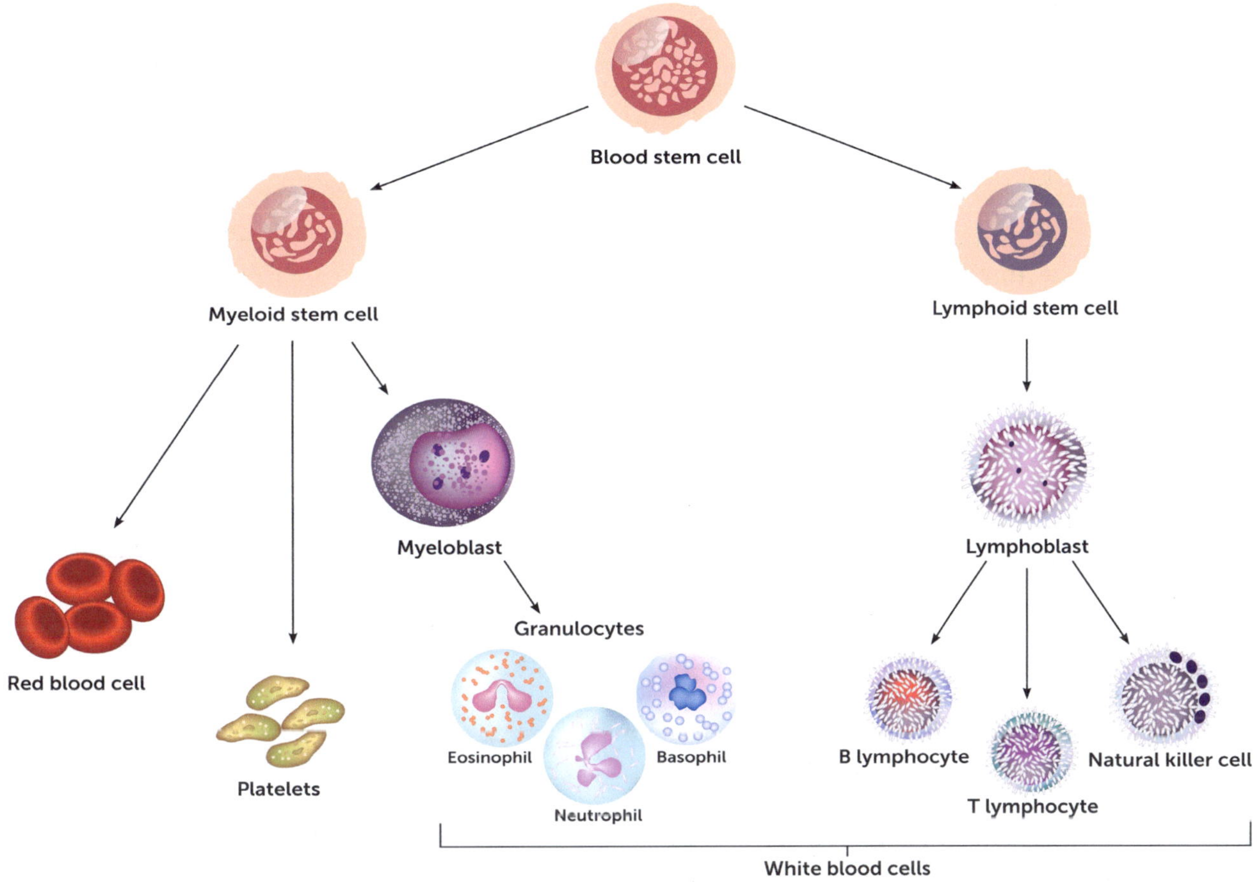

Figure 3.12. Adaptive immune response components.

Source: https://m2.healio.com/~/media/images/education-lab/learning-sites/learn-immuno-oncology/the-immune-system/learnimmunoblood.jpg.

The differentiation of these T cell subsets is often influenced by cytokine environments, which can shift the nature of the immune response toward either a protective or pathological outcome (Ałużna et al., 2022). There is a strong link between the adaptive immune system and the microbiota, and the types of microbes present can influence how the immune system functions. When microbial balance is disrupted, it can exacerbate autoimmune diseases and chronic inflammatory disorders. There is evidence that certain types of microbes can change how T cells are formed and function, which may influence the immune system of the host. Some gut microbiota can increase the number of regulatory T cells, which helps the immune system stay balanced and not overreact to harmless antigens. A lower variety of microbes in the gut may lead to stronger inflammation and problems with the regulation of the immune system. This illustrates the importance of understanding the interactions between microbial organisms and host immune components to develop novel therapeutic strategies aimed at modulating host responses to microbial infections effectively (Corriero et al., 2024) (Figure 3.12).

3.3.3. Role of Cytokines and Chemokines

The way cytokines and chemokines interact is significant for the immune system's response to microbial pathogens. Cytokines, which are produced by immune cells, regulate various aspects of inflammation and the immune system's activation. They direct the process of immune cells changing, becoming active, and moving, which helps the immune system respond to infections as a group. For example, when a virus infects, cytokines can help the immune system fight the virus in the best way. Examining how cytokines help or harm during viral infections helps us see their role in microbial pathogenesis. Such findings help create treatments that can modulate the immune system in conditions where cytokine production is imbalanced, thereby improving patient outcomes and the effectiveness of treatments. Chemokines, which are a group of cytokines, direct immune cells to places where infection or inflammation occurs. Their primary activity is chemotaxis, which enables leukocytes to move to areas where they are needed to stop pathogen invasion. When chemokines bind to their receptors on leukocytes, a series of signals is initiated within the cells, leading to cell movement and activation. The amount of chemokine produced and the number of receptors on the target cells can play a major role in determining the outcome of an infection. In viral encephalitis, some immune cells are attracted to the brain to either stop the virus or damage brain cells, which demonstrates the different roles chemokines may have. Targeting chemokine signaling pathways is a promising way to create new treatments that help the body deal better with infections. Cytokines and chemokines are important examples of how immune responses can be both helpful and harmful, mainly in inflammatory diseases. IL-17 plays a crucial role in guarding against bacteria and viruses, but excessive production can lead to harmful inflammation and tissue damage. So, the balance of IL-17 signalling reflects how cytokines can have opposing effects in the body, as has been discussed in the literature. Also, problems in cytokine and chemokine networks may cause autoimmune diseases, where the immune system attacks the body's own tissues. Understanding these complex dynamics, as evidenced by experimental models of viral diseases such as the Theiler's murine encephalomyelitis virus infection, is essential for identifying novel therapeutic strategies that can fine-tune these responses without compromising the ability to fight infections, showcasing their pivotal role in microbial pathogenesis and host response (Buchmeier et al., 1999; Das et al., 2017).

3.4. Pathogen-Host Interactions

Pathogen-host interactions are significant for studying microbial pathogenesis, since they decide the outcome of an infection. How pathogens attack the body and how the immune system responds are significant in determining if an infection becomes a disease. It is clear from a detailed look at these interactions that how well host defenses function can change a lot, depending on genetics, previous experience, and general health. For example, *Talaromyces marneffei* has developed mechanisms to evade its host's immune system, which can be particularly harmful when the host is unable to defend itself properly. This imbalance between pathogen aggressiveness and host resilience underscores the importance of studying these interactions through frameworks like the DRF, which elucidates the dual role of host immunity in microbial pathogenesis (Pruksaphon et al., 2024). Furthermore, significant progress in studying host-pathogen relationships has shown that host genetics can influence how an individual responds to certain infections. Studies indicate that host genes can cause different inflammatory reactions, which can make a person more or less susceptible to infections by Mycobacterium. Because of these genotype-specific reactions, using therapies that fit a person's genetic profile could improve the effectiveness of treatment. Examining these variations has allowed scientists to learn how the innate immune system of a host can control infections, which could lead to new personalized medicine approaches for infectious diseases. The implications of this research are profound, paving the way for targeted interventions that optimize the host's immune response while minimizing tissue damage, thus leading to more effective management of microbial infections (Rosowski, 2023). Pathogen-host interactions continually change as both entities attempt to adapt to one another. Many pathogens have methods to trick the immune system, such as altering its messages or hiding from immune cells. In the same way, hosts have created various immune systems, such as pattern recognition receptors, that spot and act against PAMPs. Because of this race, both the host and the pathogen become better adapted to each other. Because of this, scientists can develop new treatments such as vaccines that help the immune system fight particular diseases more effectively. Ultimately, continued investigation into pathogen-host interactions is essential for creating a comprehensive understanding of microbial pathogenesis and formulating effective treatment strategies that enhance host defense mechanisms while addressing pathogen threats (Rosowski, 2023; Pruksaphon et al., 2024) (Figure 3.13).

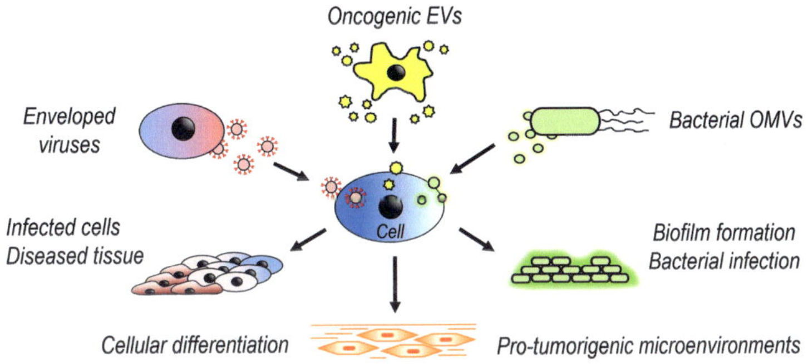

Figure 3.13. Pathogen-host interactions.

Source: https://bpb-us-w2.wpmucdn.com/sites.coecis.cornell.edu/dist/e/242/files/2019/09/pathogenic-NPs-1.jpg.

3.4.1. Molecular Interactions Between Pathogens and Host Cells

The study of pathogen-host cell interactions is crucial for understanding how diseases begin and advance. They occur in various ways, such as by interacting with host cells or by introducing toxins that alter the body's functions. The latest tools in microbial genomics and metabolomics have made it easier to see the complexity of these interactions. For instance, specific metabolites produced by microorganisms can significantly impact host metabolism, indicating that the microbiota plays an active role in disease development. This relationship highlights the need to understand microbial dynamics in contexts such as acute myeloid leukaemia (AML), where microbial-derived metabolites significantly impact host immune responses and diseases, as noted in the literature, emphasising their potential therapeutic implications in treating such conditions (Nowicka et al., 2024). Pathogens not only enter host cells, but they also affect immune responses, which may either help or hinder the progression of the disease. An example is when *Helicobacter pylori* infects the stomach, which can result in changes in the host's metabolism. The presence of *H. pylori* can prompt the immune system to act, which may alter nutrition, nutrient absorption, and metabolism. These changes point out that pathogens can alter the environment inside the host cells to help them survive, which adds more complexity to infections. Understanding these mechanistic pathways is vital for devising innovative treatment strategies aimed at metabolic diseases linked to chronic infections (Ye et al., 2023). Also, the way host cells and pathogens interact at the molecular level points to the role of the host microbiome in causing disease. When the microbiome is balanced, it can help protect from infections, but if it becomes disrupted, it can cause health problems. Changes in the microbiota have been linked to AML, and these alterations can impact the effectiveness of treatment and the likelihood of complications. It is shown by research that the variety and activities of gut microbes are vital for the host's metabolism, and microbial metabolites act as key factors in the transfer of microbial effects to host physiology. Therefore, a deeper understanding of these host-microbe interactions is essential not only for elucidating the mechanisms of disease but also for developing targeted therapies that consider both microbial and host factors in treatment regimens (Nowicka et al., 2024) (Figure 3.14).

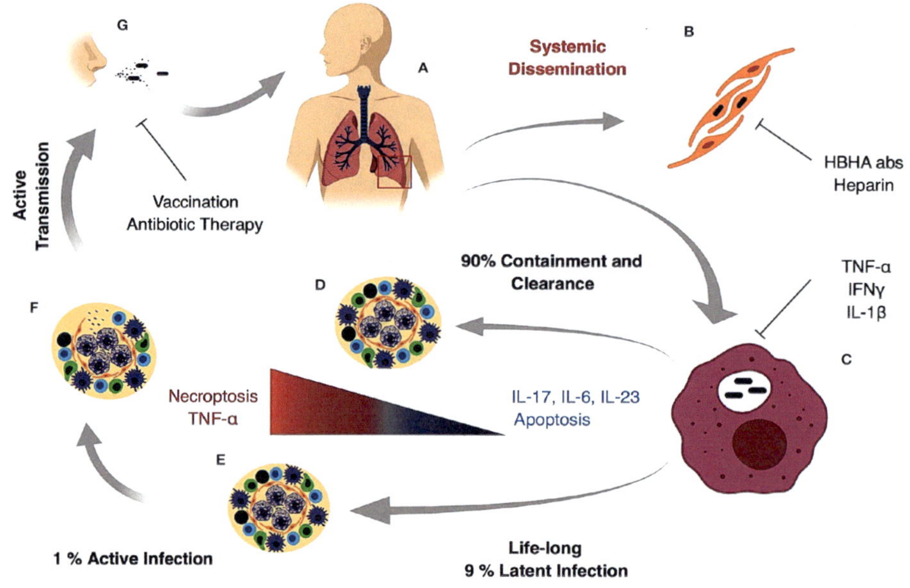

Figure 3.14. Molecular interactions between pathogens and host cells.

Source: https://www.frontiersin.org/files/Articles/513363/fimmu-11-01553-HTML/image_m/fimmu-11-01553-g001.jpg.

3.4.2. Impact of Microbial Virulence Factors

The connection between how microbes cause disease and how the body responds is vital in many diseases. Factors such as enzymes that harm host tissues, toxins that disrupt cell functions, and adhesion molecules that facilitate pathogen colonization are crucial in determining the severity of an infection and its consequences. For example, in Hidradenitis suppurativa (HS), specific bacterial strains like *Staphylococcus aureus* have been shown to express soluble virulence factors that contribute significantly to local tissue damage and chronic inflammation. Such virulence determinants not only enhance microbial persistence but also challenge the host's immune defense mechanisms, leading to a detrimental cycle of infection and inflammatory response that complicates treatment efforts (Cucu et al., 2025).

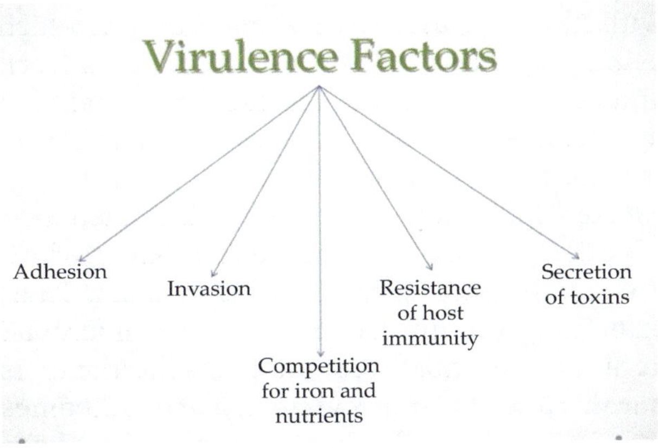

Figure 3.15. Impact of microbial virulence factors.

Source: https://image.slidesharecdn.com/bacterialvirulencefactors-150306095931-conversion-gate01/95/bacterial-virulence-factors-3-638.jpg?cb=1425636028.

Therefore, understanding these factors is crucial for developing drugs that can break this cycle and aid patients in their recovery. Emerging insights into the role of microbial virulence factors have led to a re-evaluation of traditional models of disease pathogenesis. In periodontal disease, for instance, an initial focus on bacterial infection alone has evolved into a more nuanced understanding of how microbial dysbiosis interacts with host responses and environmental factors. The shift from a purely bacterial-centric model emphasises the dynamic interplay between microbial communities and host susceptibility, wherein virulence factors can exacerbate inflammatory conditions and promote disease progression. This multifaceted perspective acknowledges the importance of host genetics, immune responses, and lifestyle choices in influencing the effects of virulent microbes and their associated pathologies (Debnath et al., 2024). Using this approach helps create strategies for diagnosis and treatment that deal with both the infection and the unique factors of the host. Also, when specific virulence factors are identified and understood, this opens up new ways to treat infections caused by pathogenic microbes. When HS is present, since biofilm formation and virulence of microbes are the primary reasons for chronic infections, interventions that address these factors can help treatment work more effectively. Disrupting the biofilm or neutralizing soluble factors that help bacteria cause infections may help reduce the seriousness of the infection and speed up recovery. Also, knowing the genetic factors behind microbial virulence can help create preventive measures for those at high risk due to their genes or the environment. Therefore, integrating knowledge of microbial virulence factors into clinical practice not only enriches the understanding of microbial pathogenesis but also offers valuable avenues for enhancing host responses and achieving better health outcomes in affected populations (Figure 3.15).

3.4.3. Consequences of Dysregulated Host Responses

The body's response to pathogens is crucial in determining the relationship between microbes and the immune system. Dysregulation may result in an immune system that is either too active or not active enough, which can have a significant effect on how diseases are managed.

An excessive immune response can lead to IBD, a chronic condition characterized by the immune system attacking gut microbes, causing tissue damage and further inflammation. Because of this, the host's inflammation makes microbial dysbiosis worse, which in turn supports the growth of harmful pathogens. Also, chronic inflammation changes the mix of microbes, which leads to pressure on the community that favors disease-causing species, making it harder to treat the disease. If the immune response is too weak, the host cannot effectively control infections, allowing pathogens to grow without resistance. As a result, immunocompromised individuals are more likely to develop opportunistic infections, as common commensals can become pathogenic. A change in the immune system can lead to serious health issues, including sepsis or infections that spread, which can be very detrimental to health. It is essential to understand how these responses become dysregulated, because this helps explain the causes of disease and the success of treatments. One example is targeted therapies that help the immune system return to normal function, which could reduce the adverse effects of these dysregulations. Besides affecting a person's health, problems in the body's responses can have wider impact on public health and medical practices. The increasing prevalence of autoimmune diseases and chronic inflammatory conditions highlights the need for a unified model to study host-microbe interactions. Research using innovative models, such as mouse-adapted human microbiota, has revealed how host inflammation fosters aggressive microbial populations that exacerbate disease severity, demonstrating that bacterial virulence can be significantly influenced by the host's immune environment (Gray et al., 2024). This evolving understanding underscores the importance of processing dysregulated immune responses not only as isolated phenomena but as integral components of the broader microbial pathogenesis landscape. Addressing these responses can ultimately lead to more effective prevention strategies and therapeutic approaches in microbial diseases.

3.5. Disease Outcomes

Understanding how microbes affect the body and how the body responds to them is crucial in determining the outcome of AML and other cancers. The diverse biology of AML underscores the importance of considering multiple factors when investigating its causes. New genetic studies are showing that the gut microbiome has a significant effect on how diseases progress and respond to therapies. The metabolism of patients with AML is related to their microbiome, which could play a role in how well treatments work and the outcome of the disease. Understanding dysbiosis—when the balance of microbes in the body is disrupted—shows that it can weaken immunity and increase the likelihood of patients developing infectious diseases, which are significant causes of illness in them. Thus, examining the interactions between microbial activity and host response mechanisms is paramount for improving disease outcomes in AML and similar malignancies (Nowicka et al., 2024). The importance of microbiota-disease interactions is shown in recent studies on recurrent ovarian cancer, which are not limited to hematological cancers. Doctors are now using pembrolizumab and bevacizumab to help T cells enter tumors, and they also give oral cyclophosphamide to lower the number of regulatory T cells. This approach in trials with patients who had been treated before showed encouraging results, such as a median progression-free survival of 10.2 months and an objective response rate of 47.5%. Further analysis revealed that specific immune features, distinct microbial patterns, and alterations in metabolism were linked. These findings suggest that the integration of immune, microbiome, and metabolic data could provide essential insights into the factors driving clinical responses, which are critical for tailoring future immunotherapy protocols and improving disease outcomes (Rosario et al., 2024). In short, understanding how microbes cause infections and how the body responds is vital for understanding the results of AML and recurrent ovarian cancer. Examining the microbiome and metabolome together can give a better understanding of the biological processes involved in these diseases. When researchers understand how microbes and their products impact the body, they can better comprehend how changes in the microbiome influence disease and its treatment. With this knowledge, it may be possible to develop strategies that adjust the microbiome or utilize the immune system to help patients and improve their chances of survival. As the evidence continues to accumulate, the integration of microbiome research into clinical practice may become a cornerstone in the quest for enhanced disease outcomes across diverse medical contexts (Nowicka et al., 2024; Rosario et al., 2024) (Figure 3.16).

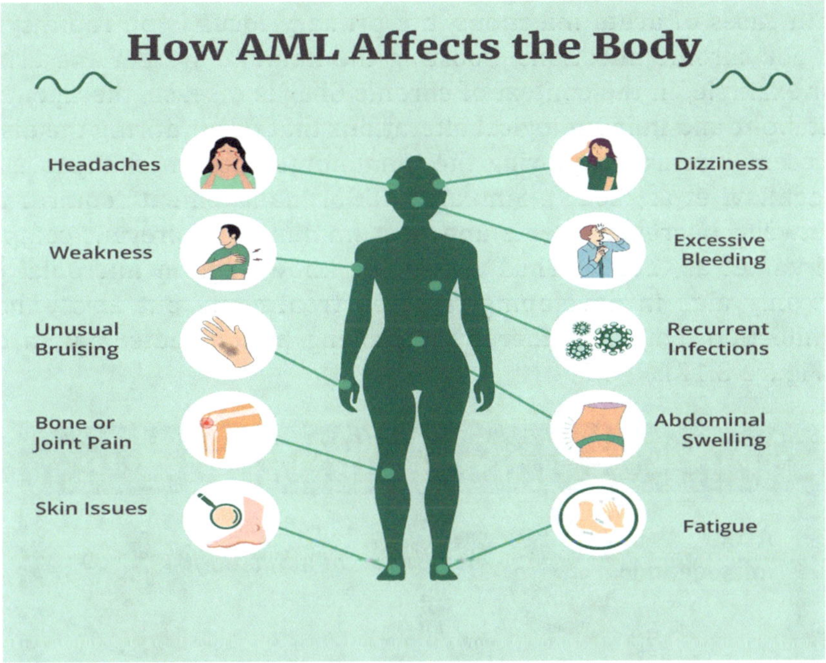

Figure 3.16. Disease outcomes: acute myeloid leukemia (AML).

Source: https://images.everydayhealth.com/images/seo-graphic-content-initiative/eh-how-aml-affects-the-body-seo-graphic.png?sfvrsn=4e260ca3_3.

3.5.1. Acute Versus Chronic Infections

It is essential to tell apart acute and chronic infections to learn about how microbes cause diseases and how the body responds. A quick development of symptoms marks acute infections because the pathogens, such as bacteria or viruses, spread fast. The immune system usually reacts strongly to this type of infection, trying to eliminate the invaders, which leads to symptoms such as fever, swelling, and pain. If a person has Chagas disease caused by Trypanosoma cruzi, the first symptoms are usually fever and fatigue, which occur because the immune system is trying to fight the parasite. If left untreated, individuals can progress into a chronic phase, where the initial symptoms subside. Still, the pathogens can remain or become inactive, which causes the immune system to react differently as it adapts to the ongoing presence of the pathogen. With chronic infections, the host and the pathogen interact for a long time, which can cause the immune system to stay active and result in damage to tissues and the development of disease. In conditions like chronic suppurative otitis media (CSOM), the prolonged presence of microbial agents has significant health implications, particularly in vulnerable populations, such as children in developing nations. Such an infection is complicated to get rid of, so pathogens can avoid being noticed by the immune system and control how the host responds. Because the immune system is always working, even if not very well, it can sometimes cause problems known as immunopathology. The chronic phase can involve times when symptoms get worse and then better which makes it harder to decide on the proper treatment. The flexibility of these pathogens makes it difficult for healthcare providers, which is why it is essential to use treatments that understand the specific ways these infections progress. Studying the differences between acute and chronic infections provides valuable insights for treating them. In cases of acute infections, the primary focus is on rapid symptom relief and pathogen removal. For chronic infections, boosting the immune system and using antibiotics are also important. For example, in the context of chronic Chagas disease, therapeutic strategies must account for the metabolic and immunological alterations that occur during the disease progression, as highlighted in recent research exploring the immunometabolism changes associated with the condition (Nasuhidehnavi et al., 2023). Similarly, CSOM management requires an understanding of the interplay between microbial agents and host immunity to prevent complications, such as hearing loss (Khairkar et al., 2023). Thus, advancing knowledge in microbial pathogenesis and host response not only aids in developing targeted treatments but also enhances the overall understanding of infection dynamics, thereby improving patient outcomes in diverse infectious disease contexts (Figure 3.17).

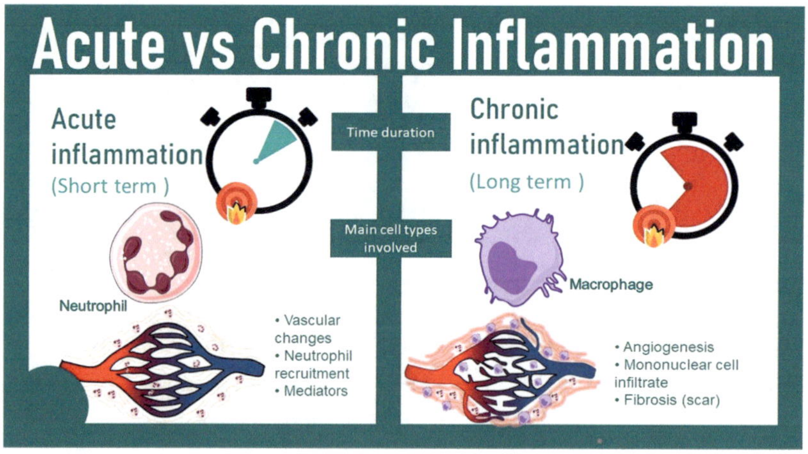

Figure 3.17. Acute versus chronic infections.

Source: https://i.ytimg.com/vi/IfVVMlm_RKU/maxresdefault.jpg.

3.5.2. Factors Influencing Disease Severity

The interplay between microbial factors and host genetics plays a crucial role in determining disease severity in various conditions. For instance, the genetic predisposition towards certain autoimmune diseases can significantly influence an individual's response to microbial stimuli. In the case of Celiac Disease (CeD), while the presence of specific human leukocyte antigen (HLA) haplotypes is necessary for disease onset, it is not solely sufficient to explain the variability in disease severity among affected individuals. The influence of non-host factors such as dietary habits and microbial interactions provides a complex layer to understanding CeD pathogenesis. Emerging studies suggest that an individual's diet and the accompanying microbial landscape play pivotal roles in modulating disease progression and inflammatory responses, emphasising the importance of these external factors in the management and prevention of CeD, as highlighted in recent reviews on the subject (Galipeau et al., 2024).

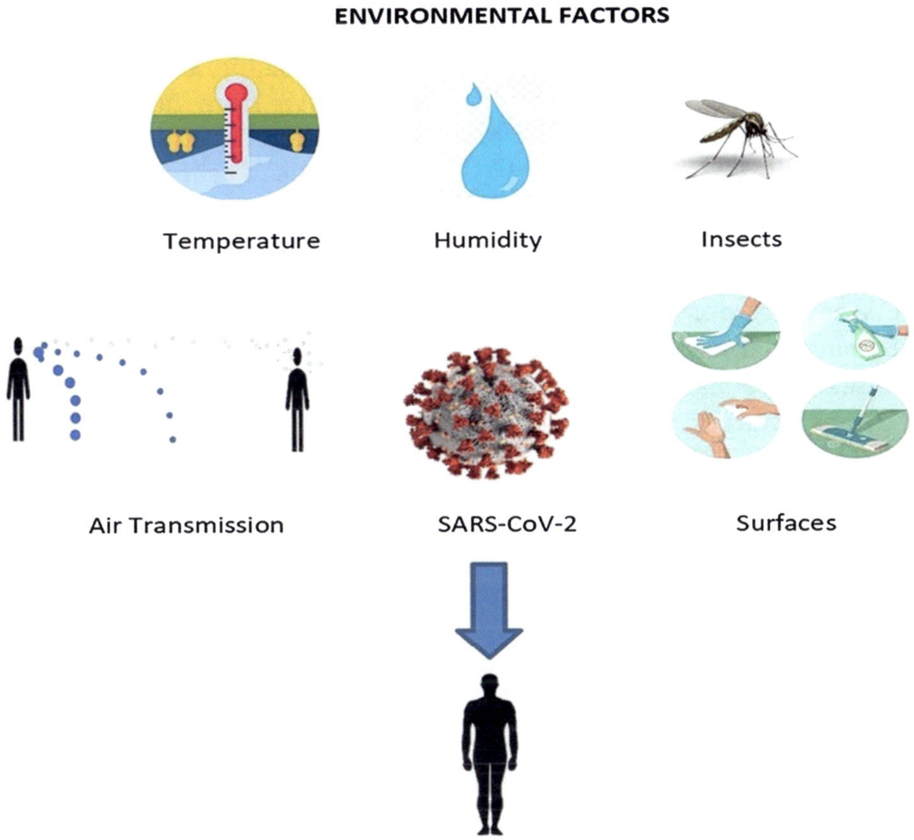

Figure 3.18. Factors influencing disease severity.

Source: https://media.springernature.com/lw1200/springer-static/image/art%3A10.1007%2Fs10311-022-01418-9/MediaObjects/10311_2022_1418_Fig1_HTML.png.

Along with genes, the makeup of the microbiome is known to play a significant role in how severe different infections become. Changes in the gut microbiota, which is known as dysbiosis, may result in a higher risk of infection and stronger inflammatory reactions. CDI is a good example, as antibiotics are often administered before dysbiosis, which can significantly impact the immune system and the patient's recovery. Certain commensal organisms, for example, *Tritrichomonas musculis*, can reduce the severity of CDI by influencing the immune system to stop inflammation and support protective responses. Such findings underscore the critical role of microbial communities not only in colonisation resistance but also in influencing the trajectory of disease severity and host reactions (Yang et al., 2024). The link between environmental conditions and the host's response to disease is also crucial when considering factors that influence disease severity. Along with genes and microbes, the way a person eats, deals with stress and looks after their health can play a significant role in how they react to pathogens. Not eating a healthy diet may make it easier for inflammatory states to develop, which can worsen the impact of infections. Stress can also alter how the immune system functions, potentially reducing the host's ability to resist infections. Being aware of these various factors is essential for managing diseases comprehensively. By integrating genetic, microbial, and environmental considerations, researchers and clinicians can better predict disease outcomes and tailor therapeutic strategies to improve patient care and disease prevention in the context of microbial pathogenesis and host response (Figure 3.18).

3.5.3. Examples of Diseases Caused by Specific Pathogens

The interaction between specific pathogens and the host can lead to a variety of diseases, illustrating the complex dynamics of microbial pathogenesis. One prominent example is the impact of *Campylobacter jejuni*, a bacterium often associated with contaminated food and water. Infection by this pathogen typically results in gastroenteritis, characterised by symptoms such as diarrhoea, abdominal pain, and fever. Such disease manifestations arise from the pathogen's ability to invade intestinal cells and trigger inflammatory responses. Importantly, the use of ozone as a biocidal agent has shown promise in inactivating this pathogen effectively, highlighting potential strategies for mitigating its public health impact. Thus, understanding the mechanisms by which *C. jejuni* causes disease, along with effective disinfection methods, is crucial for both prevention and treatment strategies in microbial pathogenesis (Anderson et al., 2003). Another notable pathogen is *Salmonella enteritidis*, which is primarily transmitted through contaminated foods, particularly poultry and eggs. Once ingested, this pathogen invades the intestinal epithelium, triggering an inflammatory response that can lead to a severe gastrointestinal illness known as salmonellosis. The disease can vary in severity, from mild flu-like symptoms to life-threatening complications in vulnerable populations. *S. enteritidis* is adept at evading host immune responses, thus enhancing its pathogenicity.

The increasing incidence of salmonellosis emphasises the need for continued research into effective food safety measures. Understanding the molecular mechanisms of *S. enteritidis* pathogenicity can shed light on strategies to minimise infection risk and improve public health outcomes regarding foodborne illnesses (Anderson et al., 2003). Furthermore, emerging evidence suggests a link between specific pathogens and autoimmune diseases, illustrating intricate relationships that extend beyond immediate illness. For instance, certain viral infections and bacterial pathogens can act as triggers for autoimmune responses through mechanisms such as molecular mimicry or bystander activation. This relationship is supported by studies that demonstrate how infections can exacerbate conditions such as rheumatoid arthritis or lupus. The triggering effect of pathogens highlights the role of the immune system in not only combating infections but also in potentially turning against the host's tissues. By elucidating these connections, researchers can gain a deeper understanding of the dynamics of microbial pathogenesis and host response, thereby paving the way for novel therapeutic approaches to manage both infectious and autoimmune diseases.

3.6. Therapeutic Approaches

Approaches to microbial infections and the body's response, particularly in periodontitis, have undergone significant improvements over time. Because periodontitis involves many factors, successful treatments should consider how bacteria and the immune system interact. Traditional therapies mainly use procedures like scaling and root planning, but these alone are usually not enough to stop the disease from progressing. Using additional therapies has become vital to improve clinical results, and new studies reveal that probiotics, antimicrobial drugs, and advanced surgery can be helpful. These strategies not only help in reducing pathogenic bacterial load but also facilitate the restoration of a balanced oral microbiome, thereby improving immune resilience against future pathogenic challenges (Acharya et al., 2025). Nanomedicine and other innovative therapies are being noticed because they can target diseases precisely at the cellular level. New delivery methods made possible by nanotechnology can enhance the effectiveness of treating periodontitis. Using nanosystems makes it possible to release medicine only when and where needed which helps the immune system and reduces overall side effects. This matters because periodontitis is caused by an overactive immune system, which often results in significant damage to the gums and bones. Research has shown that these advanced nanosystems can be utilised to deliver anti-inflammatory agents, growth factors, or antimicrobial compounds directly to the site of infection, effectively addressing both microbial dysbiosis and the excessive host inflammatory response (Cui et al., 2025). Understanding the makeup of the oral microbiome and any imbalances is essential for creating targeted therapies. Understanding the microbes involved in periodontitis helps researchers develop better treatments that address the harmful bacteria and reintroduce the helpful microorganisms needed for healthy teeth and gums. Prebiotics and certain types of probiotics are examples of treatments that can help restore healthy bacteria in the mouth, potentially improving periodontal health. Supporting a variety of microbes in the mouth is essential for reducing the inflammation caused by periodontal disease. As research evolves, future therapeutic directions may incorporate personalised medicine approaches that consider individual microbiotic profiles and host immune responses, ultimately leading to more effective management of periodontitis and its systemic implications (Acharya et al., 2025).

3.6.1. Antibiotics and Their Mechanisms of Action

Antibiotics are vital to treating bacterial infections and are important in modern medicine. They primarily function by interfering with essential functions in bacterial cells, which either prevents them from growing or causes them to die. Penicillins and cephalosporins are antibiotics that disrupt the formation of the bacterial cell wall, allowing water to enter the cell and causing it to burst. Classes such as tetracyclines and macrolides prevent bacteria from making essential proteins by sticking to their ribosomes. It is important to understand these mechanisms to design effective therapies and avoid resistance, which happens when bacteria become immune to antibiotics. Antibiotic resistance causes serious problems in the study of microbial diseases and how the body responds to them. When bacteria become resistant to antibiotics, the usual treatments become less effective, causing infections to last longer and increasing illness and mortality rates. Notably, resistance can occur through various mechanisms, such as mutations in target sites or the acquisition of resistance genes from other bacteria, often facilitated by horizontal gene transfer. This complicates the treatment landscape and necessitates the continuous development of novel antibiotics and alternative therapies. Furthermore, understanding the interplay between microbial resistance and the host immune response is crucial, as ineffective antibiotic treatment can inadvertently allow resistant strains to proliferate, further compromising patient recovery and public health initiatives. Emerging research also highlights the intricate relationship between antibiotics and the gut microbiome, emphasizing its influence on overall health and disease dynamics. Antibiotics indiscriminately target both pathogenic and beneficial bacteria, potentially leading to dysbiosis—a condition characterised by an imbalance in microbial communities. Such disturbances can affect gut health and subsequently influence systemic conditions through the brain-gut-microbiome axis, as described in recent studies that reveal shared communication pathways between gut microbes and the central nervous system. Disruptions in this axis have been implicated in various ailments, underscoring the need for a more nuanced understanding of antibiotic action beyond their immediate antimicrobial effects. Addressing these complexities could lead to better strategies that minimise collateral damage while effectively managing bacterial infections (Anderson et al., 2003; Kalani et al., 2018) (Figure 3.19).

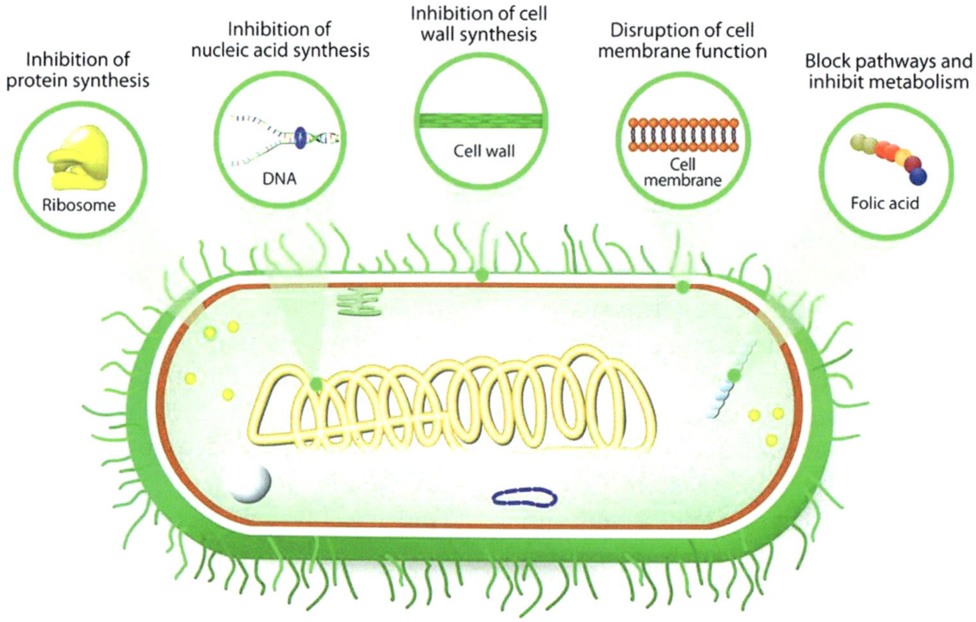

Figure 3.19. Antibiotics and their mechanisms of action.

Source: https://thumbs.dreamstime.com/z/mechanisms-action-antimicrobials-antibiotic-60642778.jpg.

3.6.2. Vaccination Strategies and Their Effectiveness

Effective vaccination strategies are crucial for controlling microbial pathogenesis and enhancing host immunity. Vaccines function by training the immune system to recognize specific pathogens, leading to the development of immunological memory that provides long-term protection. Traditional vaccines, such as inactivated or live-attenuated forms of pathogens, have effectively reduced the incidence of diseases like measles and polio. However, innovation in vaccine design has introduced novel strategies, including mRNA and viral vector vaccines, which have shown remarkable efficacy, particularly during the COVID-19 pandemic. These advanced platforms enable a more rapid response to EIDs and allow for the modulation of immune responses tailored to specific pathogens. Consequently, evaluating and adapting vaccination methodologies remains pivotal for public health initiatives aimed at controlling microbial infections and reducing morbidity and mortality related to infectious diseases. The efficacy of vaccines is influenced by various factors, including the host's immune response, age, and genetic predisposition. Individual variability in immune function can affect vaccine responsiveness, making it essential to understand and address disparities in vaccine efficacy. For instance, the efficiency of vaccines is decreased in older persons due to their frequently compromised immune responses. Furthermore, underlying medical conditions such as diabetes and autoimmune disorders can compromise immunogenicity. Studies indicate that comprehensive approaches, including the incorporation of adjuvants that boost immune responses and personalised vaccination schedules tailored to individual risk factors, can enhance overall efficacy. Additionally, public education is crucial in countering vaccine hesitancy, which poses a significant barrier to achieving herd immunity. Ultimately, recognising these variables is vital for developing optimised vaccination strategies that bolster population-wide immunity against infectious diseases. Recent findings highlight the role of inflammation in modulating vaccine responses, emphasising the interplay between the immune system and vaccination outcomes. Research suggests that acute inflammatory responses induced by vaccination can enhance the maturation of antigen-presenting cells and promote effective T-cell activation. Such mechanisms underscore the importance of understanding the inflammatory pathways involved during vaccination and their potential effects on long-term immunity. For example, microbial challenges that stimulate the immune system can enhance sleep quality, further suggesting a bidirectional relationship between immune responses and physiological states that support vaccine efficacy (Besedovsky et al., 2019). In this context, it is essential for future vaccination strategies to consider not only the antigenic components but also the host's inflammatory milieu, as harnessing these interactions might lead to improved protective responses. Therefore, integrating insights from microbial pathogenesis and host response into vaccination strategies will be critical for advancing public health goals and achieving effective disease control measures.

3.6.3. Emerging Therapies and Future Directions

Emerging therapies targeting microbial pathogenesis and host responses are critical in advancing treatment options for infectious diseases. Current research emphasizes the role of exosomes, which are small EVs that facilitate intercellular communication, in mediating therapeutic effects. Recent studies have highlighted the potential of exosomes derived from human mesenchymal stem cells (hMSCs) in regenerative medicine, owing to their bioactive cargo, including tRNA-derived fragments (tRFs) and tRNA-derived internal fragments (tiRNAs). It is suggested that these molecules may influence the capacity of exosomes to promote tissue regeneration, thereby acting as a novel approach to manage pathologies resulting from microbial infections (San et al., 2018). As researchers continue to explore the complexities of exosomal cargo, therapies leveraging these vesicles could revolutionize how we approach cellular repair and response to microbial challenges. Another promising direction emerges from the modulation of gut microbiota, particularly in relation to metabolic disorders such as Type 2 diabetes mellitus (T2DM). Recent findings indicate that altering the composition of gut microbiota through strategies like probiotics, prebiotics, and dietary adjustments may enhance metabolic outcomes in T2DM management. These interventions demonstrate the capacity to improve glycemic control and insulin sensitivity, while also exhibiting anti-inflammatory effects (Akhtar et al., 2024). This highlights the interconnectedness of microbial health and overall metabolic processes, offering a multidimensional approach to tackling chronic diseases influenced by microbial imbalance. Consequently, integrating gut microbiota modulation into clinical practice could pave the way for innovative therapies that address both microbial pathogenesis and its repercussions on host health. Looking to the future, the combination of emerging therapeutic strategies could yield substantial benefits in managing infections and their systemic effects on host responses. Developing an integrative framework that encompasses exosome-based therapies alongside microbiota modulation may yield synergistic effects, leading to enhanced efficacy compared to conventional treatments. This holistic approach recognizes the complexity of host-microbe interactions and their implications for health and disease. For instance, understanding how tRFs and tiRNAs delivered via exosomes can influence gut microbiota dynamics may create a dialogue between cellular therapy and microbial health. As research continues to unveil these intricate relationships, the potential to harness these interactions for therapeutic purposes becomes increasingly attainable, promising a future where targeted interventions revolutionise our approach to microbial pathogenesis and host responses.

SUMMARY

In conclusion, the intricate relationship between microbial pathogenesis and host response underscores the dynamic interplay that shapes the outcomes of infections. Understanding this relationship is vital for developing targeted therapeutic strategies and preventive measures. For instance, the examination of enteric diseases in pigs, particularly those caused by *Brachyspira hyodysenteriae* and *Lawsonia intracellularis*, reveals the significance of microorganism's mechanisms of infection and the hosts reactions to these pathogens. The identification of key pathogens through advanced diagnostic methods has facilitated a deeper understanding of disease progression, allowing for more effective interventions in both veterinary and human medicine. As a result, improved management practices and preventative strategies can mitigate the impacts of these diseases on livestock and public health (Jacobson et al., 2003). Furthermore, the role of post-translational modifications, such as *glutathionylation*, highlights the complexities involved in microbial infections and the host's immune response. *Glutathionylation* modifies the functional characteristics of both microbial and host proteins, influencing their roles in the immune/inflammatory responses to infection. This modification represents a critical signaling mechanism that contributes to the outcome of infections by modulating the redox state within cells. The growing body of evidence illustrating the significance of glutathionylated proteins in both pathogens and hosts suggests that these modifications could serve as potential therapeutic targets. By manipulating the *glutathionylation* process, researchers could develop novel strategies to combat microbial infections and enhance the host's response (Baldelli et al., 2019). Overall, the conclusion drawn from the studies of microbial pathogenesis and host responses emphasizes the necessity of a multidisciplinary approach in addressing infectious diseases. Advances in molecular biology techniques have improved our ability to dissect the mechanisms of pathogenesis and the hosts defensive strategies. The integration of such knowledge allows for the exploration of innovative methodologies for disease management and treatment. As we continue to unravel the complexities of microbial interactions with hosts, our enhanced understanding will inform public health policies, veterinary practices, and the design of effective vaccines, ultimately contributing to a healthier population and improved animal welfare (Jacobson et al., 2003; Baldelli et al., 2019).

The intricate relationship between microbial pathogenesis and host response emerges as a crucial area of study, with far-reaching implications for health and disease. Within this context, research has illuminated the essential role of the gut microbiota in mediating interactions between microbes and the host's immune system. Recent studies highlight the microbiota-gut-brain axis as a significant pathway through which microbial composition can influence neurological and psychological outcomes. Factors such as diet, antibiotic use, and environmental stressors influence the diversity and functionality of the microbiota, thereby affecting the host's responses to pathogens. For instance, disruptions in microbiota due to early-life infections can lead to lasting consequences, potentially increasing susceptibility to neurodevelopmental disorders. Understanding these dynamics is paramount in addressing conditions ranging from anxiety to Alzheimer's disease, showcasing the profound impact of microbial interactions on human health and disease progression (Cryan et al., 2019). Advancements in clinical metagenomic next-generation sequencing (mNGS) have revolutionised our approach to diagnosing microbial infections. This innovative technique allows for the comprehensive characterisation of microbial communities and host responses directly from patient samples. By analysing both microbial and host genetic material, mNGS enhances our capability to identify pathogens with precision, paving the way for tailored therapeutic strategies. Notably, the integration of mNGS into clinical practice raises challenges that hospitals must address, including the need for standardised protocols and interoperability with existing diagnostic systems. However, the potential benefits, including targeted treatments and insights into AMR, underscore the importance of overcoming these hurdles. As mNGS continues to establish its presence in clinical laboratories, it has the potential to significantly transform the landscape of infectious disease management and provide deeper insights into host-microbe interactions (Chiu et al., 2019). Furthermore, ongoing research into microbial pathogenesis emphasizes the critical need for perpetual exploration of host-microbe dynamics throughout the human lifespan. According to new research, microbial diversity declines with age, which may increase an older person's susceptibility to infections and inflammatory illnesses. The interplay between stress and the microbiota-gut-brain axis is particularly noteworthy; chronic stress can exacerbate dysbiosis, further impacting mental health and disease susceptibility. As scientists seek to elucidate the underlying mechanisms governing these processes, future studies will undoubtedly focus on microbial-based interventions as therapeutic strategies. Such interventions may not only bolster immune response but also hold promise for preventing or mitigating the repercussions of various pathologies. The insights gleaned from these investigations will pave the way for innovative approaches in translational medicine, ultimately enhancing our understanding of microbial pathogenesis and its profound effects on host responses across all stages of life (Cryan et al., 2019).

CLOSER LOOK:

BECAUSE OF ANTIGENIC VARIATION:

Antigenic variation is one of the most powerful survival strategies used by pathogens, allowing them to evade host immune defenses and persist within populations. Taking a closer look at this phenomenon reveals how subtle genetic alterations can reshape the course of infections, influence vaccine development, and complicate global public health efforts. Because of antigenic variation, pathogens are able to remain a step ahead of the immune system, transforming what might otherwise be short-lived infections into ongoing challenges.

At its core, antigenic variation refers to changes in the surface molecules—antigens—that the host immune system recognizes. When these markers shift, previously generated antibodies or memory immune cells may no longer recognize the pathogen effectively. This forces the immune system to start from scratch, granting the pathogen additional time to replicate, spread, or establish chronic infection. Some organisms achieve this through rapid mutation, while others use gene conversion, recombination, or phase variation to alter the expression of key surface proteins.

A classic consequence of antigenic variation is the recurring nature of certain diseases. Influenza viruses, for example, undergo frequent antigenic drift, producing seasonal strains that differ enough from previous versions to escape immunity. Other pathogens, such as HIV, mutate so rapidly that they generate countless variants within a single host, undermining the effectiveness of immune responses and complicating therapeutic strategies. Still others, including malaria parasites and *Neisseria* species, employ structured genetic programs to switch between antigenic forms, creating waves of immune evasion that prolong infection.

Because of antigenic variation, vaccine design becomes significantly more challenging. Vaccines typically aim to train the immune system to recognize a stable target. When pathogens continually change that target, vaccines must either be updated regularly or engineered to elicit broader, cross-reactive immunity. This is why some vaccines are highly effective and long-lasting, while others require frequent reformulation or fail to provide complete protection.

Antigenic variation also shapes epidemiology. It influences patterns of reinfection, the persistence of pathogens within communities, and the emergence of new outbreaks. Understanding how and why these changes occur helps researchers anticipate future variants, refine surveillance systems, and design better interventions.

In essence, because of antigenic variation, the relationship between pathogens and hosts is dynamic and ongoing. It underscores the adaptive ingenuity of microbes and the need for equally adaptive scientific strategies to combat them.

REFERENCES

1. Acharya, A. B., Hegde, U., & Acharya, S. (2025). Nanosystems for modulation of immune responses in periodontal therapy: a mini-review. *Frontiers in Dental Medicine, 5*. https://doi.org/10.3389/fdmed.2024.1509775Adam, A., Alexopoulou, L., Blander, J., Brightbill, H., Busch, D., Coley, R., Coley, M., et al. (2012). *Innate Immunity: Ignored for Decades, But not Forgotten.* https://core.ac.uk/download/323076512.pdf (accessed on 30th May 2025).

2. Ahmed, M. M. (2024). Interferon lambda: An anonymous warrior of host-microbial fray in the pathogenesis of periodontal diseases. *Bangladesh Journal of Medical Science*. https://www.semanticscholar.org/paper/1c0384c2197ede34f92a31cdc8f789f5c3178e25 (accessed on 30th May 2025).

3. Akhtar, M., & Tousif, M. (2024). *Modulating Gut Microbiota in the Management of Type 2 Diabetes Mellitus: A Narrative Review*. https://core.ac.uk/download/613230059.pdf (accessed on 30th May 2025).

4. Anderson, J. G., Goudie, A. C., MacGregor, S. J., & Olateju, M. (2003). *Inactivation of Pathogens on Food and Contact Surfaces Using Ozone as a Biocidal Agent*. https://core.ac.uk/download/9020578.pdf (accessed on 30th May 2025).

5. Baldelli, S., Checconi, P., Ciriolo, M. R., & Limongi, D. (2019). *Role of Glutathionylation in Infection and Inflammation*. https://core.ac.uk/download/231746825.pdf (accessed on 30th May 2025).

6. Besedovsky, L., Lange, T., & Haack, M. (2019). The sleep-immune crosstalk in health and disease. *Physiological Reviews, 99*, 1325–1380. https://doi.org/10.1152/physrev.00010.2018.

7. Buchmeier, M. J., & Lane, T. E. (1999). *Viral-Induced Neurodegenerative Disease*. https://core.ac.uk/download/323075723.pdf (accessed on 30th May 2025).

8. Cacciotti, F., Cicerone, C., Corazziari, E. S., Gagliardi, A., et al. (2016*). Eubiosis and Dysbiosis: The Two Sides of the Microbiota*. https://core.ac.uk/download/54532058.pdf (accessed on 30th May 2025).

9. Chiu, C. Y., & Miller, S. A. (2019). Clinical metagenomics. *Nature Reviews Genetics, 20*, 341–355. https://doi.org/10.1038/s41576-019-0113-7.

10. Cicerone, C., Nenna, R., & Pontone, S. (2015). *Th17, Intestinal Microbiota and the Abnormal Immune Response in the Pathogenesis of Celiac Disease*. https://core.ac.uk/download/54248894.pdf (accessed on 30th May 2025).

11. Corriero, A., Giglio, M., Soloperto, R., Inchingolo, F., Varrassi, G., & Puntillo, F. (2024). Microbial symphony: Exploring the role of the gut in osteoarthritis-related pain. A narrative review. *Pain and Therapy, 13*, 409–433. https://www.semanticscholar.org/paper/ba9f93233321f5e320a244c5ba9fe2124108b3a6 (accessed on 30th May 2025).

12. Costa, E. N. De. O. Q. (2011). *Viral Modulation of Interferon (IFN) Responses to African Swine Fever Virus (ASFV)*. https://core.ac.uk/download/12424877.pdf (accessed on 30th May 2025).

13. Cryan, J. F., O'Riordan, K. J., Cowan, C. S. M., Sandhu, K. V., Bastiaanssen, T. F. S., Boehme, M., Codagnone, M. G., et al. (2019). The microbiota-gut-brain axis. *Physiological Reviews, 99*, 1877–2013. https://doi.org/10.1152/physrev.00018.2018.

14. Cucu, C., Giurcaneanu, C., Poenaru, E., Popa, L. G., Popa, M., Chifiriuc, M., Lazăr, V., et al.

(2025). Phenotypic and genotypic bacterial virulence and resistance profiles in hidradenitis suppurativa. *International Journal of Molecular Sciences, 26.* https://www.semanticscholar.org/paper/67ed62da9512d5b2dde171a6260889ead74c9a7b (accessed on 30th May 2025).

15. Cui, Z., Wang, P., & Gao, W. (2025). Microbial dysbiosis in periodontitis and peri-implantitis: Pathogenesis, immune responses, and therapeutic. *Frontiers in Cellular and Infection Microbiology, 15.* https://www.semanticscholar.org/paper/db5b45d8c8571c36d11a826329fc45d2668bdea8 (accessed on 30th May 2025).

16. Das, S., & Khader, S. (2017). *Yin and Yang of Interleukin-17 in Host Immunity to Infection [Version 1; Referees: 2 Approved].* https://core.ac.uk/download/84911322.pdf (accessed on 30th May 2025).

17. Debnath, D., Tatuskar, P., & Attar, S. M. F. (2024). From bacterial origins to multifactorial complexity: Tracing the evolution of periodontitis pathogenesis from early era to 2017: A review article. *International Journal of Oral Health Sciences.* https://www.semanticscholar.org/paper/da2dc0111319126f233e5b9ca074eba3d9561b38 (accessed on 30th May 2025).

18. Deidda, S., Delitala, G., Delogu, L. G., & Manetti, R. (2011). *Infectious Diseases and Autoimmunity.* https://core.ac.uk/download/11692556.pdf (accessed on 30th May 2025).

19. Diaz-Ochoa, V. E., Jellbauer, S., Klaus, S., & Raffatellu, M. (2014). *Transition Metal Ions at the Crossroads of Mucosal Immunity and Microbial Pathogenesis.* https://core.ac.uk/download/323064423.pdf (accessed on 30th May 2025).

20. Galipeau, H., Hinterleitner, R., Leonard, M. M., & Caminero, A. (2024). Non-host factors influencing onset and severity of celiac disease. *Gastroenterology.* https://www.semanticscholar.org/paper/b23b4a9b521fb329fe570bc5f465b35ee42c42c9 (accessed on 30th May 2025).

21. Gao, L., Ho, S. P., Kamarajan, P., Kang, W., et al. (2020). *Polymicrobial Periodontal Disease Triggers a Wide Radius of Effect and Unique Virome.* https://core.ac.uk/download/288432854.pdf (accessed on 30th May 2025).

22. Gray, S. M., Moss, A. D., Herzog, J., Kashiwagi, S., Liu, B., Young, J. B., Sun, S., et al. (2024). Mouse adaptation of human inflammatory bowel diseases microbiota enhances colonization efficiency and alters microbiome aggressiveness depending on recipient colonic inflammatory environment. *bioRxiv.* https://www.semanticscholar.org/paper/3b5e610879fbe8caf96f0bd87bade690e37873dd (accessed on 30th May 2025).

23. Gray, S. M., Moss, A. D., Herzog, J., Kashiwagi, S., Liu, B., Young, J. B., Sun, S., et al. (2024). Mouse adaptation of human inflammatory bowel diseases microbiota enhances colonization efficiency and alters microbiome aggressiveness depending on the recipient colonic inflammatory environment. *Microbiome, 12.* https://www.semanticscholar.org/paper/16fc5f8025babe5986b422f27a303b3b3bf854a8 (accessed on 30th May 2025).

24. Grondin, J., Jamal, A., Mowna, S., Seto, T., & Khan, W. (2024). Interaction between intestinal parasites and the gut microbiota: Implications for the intestinal immune response and host defense. *Pathogens, 13.* https://www.semanticscholar.org/paper/23a4a64c23bc88c03714346dd4e9868be3298aa6 (accessed on 30th May 2025).

25. He, X., Jiang, X., Guo, J., Sun, H., & Yang, J. (2025). PANoptosis in bacterial infections: A double-edged sword balancing host immunity and pathogenesis. *Pathogens, 14.* https://www.semanticscholar.org/paper/e73ddd151fdffd131d01a5b601b0ecc2a98f9094 (accessed on 30th May 2025).

26. Jacobson, M. (2003). *Enteric Diseases in Pigs from Weaning to Slaughter.* https://core.ac.uk/download/11694636.pdf (accessed on 30th May 2025).

27. Jiang, H., & Wang, D. (2016). *The Microbial Zoo in the C. Elegans Intestine: Bacteria, Fungi and Viruses.* https://core.ac.uk/download/212858942.pdf (accessed on 30th May 2025).

28. Kalani, A., Martin, C. R., Mayer, E. A., & Osadchiy, et al. (2018). *The Brain-Gut-Microbiome Axis.* https://core.ac.uk/download/323079891.pdf (accessed on 30th May 2025).

29. Kałużna, A., Olczyk, P., & Komosińska-Vassev, K. (2022). The role of innate and adaptive immune cells in the pathogenesis and development of the inflammatory response in ulcerative colitis. *Journal of Clinical Medicine, 11.* https://www.semanticscholar.org/paper/0b007cef01dbbf3934f734b39b9af7e472348d3b (accessed on 30th May 2025).

30. Khairkar, M., Deshmukh, P., Maity, H., & Deotale, V. (2023). Chronic suppurative otitis media: A comprehensive review of epidemiology, pathogenesis, microbiology, and complications. *Cureus, 15.* https://www.semanticscholar.org/paper/3c971c6334c0e65863ae687664e35d845383585a (accessed on 30th May 2025).

31. Köhl, J., Kolnaar, R., & Ravensberg, W. J. (2019). Mode of action of microbial biological control agents against plant diseases: Relevance beyond efficacy. *Frontiers in Plant Science, 10.* https://doi.org/10.3389/fpls.2019.00845.

32. Masters, E., Ricciardi, B., Bentley, K., Moriarty, T. F., Schwarz, E., & Muthukrishnan, G. (2022). Skeletal infections: Microbial pathogenesis, immunity and clinical management. *Nature Reviews Microbiology, 20,* 385–400. https://www.semanticscholar.org/paper/fea546c64bde2b8b3e8f7ba8b09894e8cabde064 (accessed on 30th May 2025).

33. N/A. (2024). *Innate Immune Cells in the Pathogenesis of Inflammatory Bowel Disease – from Microbial Metabolites to Immune Modulation.* https://core.ac.uk/download/630284543.pdf (accessed on 30th May 2025).

34. Nasuhidehnavi, A., & McCall, L. I. (2023). It takes two to tango: How immune responses and metabolic changes jointly shape cardiac Chagas disease. *PLOS Pathogens, 19.* https://www.semanticscholar.org/paper/000c94c7a40213fd129fc06bc337f171194d3c7f (accessed on 30th May 2025).

35. Nowicka, A., & Gil, L. (2024). Microbial metabolomics in acute myeloid leukemia: From pathogenesis to treatment. *Advances in Clinical and Experimental Medicine: Official Organ Wroclaw Medical University.* https://www.semanticscholar.org/paper/d2dc88c0641744800ae50077ab14e9c64cb718e6 (accessed on 30th May 2025).

36. Olebo, D. F., & Igwe, M. C. (2025). Comparative analysis of virology and pathogenesis of SARS-CoV-2 and HIV infections: Implications for public health and treatment strategies. *Infection and Drug Resistance, 18,* 269–283. https://www.semanticscholar.org/paper/f30820e06415bf4589dfc64e55689c18df6e370a (accessed on 30th May 2025).

37. Parada, V. D., De La Fuente, M. K., Landskron, G., González, M. J., Quera, R., Dijkstra, G., Harmsen, H. J. M., et al. (2019). Short chain fatty acids (SCFAs)-mediated gut epithelial and immune regulation and its relevance for inflammatory bowel diseases. *Frontiers in Immunology, 10.* https://doi.org/10.3389/fimmu.2019.00277.

38. Peregrino, E. S., Castañeda-Casimiro, J., Vázquez-Flores, L., Estrada-Parra, S., Wong-Baeza, C., Serafín-López, J., & Wong-Baeza, I. (2024). The role of bacterial extracellular

vesicles in the immune response to pathogens, and therapeutic opportunities. *International Journal of Molecular Sciences, 25*. https://www.semanticscholar.org/paper/d019abe386f99bd1719c73d8b8e712babc11d0f2 (accessed on 30th May 2025).

39. Pruksaphon, K., Amsri, A., Jeenkeawpieam, J., Thammasit, P., Nosanchuk, J., & Youngchim, S. (2024). The microbial damage and host response framework: Lesson learned from pathogenic survival trajectories and immunoinflammatory responses of *Talaromyces marneffei* infection. *Frontiers in Immunology, 15*. https://www.semanticscholar.org/paper/6d1198e999b8ddb7abbbcc0c6e79451b814dd228 (accessed on 30th May 2025).
40. Rosario, S. R., Long, M. D., Chilakapati, S., Gomez, E. C., Battaglia, S., Singh, P., Wang, J., et al. (2024). Integrative multi-omics analysis uncovers tumor-immune-gut axis influencing immunotherapy outcomes in ovarian cancer. *Nature Communications, 15*. https://www.semanticscholar.org/paper/3c4dab2a0c659bc66709b85ead816d931f6b087f (accessed on 30th May 2025).
41. Rosowski, E. (2023). mSphere of influence: How host genetics impact microbial pathogenesis and treatment of infectious disease. *mSphere, 9*. https://www.semanticscholar.org/paper/40e92301569b368ffef44ac1095b2571622a71ba (accessed on 30th May 2025).
42. San, K. M. M. (2018). *tRNA Profiling of Mesenchymal Stem Cell Exosome*. https://core.ac.uk/download/215485366.pdf (accessed on 30th May 2025).
43. Shreiner, A. B., Kao, J. Y., & Young, V. B. (2014). The gut microbiome in health and in disease. *Current Opinion in Gastroenterology, 31*, 69–75. https://doi.org/10.1097/mog.0000000000000139.
44. Taylor, J. W., & Whiston, E. (2015). *Comparative Phylogenomics of Pathogenic and Nonpathogenic Species*. https://core.ac.uk/download/323082172.pdf (accessed on 30th May 2025).
45. Yang, H., Wu, X., Li, X., Zang, W., Zhou, Z., Zhou, Y., Cui, W., et al. (2024). A commensal protozoan attenuates *Clostridioides difficile* pathogenesis in mice via arginine-ornithine metabolism and host intestinal immune response. *Nature Communications, 15*. https://www.semanticscholar.org/paper/03be54751f0a18c5198142c6919243e82754afe5 (accessed on 30th May 2025).
46. Ye, J., Feng, T., Su, L., Li, J., Gong, Y., & Ma, X. (2023). Interactions between *Helicobacter pylori* infection and host metabolic homeostasis: A comprehensive review. *Helicobacter, 28*. https://www.semanticscholar.org/paper/03f56cf18801ac18e43e7e4ba6f3ebb8ee2dac70 (accessed on 30th May 2025).
47. Younes, N., & Nasrallah, G. K. (2021). Editorial: Unconventional animal models in infectious disease research – Part I. *Frontiers in Cellular and Infection Microbiology, 11*. https://www.semanticscholar.org/paper/bd9080d7b49f6ceb3862dcef8f5518e3f109b204 (accessed on 30th May 2025).
48. Zhao, H., Wu, L., Yan, G., Chen, Y., Zhou, M., Wu, Y., & Li, Y. (2021). Inflammation and tumor progression: Signaling pathways and targeted intervention. *Signal Transduction and Targeted Therapy, 6*. https://doi.org/10.1038/s41392-021-00658-5.

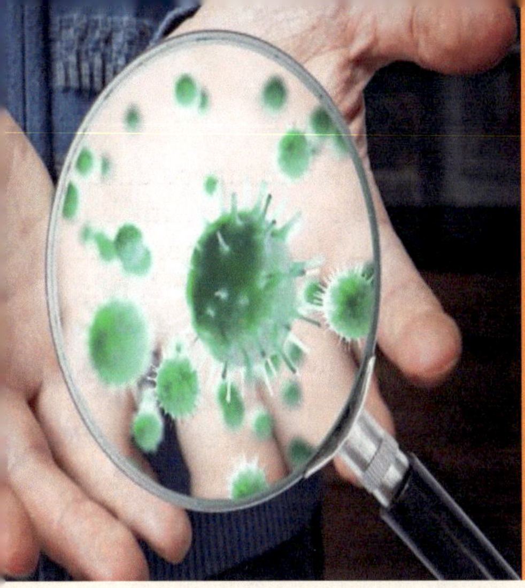

Chapter 4

TRANSMISSION OF INFECTIOUS DISEASES

Contents

Introduction

Currently, the spread of infectious diseases is a significant public health problem that needs to be dealt with right away. Some infectious diseases are caused by bacteria, viruses, and fungi, and their spread can be affected by how many people live together, how clean people are, and the quality of healthcare services. The consequences of unchecked transmission are often compounded by antimicrobial resistance (AMR), which renders common treatments ineffective and escalates the burden on healthcare systems. For instance, a recent study estimated that bacterial AMR was responsible for approximately 4.95 million deaths globally in 2019, with significant regional variations in its impact (Murray et al., 2022). It is crucial to understand these dynamics to develop strategies that control outbreaks and protect vulnerable individuals from the severe consequences of infectious diseases. Also, the emergence of new pathogens, such as SARS-CoV-2, highlights the complexity of infectious diseases spreading. The coronavirus disease 19 (COVID-19), which originated in Wuhan, China, exemplifies how rapidly contagious diseases can spread across borders, highlighting the interconnectedness of global health. Research indicates that the virus has a strong genetic relationship with bat coronaviruses, suggesting that zoonotic transmission remains a critical pathway for the emergence of new infectious threats (Shereen et al., 2020). A lack of early antiviral drugs and vaccines during COVID-19 led to many people getting infected and many deaths. It is crucial to understand what facilitates such rapid transmission, as this knowledge supports public health actions during future outbreaks. Additionally, the spread of diseases is influenced by social and economic conditions, as well as biological factors. Socioeconomic status, education, and access to healthcare play a significant role in determining how easily a population can be infected and how effectively it can respond to infectious diseases. Marginalized groups can have more contagious diseases because they face difficulties in getting preventive healthcare and in living healthily. The intersection of poverty and health complicates efforts to mitigate transmission, especially in resource-limited settings where the burden of diseases like AMR is disproportionately high (Murray et al., 2022). A comprehensive understanding of these social determinants is integral to developing tailored interventions aimed at reducing transmission rates and ensuring equitable health outcomes in diverse populations (Figure 4.1).

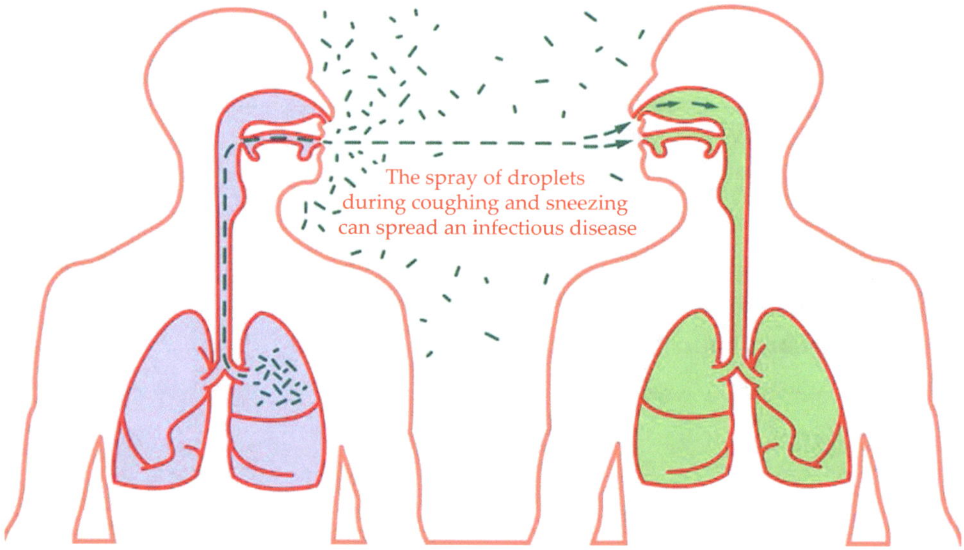

Figure 4.1. Transmission of infectious diseases.

Source: https://cdn3.vectorstock.com/i/1000x1000/99/37/infectious-disease-transmission-vector-31569937.jpg.

Definition of Infectious Diseases

Infectious diseases occur when pathogenic microorganisms, including bacteria, viruses, fungi, and parasites, are transmitted from one person to another. They may show up in many ways, from mild to serious, and these diseases are a significant concern for global public health. Most infectious diseases are spread through direct contact, inhalation of droplets, bites from infected insects, or contact with contaminated surfaces, which can lead to outbreaks, epidemics, or pandemics. Learning about these pathogens and their methods of transmission is essential to prevent the spread of diseases and implement effective control measures. Because these interactions can be so complex, it is clear that effective surveillance and response are needed to control and reduce the impact of infectious diseases in communities, as is shown by ongoing studies of their spread and rates. Improvements in public health and environmental sanitation have influenced the way infectious diseases spread over time and are now handled. The sanitary revolution in the 19th century demonstrated how public health policy transformed cities to reduce the incidence of diseases by controlling the main factors that spread them. At this point, people began to see how different environmental factors, such as waste management and population density, can lead to more infections. As a result of this revolution, we now recognise that better sanitation and hygiene depend on robust infrastructure for health. The interaction between human behavior, environmental factors, and microbial pathogens creates a complex scenario that necessitates a multifaceted approach to managing infectious diseases, as highlighted in ongoing research and public health discussions (Budge et al., 2022). Both people and communities are still encouraged to play a role in preventing the spread of infectious diseases. Vaccination, better sanitation, and public awareness efforts play a significant role in stopping the spread of contagious diseases. It appears that environmental factors play a significant role in the spread of diseases, and this is further complicated by emerging issues such as climate change and urban growth. The coronavirus pandemic clearly demonstrates the strong link between health, the environment, and social and economic factors. Notably, studies have indicated potential relations between public health interventions and changes in disease prevalence, as seen with strictly enforced lockdowns during the pandemic (Nomden et al., 2023). It highlights the need for experts from various fields to collaborate and develop strategies to combat infectious diseases and their transmission.

Importance of Understanding Transmission

Knowing how infections are spread is necessary to prevent them, since it guides public health actions. Understanding how pathogens, such as bacteria and viruses, spread through direct contact, aerosol transmission, or vectors enables health officials to design targeted interventions. In places where many people are gathered, such as schools, knowing the ways diseases spread can result in campaigns for vaccination, stricter hygiene, and educational efforts. They are crucial for both managing outbreaks and encouraging people to be more aware of their health, which over time leads to fewer infections, illustrating the direct link between learning about transmission and improved public health. Also, studying sapronotic diseases, which are caused by pathogens in the environment, underlines the need to know how these diseases are transmitted. Recent studies have shown that a significant number of infectious diseases are caused by these agents which can survive alone in soil or water and keep threatening people's health. Studies on *Mycobacterium ulcerans,* which causes Buruli ulcer, highlight how the environment and the behavior of these pathogens are connected. By recognising these complexities and addressing the gaps in our knowledge regarding sapronosis, researchers can develop refined epidemiological models that not only represent the nuances of transmission but also guide effective management and prevention strategies, ultimately saving lives and resources (Sylla et al., 2024). It is also essential for people to know how infectious diseases can be spread which helps communities respond to outbreaks. When people learn about pathogens and hygiene, they often change their habits, as evidenced by school education about microbiology. In addition to helping people understand, such programs teach them useful habits, such as washing their hands frequently and covering their mouths when coughing, which are essential for preventing outbreaks. The effectiveness of these educational strategies reveals the profound impact of informed communities on public health, highlighting that understanding transmission does not merely reside within academic discourse but is fundamental for empowering populations to combat infectious diseases at a grassroots level (Fahdi et al., 2024) (Figure 4.2).

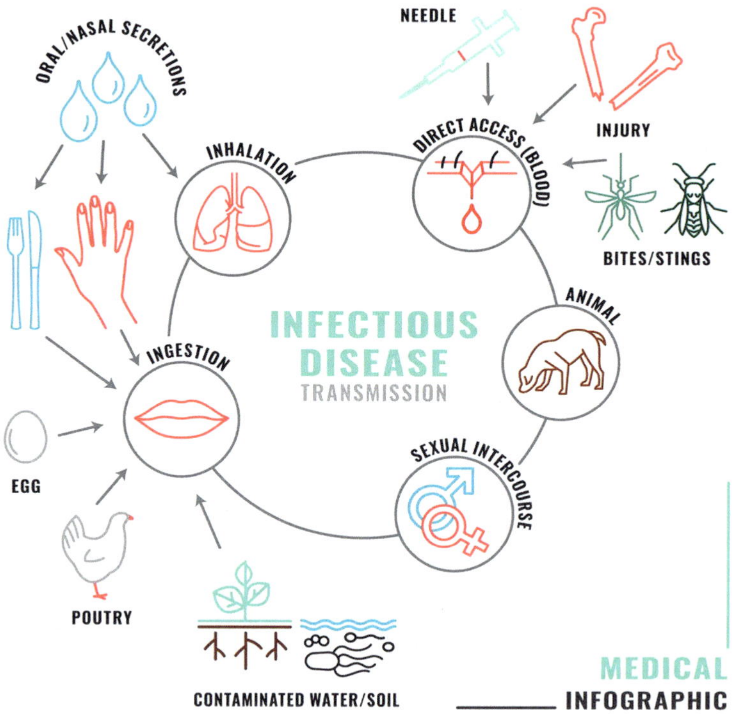

Figure 4.2. Transmission dynamics is crucial in mitigating the spread of infectious diseases.

Source: https://cdn2.vectorstock.com/i/1000x1000/34/36/infectious-disease-transmission-vector-32443436.jpg.

Overview of Transmission Methods

A variety of methods allow infectious diseases to be transmitted from one individual to another, which helps the illness spread. It is essential to understand these methods to create good public health strategies and interventions. If an infected person comes into direct contact with a healthy person, such as by touching, kissing, or engaging in sexual activity, it is called direct transmission. Sometimes, the pathogen is spread when a vector, such as contaminated surfaces, airborne droplets, or mosquitoes, carries it to the host. Every way the virus spreads adds something unique to the epidemic, and the right ways to stop the infection are determined by the method of spread. Within the framework of indirect transmission, vectors play an essential role, particularly in the case of vector-borne diseases (VBDs). An example is mosquitoes, which can spread several pathogens, including those that cause malaria, dengue fever, and West Nile virus. The connection between mosquitoes and the diseases they carry is complex, as it depends on many species-specific and environmental aspects that facilitate their reproduction. New research highlights that successful control and prevention of these diseases depend on understanding the environment and the diseases carried by these vectors. Therefore, integrating quantitative models that consider both the identity of mosquito species and pathogen dynamics is critical for predicting outbreaks and managing public health threats effectively (Ferraguti, 2024). More research is also showing that the contact between wildlife and domestic animals can create more complex ways for zoonotic diseases to spread. Where wild and domestic animals coexist, the risk of disease transmission between species increases significantly. Rabies transmission among wild and domestic dogs in northern Australia is examined in a case study, which highlights the need to study how the two groups contact each other and their behaviours. Any approach to reduce this risk should take into account how wildlife behaviour changes with the seasons and how that might affect disease spread when animals interact. Thus, the models capturing this wildlife-domestic interface not only enhance our comprehension of transmission methods but will also inform policies aimed at disease control and prevention (Ward et al., 2024) (Figure 4.3).

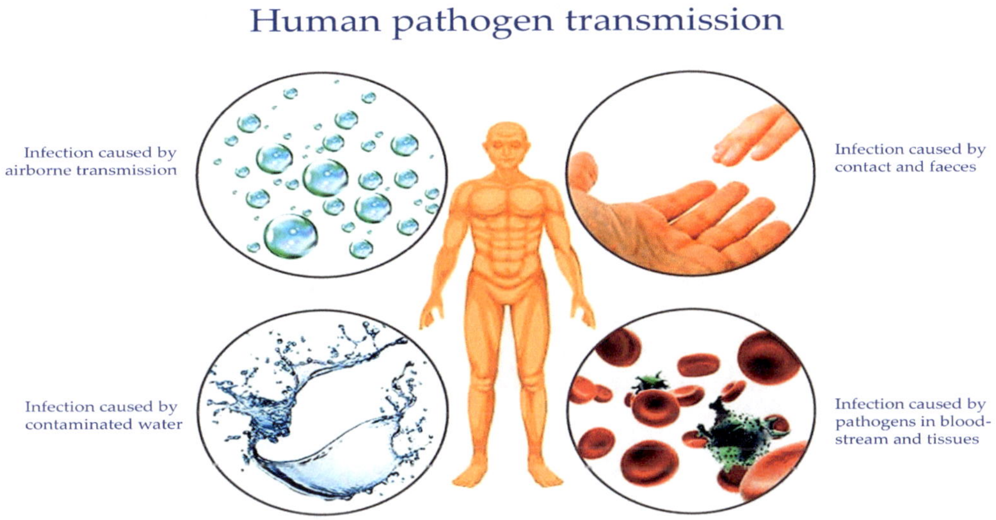

Figure 4.3. Transmission methods.

Source: https://www.hartmann-science-center.com/-/media/country/hsc/glossary-s-v/transmission-paths_730x516.jpg?h=516&iar=0&mw=840&w=730&rev=41d009ae8694496c9f052210e5248027&sc_lang=en&hash=59F4584D21B56FF2100A5A13DD26802B.

4.1. Types of Infectious Diseases

Infectious diseases can be categorized into several types based on their causative agents, transmission modes, and reservoirs. Among these categories, bacterial infections pose significant public health challenges due to their diverse mechanisms of pathogenicity and ability to develop resistance to treatment. Examples of how bacteria can impact health include tuberculosis and streptococcal infections, which can be contracted through respiratory droplets or direct contact with infected individuals. Furthermore, bacterial pathogens can be resilient, often persisting in the environment as fomites, which contributes to their transmission dynamics (Guleria, 2024). Recognising how bacteria are spread supports the creation of public health measures, including vaccinations and improved hygiene, to prevent the spread of bacterial infections. A major group of infectious diseases is viral infections, which use host cells to replicate and survive. A noteworthy example of this is the emergence of non-polio enteroviruses, which have been shown to have a high prevalence among children with acute intestinal infections (Selivanova et al., 2024). Many cases of diarrhoea are passed on through the faecal-oral route, mainly when sanitation is not adequate. During the COVID-19 pandemic, significant shifts were observed in the types of enterovirus affecting children, suggesting that changes in human behavior and public health measures can profoundly impact viral transmission patterns (Selivanova et al., 2024). It emphasises the importance of regular monitoring and understanding the biological and environmental factors that can lead to viral infections, which supports the development of more effective control measures for outbreaks. Parasitic infections, which are the third major kind of infectious diseases, are also a significant issue. Parasites can affect numerous body systems and often require complex life cycles involving multiple hosts, which can complicate their transmission. Diseases like malaria and schistosomiasis are primarily spread through vectors such as mosquitoes and contaminated water sources, respectively. The transmission dynamics are heavily influenced by environmental conditions, including climate change, which can expand the habitat ranges for these vectors and increase the risk of infection in human populations. Furthermore, understanding the various types of parasites and the ecological niches they inhabit is essential for developing targeted interventions aimed at reducing transmission rates. Such insights contribute to a broader public health strategy, integrating epidemiological research with practical measures to combat parasitic diseases (Guleria, 2024) (Figure 4.4).

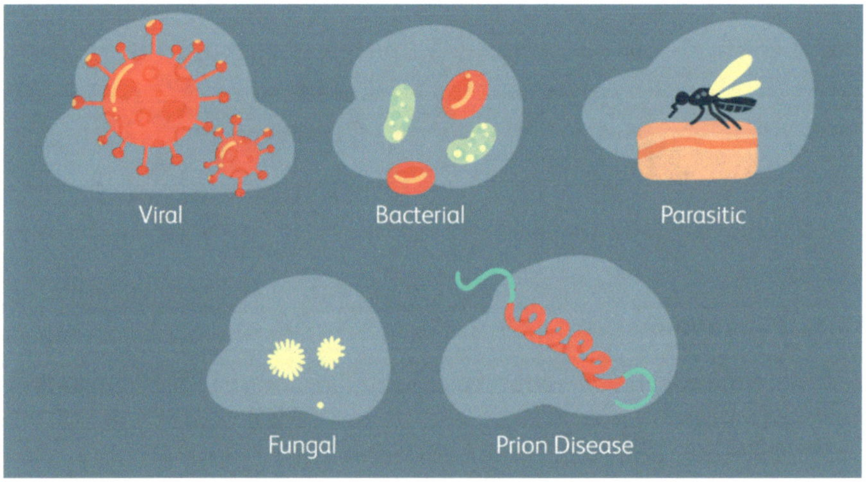

Figure 4.4. Types of infectious diseases.

Source: https://www.verywellhealth.com/thmb/jh_Nd_U7R0i5_4AtGSW9mr3K_II=/1500x1000/filters:no_upscale():max_bytes(150000):strip_icc()/infection-5096014-Final-eaf7a90b39fd4eb69b3a1776b721d975.gif.

4.1.1. Bacterial Infections

Bacterial infections represent a significant facet of infectious disease transmission, often following viral infections or occurring independently through various pathways. The mechanics of these transmissions are influenced by a range of factors, including direct contact with infected individuals, contaminated surfaces, and foodborne routes. For instance, bacterial pathogens such as *Streptococcus pneumoniae* and *Staphylococcus aureus* frequently thrive in environments compromised by a preceding viral infection, like influenza. Individuals infected with influenza are particularly at risk of developing bacterial pneumonia, as the viral illness can compromise the immune system, making it easier for bacteria to establish an infection (Goradwar et al., 2024). Because viral and bacterial infections are connected, it is necessary to use prevention strategies that target both types of pathogens. Because of bacterial biofilms, infections can be more complicated to transmit and treat. Biofilms are groups of bacteria sticking to each other and to surfaces which makes them more challenging to treat with antibiotics. Both environmental and clinical settings can foster biofilm formation, particularly in chronic infections or on medical devices (Tavares et al., 2024). If someone has a weak immune system, such as after an influenza infection, the presence of bacterial biofilms greatly increases the risk of severe complications. They carry bacteria that are resistant to many drugs, which can complicate the treatment of the infection and prolong the healing process. It is crucial to address biofilms in both medical and community settings to mitigate the impact of bacterial infections, particularly as antibiotic resistance increases. AMR plays a crucial role in the transmission of bacterial infections. When antibiotics are used too frequently or incorrectly, resistant strains emerge and can be easily passed among people. Data indicate that multidrug-resistant strains, particularly those capable of biofilm formation, pose significant threats to public health (Tavares et al., 2024). Their transmission through animal products or direct contact with contaminated surfaces in agricultural settings illustrates the intricate connections between human health, animal health, and the environment. Raising awareness and promoting responsible antibiotic usage are critical components of infection control strategies. These efforts not only mitigate the risk of bacterial infections but also ensure that effective treatment options remain available, ultimately supporting larger public health initiatives aimed at curbing the transmission of infectious diseases (Figure 4.5).

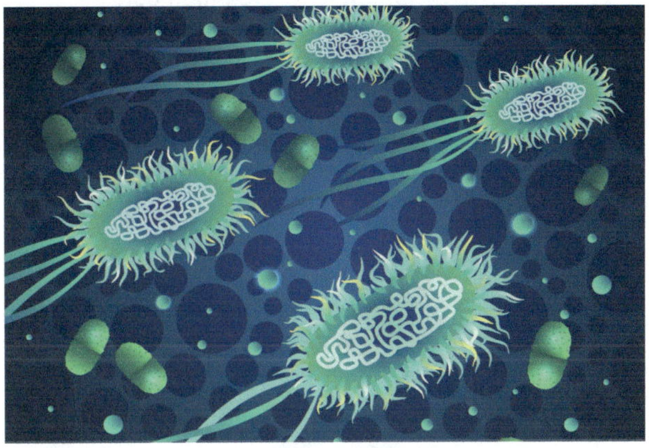

Figure 4.5. Bacterial infections.

Source: https://gradschool.weill.cornell.edu/sites/default/files/news_images/shutterstock_1037009701.png.

4.1.2. Viral Infections

Viral infections are a type of infectious disease because they can easily be passed from one person to another and can seriously affect health. Viruses can be transmitted through contact, inhalation of airborne droplets, or by vectors such as insects. An example is that influenza can be spread by an infected person coughing or sneezing, which can reach those close by. Also, viruses such as HIV mainly spread through sexual contact, which makes it harder to control the spread of infection in the public health system. It is crucial to understand how diseases spread in order to create practical ways to prevent them, especially in the aftermath of the COVID-19 pandemic. The pandemic made it clear that viral infections can spread rapidly in places where people are in close contact which is why strong public health measures are needed to reduce the spread. The spread of viral infections through social and environmental factors is being examined more closely. Natural disasters and global pandemics can alter the way people behave, which can inadvertently facilitate the spread of disease. During the COVID-19 lockdowns, some diseases typically caused by viral infections experienced a noticeable increase.

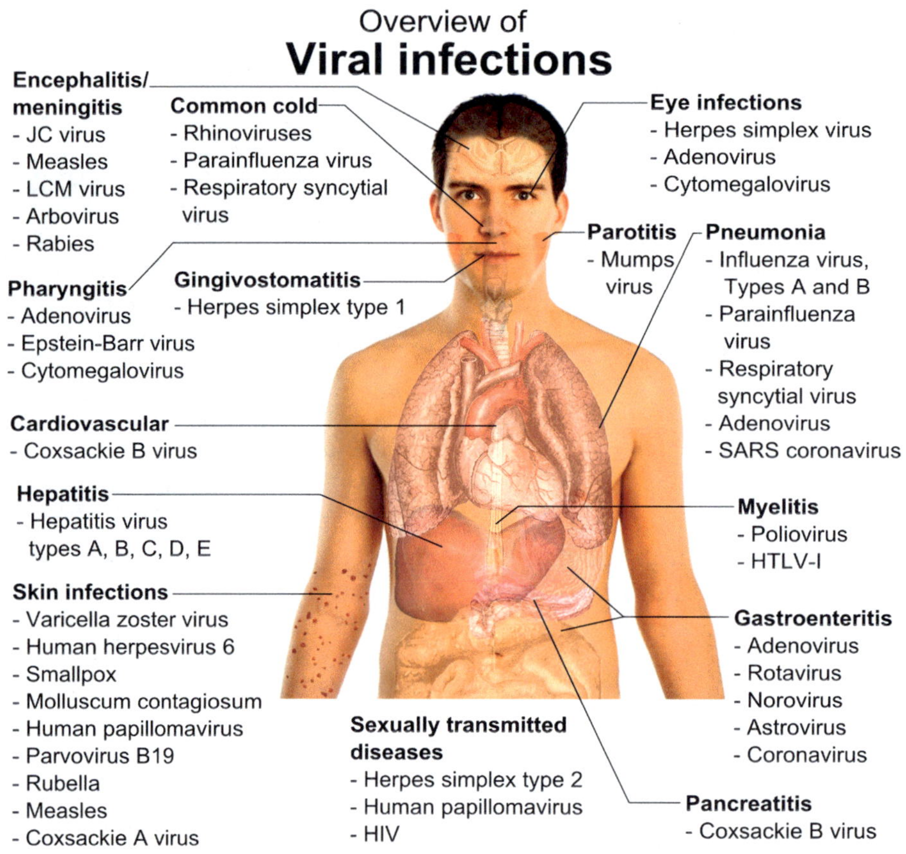

Figure 4.6. Viral infections represent a significant category of infectious diseases.

Source: https://www.healthhype.com/wp-content/uploads/Viral_infections.png.

A study found that the strictness of lockdowns was associated with a decrease in the number of isolated biliary atresia cases in Europe each month. Due to the inverse relationship, it was observed that limited mobility could prevent people from coming into contact with certain viral pathogens. Such findings underscore the importance of context when evaluating infection rates and highlight the varied influence of external factors on the epidemiology of viral diseases (Nomden et al., 2023). When viral infections are chronic such as HIV, viral mutations and drug resistance can cause more complications in their spread. Studies have found that some treatments do not fully control the viral load in all patients, allowing some resistant strains to persist and evolve within the host. When resistant variants are present in the community, it becomes tough for public health systems to keep infections under control. It has been found that spreading resistant strains can make it harder for new patients to be effectively treated which increases the spread of the disease and complicates how it is managed. Thus, incorporating the monitoring of drug resistance emerges as a crucial component in managing viral infections effectively, prompting a reconsideration of existing protocols in infectious disease treatment (Sönnerborg, 2003) (Figure 4.6).

4.1.3. Fungal Infections

Fungal infections are a significant type of infectious disease that can affect people in various ways, from minor skin infections to more serious diseases that spread throughout the body. Many fungi, such as yeasts, molds, and dermatophytes, can cause these infections. Each type has its own transmission methods and levels of harm. These infections often spread in areas that are warm, moist, and rich in organic matter, which highlights the key role of the environment in fungal pathogen transmission. Because of health conditions like diabetes or HIV/AIDS, people with weakened immune systems are more likely to suffer from these fungal infections and serious health problems. Being aware of the causes and risk factors of fungal infections helps in designing good preventive and treatment options. affect how fungal infections are transmitted, such as the health of the host and the amount of exposure to the environment. Infection can occur by touching objects or people who have fungi, by breathing in airborne spores, or through contact with soil or water that contains the fungi. An example is the inhalation of *Histoplasma capsulatum* spores, which can cause lung infections in people whose immune systems are compromised. Even though some fungi live on the skin or mucous membranes without causing illness, antibiotics or a weakened immune system can allow these opportunistic fungi to cause infections. So, the ways fungal infections spread highlight the importance of being more aware, especially in places where these pathogens may be more likely to spread. Recent findings suggest that fungal pathogens and the host's immune system interact in numerous ways, and when this interaction goes awry, the consequences can be severe for the patient. Due to COVID-19, a known link has been established between viral and fungal infections, indicating that a weakened immune system increases the likelihood of fungal infections. Severe cases of viral infections may lead to cytokine storms that do not eliminate the virus and, in fact, help fungal infections to develop. As noted in recent investigations into SARS-CoV-2, the activation of immune responses can contribute to the pathophysiology of both viral and fungal infections, necessitating an integrative approach to understanding transmission dynamics of infectious diseases to enhance treatment and prevention strategies (Tay et al., 2020; Xu et al., 2020) (Figure 4.7).

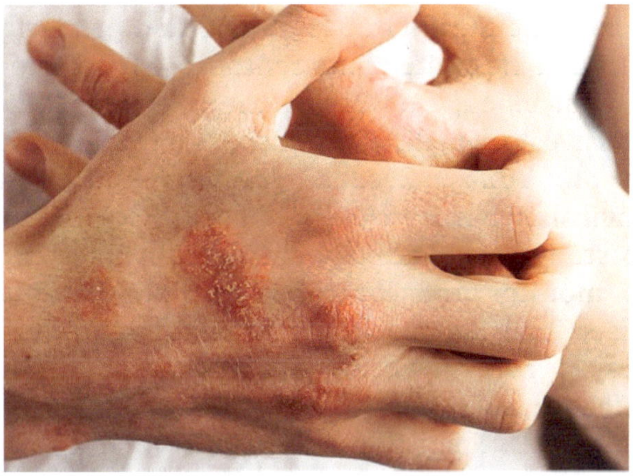

Figure 4.7. Fungal infections.

Source: https://www.cosmeticdermamedicine.gr/wp-content/uploads/mykitiasi-hero.jpg.

4.2. Modes of Transmission

It is essential to know how infectious diseases are spread, as this guides practical public health actions. Several ways exist for transmission, such as direct contact, airborne routes, infections spread by insects, and contact with objects. In direct contact transmission, pathogens are transmitted when people come into physical contact, which is common in the flu and COVID-19. Because droplets or aerosols carrying infectious agents can stay suspended in the air, they can infect others who are nearby. The realization of asymptomatic transmission, particularly during the COVID-19 pandemic, highlights the need for vigilance in monitoring health behavior, as carriers may unknowingly spread infections without presenting symptoms, complicating traditional understanding of disease management (Ogbunugafor, 2024). Vector-borne transmission presents unique challenges in the study of infectious diseases. Ticks and mosquitoes help carry pathogens from infected animals to people. An illustrative case is Crimean-Congo Hemorrhagic Fever (CCHF), where the CCHF virus is transmitted primarily through tick bites and contact with infected animal blood, showcasing the role of wildlife and livestock in disease transmission (Srivastava et al., 2024). Because humans and their environments are closely linked, it is essential to study vector ecology and establish systems to monitor and control vector populations. Also, realising that environmental conditions play a role in vector behaviour can direct effective public health actions to stop disease outbreaks. Fomite transmission, which is not always considered, points out how important it is to focus on hygiene and sanitation to control infectious diseases. With this type of spread, germs can live on inanimate objects, and when people touch these things and then touch their face, mouth, or eyes, the germs can be transferred. The COVID-19 pandemic has made people more aware that viruses spread on surfaces, which led to many infections. They make it clear that strong cleaning and disinfection measures are needed in public areas. Ongoing research further emphasizes the role of personal habits and community practices in modulating transmission rates, reinforcing the importance of education and public awareness in mitigating the spread of infectious diseases across multiple transmission pathways (Ogbunugafor, 2024; Srivastava et al., 2024) (Figure 4.8).

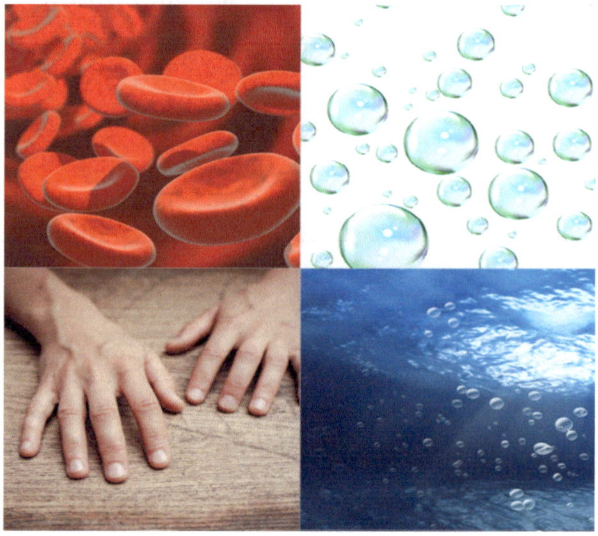

Figure 4.8. Modes of transmission.

Source: https://www.hartmann-science-center.com/en/-/media/country/hsc/top-issues/modes-of-transmission-article_677x711.jpg?rev=c50b697ed0bf4ddea266380962a43f55&sc_lang=en&hash=1BF16167D81EFB25FB332635D9D7E417.

4.2.1. Direct Contact Transmission

Direct contact transmission occurs when an infected person transfers infectious agents to a susceptible individual through physical contact. Many communicable diseases, for instance influenza, norovirus, and various respiratory infections, are mainly spread through this method. Shaking hands, hugging, and caring for the sick can significantly increase the chance of spreading pathogens. If a healthy person touches something that has infectious agents, they can become infected. It is crucial to understand how diseases are spread through direct contact to develop effective methods for controlling them and preserving public health. Identifying the ways people interact in direct contact is very important for creating effective epidemiological models to understand disease outbreaks. Direct contact transmission is a concern because it can occur in healthcare settings, schools, and public areas. Failing to follow proper hygiene rules in healthcare settings can lead to nosocomial infections, posing a threat to both patients and staff. Therefore, organizations put in place strict infection prevention measures that emphasize handwashing and the use of personal protective gear. Also, touching and exchanging personal items can help the virus spread in groups, mainly among children who might not wash their hands properly. For this reason, teaching people about direct contact transmission and why it is important to take preventive actions is crucial. They can be very successful in preventing diseases from spreading within close-knit communities.

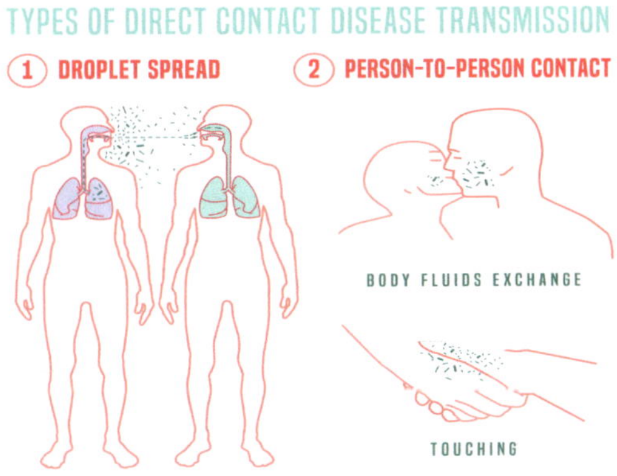

Figure 4.9. Direct contact transmission.

Source: https://thumbs.dreamstime.com/z/infectious-disease-transmission-infectious-disease-transmission-landscape-poster-virus-pandemic-transfer-direct-contact-types-187489566.jpg.

To further illustrate the impact of direct contact transmission, consider NASAs efforts to mitigate infectious diseases within its Human Space Flight Program (HSP). Because living conditions in space are limited and confined, maintaining the health of astronauts is crucial for a mission to succeed. The HSP uses several measures to reduce exposure, such as medical checks and restricted access among the crew, to avoid bringing in infectious agents. Also, informing contacts about the possibility of direct transmission improves the overall safety measures. It clearly points out that direct contact transmission is essential to understand in specialized environments. The insights gained from these practices not only facilitate safe missions but also contribute to broader public health strategies aimed at controlling infectious diseases in various sectors of society (Min et al., 2018; Johnston et al., 2025) (Figure 4.9).

4.2.2. Indirect Contact Transmission

Among the different ways pathogens spread, indirect contact transmission is significant in infecting people. It occurs when pathogens enter a host by touching contaminated objects, walking on contaminated surfaces, or inhaling contaminated air, rather than through direct contact with another person. Doorknobs, light switches, and utensils are examples of surfaces that individuals frequently touch, and these surfaces may carry bacteria or viruses for varying periods. If a person comes into contact with a contaminated surface and then touches their mouth, nose, or eyes, transmission is possible, which can result in outbreaks of diseases. These ways of spread underline the need for proper sanitation and hygiene in communities to prevent risks from indirect contact. Indirect contact transmission is made more complicated by the fact that zoonotic pathogens that pass from animals to humans play a significant role. Many of these pathogens are found on surfaces contaminated by animal secretions or wastes, increasing the risk of infection through contact. A significant proportion, approximately 70%, of all emerging infectious diseases (EIDs) have a zoonotic origin, highlighting the critical link between animal reservoirs and human health. This often occurs in areas where humans and animals coexist, increasing the risk of contracting diseases from pathogens that can be harmful. Mechanisms such as contaminated food or water, which are vehicles for indirect transmissions, further exacerbate the situation, making comprehensive strategies to control zoonotic diseases essential for public health (Sizikova et al., 2024). We can prevent indirect contact transmission by educating people and promoting good hygiene practices. Telling people to wash their hands often and use disinfectants reduces the chances of spreading germs from contaminated things. Recent studies have shown that biosensors detecting pathogens can quickly help identify and control contaminated areas. Innovations such as DNAzyme-based biosensors show promise in enhancing detection efficiency, thereby addressing the shortcomings of traditional pathogen detection methods (Liu et al., 2024). All of these measures help reduce the spread of diseases and also teach us how human actions, the environment, and infectious diseases are interconnected, which is why we must stay vigilant in healthcare.

4.2.3. Vector-Borne Transmission

Through vector-borne transmission, infectious diseases can spread rapidly because pathogens are passed from one host to another via intermediary arthropods. Mosquitoes, ticks, and flies are examples of hematophagous arthropods that spread diseases by biting animals and humans. By eating in this way, animals help themselves get infected and spread the pathogens to others. Examples of such diseases include malaria, dengue, and Lyme disease, which illustrate the dangers of such transmissions to public health. The challenges presented by VBDs are further compounded by their complex life cycles and the ability of vectors to adapt to various ecological niches, making control and prevention efforts particularly difficult (Wang et al., 2024). It is crucial to understand the interactions between vectors, hosts, and pathogens to address these public health issues effectively. We should not forget the impact of environmental conditions on vector-borne diseases, as they determine both the presence and survival of both vectors and pathogens. Changes in temperature and rainfall can change the life cycles of vectors, which in turn affects how infectious diseases are spread. For instance, studies have indicated that very low temperatures tend to correlate with increased incidences of influenza and invasive bacterial infections. In contrast, elevated temperatures can facilitate the spread of gastrointestinal pathogens and vector-borne infections (Yin et al., 2024).

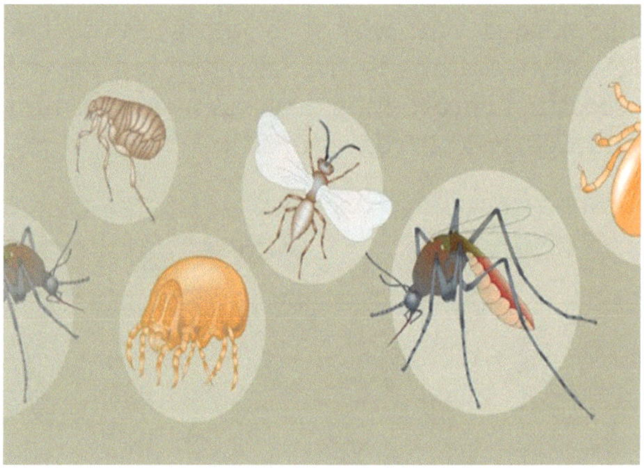

Figure 4.10. Vector-borne transmission.

Source: https://media.springernature.com/w580h326/nature-cms/uploads/collections/Vector-borne_disease_hero-93b52801cf986e92c30b7e364c7ab975.jpg.

Because of these interactions, it is essential to have surveillance systems that use both meteorological and epidemiological data. If we notice these relationships, public health strategies can be improved to respond to and control the spread of vector-borne diseases during extreme weather. Vaccination remains an effective way to prevent VBDs, but developing vaccines that work well is challenging. Since vectors and pathogens are distinct and complex, creating vaccines can be challenging. New findings have made it possible to focus on antigens derived from vectors, primarily found in the saliva of arthropods. These salivary proteins not only facilitate pathogen transmission but also modulate the host's immune responses (Wang et al., 2024). Science is focused on making vaccines that boost the body's immunity against mosquito antigens to help prevent various VBDs. Consequently, the integration of vector biology with immunology represents a transformative approach to vaccine development, potentially paving the way for novel interventions that can significantly reduce the burden of infectious diseases transmitted by vectors (Figure 4.10).

4.3. Environmental Factors Influencing Transmission

The transmission of infectious diseases is profoundly influenced by environmental factors that shape the interactions among pathogens, hosts, and the surrounding ecosystem. Because these issues are now better understood, attention has shifted to examining the entire environment, rather than just individual factors. Climate, urbanization, and land use are among the factors that significantly impact how diseases spread. The closer living conditions in cities make it much simpler for diseases to be shared. Both temperature and humidity help pathogens stay alive and reproduce. Recent research emphasizes the intricate relationships between built environments and health outcomes, suggesting that a thorough understanding of these spatial determinants is vital when devising strategies for disease prevention and control (Lakes et al., 2025). Air quality, now being a major environmental issue, highlights the connection among the environment, society, and health. Exposure to air pollution has been identified as a risk factor not only for respiratory diseases but also for various infectious diseases, including COVID-19 and tuberculosis (TB). According to studies, pollutants may weaken the immune system which increases a person's chances of getting sick and worsens their health condition. Since environmental health affects the spread of infections, it is essential to have health policies that address both environmental factors and public health measures together. As indicated in recent literature, socioeconomic factors further exacerbate these challenges, presenting a complex interplay that necessitates comprehensive approaches to mitigate disease transmission effectively (Othman et al., 2024). Taking into account both biological and social factors, public health can respond more effectively to the way diseases develop. Learning about environmental causes of disease spread is very important for global health, especially following recent pandemics. Activities like deforestation and city growth have brought people and wildlife closer, which has raised the chance of zoonotic diseases being transmitted. Climate change caused by global warming is altering the habitats of many pathogens and vectors, such as mosquitoes, which is contributing to the emergence of diseases like malaria and dengue. To prevent diseases effectively, strategies should involve checking the environment and implementing practices that protect it. As communities grapple with the dual challenges of infectious diseases and environmental degradation, interdisciplinary collaboration is essential for developing robust, innovative public health strategies that address both immediate health concerns and long-term ecological sustainability (Lakes et al., 2025; Othman et al., 2024).

4.3.1. Climate and Weather Conditions

The intricate relationship between climate and weather conditions plays a crucial role in the transmission of infectious diseases. Due to climate change, the rise in temperatures and increased weather extremes often make it easier for pathogens to thrive. Higher temperatures can cause mosquitoes to breed longer, increasing the risk of diseases such as malaria and dengue fever. More vectors in the area result in more people getting infected, which is a significant problem for public health. Additionally, when climates change, rainfall patterns can shift, leading to the formation of water pools that facilitate mosquito reproduction. Such environmental shifts not only enhance the life cycle of infectious agents but also increase human exposure to these pathogens, especially in populations already vulnerable due to underlying health conditions (Ratter-Rieck et al., 2023). Furthermore, floods and heatwaves, which are types of extreme weather events, can help spread infectious diseases more easily.

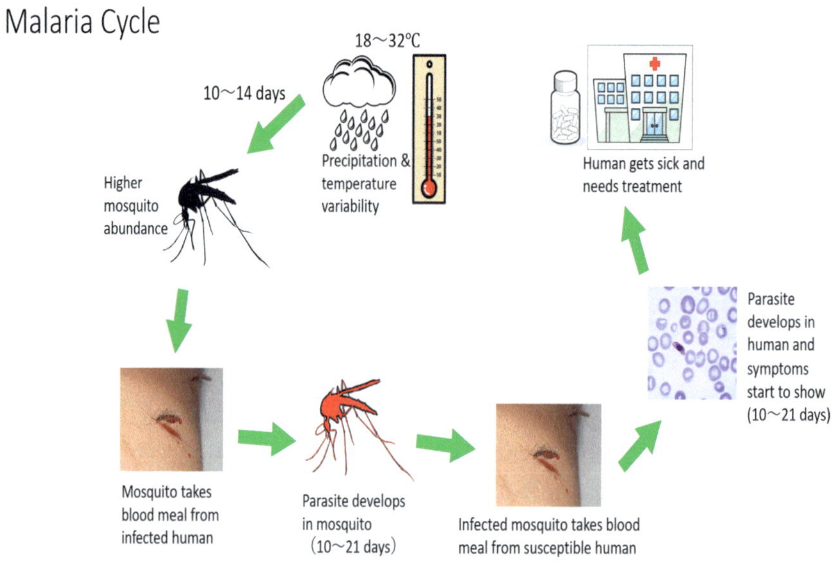

Figure 4.11. Climate and weather conditions.

Source: https://www.jamstec.go.jp/sdgs/e/case/img/013_01.png.

A flood can contaminate drinking water, increasing the risk of diseases such as cholera. At the same time, heatwaves can negatively affect people's health, mainly those who already have health problems, and make them more vulnerable to infections. Air quality worsening due to climate-related events such as wildfires can result in breathing difficulties, which makes people more at risk of infectious diseases. As these conditions evolve, public health systems must adopt climate-smart strategies to mitigate the adverse effects of extreme weather on disease transmission (Napoli et al., 2023). New evidence about health outcomes linked to climate change shows that we must act now. Integrating information about climate and health is demonstrated by studies to significantly improve the public health sector's response to infectious diseases. If climate services utilise reanalysis data to track health indicators, they can provide important insights into how climate change is affecting the risk of diseases. They can be used to observe how environmental hazards affect mortality rates, the workforce, and food supply, which are all critical for disease transmission. Therefore, establishing a comprehensive understanding of these relationships can facilitate the development of targeted interventions, ultimately lowering the incidence of infectious diseases in a changing climate (Napoli et al., 2023; Ratter-Rieck et al., 2023) (Figure 4.11).

4.3.2. Urbanization and Population Density

The way infectious diseases are spread is strongly affected by the interaction between urbanization and population density. With more people living in cities, there are more chances for people to interact and travel, which helps diseases spread faster. Because people in crowded areas are in close proximity, the spread of pathogens can occur very quickly. It was obvious during the COVID-19 pandemic, as urban areas saw faster outbreaks than less crowded areas. The findings of Patil et al. (2021) underline that typical epidemiological models overlook the complexities of urban mobility and social contact networks, highlighting the need for more nuanced frameworks to understand disease propagation in urban landscapes. Due to the large number of people and complex social systems in cities, specialised public health strategies are necessary to control the spread of infectious diseases.

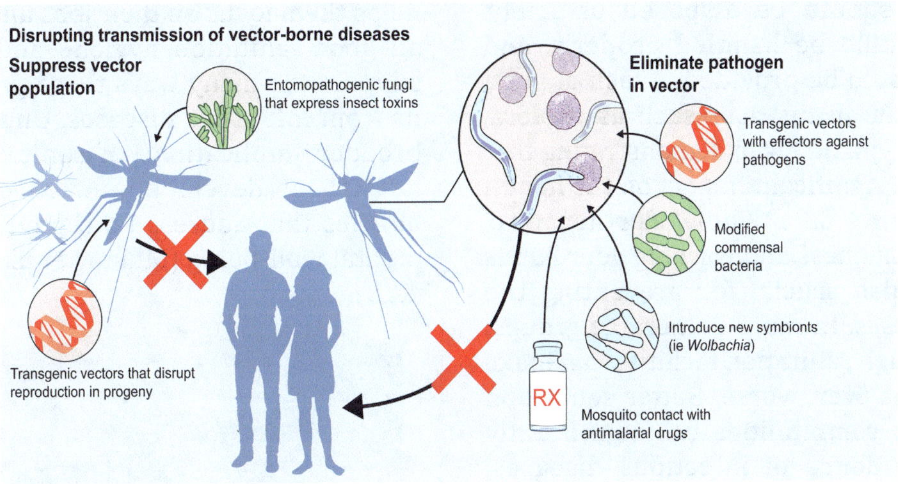

Figure 4.12. Urbanization and population density.

Source: https://www.science.org/cms/10.1126/science.abc2757/asset/c0506249-8ed4-4834-acba-93fdecc04035/assets/images/large/science.abc2757-f3.jpg.

As a result of these dynamics, it is clear that urbanization brings special problems for managing public health. Especially, the COVID-19 pandemic highlighted that highly populated cities can quickly spread infectious diseases. Higher mobility and increased social events in cities can facilitate the spread of infectious diseases. According to research, understanding varying disease transmission rates across different urban environments requires a critical examination of social connectivity and area-specific factors, as detailed in Patil et al. (2021). Therefore, urban planners and public health officials should collaborate to develop solutions that address the impact of population density and social mobility, thereby enhancing community health. In addition, vaccination in cities adds more challenges to the debate about how diseases are spread. It has been found that prosocial concern plays a significant role in vaccination decisions, particularly in less densely populated areas. According to, individuals are more likely to care about vaccination in rural areas than in urban areas, where anonymity can make people feel less responsible for others. It points out that public health messages should be designed to appeal to what motivates people in cities. By emphasizing community benefits and collective responsibility in vaccination campaigns, public health officials can foster a stronger sense of cooperation and engagement among urban populations, ultimately contributing to reduced transmission rates of infectious diseases throughout these densely populated areas (Figure 4.12).

4.3.3. Sanitation and Hygiene Practices

Good sanitation and hygiene prevent the spread of infectious diseases, which has a direct effect on public health. To have good sanitation, human waste should be disposed of safely, solid waste should be handled properly, and clean water should be provided. A lack of good sanitation results in diseases such as cholera, dysentery, and typhoid fever, demonstrating that sanitation has a significant impact on the health of the community as a whole. Furthermore, maintaining cleanliness and washing your hands frequently is also crucial for preventing the spread of diseases. In more vulnerable groups, not having enough sanitation facilities can make health problems even worse. Better sanitation and hygiene in communities can significantly reduce the incidence of infectious diseases, leading to a better quality of life and reduced spending on preventable illnesses. Additionally, research suggests that modifying sanitation and hygiene habits can have a significant impact on health, although the effectiveness of these changes can vary. For instance, a study assessed the Andilaye intervention, which aimed to enhance water, sanitation, and hygiene (WASH) practices in Ethiopia through a multi-level community approach. Although the program was well-structured, it did not lead to significant improvements in building latrines or washing hands, which shows how hard it is to change behaviors in sanitation and hygiene. Mainly, the limited impact was caused by problems in how the intervention was carried out, highlighting how hard it is to change behavior. The findings emphasize that while such programs are crucial, their design must consider local contexts, existing practices, and the socio-cultural factors that influence adherence to improved sanitation and hygiene practices (Freeman et al., 2022). Besides making people healthier, improved sanitation and hygiene can also enhance the mental health of communities. The threat of safe. Disease transmission can cause people to worry more about maintaining cleanliness and safety. Maintaining good sanitation can calm such worries by making people feel more secure and stable, which is good for mental health. When clean facilities are available, people do not have to worry about poor hygiene, which helps them focus on their jobs and studies. All in all, good sanitation, hygiene, and mental health support the many ways these practices protect us from infectious diseases. Understanding the broader implications of sanitation initiatives is vital for developing effective public health policies that address both physical health and mental well-being (Murray et al., 2022) (Figure 4.13).

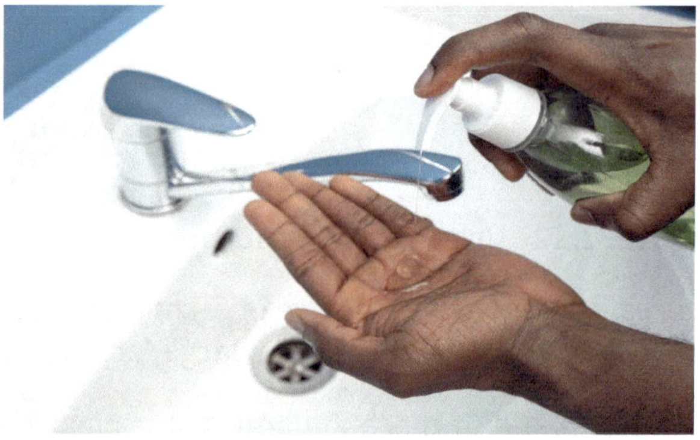

Figure 4.13. Sanitation and hygiene practices.

Source: https://humanitarianglobal.com/wp-content/uploads/2022/02/A-person-washing-their-hands.jpg.

4.4. Role of Human Behaviour

Infectious diseases can spread more easily during crises like the COVID-19 pandemic because of human behaviour. People's habits, such as whether they smoke or what they eat, can make them more likely to get infections. For example, research indicates that the lockdowns during the pandemic led to significant changes in people's behaviour. Smoking rates have generally decreased, but this change warrants careful examination. The complexity of human behaviour reveals that while some individuals may have reduced smoking, others may have turned to it as a coping mechanism amid increased stress and anxiety, potentially exacerbating their health risks (Sabbah et al., 2022). Because people respond differently, we should realise that changes in behaviour can lead to different health outcomes. Social interactions and the actions of communities play a significant role in the transmission of infectious diseases. Because of the COVID-19 lockdowns, how people interacted with each other changed, which influenced disease transmission. Data collected indicated that following the lockdown decree, the demographics of new COVID-19 cases changed, reflecting the differential impact of social and economic factors on susceptibility (Stivanello et al., 2020). For instance, the number of cases went up among elderly people, which suggests that some groups are more at risk because of their living situations and social ties. It demonstrates that addressing how people behave is a crucial component of public health interventions. Targeted strategies based on what makes a community unique can help control and prevent diseases more effectively. Besides personal habits, how society as a whole views health is also essential in spreading diseases. Encouraging people to be proactive about their health should be a primary goal of public health campaigns, since community attitudes can help or hinder efforts to control infection outbreaks. When people in a community consider their health and well-being together, they are more likely to comply with preventive actions, such as vaccination or social distancing. The varying educational levels of the population, as illustrated in studies involving smoking cessation during the pandemic, demonstrate that informed and engaged communities are more likely to resist unhealthy habits and reduce disease transmission rates (Sabbah et al., 2022). Therefore, it is essential to comprehend how human actions, social life, and public health strategies interact to manage infectious diseases.

4.4.1. Personal Hygiene Practices

Good personal hygiene helps reduce the spread of infectious diseases, especially in places where large numbers of people gather, such as schools. Improving hygiene practices can significantly lower the rate of diseases, which helps students stay healthy and perform better in school. In the Amravati district, providing students with access to clean water and encouraging handwashing with soap helped decrease the number of primary school students missing school due to illness. When students are taught to wash their hands properly and there is clean water available, schools become essential places for encouraging habits that keep children safe from enteric infections. Emphasising personal hygiene helps young learners stay healthy now and also promotes a healthy lifestyle, which is essential for public health. In addition, maintaining cleanliness is vital for numerous health reasons, not just to prevent infections. UNICEF shows that better WASH can positively affect school attendance, the health of mothers and newborns, and nutrition. When schools include hygiene education, it can directly help students avoid gastrointestinal infections. Focusing on these areas enables health intervention programs to impact public health in multiple ways, demonstrating the importance of proper hygiene in preventing diseases and improving life. It highlights that good hygiene is a crucial component in public health measures aimed at reducing the spread of infectious diseases. Personal hygiene should be part of public health efforts to reduce the impact of infectious diseases everywhere. Improving hygiene education and building safe water and sanitation facilities can significantly enhance the health of those who are at risk. The study in Amravati found that illness absenteeism was reduced by 20% which suggests that good hygiene practices can help maintain better health. Additionally, paying attention to hygiene helps address issues related to neglected tropical diseases, stress among children, and overall well-being. Thus, making personal hygiene a regular habit helps individuals and strengthens communities against easily spread diseases. Through comprehensive hygiene promotion, public health initiatives can boost community health frameworks, ultimately reducing the transmission of infectious diseases and fostering a healthier future (Figure 4.14).

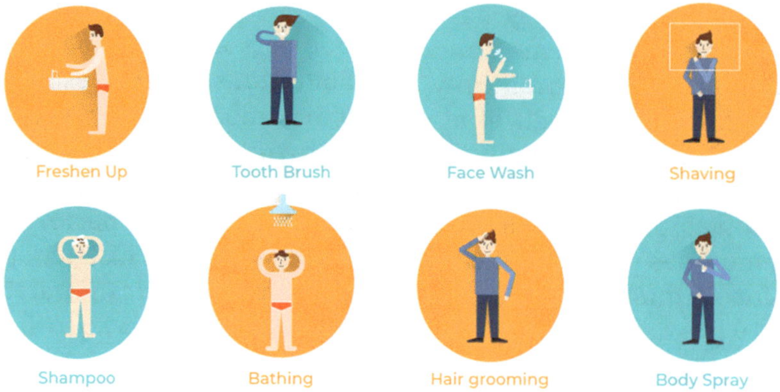

Figure 4.14. Personal hygiene practices.

Source: https://blogger.googleusercontent.com/img/b/R29vZ2xl/AVvXsEhEKDEnb8k-aNRv2GvTBvXPBs2MzxZBX6X3tV0NPscsoza90JK4n1GCVSnS_2sGhma3tri93eX9nt36kOuYt4HiqQLCMClHi_H69YIymKY_tQcE1rKE5IuEJKQEid1KfeOFA0DjhG0Onjd9Ojid9F8dlkBA3dp-xiEV9sbLGXktaJkJ8dhrRQEUW-dt/w1200-h630-p-k-no-nu/The%20Importance%20of%20Personal%20Hygiene%20in%20Preventing%20Illness%20and%20Disease.png.

4.4.2. Travel and Migration Patterns

Travel and migration have always been essential in spreading infectious diseases. Travellers may transport pathogens from one place to another, which can cause local outbreaks that could become global pandemics. The example of COVID-19 clearly demonstrates how international travel facilitated the rapid spread of the virus from one region to many others in a short period. Because of the way modern transportation links places, diseases now spread much quicker than they used to. Public health actions are better guided by travel data, which provides information on migration and movement patterns. Such analyses allow for timely interventions, particularly in areas identified as high-risk based on population density and travel frequency, which are closely correlated with disease outbreaks (Hill et al., 2021). Urbanization plays a significant part in determining how people travel and migrate. Due to their high population and frequent movement, cities are the primary locations where infectious diseases spread. When many migrants live in cities, it becomes easier for different groups to interact, which can allow pathogens to spread more quickly. For this reason, urban health strategies should consider both the demographic composition of the population and the unique patterns of movement within cities. For example, when many people use public transport for daily commutes, it can become a significant way for diseases to spread in crowded areas. Therefore, public health actions should be supported by city planning and transportation to deal with these risks ahead of time. By aligning health interventions with migration patterns, city planners and public health officials can reduce vulnerability to outbreaks and enhance overall community resilience (Kapitsinis, 2020). The meeting of travel, migration and infectious diseases in global health brings both issues and possibilities. Policymakers must manage international travel rules and public health advice to prevent outbreaks from worsening through migration. By examining past migration trends, we can identify similar patterns that may lead to increased disease transmission, highlighting the importance of genomic epidemiology, as reported in studies on the spread of diseases during past pandemics. As genomic sequencing becomes easier to use, researchers can follow the routes of infectious agents and see which demographic factors play a role in their spread. By effectively integrating this information with travel and migration data, health authorities can develop targeted interventions that are responsive to the ever-changing landscape of global disease transmission (Hill et al., 2021).

4.4.3. Public Health Compliance

Following public health rules means people and organizations obey the laws and guidelines that aim to stop the spread of infectious diseases. During outbreaks, following the rules quickly can help stop the spread of pathogens. As an example, the Public Health Unit of Albufeira took practical steps to follow compliance measures when influenza B broke out in a local school. When some students showed flu-like symptoms, the Public Health Unit told school officials, gave out helpful information and provided masks and sanitisers to all. Such proactive measures emphasize the necessity of collaboration between public health entities and educational institutions to ensure the protective measures are effectively communicated and enforced, ultimately mitigating the impact of infectious diseases on vulnerable populations like school-aged children (the nationwide et al., 2023). Responding fast and having detailed plans are essential for good public health compliance during outbreaks. When the flu outbreak happened in Albufeira, there were no guidelines for schools to follow which showed the need for clear rules during such events. They should include simple methods for everyone to inform each other, collect details and organize the response. Building these structures helps public health agencies prepare for future outbreaks. It is also very important to make sure school staff and students are well-trained in following these emergency procedures. When schools are equipped with well-defined response plans, they contribute to the broader public health goal of controlling infectious disease transmission within the community (the nationwide et al., 2023). The COVID-19 pandemic makes it clear that following public health rules is important for all groups. Before and after the I stay at home decree in Italy, analysis of transmission profiles showed significant changes in infection rates and the group of people affected. The way people followed lockdown rules demonstrated that the pandemic affected different age groups, social classes, and individuals with various occupations in various ways. This research emphasizes that public health strategies should be equitable to meet the needs of all communities. As the pandemic continued, following public health rules was shown to play a bigger role in controlling the spread of the virus, making it more important for everyone to comply. Understanding the implications of compliance on infectious disease transmission can guide future policy decisions and preparedness efforts to manage similar public health crises (Figure 4.15) effectively.

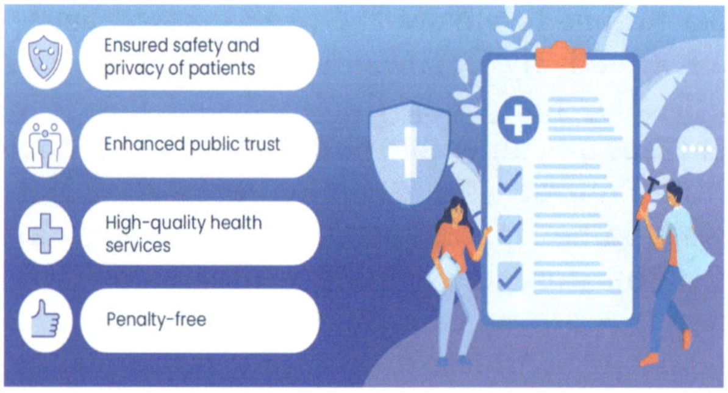

Figure 4.15. Public health compliance.

Source: https://cdn.azeusconvene.com/wp-content/uploads/Image-1-1.png.

4.5. Impact of Technology on Disease Transmission

The link between technology and health has dramatically changed the way infectious diseases are spread, mainly by improving surveillance and communication. New technology has made it possible to track disease outbreaks as they occur, enabling faster responses to public health emergencies. For example, data analytics platforms bring together data from various sources, such as hospitals and laboratories, to identify patterns in the spread of diseases. Such models have proven their worth in the COVID-19 pandemic by allowing experts to monitor and anticipate infection rates, which supports quick actions. Also, the ability to share data internationally has made it easier for health organisations to work together with others in different countries, which has improved global coordination.

However, using technology more can also raise concerns about privacy and ensuring equal access for everyone. Along with helping to monitor disease, technology has also affected both public understanding and actions related to the spread of diseases. Many people rely on digital platforms for health information, which affects how the public sees and follows health guidelines. For instance, applications that provide information about infections and safety measures in the area may encourage users to adopt safer habits, such as social distancing and wearing masks. Telehealth services became very popular during the COVID-19 pandemic, giving patients a way to get care without risking infection.

It helps people take care of their health and also decreases the strain on hospitals. Even so, the move to digital services means we must consider differences in access, as people without dependable internet or devices may be left behind in accessing health information and support on time. Even though technology helps decrease the spread of infectious diseases, it also introduces new issues and risks. For example, false news and rumors spreading fast on social media can weaken public health campaigns. Because of the COVID-19 pandemic, it became clear that misconceptions can quickly spread, which led to harmful actions and a refusal to follow health advice supported by science. Additionally, the use of technology for health management raises concerns about the safety of our personal data and the extent to which we can maintain our privacy. The growth of digital health initiatives necessitates the design of robust systems to safeguard personal data and encourage individuals to participate in health-related decisions. Continuous evaluation of technological impacts on disease transmission, as evidenced by studies examining behavioral changes during lockdowns (Nomden et al., 2023) and smoking habits during the pandemic (Sabbah et al., 2022), will be essential for addressing these emerging challenges in health communication and policy formulation (Figure 4.16).

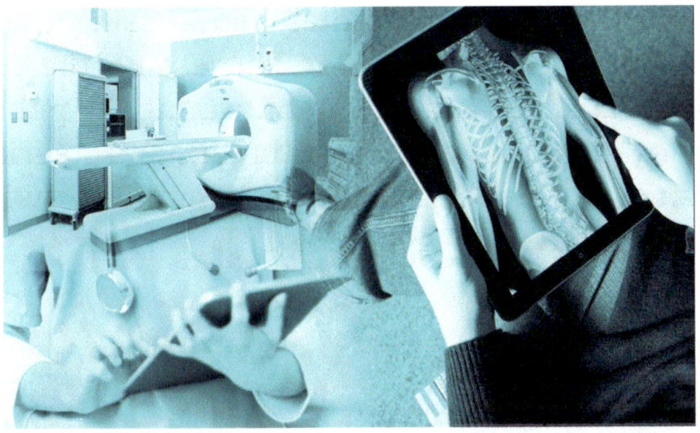

Figure 4.16. Impact of technology on disease transmission.

Source: https://www.instantconsult.com.au/wp-content/uploads/2017/08/The-Impact-of-Technology-in-the-Healthcare-Industry.jpg.

4.5.1. Advances in Medical Technology

The field of infectious disease transmission has undergone significant changes due to new developments in medical technology, particularly in diagnostics and treatment. Innovations in diagnostic tools, such as polymerase chain reaction (PCR) and next-generation sequencing, allow healthcare professionals to identify pathogens with greater speed and accuracy. Such technologies assist in detecting microbes that are often present but difficult to find, such as *Helicobacter pylori,* which is connected to several gastric diseases. Being able to identify different strains and their resistance to antibiotics enables doctors to use the right treatments and design more effective interventions for each patient, thereby improving infection control in hospitals. By integrating advanced diagnostics into routine practice, medical practitioners can significantly alter the trajectory of disease management and reduce the overall burden of infectious diseases, as evidenced by successful antimicrobial stewardship initiatives (Hsu et al., 2025). Also, as new antibiotics and alternative treatments are introduced, the fight against infectious diseases is improved. Because *Helicobacter pylori* and other pathogens are becoming increasingly resistant to antibiotics, new strategies are needed to deal with this problem. Through antimicrobial stewardship, doctors are encouraged to select the most effective antibiotics and avoid unnecessary prescriptions, which can help prevent resistance. Strategies like using potassium-competitive acid blockers are an example of how medicine is becoming more precise. At the same time, healthcare organizations are starting to focus on using different medical fields together to make sure both harmful germs are eliminated and treatments are sustainable in the future. Therefore, advances in treatment methodologies are crucial in limiting the transmission and impact of infectious diseases (Hsu et al., 2025). Besides diagnostics and treatment, nanotechnology is providing new ways to monitor and control the spread of contagious diseases. Due to plasmonic sensing, we can now utilise small and highly sensitive tools to detect biomarkers with exceptional accuracy. If nanoscale electromagnetic communication systems are built, healthcare providers may be able to send data in real-time, which could transform the way patient data is handled. They are expected to facilitate the detection of infections and enable quick responses by utilizing intra-body networks. Such small bio-sensing devices could significantly reduce the pressure on regular medical systems, making it simpler to monitor and control diseases. All in all, using advanced medical technologies improves our understanding of infections and helps international efforts to reduce the spread of diseases and improve the health of patients.

4.5.2. Role of Social Media in Spreading Information

Social media has become very important for sharing information about epidemics, mainly regarding infectious diseases. Social media enables people to access current news and advice on outbreaks, learn how to stay safe, and stay informed about the government's response.

Because information spreads so quickly on these platforms, it can shape public behaviour since users often look at content shared by others as well as official messages. According to the research, increased psychological fear generated by social media can help maintain steady disease transmission, thereby lowering the rate of infection fluctuations. This relationship between media influence and public response elucidates how social media acts as both a tool for information dissemination and a factor that shapes collective attitudes toward health interventions (Pal et al., 2024). Additionally, the way social media is structured makes it more challenging for information about infectious diseases to be understood and shared. Especially, those with numerous connections can help disseminate specific messages, which may lead more people to adopt safety measures. Studies have shown that by examining the interplay between opinions and diseases, researchers can model public reactions to crises using a model that includes social behaviour. The findings indicate that the behaviour of highly connected individuals can significantly shape epidemic outcomes, underscoring the need for a nuanced understanding of social influences in public health communications (Albi et al., 2024). Therefore, social media allows people to share information and also influences how groups act, which can help or harm the spread of diseases. Still, social media does not always do a good job of sharing accurate information. Information that is not true and overly dramatic stories are shared at the same time as real health messages, which can confuse people and lead to adverse reactions. Because social media can spread correct information as well as incorrect information, it adds challenges to public health strategies. Awareness campaigns about healthy actions often have to contend with misinformation that can undermine the effectiveness of safety efforts. Also, the constant changes in social media, such as how people interact and the way algorithms work, make it harder to get the correct information to the right people. Ultimately, addressing these challenges is essential for harnessing the full potential of social media in informing the public during infectious disease outbreaks and steering community behavior toward compliance with health guidelines (Figure 4.17).

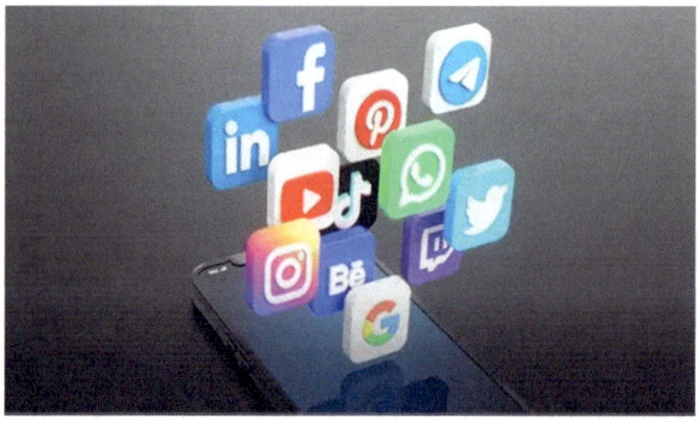

Figure 4.17. Role of social media in spreading information.

Source: https://cleverlight.com/wp-content/uploads/The-Role-of-Social-Media-in-Digital-Marketing.webp.

4.5.3. Use of Telemedicine During Outbreaks

Telemedicine has become very important in responding to infectious disease outbreaks, changing the way healthcare is delivered. Telemedicine enables patients to consult doctors from home, thereby reducing the risk of contracting illnesses from others in healthcare settings. It helps people access medical advice and treatment, and it also facilitates the handling of patient care in emergency situations. When diseases such as Ebola spread quickly, telemedicine enables doctors to monitor symptoms, conduct rapid assessments, and provide helpful advice to people in quarantine or with mild illness. When new diseases appear, using telemedicine in public health will help slow the spread of the disease and maintain the operation of healthcare systems. In addition, telemedicine platforms can easily adapt, which makes them essential during public health emergencies. For instance, during the Ebola outbreak, health agencies utilised telemedicine to distribute accurate information, engage in contact tracing, and provide timely updates to communities (Aguzzi et al., 2015). This approach helped people prioritise their health and also enhanced the management of public health. Telemedicine helps by allowing real-time data gathering, which is crucial for identifying disease trends and determining ways to prevent their spread. Virtual assessments enable a quick response to potential cases, helping to prevent the virus from spreading further. Therefore, telemedicine goes further than just seeing patients; it encourages informed decisions in public health, which is crucial during outbreaks. Telemedicine is expected to continue developing and gaining acceptance, which will significantly influence how future infectious disease outbreaks are managed. With travel and health habits changing, healthcare systems must be ready to respond.

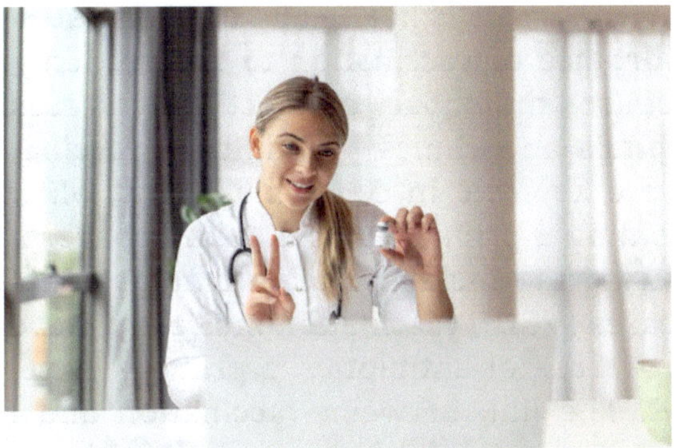

Figure 4.18. Use of telemedicine during outbreaks.

Source: https://img.freepik.com/premium-photo/female-doctor-having-online-therapy-with-her-patient-s-giving-them-advice-while-using-telemedicine-as-new-normal-covid19-pandemic-outbreak_1212-8328.jpg.

Telemedicine offers a scalable solution that can be adapted to varying disease contexts, such as the need for vaccinations in travel medicine, where services can be rendered remotely to reassure travelers about their health risks based on destination (Akele et al., 2024). As telehealth technologies continue to improve with the integration of AI and health monitoring, they open doors to both preventive and reactive actions against emerging infectious diseases. Hence, the synergy between telemedicine and public health strategies is critical, as it not only enhances healthcare delivery during outbreaks but also fortifies the resilience of health systems worldwide against future challenges (Figure 4.18).

4.6. Prevention and Control Measures

Managing the spread of infectious diseases depends on strong prevention and control measures, mainly to prevent outbreaks from growing into epidemics. Vigorous testing and tracing help healthcare systems quickly find and isolate people who are infected. It is crucial to act quickly; during the COVID-19 pandemic, areas that employed these methods had significantly lower infection rates than those that did not. This way, the risk of transmission is lowered and it becomes easier to track the disease and evaluate how public health responses are working, so reactions can be changed when needed. Additionally, incorporating community involvement into these strategies enhances the effectiveness of public health recommendations and increases the number of people who actively participate in reducing the risk of infection. Besides testing and tracing, social factors that can spread the disease must be controlled as well. Recent agent-based models suggest that where people live can either facilitate or hinder the transmission of infectious diseases. If places are sorted by their likelihood of spreading the disease, such as public transport, workplaces, and social gathering sites, strategies can be created to focus on these areas. Using this method, resources are used more efficiently and preventive measures are followed better, since it highlights the need to change behaviors in key situations. Moreover, simulation models have demonstrated that adjusting individual isolation intensity and controlling access to high-risk locations can significantly alter the trajectory of disease spread, reinforcing the need for interventions that consider the multifaceted roles of personal behaviors and environmental factors (Zhang et al., 2024). The effectiveness of any prevention and control measure depends on being able to use and change interventions quickly as the disease situation evolves. Evidence from the COVID-19 pandemic demonstrates how rapidly implemented test-trace-isolate measures can significantly reduce infection rates, underscoring the need for a proactive rather than reactive approach (Deng et al., 2024).

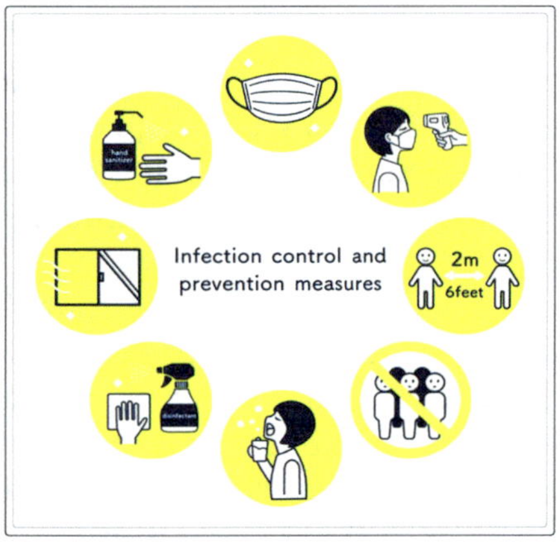

Figure 4.19. Prevention and control measures.

Source: https://engiomed.ae/wp-content/uploads/2022/04/IPC.jpg.

Additionally, regularly monitoring and reviewing the situation enables public health officials to make necessary adjustments based on current developments. Adjusting the number of contacts allowed per person, like during a rise in cases, can support efforts to control infections and stop the spread. By promoting an integrated framework that encompasses individual behaviors, social environments, and systematic responses, public health initiatives can more effectively navigate and control the complex dynamics of infectious disease transmission (Figure 4.19).

4.6.1. Vaccination Programs

The use of vaccination programs is essential in controlling the spread of infectious diseases. Because these programs help people build immunity, the chances of disease spreading are reduced. This phenomenon is particularly evident in the case of hepatitis B virus (HBV) vaccination initiatives globally. Studies have shown that countries that have established national vaccination programs for HBV have seen significant drops in chronic cases, proving the need for organised vaccination. For instance, between 1990 and 2020, the prevalence of chronic HBV infections in China decreased markedly, illustrating the long-term benefits of sustained vaccination strategies (Liu et al., 2022). It improves public health and demonstrates the importance of vaccination to the economy, as it reduces the impact of infectious diseases on hospitals and clinics. In addition, vaccination plays a key role in controlling AMR, which is becoming a primary global health concern. By lowering the incidence of vaccine-preventable diseases (VPD), vaccination indirectly prevents the overuse of antibiotics, a primary driver of AMR. The link between vaccination and less antibiotic use is vital; by lowering infection rates with vaccines, healthcare facilities can better control their antibiotic supplies. Data suggest that regions with robust vaccination initiatives experience lower rates of disease caused by antibiotic-resistant pathogens, highlighting the interconnectedness between effective vaccination strategies and the broader context of AMR management (Murray et al., 2022). Thus, vaccination is essential for stopping diseases and for protecting the effectiveness of current antibiotics. Additionally, ensuring that vaccines are distributed fairly is a crucial issue that can impact the spread of infectious diseases. Herd immunity can only be reached if marginalized and under-resourced people are given access to vaccinations. As seen in the success of HBV vaccination programs in high-burden areas, giving everyone equal access to health services can significantly improve health and reduce many kinds of diseases. Focusing on vaccinating vulnerable groups is crucial for achieving better health equity and reducing the spread of disease. Without a collective commitment to equitable vaccine distribution, the potential benefits of vaccination programs may be undermined, compromising global efforts to control infectious diseases (Liu et al., 2022; Murray et al., 2022).

4.6.2. Public Health Campaigns

Public health campaigns play a crucial role in controlling the spread of infectious diseases, particularly among individuals in conflict-affected and health emergency zones. They are designed to provide people with information on how to prevent diseases, modify their habits, and utilise preventive methods that help reduce the spread of infectious diseases. It was shown in a systematic review that armed conflicts cause significant problems for healthcare systems and increase the number of tuberculosis and cholera cases. To be successful, public health campaigns should be flexible and employ community-focused strategies that utilise messages understood by the culture. By addressing specific needs and leveraging local networks, campaigns can significantly enhance community resilience and adapt public health infrastructure, ultimately curbing the transmission of infectious diseases in conflict-affected regions (Alfaleh et al., 2025). The recent emergence of diseases such as Mpox underscores the importance of responsive public health campaigns that can quickly address new threats. When cases of Mpox were reported outside endemic regions in 2022, it became imperative for health authorities to inform the public about symptoms, transmission methods, and preventive measures. Vaccination campaigns, in particular, have proven essential in controlling outbreaks of infectious diseases. Following the historical eradication of smallpox through coordinated vaccination efforts, similar campaigns can be adapted to combat the spread of Mpox. The World Health Organisation's (WHO) decision to rebrand Monkeypox as Mpox reflects ongoing efforts to reduce stigma while promoting public awareness and education regarding the disease. By enhancing surveillance and implementing targeted campaigns, policymakers can significantly mitigate the risks associated with new infectious diseases in a globalized world (Martini et al., 2023). Public health campaigns are not only about disseminating information but also about fostering an environment conducive to healthy behaviors. Combining traditional health messaging with modern communication technologies can increase reach and effectiveness.

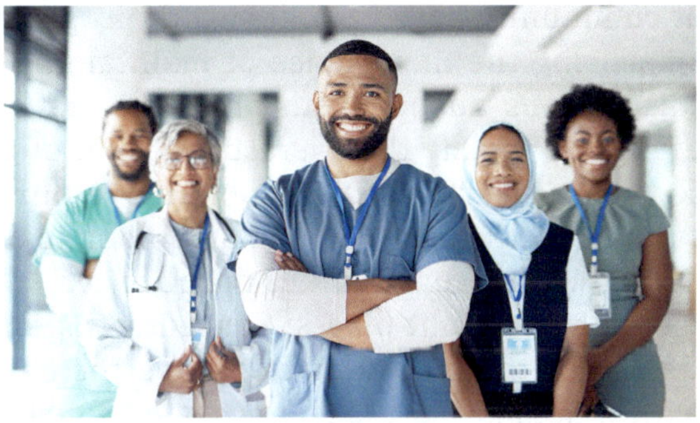

Figure 4.20. Public health campaigns.

Source: https://www.chenmed.com/sites/default/files/2023-12/The%20Role%20of%20Public%20Health%20Campaigns%20in%20Advancing%20Health%20Equity.jpg.

Social media platforms, for instance, present new opportunities for engaging younger populations, who are often key players in disease transmission networks. Campaigns that involve interactive content, such as quizzes or challenges, can further amplify their impact. Additionally, leveraging partnerships with community organizations can bring credibility and improve trust in public health messages.

Ultimately, addressing the multifaceted dimensions of infectious disease transmission requires innovative public health campaigns that not only inform but also motivate communities to take proactive steps against disease spread. By strategically implementing these campaigns, public health officials can create a more informed society capable of responding to infectious disease threats efficiently (Alfaleh et al., 2025) (Figure 4.20).

4.6.3. Quarantine and Isolation Protocols

The use of quarantine and isolation measures is crucial in preventing the spread of infectious diseases, particularly during pandemics like COVID-19. Quarantine is used to separate people who might have been exposed to the disease from those who have not, so that the disease does not spread when people start to show symptoms. People who have tested positive are placed in isolation. They help keep people healthy and reduce the likelihood of the health system becoming overburdened. New studies have found that limiting people's movement in cities is crucial for managing local cases. However, these strategies must be complemented by rigorous community engagement to ensure compliance and understanding of the protocols implemented during such health crises (Wang et al., 2023). The success of quarantine and isolation depends on how quickly and correctly people are informed about the nature of the disease. For example, the actions of residents play a significant role in determining the effectiveness of these measures; those who believe the disease is dangerous are more likely to follow the quarantine rules. Studies indicate that community-based public health programs can help people adhere to guidelines, especially by emphasising the importance of maintaining good health during isolation. Engaging communities in discussions about health protocols fosters a sense of collective responsibility and resilience, thereby supporting the overarching goal of breaking transmission chains (Soniawan et al., 2021). Also, being aware of how people move during a quarantine can help improve the planning and results of such steps. The Wuhan epidemic demonstrated that, after a lockdown, more cases were observed within communities than between them, suggesting that restrictions should be flexible and targeted at the right places. Concentrating on high-risk areas and implementing local quarantines enables health authorities to reduce the spread of the virus. This approach focuses on both the practical details and the feelings and thoughts of people in the community, ensuring they continue to support the strict health measures. Proper use of quarantine and isolation measures is essential to control diseases and protect the community's health.

SUMMARY

It is essential to understand the various factors that influence the spread of infectious diseases, particularly among more vulnerable populations. Warfare and instability significantly contribute to the spread and increase of infectious diseases, as demonstrated by several studies. In these situations, people being moved, health services being interrupted, and damaged infrastructure open the way for Cholera, Tuberculosis, and Measles to appear. As Marou et al. (2024) note, the consequences of armed conflict often exacerbate existing vulnerabilities, leading to increased morbidity and mortality rates among affected populations. For this reason, understanding these dynamics is crucial for developing public health measures that mitigate the harmful effects of infectious diseases in conflict zones. Moreover, the examination of VPD illustrates the challenges faced in controlling infectious disease transmission in low- and middle-income countries (LMICs). Although vaccines have advanced a lot, the number of people who die from diseases is still high, mainly among children younger than five. As indicated in Frenkel (2021), 700,000 children died from VPD in 2018 alone, highlighting the urgent need for effective immunisation strategies. The introduction of vaccines for *Streptococcus pneumoniae* and Measles has been essential for future public health strategies, especially during emergencies such as COVID-19. Lessons from past experiences guide policymakers in improving vaccine distribution, enabling more people in these groups to access and utilise them, which in turn helps reduce the spread of disease. In short, addressing the spread of infectious diseases in conflict zones requires consideration of the unique challenges posed by war, inadequate health systems, and limited vaccine availability. It is important to have preparedness and response plans, such as more immunization and teamwork among different sectors, to control infectious diseases in high-risk areas. The insights gleaned from Frenkel (2021) and Marou et al. (2024) emphasize the importance of adapting public health strategies to meet the specific needs of affected populations. In the future, international work should focus on solutions backed by evidence to help health systems and communities prevent the spread of infectious diseases, thereby protecting public health and benefiting those most at risk. Such efforts help people understand how diseases are spread, which supports the health and resilience of the global community.

Public health places great importance on the transmission of infectious diseases, which requires regular study and assessment. Pharmacotherapy for different infectious diseases has become a primary focus, mainly because of the COVID-19 pandemic. The Houston Infectious Diseases Network (HIDN) identified 35 influential articles in 2021, which included significant contributions to general infectious disease pharmacotherapy and specific concerns related to HIV/AIDS. With more complex treatments, it is now essential to use antimicrobial stewardship to help patients and lower the risk of resistance. Thus, understanding these key contributions not only enhances clinical knowledge but also guides mitigating the spread of infectious diseases through informed pharmacological interventions (Nguyen et al., 2022). In addition, how a disease is communicated depends a lot on tailoring the message. Surveys of members of the Infectious Diseases Society of America showed that physicians have different ways of diagnosing infections caused by poxviruses such as monkeypox and orf. It was found that there are significant differences in the frequency of diagnostic tests requested and the use of appropriate precautions during transmission. Knowing about these differences allows public health officials to guide education better, so practitioners are ready to address infectious disease cases. This highlights the importance of ongoing dialogue and resource availability in bridging potential knowledge gaps among healthcare providers (Hughes et al., 2010). To sum up, dealing well with infectious diseases depends on the development of new drugs and the provision of better training and awareness for doctors. The key points from the HIDN stress the need for ongoing professional growth, and the Infectious Diseases Society of America survey points out some areas where practice could be improved. These points demonstrate that effective treatment and disease prevention are closely linked. By fostering a comprehensive understanding among healthcare providers and incorporating evidence-based practices, the transmission of infectious diseases can be better managed, ultimately safeguarding public health and enhancing patient care (Hughes et al., 2010; Nguyen et al., 2022).

CLOSER LOOK:

HUMAN SPACE FLIGHT PROGRAM (HSP):

The Human Space Flight Program (HSP) stands as one of humanity's most ambitious, complex, and inspiring endeavors. Taking a closer look at the HSP reveals how decades of scientific innovation, engineering achievement, and global collaboration have enabled humans to live and work beyond Earth. More than a collection of spacecraft and missions, the program represents a sustained commitment to expanding the boundaries of human capability and understanding.

At its core, the HSP focuses on safely sending humans into space, supporting them in the harsh environment beyond Earth's atmosphere, and bringing them home. This requires a sophisticated integration of subsystems: launch vehicles that can overcome Earth's gravity, spacecraft capable of sustaining life in microgravity, and mission control centers that coordinate every moment from liftoff to landing. Each mission draws upon thousands of experts—engineers, medical teams, scientists, analysts, and technicians—who work together to reduce risk while maximizing the scientific and exploratory benefits.

One defining feature of modern human spaceflight is the emphasis on long-duration missions. With the International Space Station (ISS) as a continuous laboratory in orbit, astronauts conduct experiments on human physiology, materials science, fluid dynamics, plant biology, radiation exposure, and more. These studies generate insights that support life on Earth, such as innovations in medical imaging and water purification, while also preparing humanity for future journeys deeper into the solar system. Living in microgravity provides a unique setting to understand how the human body adapts, revealing challenges such as muscle atrophy, bone loss, and shifts in cardiovascular function.

The HSP also serves as a platform for international cooperation. Agencies such as NASA, ESA, Roscosmos, JAXA, and CSA contribute hardware, expertise, and astronauts, demonstrating that human space exploration is most powerful when nations work together. This collaborative spirit extends into the commercial sector, where private companies increasingly support crew transportation, cargo delivery, and technology development.

Looking ahead, the Human Space Flight Program continues to evolve toward deeper exploration. Programs aimed at returning humans to the Moon, establishing sustainable lunar operations, and eventually sending crews to Mars reflect a long-term vision of expanding human presence beyond low Earth orbit. These missions will rely on advances in propulsion, habitat design, radiation protection, and autonomous systems.

Ultimately, a closer look at the HSP reveals a program driven by curiosity, cooperation, and the enduring human desire to explore. It stands as a testament to what humanity can achieve when imagination and science unite.

REFERENCES

1. Chiappelli, F., Bakhordarian, A., Thames, A. D., Du, A. M., Jan, A. L., Nahcivan, M., Nguyen, M. T., Sama, N., Manfrini, E., Piva, F., Rocha, R., & Maida, C. A. (2015). Ebola: translational science considerations. *Journal of Translational Medicine, 13*(1), 11. https://doi.org/10.1186/s12967-014-0362-3Akele, R. Y., Akinpelu, R. T., Dada, M. O., Edafetanure-Ibeh, et al. (2024). The role of travel medicine in managing future pandemics: Lessons learned from global infectious disease outbreaks. https://core.ac.uk/download/604373473.pdf (accessed on 30th May 2025).
2. Al Sabbah, H., Assaf, E. A., Taha, Z., Qasrawi, R., Cheikh, I. L., Al Dhaheri, A. A., Hoteit, M., et al. (2022). Impact of COVID-19 lockdown on smoking (waterpipe and cigarette) and participants' BMI across various sociodemographic groups in Arab countries in the Mediterranean Region. *Tobacco Induced Diseases, 20.* https://www.semanticscholar.org/paper/6d5c240f4cf863b3cb3ded31e3553693c87ef30b (accessed on 30th May 2025).
3. Albi, G., Calzola, E., Dimarco, G., & Zanella, M. (2024). *Impact of Opinion Formation Phenomena in Epidemic Dynamics: Kinetic Modeling on Networks.* ArXiv, abs/2409.17669. https://www.semanticscholar.org/paper/e64ed5912e2cfd38ea278e84638d637f59a53c6f (accessed on 30th May 2025).
4. Alfaleh, R., Alsuwailem, W. A., Almazyad, R. T., Alanazi, F. F., & Alanazi, L. T. (2025). The impact of armed conflicts on the prevalence, transmission, and management of infectious diseases: A systematic review. *Cureus, 17.* https://www.semanticscholar.org/paper/2411296fe579b1e32c11d76d47e2150bc4e16a47 (accessed on 30th May 2025).
5. Budge, S., Ambelu, A., Bartram, J., Brown, J., & Hutchings, P. (2022). Environmental sanitation and the evolution of water, sanitation and hygiene. *Bulletin of the World Health Organization, 100*, 286–288. https://www.semanticscholar.org/paper/41e671100c97c00c6ceda37301017dca3ad8a03b (accessed on 30th May 2025).
6. Burton, M. J., Ramke, J., Marques, A. P., Bourne, R., Congdon, N., Jones, I., Ah Tong, B. A. M., et al. (2021). The Lancet Global Health Commission on Global Eye Health: Vision beyond 2020. *The Lancet Global Health, 9*, e489–e551. https://doi.org/10.1016/s2214-109x(20)30488-5.
7. Combs, B. G., Giele, C. M., Kwan, K. S. H., Mak, et al. (2008). *Audit of Antenatal Testing of Sexually Transmissible Infections and Blood Borne Viruses at Western Australian Hospitals.* https://core.ac.uk/download/61303469.pdf (accessed on 30th May 2025).
8. Deng, Y., Li, M., & Lei, J. (2024). Evaluation of infectious diseases control using an individual model under the test-trace-isolate program. *Medical Research Archives.* https://www.semanticscholar.org/paper/932a19a6f368fa0f8576e68908983bb4fb048f39 (accessed on 30th May 2025).
9. Di Napoli, C., Romanello, M., Minor, K., Chambers, J., Dasgupta, S., Escobar, L. E., Hang, Y., et al. (2023). The role of global reanalyzes in climate services for health: Insights from the *Lancet* Countdown. *Meteorological Applications, 30.* https://doi.org/10.1002/met.2122.
10. Esteves, M. J., & Cumming, O. (2016). *The Impact of Water, Sanitation, and Hygiene on Key Health and Social Outcomes: Review of Evidenc*e. https://core.ac.uk/download/75761114.pdf (accessed on 30th May 2025).
11. Fahdi, F., & Sari, H. (2024). Introduction to basic microbiology concepts in the prevention of infectious diseases at YAPIM Biru-Biru Private High School. *Jurnal Pengabdian Masyarakat*

Putri Hijau. https://www.semanticscholar.org/paper/3c0ba05bf2960cbab82f682380da240b701632c1 (accessed on 30th May 2025).

12. Ferraguti, M. (2024). Mosquito species identity matters: Unraveling the complex interplay in vector-borne diseases. *Infectious Diseases*. https://www.semanticscholar.org/paper/5123f987cb60003c3142955a905c904d0b0a2f5e (accessed on 30th May 2025).
13. Freeman, M. C., Delea, M. G., Snyder, J. S., Garn, J. V., Belew, M. L., Caruso, B. A., Clasen, T., et al. (2022). The impact of a demand-side sanitation and hygiene promotion intervention on sustained behavior change and health in Amhara, Ethiopia: A cluster-randomized trial. *PLOS Global Public Health, 2*, e0000056–e0000056. https://doi.org/10.1371/journal.pgph.0000056.
14. Frenkel, L. D. (2021). The global burden of vaccine-preventable infectious diseases in children less than 5 years of age: Implications for COVID-19 vaccination. How can we do better? *Allergy and Asthma Proceedings, 42*, 378–385. https://doi.org/10.2500/aap.2021.42.210065.
15. Goradwar, V. U., & Anjankar, A. (2024). H3N2 influenza virus pathogenesis, transmission and complications: A narrative review. *Journal of Clinical and Diagnostic Research*. https://www.semanticscholar.org/paper/b8f8984950b22474ebe9c925da403926d9541940 (accessed on 30th May 2025).
16. Guleria, A. (2024). Spread of infectious diseases by microorganisms present in fomites. *World Journal of Advanced Research and Reviews*. https://www.semanticscholar.org/paper/be18d8e3d8bb15ef21240aaa6aa7a4eee15a4792 (accessed on 30th May 2025).
17. Hill, V., Ruis, C., Bajaj, S., Pybus, O. G., & Kraemer, M. U. G. (2021). Progress and challenges in virus genomic epidemiology. *Trends in Parasitology, 37*, 1038–1049. https://doi.org/10.1016/j.pt.2021.08.007.
18. Hsu, J. Y., Wu, U. I., Wang, J. T., Sheng, W. H., Chen, Y. C., & Chang, S. C. (2025). Managing *Helicobacter pylori* as an infectious disease: Implementation of antimicrobial stewardship. *Helicobacter, 30*(1), e70013. https://www.semanticscholar.org/paper/a6a8475303d838cdda86b1793dd997e2d16257a6 (accessed on 30th May 2025).
19. Hughes, C., Lederman, E., Reynolds, M., Damon, I., Lash, R., Beekmann, S., Polgreen, P., et al. (2010). Clinical experience, infection control practices and diagnostic algorithms for poxvirus infections – an Emerging Infections Network survey. *BMC Research Notes, 3*, 46. https://www.semanticscholar.org/paper/f5283f564b299bdf18d848fcbab8039e9b205e72 (accessed on 30th May 2025).
20. Johnston, S. L. (2025). *Flight Crew Health Stabilization Program*. https://core.ac.uk/download/pdf/10572163.pdf (accessed on 30th May 2025).
21. Jung, H., & Albarracín, D. (2020). Concerns for others increase the likelihood of vaccination against influenza and COVID-19 more in sparsely rather than densely populated areas. *Proceedings of the National Academy of Sciences, 118*. https://doi.org/10.1073/pnas.2007538118 (accessed on 30th May 2025).
22. Kapitsinis, N. (2020). The underlying factors of the COVID-19 spatially uneven spread: Initial evidence from regions in nine EU countries. *Regional Science Policy & Practice, 12*, 1027–1046. https://doi.org/10.1111/rsp3.12340.
23. Lakes, T., Schmitz, T., & Füller, H. (2025). Pathogenic built environment? Reflections on modeling spatial determinants of health in urban settings considering the example of COVID-19

studies. *Frontiers in Public Health, 13.* https://www.semanticscholar.org/paper/87ef99b3ee0d1a1d895570f2ed65084a8ef79ca0 (accessed on 30th May 2025).

24. Lara, 1. P., Health, Instituto de, et al. (2023). Addressing influenza outbreaks in schools. *The European Journal of Public Health, 33.* https://www.semanticscholar.org/paper/2729fd4a5e8574b1dc0cc2df0ecf514a22158d7b (accessed on 30th May 2025).

25. Liu, X., Yuan, W., & Xiao, H. (2024). Recent progress on DNAzyme-based biosensors for pathogen detection. *Analytical Methods: Advancing Methods and Applications.* https://www.semanticscholar.org/paper/858298a5e6c9c2ee5740c06a169b684eccf873c5 (accessed on 30th May 2025).

26. Liu, Z., Li, M., Hutton, D. W., Wagner, A. L., Yao, Y., Zhu, W., Cao, L., et al. (2022). Impact of the national hepatitis B immunization program in China: A modeling study. *Infectious Diseases of Poverty, 11.* https://doi.org/10.1186/s40249-022-01032-5.

27. Marou, V., Vardavas, C., Aslanoglou, K., Nikitara, K., Plyta, Z., Leonardi-Bee, J., Atkins, K., et al. (2024). The impact of conflict on infectious disease: A systematic literature review. *Conflict and Health, 18.* https://doi.org/10.1186/s13031-023-00568-z.

28. Martini, M., Behzadifar, M., Bragazzi, N., & Orsini, D. (2023). Poc (Pox), a term for various infectious diseases in the history of public health and epidemiology: The dreaded smallpox, the almost unknown alastrim and the mpox. *Journal of Preventive Medicine and Hygiene, 64,* E209–E214. https://www.semanticscholar.org/paper/6ee62760c3b214e7c389df845d1f700fdde11e09 (accessed on 30th May 2025).

29. Min, B., Issarow, C. M., Brenner, F., Chowell, G., Stehlé, J., Shirley, M. D. F., Zhang, N., et al. (2018). *Impact of Indirect Contacts in Emerging Infectious Disease on Social Networks.* http://arxiv.org/abs/1803.07968 (accessed on 30th May 2025).

30. Murray, C. J. L., Ikuta, K. S., Sharara, F., Swetschinski, L. R., Robles, A. G., Gray, A. P., Han, C., et al. (2022). Global burden of bacterial antimicrobial resistance in 2019: A systematic analysis. *The Lancet, 399,* 629–655. https://doi.org/10.1016/s0140-6736(21)02724-0.

31. Mutima, N. (2004). *Funding for Health in Africa: Mapping the U. S. Foundation Landscape, 2000–2002.* https://core.ac.uk/download/75779536.pdf (accessed on 30th May 2025).

32. Nguyen, N., Chua, H. C., Drake, T., Jo, J. U., Stramel, S., Vuong, N., Gonzales-Luna, A., et al. (2022). Significant publications on infectious diseases pharmacotherapy in 2021. *Journal of Pharmacy Practice, 37,* 198–211. https://www.semanticscholar.org/paper/ed8d15c2c18ed5aa471b96c4f3d579fc2c41f774 (accessed on 30th May 2025).

33. Nomden, M., Alizai, N., Betalli, P., Bruggink, J., Cananzi, M., Christensen, V., D'Antiga, L., et al. (2023). Incidence of isolated biliary atresia during the COVID lockdown in Europe: Results from a collaborative project by RARE-Liver. *Journal of Clinical Medicine, 12.* https://www.semanticscholar.org/paper/5b0bdc32ac581102d5702ea410ab027ac1a11d4e (accessed on 30th May 2025).

34. Ogbunugafor, C. B. (2024). On modes of disease transmission and the hidden shape of pandemics: A review of *Asymptomatic* by Joshua Weitz. *Virus Evolution, 10.* https://www.semanticscholar.org/paper/aa4b16a11543d29caa6fcf3cfb9cd0cfbaacf81f (accessed on 30th May 2025).

35. Othman, R., Safian, N., & Hassan, M. R. (2024). The roles of socio-environmental factors

influencing the transmission, prevention, and control of COVID-19 and tuberculosis disease: A review. *International Journal of Public Health Research*. https://www.semanticscholar.org/paper/faffe0c97866db0c26b34b1bebe7a5f59bdfa663 (accessed on 30th May 2025).

36. Pal, K., Rai, R. K., & Tiwari, P. K. (2024). Impact of psychological fear and media on infectious diseases induced by carriers. *Chaos, 34*(12). https://www.semanticscholar.org/paper/cf31362b354566ec97090d620d1cb210e73bed02 (accessed on 30th May 2025).

37. Patil, R., Dave, R., Patel, H. K., Shah, V., Chakrabarti, D., & Bhatia, U. (2021). Assessing the interplay between travel patterns and SARS-CoV-2 outbreak in realistic urban setting. *Applied Network Science, 6*. https://doi.org/10.1007/s41109-020-00346-3.

38. Ratter-Rieck, J. M., Roden, M., & Herder, C. (2023). Diabetes and climate change: Current evidence and implications for people with diabetes, clinicians and policy stakeholders. *Diabetologia, 66*, 1003–1015. https://doi.org/10.1007/s00125-023-05901-y.

39. Sangwan, A., & Jornet, J. (2022). Joint communication and bio-sensing with plasmonic nano-systems to prevent the spread of infectious diseases in the internet of nano-bio things. *IEEE Journal on Selected Areas in Communications, 40*, 3271–3284. https://www.semanticscholar.org/paper/caf26731f3b6b379866793abd8978e4fcdbc7b28 (accessed on 30th May 2025).

40. Selivanova, S., Zverev, V. V., Ponomareva, N., Leonov, A. V., Kashnikov, A. Y., Epifanova, N. V., Polyanina, A. V., et al. (2024). Detection and type identification of non-polio enteroviruses in children against the background of acute intestinal infections of various etiologies: 2018–2023. *Journal of Microbiology, Epidemiology and Immunobiology*. https://www.semanticscholar.org/paper/58016ac39fa55acd4649b5eac68acd2b894a98ae (accessed on 30th May 2025).

41. Shereen, M. A., Khan, S., Kazmi, A., Bashir, N., & Siddique, R. (2020). COVID-19 infection: Emergence, transmission, and characteristics of human coronaviruses. *Journal of Advanced Research, 24*, 91–98. https://doi.org/10.1016/j.jare.2020.03.005.

42. Shirsat, S. D., & Tambekar, D. H. (2012). *Minimization of Illness Absenteeism in Primary School Students Using Low-Cost Hygiene Interventions*. https://core.ac.uk/download/pdf/13598746.pdf (accessed on 30th May 2025).

43. Sizikova, T. E., Lebedev, V. N., & Borisevich, S. (2024). The assessment of the danger of pathogens of zoonotic viral infections as potential agents of pandemics. *Journal of NBC Protection Corps*. https://www.semanticscholar.org/paper/9129e145edce7eac797b1e7c12e778e5d49e164d (accessed on 30th May 2025).

44. Soniawan, V., Adnan, A., Haryanto, J., Lesmana, H. S., Arifan, I., Purnomo, E., & Pratama, D. S. (2021). Tingkat kesadaran masyarakat akan pentingnya beraktivitas fisik selama pandemi COVID-19. *Jurnal Performa Olahraga*. https://www.semanticscholar.org/paper/caff4c865d1c8c8021807fe94b29ea6e9337b9a6 (accessed on 30th May 2025).

45. Sönnerborg, A. (2003). Genotypic resistance tests for the management of the patient failing highly active antiretroviral therapy: The resistance pattern in different biological compartments. https://www.semanticscholar.org/paper/720578a1cb8c61c9c9eb4d1442911e7f3c15269c (accessed on 30th May 2025).

46. Srivastava, S., Kumar, S., Sharma, P. K., Rustagi, S., Mohanty, A., Donovan, S., Henao-Martínez, A., et al. (2024). Control strategies for emerging infectious diseases: Crimean-Congo hemorrhagic fever management. *Health Science Reports, 7*. https://www.semanticscholar.org/paper/0070505be9f28cb5bfef53d331b24da065a5ce2c (accessed on 30th May 2025).

47. Stivanello, E., Perlangeli, V., Resi, D., Marzaroli, P., Pizzi, L., Pandolfi, P. on behalf of the Bologna Public Health Authority. (2020). COVID-19 cases before and after the "I stay at home" decree, Bologna Local Health Authority, Italy. *Acta Bio Medica: Atenei Parmensis, 91*, e2020001–e2020001. https://www.semanticscholar.org/paper/2293ba992e59cd5fcf845df70047505bcdb3f3f9 (accessed on 30th May 2025).

48. Sylla, A., Chevillon, C., Djidjiou-Demasse, R., Seydi, O., Campos, C. A. V., Dogbe, M., Fast, K. M., et al. (2024). Understanding the transmission of bacterial agents of sapronotic diseases using an ecosystem-based approach: A first spatially realistic metacommunity model. *PLOS Computational Biology, 20*. https://www.semanticscholar.org/paper/9ee9a5e21553d6643745fbaeccfbf8326cf1cb80 (accessed on 30th May 2025).

49. Tavares, A. M. de F., Souza, C. N., Carvalho, C. M. C., Sanglard, D., & de Almeida, A. C. (2024). Multidrug resistance and phenotypic characterization of biofilm formation by *Staphylococcus aureus*: Contributions to public health. *IOSR Journal of Humanities and Social Science*. https://www.semanticscholar.org/paper/7df1ff87e27eca443232f2562a34fbd6cb7590c0 (accessed on 30th May 2025).

50. Tay, M. Z., Poh, C. M., Rénia, L., MacAry, P. A., & Ng, L. F. P. (2020). The trinity of COVID-19: Immunity, inflammation and intervention. *Nature Reviews Immunology, 20*, 363–374. https://doi.org/10.1038/s41577-020-0311-8.

51. Wang, J., Shi, H., Ji, J., Lin, X., & Tian, H. (2023). High-resolution data on human behavior for effective COVID-19 policy-making — Wuhan City, Hubei Province, China, January 1–February 29, 2020. *China CDC Weekly, 5*, 76–81. https://www.semanticscholar.org/paper/516d7f690c14a718f8fb429df5fb8e54bd88554f (accessed on 30th May 2025).

52. Wang, Y., Ling, L., Jiang, L., & Marín-López, A. (2024). Research progress toward arthropod salivary protein vaccine development for vector-borne infectious diseases. *PLOS Neglected Tropical Diseases, 18*. https://www.semanticscholar.org/paper/bcf646362d79de65528072b3a51a2288ccd57288 (accessed on 30th May 2025).

53. Ward, M. P., & Brookes, V. (2024). An overview of the challenges and methods for defining the wildlife-disease interface in the context of disease spread modeling, including concepts of infectious diseases epidemiology. *Australian Zoologist*. https://www.semanticscholar.org/paper/1f864dda93a2b01a9de5602856bc305161c2f3af (accessed on 30th May 2025).

54. Xu, X., Han, M., Li, T., Wei, S., Wang, D., Fu, B., Zhou, Y., et al. (2020). Effective treatment of severe COVID-19 patients with tocilizumab. *Proceedings of the National Academy of Sciences, 117*, 10970–10975. https://doi.org/10.1073/pnas.2005615117.

55. Yin, N., Fachqoul, Z., van Cauteren, D., Van Den, W. S., Martiny, D., Hallin, M., & Vandenberg, O. (2024). Impact of extreme weather events on the occurrence of infectious diseases in Belgium from 2011 to 2021. *Journal of Medical Microbiology, 73*(7). https://www.semanticscholar.org/paper/b552f234ffd34ea2c514390a1508610dae54ce36 (accessed on 30th May 2025).

56. Zhang, J., Rong, L., & Gong, Y. (2024). An agent-based transmission model of major infectious diseases considering places: Forecast and control. *Mathematics*. https://www.semanticscholar.org/paper/a8299adb8fd8a6753678d29a7b81fec035d0fe05 (accessed on 30th May 2025).

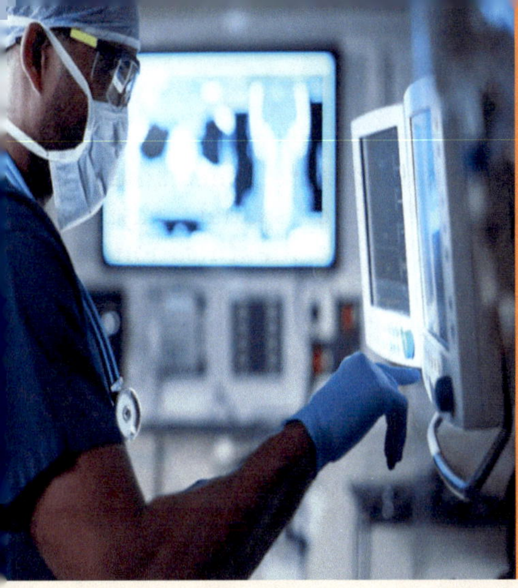

Chapter 5

SURVEILLANCE AND MONITORING OF INFECTIOUS DISEASES

Contents

Introduction

The epidemiology of infectious diseases has long presented a significant challenge to global public health systems, demanding robust mechanisms for surveillance and monitoring. With increased global interlinkage through travel and business, so is the spread of diseases across borders at high velocity. This observation once again underscores the importance of effective surveillance systems that not only facilitate early case detection during outbreaks but also track disease patterns over time. Such systems can aid health authorities in identifying populations at risk, deploying resources, and implementing preventive measures that can retard the transmission of infection. These surveillance activities involve the combining of vast amounts of information from several sources, including healthcare settings, laboratories, and community reporting, which in their turn guide decision-making and response to the prospect of emerging health risks (Bernstein et al., 2016). Advances in technology are at the center of enhancing surveillance for infectious disease control. The use of digital health tools, including mobile apps and online reporting, has transformed the way disease statistics are collected and analysed. In addition, geographical information systems (GIS) have also facilitated spatial analysis, providing insights into the geographic patterns of disease and aiding in the identification of outbreak hotspots. When these technologies are used together, data can be collected in real time and threats can be handled more quickly. However, these innovations also raise ethical concerns regarding data privacy and security, necessitating a regulatory approach to safeguard against the exposure of sensitive information (Habib et al., 2015).

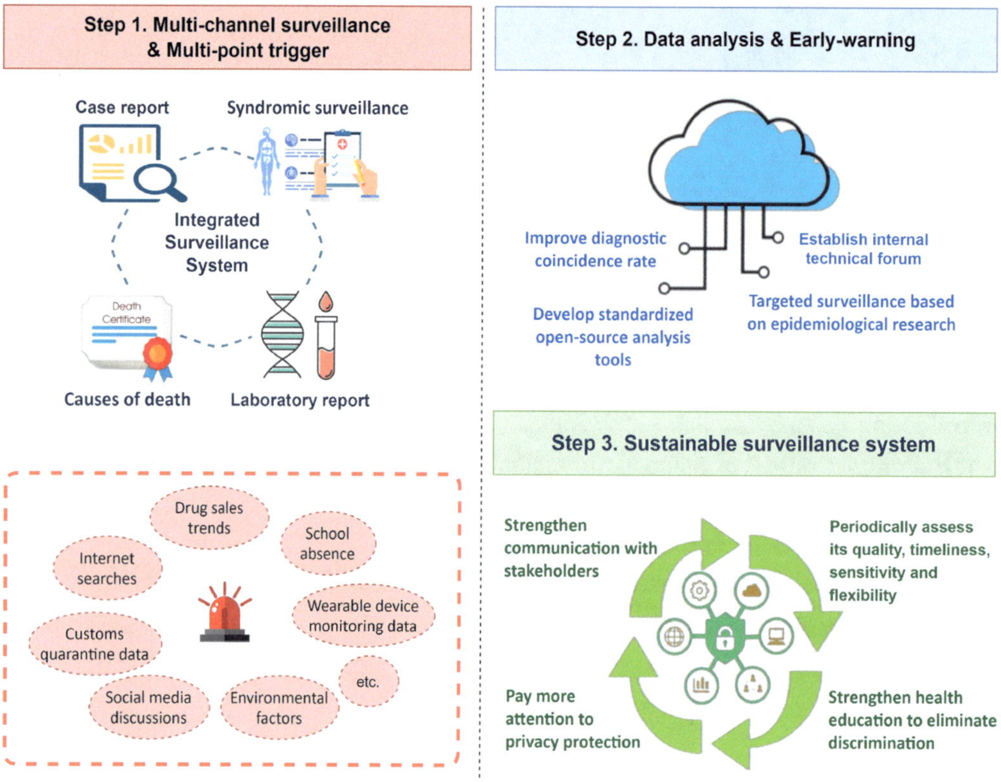

Figure 5.1. Surveillance and monitoring of infectious diseases.

Source: https://www.thelancet.com/cms/10.1016/j.lanwpc.2022.100485/asset/df0eccc7-1691-4c69-8fe6-47288236ea36/main.assets/gr1_lrg.jpg.

As public health agencies address these challenges, they must ensure surveillance is effective yet respectful of individuals' rights. Working together globally helps improve the effectiveness of systems that watch for infectious diseases. Global health organizations, such as the World Health Organization (WHO), play a crucial role in facilitating data and best practice exchange between nations, thereby fostering collaborative disease control activities. They also give training and technical assistance to help countries improve their surveillance, especially those that cannot afford it. When nations have strong partnerships and good communication, they can respond to outbreaks as a team and share details that help everyone. Hence, with infectious diseases still evolving and posing threats at all-time highs, integration of surveillance systems with technological advancements and international collaborations will be a key factor in upholding public health measures and protection of populations from infectious disease spread (Bernstein et al., 2016) (Figure 5.1).

Definition of Surveillance and Monitoring

Surveillance and monitoring are essential elements in the proper control of infectious diseases, with a systematic means of following health events. Information on surveillance is most often described as the ongoing, systematic acquisition, analysis, and interpretation of health-related information used to drive public health interventions. This is required for identifying trends, outbreaks, and overall rates of infection within populations. Monitoring involves the ongoing observation of disease occurrence and the efficacy of interventions. Use of surveillance and monitoring enables public health officials to deploy more effectively, building targeted responses to new threats. All in all, the implementation of these two practices is what constitutes effective disease prevention, further enabling the capability to respond pre-emptively to public health emergencies. Surveillance encompasses more than just data collection; it is a comprehensive system that brings together many people to support health security. An example is the Basic Surveillance Network created by the European Commission, which works to unite information on infectious diseases from all member states. In addition to sharing data, the network ensures that cases are reported and classified in a consistent manner. Expanding from 10 to over 40 diseases demonstrates the networkis commitment to tracking a broader range of infectious diseases. This activity emphasizes the value of an integrative effort in surveillance, as it enhances the likelihood of monitoring disease incidence trends and informing public health policy (Ternhag et al., 2004). In other words, monitoring involves checking the data to see how interventions have affected the situation and to find places that require improvement. This becomes very important when looking at the long-term effects of infectious diseases. Analysis of worldwide health statistics reveals large patterns in child mortality due to diseases such as lower respiratory tract infections, underscoring the need for ongoing monitoring (Kyu et al., 2016). By reviewing the effectiveness of interventions throughout history, public health practitioners can identify effective approaches and where resources are needed most. Therefore, an ongoing commitment to strict surveillance and monitoring systems is vital in combating the nuances of infectious diseases so that more efficient public health responses can be made and, ultimately, improved health outcomes within populations (Figure 5.2).

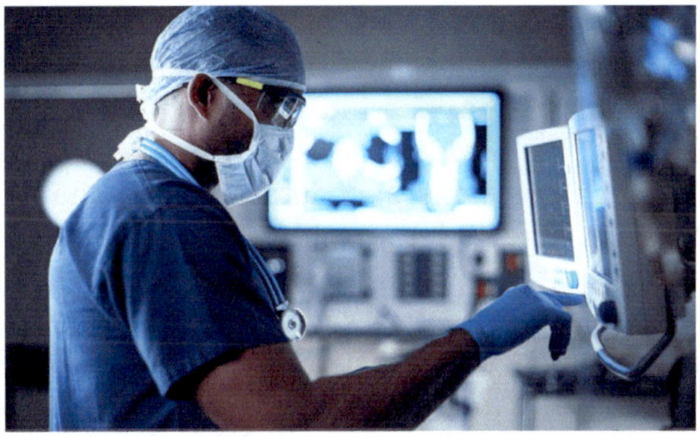

Figure 5.2. Surveillance and monitoring.

Source: https://images.ctfassets.net/9mz5xx7mqy8x/29FQEwjFipXRG7IrMo1TNW/37f43a87738ee18a087f9b0bb32656ed/surveillance-solutions-for-hospitals-remote-video-monitoring_1552x968.png.

Importance of Infectious Disease Tracking

The importance of infectious disease surveillance lies in its role as a pillar of public health policy and community protection. Through routine surveillance of disease outbreaks, health organizations can detect trends, assess risks, and intervene at the appropriate time. Not only does this proactive strategy enable quick detection of novel pathogens, but it also informs resource planning and public health activities that break disease transmission chains. An increased emphasis on notifiable disease lists and surveillance standards is required to simplify the monitoring process and ensure the optimal use of public health resources. Such improvement in strategic surveillance systems can significantly enhance the ability to react promptly to infectious threats, ultimately safeguarding populations and optimizing health security at national and international levels (Zucs et al., 2024). Communicable disease surveillance is vital because it helps the world get ready for pandemics and outbreaks. The interconnectivity of human, animal, and environmental health emphasises the need for comprehensively integrated concepts, such as the One Health paradigm. One Health promotes inter-disciplinary collaboration and geographic cooperation to facilitate early warning of potential outbreaks. The use of high-tech solutions and data analysis enables scientists and public health administrators to predict better and counter threats. Through the utilization of integrated sources of data, genomic surveillance, and electronic health records, public health infrastructure can be upgraded to respond effectively to new health threats. Ultimately, all this unifies efforts to strengthen community resilience and equip global health actors to address emerging challenges more effectively (Singh et al., 2024). In addition, the consequences of infectious disease tracking spill over to broader economic and social welfare. Effective surveillance programs can prevent the substantial expenses associated with large-scale outbreaks, including healthcare costs, lost work productivity, and disruptions to livelihoods. Having strong tracking systems, therefore, plays a key part in making economies more resilient, especially as the world becomes more connected. The upgrades in surveillance systems outlined in European plans show a commitment to being more vigilant and tough against diseases. Such frameworks should yield not only more effective disease surveillance systems but also a collaborative environment that encourages knowledge sharing and situational awareness among nations, ultimately enhancing global health security (Zucs et al., 2024).

5.1. Historical Context of Disease Surveillance

The historical evolution of disease surveillance goes back to ancient civilizations, in which simple health pattern observations formed the foundation for contemporary methods. Most significantly, quarantine efforts during outbreaks, such as the Black Death outbreak in the 14th century, demonstrated early attempts to monitor infectious diseases and control their spread. Cities began adopting a systematic approach to collecting data on mortality rates and disease prevalence in a straightforward manner. These measures not only reflected reactions to short-term health emergencies but also marked the start of organized epidemiological observations that would become modern-day surveillance systems. As people advanced in civilization, using statistics became important for tracking diseases, which led to more advanced ways of managing and understanding health information. The progress of science and technology in the 19th century played a significant role in how disease surveillance was carried out. The development of vital statistics, spearheaded by the likes of Edwin Chadwick, enabled the organised reporting of health information to inform and target the work of public health initiatives. During this time, the germ theory of disease also emerged, leading to a shift in emphasis towards the causes of outbreaks at the microscopic level. Backing up this scientific change, the formation of disease-reporting institutions was a turning point in the institutionalization of health surveillance. These events created an environment in which decision-making based on data was necessary in both infectious disease management and the formulation of public health policy, laying the groundwork for our organized systems as we now understand them. The modern disease surveillance landscape is the result of a culmination of historical events mixed with the appearance of emerging challenges. The emergence of EIDs has underscored the importance of robust surveillance systems, particularly in low- and middle-income countries (LMICs), where capacity is often limited. Local surveillance capacities need to be strengthened because local outbreaks can spread rapidly and become public health threats at large. Addressing LMIC-specific needs not only improves the capacity to identify and respond to EIDs but also reduces current inequalities in global health systems. Additionally, the history of disease surveillance offers valuable lessons on the need to evolve surveillance strategies to suit new epidemiological challenges while still drawing from previous experiences for better and more equitable health interventions (Cleaveland et al., 2017; Held et al., 2007) (Figure 5.3).

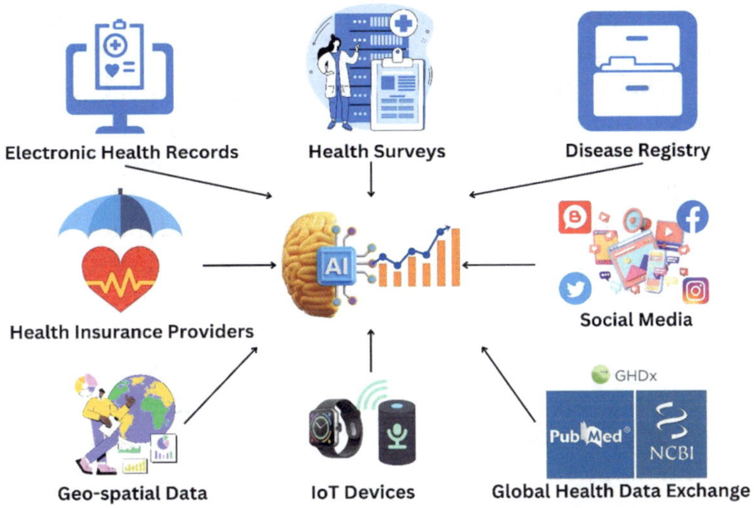

Figure 5.3. Historical development of disease surveillance has roots tracing back to ancient civilizations.

Source: https://www.pashudhanpraharee.com/wp-content/uploads/2024/08/Picture4-4.png.

5.1.1. Early Methods of Disease Tracking

In the history of public health, early disease tracking has been crucial in containing infectious diseases. Conventional surveillance methods relied on clinical reports, where doctors notified health officials of diagnosed cases. This tended to create a response delay due to inaccurate and incomplete information. Despite this, historical records indicate the worth of organized surveillance that arose during outbreaks. For example, John Snow's efforts during the mid-19th-century cholera epidemic in London best illustrated the dynamic of geographic disease mapping, and it formed the basis of what has come to be known as spatial epidemiology. By examining mortality statistics in conjunction with water source distribution, Snow effectively highlighted contaminated water as a significant vehicle for disease transmission, thereby underscoring the value of precise tracking of outbreaks to guide public health interventions. Because of new trends in monitoring, statistical models and data visualization played a significant role in understanding how diseases develop. The use of an epidemic curve, which charts the spread of an outbreak over time, helped epidemiologists find out the reasons and patterns of infection more clearly. Thanks to using statistics, the first approaches showed that epidemics tend to follow a pattern, which made it simpler for public health officials to plan their actions. Also, surveillance systems now include laboratory findings to confirm the pathogens that caused the outbreaks. With the help of clinical, spatial, and laboratory data collection, the infectious disease surveillance environment was improved, so that it could respond proactively to upcoming threats. Additionally, community involvement in healthcare facilitated early disease detection. Local health authorities involved communities in surveillance and they encouraged people to report any symptoms or cases through outreach. Due to this model, officials were able to identify more cases and detect outbreaks more quickly. Additionally, the advent of such technology as telegraphs and later radio communication facilitated the dissemination of information among health units more effectively. For example, during the early 20th century, building national surveillance networks provided a more integrated system for tracking disease transmission across borders. Taken collectively, these early disease-tracking technologies established the fundamental basis for today's surveillance systems, as exemplified in recent innovations like wastewater monitoring, which applies these basic principles to track disease patterns with unprecedented success (Tiwari et al., 2023) and is integrated with advanced technologies like AI (Olaboye et al., 2024).

5.1.2. Development of Modern Surveillance Systems

The use of modern surveillance systems has significantly enhanced the ability to detect and control infectious diseases. Earlier, disease surveillance depended on people reporting and collecting information, which usually meant that responses to outbreaks were slow. With the creation of modern technologies such as the Internet of Things (IoT) and machine learning (ML), the process has been revolutionized. For instance, IoT inclusion, such as that enabled by smart thermometers and wearable sensors, facilitates the continuous collection of health-related information, allowing for real-time monitoring of potential outbreaks. By using deep learning methods, more specifically recurrent neural networks (RNNs), health authorities can identify temporal patterns that would be characteristic of infectious disease outbreaks, thereby enabling early intervention. This technological innovation highlights the importance of rapid identification and effective response measures, which are especially important in the event of public health crises, particularly within the context of EIDs and pandemics (Sumithra et al., 2025). The integration of genomic surveillance into contemporary infectious disease monitoring shows a significant improvement in public health readiness. The international reaction to the COVID-19 pandemic underscored the importance of pathogen genomic monitoring, particularly in tracking and controlling the emergence of SARS-CoV-2 strains. Through a One Health strategy, health systems can close the loop between human, animal, and environmental health, optimising their capacity to respond to complex health challenges. The integration of real-time whole genome sequence (WGS) data enables public health officials to guide clinical practice, inform infection control interventions, and inform vaccine strategies efficiently. This holistic method of data integration not only enhances the transmission dynamics insight but also promotes coordinated action across disciplines, which is critical in containing infectious diseases in our globalised world (Struelens et al., 2024). Additionally, the multi-agency nature of these contemporary surveillance systems highlights the importance of inter-sectoral alliances and information exchange. Surveillance of infectious diseases is only effective when there is collaboration of efforts across the healthcare, public health, veterinary, and environmental sectors to build a comprehensive appreciation for health threats. As demonstrated during the COVID-19 pandemic, intersectoral collaboration establishes a robust response network with the potential to combat the complexities of AMR and emerging pathogens. The implementation of standards such as FAIR (findability, accessibility, interoperability, and reusability) emphasises the importance of responsible data exchange between global surveillance networks. By focusing on international collaboration and standardising laboratory practices, actors can streamline reporting processes, ultimately making global public health more resilient to infectious diseases. These constant advancements in surveillance systems are indicative of an anticipatory move towards protecting human, animal, and environmental health during the age of fast-paced technological progress (Struelens et al., 2024) (Figure 5.4).

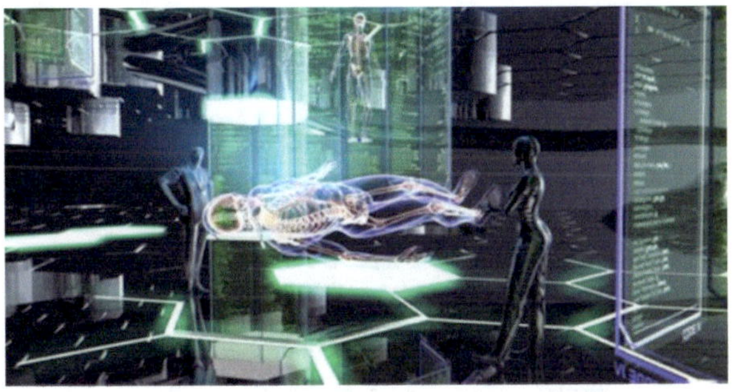

Figure 5.4. Development of modern surveillance systems.

Source: https://external-content.duckduckgo.com/iu/?u=https%3A%2F%2Ftse3.mm.bing.net%2Fth%3Fid%3DOIP.Ue9xYfetes1lOCf-QegSmAHaD8%26pid%3DApi&f=1&ipt=4cab844799d9b6b4c3e47b8407d18e5c20a9ce68f54adef78da384f4150d0fab.

5.1.3. Key Historical Outbreaks and Their Impact on Surveillance

The historical background of infectious disease epidemic occurrence has had a very significant impact on the development of disease surveillance systems. Severe outbreaks, like the influenza pandemic of 1918 and the onset of HIV/AIDS in the latter half of the 20th century, have led public health agencies to evolve their data collection and analysis techniques. Due to these events, it became clear that swift action is necessary to prevent epidemics and that a more effective system is required to monitor and track diseases. As a result, building detailed surveillance systems became necessary, since they help both with current cases and with predicting future outbreaks. Experience from past epidemics helps guide decisions that can prevent such events from happening again and also aid in adapting to new challenges in infectious disease epidemiology. The COVID-19 pandemic in recent years has shed light on the role of surveillance in preventing infectious disease epidemics. Data collected during the period revealed pervasive shifts in epidemiological trends, particularly following the introduction and lifting of non-pharmaceutical interventions (NPIs). A study in Bavaria revealed that relaxation of NPIs resulted in variable epidemiological responses among diseases, for example, a rapid rise in influenza cases over pre-pandemic trends. The catch-up effect strongly reminded us of the interconnectivity of disease patterns, necessitating a reconsideration of accessible surveillance strategies. The study showed that dynamic and continuous monitoring systems played a pivotal role in reaction to the unstable nature of infectious diseases, which had been affected not only by natural viral behaviors but also by public health interventions. The retrospective analysis of outbreaks such as brucellosis and tuberculosis in Saudi Arabia also demonstrates the continued value of high-quality surveillance mechanisms. Surveillance indicates that there are significant trends related to gender and nationality for these infections, requiring specific public health approaches to deal with particular groups. In the context of the COVID-19 pandemic, the rates of many bacterial infections declined, requiring a reappraisal of how surveillance systems can increase sensitivity and specificity. Upcoming developments in disease surveillance should incorporate the integration of various factors, including travel history and hospitalisation rates. Through the modification of lessons derived from past outbreaks, public health officials can enhance responses to upcoming infectious disease crises, in the end, prioritising the most urgent health threats as revealed by information from previous epidemics (Alhumaid et al., 2024; Hausmann et al., 2024).

5.2. Types of Surveillance Systems

Surveillance systems are essential for infectious disease monitoring and control, as they enable the collection, analysis, and dissemination of health information. Surveillance systems can be broadly categorized into various types that serve different functions in public health systems. The most commonly used is passive surveillance, where healthcare providers report infectious disease cases to public health officials. The method relies on routine data collection, which traditionally results in underreporting due to its reliance on clinical diagnosis and voluntary reporting. Active surveillance, however, involves active case finding where the public health authorities go out of their way to seek out cases by means of surveys, interviews, or laboratory tests, ensuring wider collection of data and higher accuracy in the detection of disease outbreaks. Syndromic surveillance is another significant type of surveillance that monitors health-related information to identify potential outbreaks before actual diagnosis.

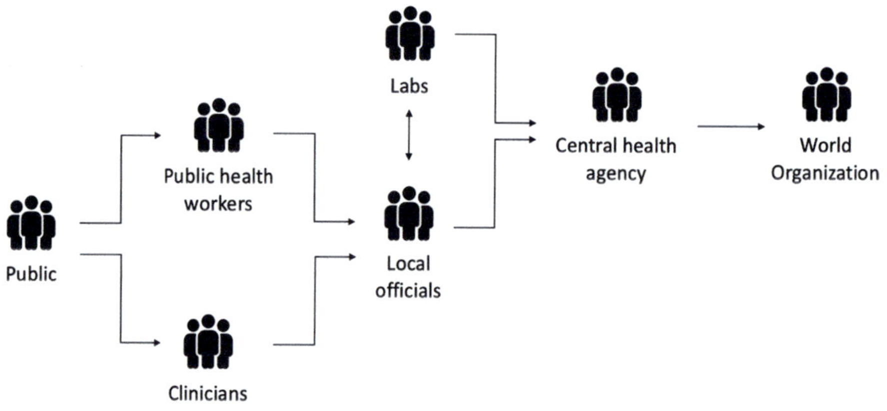

Figure 5.5. Types of surveillance systems.

Source: https://emergencies.pubpub.org/pub/surveillance-and-early-warning/release/3.

Syndromic surveillance utilises various data sources, including emergency department visits, pharmacy sales, and over-the-counter drug purchases, to identify unusual patterns of symptoms. Syndromic surveillance has also become extremely relevant in the event of public health emergencies, such as the COVID-19 pandemic, where early detection can facilitate timely intervention. Further, geospatial surveillance integrates geographic information systems (GIS) and epidemiological data, providing information on environmental determinants and population distribution as they aid the transmission of infectious diseases.

These new surveillance tools enhance the response to public health emergencies and enable more effective interventions among specific groups. Due to technological advances, digital surveillance now utilizes electronic health records, mobile apps, and social media. Thanks to these systems, health authorities can get and analyze data in real time, which helps them act rapidly when EIDs occur. For instance, contact tracing applications enable the identification of potential exposure in minutes, allowing for prompt quarantining of affected individuals. Moreover, artificial intelligence (AI) applications in surveillance systems can aid in predictive modelling capabilities to forecast outbreaks and efficiently distribute resources. Although digital surveillance systems are helpful, there is concern about the privacy and safety of patients' data.

Ensuring the ethical application of such systems is most critical as public health organisations continue to streamline their strategies for epidemic control and disease prevention, as exemplified by the emergent need for data expansion in low-resource settings to address antimicrobial resistance (AMR), as reported in recent literature (Roth et al., 2020; Murray et al., 2022) (Figure 5.5).

5.2.1. Passive Surveillance

Passive surveillance is a cornerstone of infectious disease surveillance and monitoring, providing a systematic way to track and identify trends in disease occurrence over time. Passive surveillance uses information from existing healthcare systems, which get data from healthcare providers, laboratories, and institutions. Since this system is decentralized, information is constantly being gathered, letting public health workers spot trends in specific groups or areas. Even so, passive surveillance provides a clear picture of disease rates, but it is influenced by reporting biases and disparities in healthcare access, which can render the data unreliable.

This means that different approaches are needed, particularly when it comes to eliminating diseases, as research and planning indicate. It is evident from evidence that the weaknesses of passive surveillance are most noticeable when trying to eradicate malaria. When the goal of public health is to eliminate diseases, the systems must be more active, so active surveillance is needed. Active surveillance involves taking steps to identify new cases, primarily in areas with a high risk of infection or where infection rates are increasing, to compensate for the limitations of traditional passive systems. For instance, a study evaluating the patterns of malaria transmission in southern China identified trends that necessitated enhanced surveillance systems to effectively control disease foci, illustrating that passive surveillance is inadequate for evidence-based decision-making in elimination settings (Shi et al., 2021). This understanding demonstrates a broader perception of disease dynamics, displaying the need for flexible surveillance systems that combine both passive and active components to provide strong monitoring of infectious disease threat.

Additionally, the development of public health surveillance indicates the need for an association between environmental data and disease incidence, further adding to the complexity of passive surveillance. The U.S. Centers for Disease Control and Prevention's program to create the Environmental Public Health Tracking (EPHT) network illustrates the need to develop further surveillance methods to get better a picture of health threats, including those environmental factors that have an impact on disease prevalence (Balmes et al., 2004). This effort underscores the importance of recognising that passive surveillance is not a standalone solution; to be effective, it must be complemented by new data integration initiatives that further expand our understanding of disease patterns and risk factors. As we move toward advanced monitoring systems, the challenge is to balance resource management while ensuring that such hybrid models assess exposure pathways and effectively address emerging public health challenges in real time (Figure 5.6).

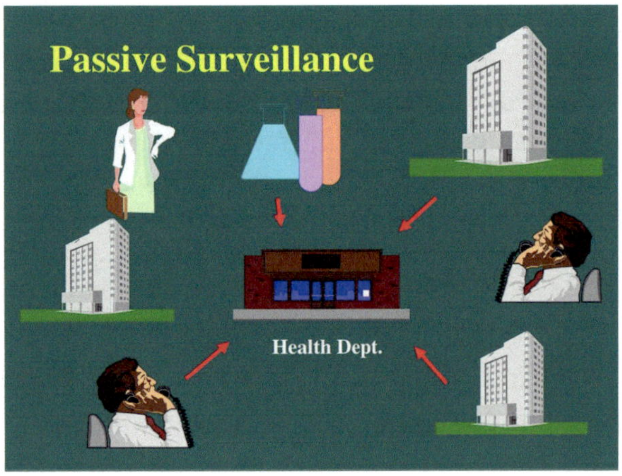

Figure 5.6. Passive surveillance.

Source: https://image.slideserve.com/247395/passive-surveillance12-l.jpg.

5.2.2. Active Surveillance

Active surveillance is a crucial component in public health policies for monitoring and regulating infectious diseases. Active surveillance is a systematic process for disease incidence and prevalence collection, usually through direct contact with healthcare practitioners and laboratories. It differs from passive surveillance, which depends on voluntary reporting of information, as active surveillance actively solicits data for a better understanding of disease dynamics in a population.

Such techniques significantly enhance epidemiologic insight, enabling health agencies to quickly detect outbreaks and allocate appropriate resources for prevention and care. Public health organizations can utilize active surveillance to engage health care providers, fostering collaboration and ensuring high-quality data collection. Such collaboration is essential during epidemics when information must be made available urgently to make evidence-based decisions and contain disease transmission. The impact of active surveillance is better understood when considering its application in individual infectious diseases, like hepatitis C virus (HCV) infection. The AASLD-IDSA HCV guidance project is an example of how active surveillance works in real-life settings, providing up-to-date information and guidance for the management of HCV infections worldwide. The project collects information from different healthcare facilities which helps us spot patterns in HCV cases and their treatment outcomes. It is in agreement with the WHO's goals to eliminate hepatitis C as a public health risk by 2030. In fact, the multidimensional extent of active surveillance ensures that the data acquired are not only plentiful but also meaningful, thereby guiding well-focused interventions that eventually yield better health outcomes among targeted populations (Ghany et al., 2019). In addition, active surveillance encompasses various techniques and methodologies for managing different infectious diseases, including those that present challenges due to antibiotic resistance.

The rise of antibiotic-resistant bacteria is a significant threat to public health, especially in the developing world where surveillance infrastructures might not be well developed. It is crucial to monitor antibiotic use and resistance in these areas, particularly in agriculture, as antibiotic residues can contaminate food. Antibiotic surveillance and resistance should be improved by collaboration between local, regional, and global stakeholders. Sustaining strong surveillance systems fosters effective monitoring, which finally leads to curbing the transmission of antibiotic resistance and safeguarding the effectiveness of current treatment regimens. This emphasizes the need to spread correct information and ensure responsible antibiotic stewardship in many areas of health and agriculture (Manyi-Loh et al., 2018) (Figure 5.7).

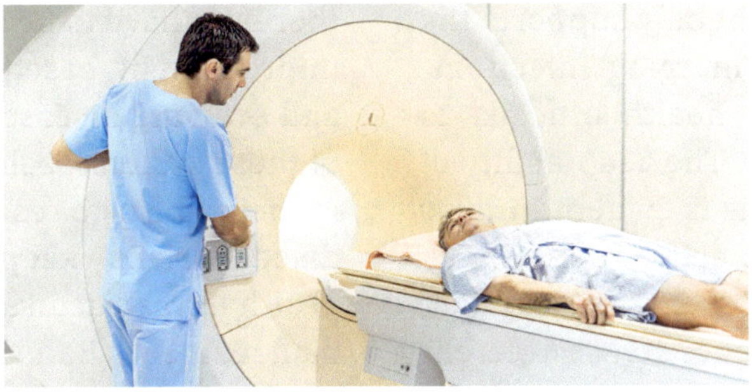

Figure 5.7. Active surveillance.

Source: https://external-content.duckduckgo.com/iu/?u=https%3A%2F%2Fstatic.inspire.com%2Fsponsored-resource-center%2Fimages%2Fgb21x26ak63g_6FxZ97Z74SbdZY8GDzuTTK_d322c1518270ecd84709ba4cdcd57049_Prostate_Cancer_Active_Surveillance__OG_.jpg&f=1&nofb=1&ipt=8e2965c5339fad615b38ed4cf3c6d6d0437404dd6a66980bd866495fd8ba3d6f.

5.2.3. Sentinel Surveillance

Sentinel surveillance is a crucial component of the broader context of infectious disease monitoring, serving as a strategic system for the early detection and control of disease outbreaks. Sentinel surveillance is distinct from conventional methods that may necessitate extensive, across-the-board testing in many geographic locales, as sentinel surveillance targets select sites or populations that are especially representative or at high risk.

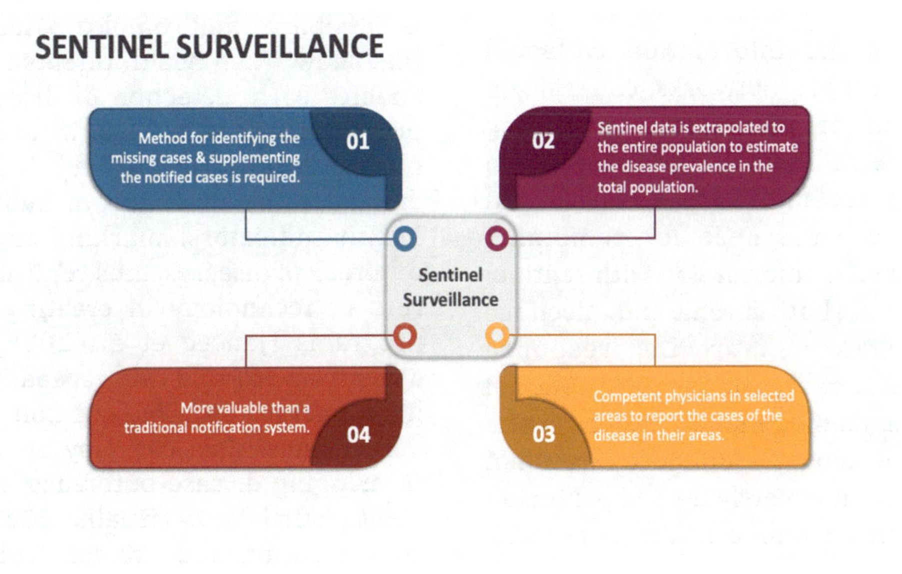

Figure 5.8. Sentinel surveillance.

Source: https://www.collidu.com/media/catalog/product/img/1/d/1d811c3d29b480a66ff7063518cd1b124c6b3dd2cdb96e7d30d8c8843092d0c2/sentinel-surveillance-slide1.png.

This focused strategy not only supports the early detection of newly emerging infections, but it also enables public health officials to manage resources optimally. The adaptability of sentinel surveillance systems is evident in their design, which often involves active reporting by healthcare providers, making them robust against fluctuations in disease incidence across different settings. As emphasised by recent research on animal disease, as in the case of Bluetongue Virus management, targeted surveillance interventions can drastically reduce the likelihood of outbreaks (Carrasco et al., 2025). Sentinel surveillance is effective in that it both involves real-time data generation and purposeful public health intervention. Through sentinel sites available—whether in clinics, hospitals, or in agricultural environments—health authorities can monitor trends and infections that pose a risk to public health. These can be implemented immediately, such as vaccination campaigns in high-risk areas, thereby halting the transmission of infectious diseases.

Additionally, the information collected through these expert networks can inform broader systems of surveillance, providing policymakers with insights into trends in disease emergence and spread. Successful cases demonstrate the need for combining environmental health information with sentinel surveillance to meet both chronic and infectious diseases, ultimately improving response measures (Balmes et al., 2004). While sentinel surveillance has many benefits, it also has its limitations. The need for stable operational infrastructure and adequately trained personnel can put a strain on public health resources, especially in health systems that are not well-resourced. In addition, its effectiveness can be compromised by factors like underreporting, unstable population health care access, and variability in the criteria for case identification. An effective sentinel surveillance system will therefore have to be adaptive and permit system improvement based on information collected and evolving disease trends. The final yardstick of these systems' achievement, nonetheless, lies in their ability to respond to incoming infectious disease risks, keeping them part of public health infrastructure for prevention and disease management (Balmes et al., 2004; Carrasco et al., 2025) (Figure 5.8).

5.3. Technologies Used in Disease Monitoring

Now that the latest technologies are available, disease surveillance is significantly improved at detecting infectious diseases quickly and accurately. The technology that combines the Internet of Things (IoT) and deep learning algorithms is really revolutionary. The use of smart thermometers and wearables allows healthcare professionals to track health data from many people in real time. With RNNs, it is possible to find complex patterns in the data that show when health threats might appear. It enables early detection of diseases and helps prevent large outbreaks. In addition, the use of long short-term memory (LSTM) networks enhances the detection of subtle changes in health indicators, marking the onset of an outbreak of diseases, thus confirming the pivotal role of technology in creating public health programs (Jancee et al., 2025). In addition, aside from IoT and ML, geospatial technologies have emerged as a sine qua non tool for disease surveillance. GISs can play an important role in mapping disease outbreaks, enabling public health officials to visualize areas of infection concentration and project probable areas of future outbreaks. By integrating health data and geographic information, officials can monitor trends and allocate resources more effectively, targeting interventions to specific areas of disease occurrence. In addition, examining spatial patterns helps trace the movement of people during an outbreak, facilitating targeted testing and effective contact tracing activities. Grasping the spatial dynamics of disease spread is crucial for an effective public health response, providing key insights into containing and preventing the risks associated with infectious diseases (Ekirapa et al., 2011). To support these technological efforts, collaborative structures are critical to developing improved disease surveillance capacities at the local and global levels. Efforts like the Disease Surveillance Networks (DSN) place a strong emphasis on traditional partnerships between multifaceted stakeholders, such as the government and private sectors. DSN emphasizes building technical capacity in countries to enhance response systems during outbreaks and promotes sharing the best practices across networks across borders. The addition of multidisciplinary methodologies follows an increased awareness that health problems frequently overlap across single sectors, thereby employing One Health strategies that incorporate environmental and animal health considerations. Through successful enhanced access to better monitoring equipment and driving innovation via collaboration, these networks establish the platform necessary for intense disease surveillance, eventually aiding in global health security (Ekirapa et al., 2011) (Figure 5.9).

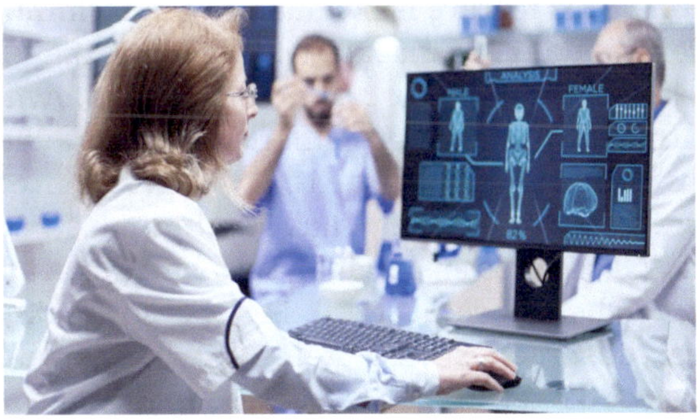

Figure 5.9. Technologies used in disease monitoring.

Source: https://drkumo.com/wp-content/uploads/2023/02/doctor-analyzing-patient-data-using-ai-in-healthcare.webp.

5.3.1. Data Collection Tools and Software

Using data collection software and tools is crucial for monitoring and surveillance of infectious diseases, as it enables public health officials to efficiently handle and interpret large amounts of health information. The tools allow the systematic gathering of information on disease incidence, demographic features, and possible risk factors, which eventually strengthens response strategies. For instance, Laboratory Information Management Systems (LIMS) have played a crucial role in laboratory sample handling, tracking test results, and integrating genomic information for a comprehensive understanding of pathogens. Due to these technologies, health agencies can handle procedures more efficiently, which enables them to spot outbreaks and respond more quickly. Advanced methods of data collection are primarily used to combat infectious diseases and maintain public safety and health. Advanced software systems such as SIEGA have significantly changed how contagious diseases are monitored. The tool is a good example of the One Health concept because it uses health information from people, animals, and the environment. It has managed to sequence over 1900 bacterial genomes, which helps explain how pathogens and their resistance change. SIEGA's ability to generate personalised reports and rapidly identify transmission chains is critical in responding to emerging health threats. SIEGA helps health authorities be more ready to respond to potential genetic threats. With these advanced data collection methods, the accuracy of following disease trends is improved, and stakeholders have the facts needed to create effective policies and actions. In addition, the potential for genomic data in surveillance systems cannot be overemphasised. Instruments based on raw whole-genome sequencing are vital to the discovery of genes associated with AMR and virulence, essential for solving modern health issues such as zoonotic diseases and antibiotic resistance (Casimiro-Soriguer et al., 2024). Bioinformatics integration into these data-gathering tools offers an analytical system for deciphering intricate biological data and determining pathways of infection transmission. With researchers and health practitioners increasingly using a data-based model, the importance of collaboration and sharing information grows stronger. In the end, the use of sophisticated data collection software creates a more comprehensive picture in the surveillance of infectious diseases, highlighting the relevance of a union-wide response plan across all the different areas of health (Casimiro-Soriguer et al., 2024) (Figure 5.10).

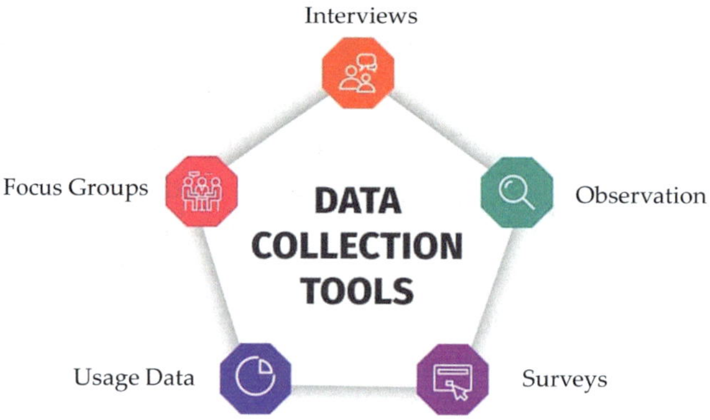

Figure 5.10. Data collection tools and software.

Source: https://www.questionpro.com/blog/wp-content/uploads/2019/06/DataCollectionTools.jpg.

5.3.2. Geographic Information Systems (GIS)

GIS are essential tools of contemporary epidemiology, especially in infectious disease surveillance and monitoring. GIS allows public health experts to combine information about health and geography which helps them study outbreaks across different regions. This feature is invaluable in determining outbreak "hot spots" and elucidating environmental determinants of disease spread. For example, mapping vector-borne diseases on geographic maps helps assess where the risks are, allowing interventions to be directed accordingly. Additionally, the ability to merge different types of data, such as population coverage or health access, enhances GIS's capacity to identify vulnerable areas during outbreaks. The combination of GIS with conventional epidemiology has revolutionized our infectious disease control strategy. Advanced GIS software facilitates easier analysis by public health professionals of spatial data, eliminating the need for specialised technical training, thereby making these tools more accessible and democratic. As has been observed, such systems provide new and growing possibilities for epidemiology since they enable an educated user to select among alternatives when geographic patterns are involved in the issue (Clarke et al., 1996). Thus, health officials can create actionable information that directs policy and resource decisions, so they can take action before problems arise. With this shift, the way diseases spread can be understood more clearly, which helps public health efforts succeed. Besides displaying data, GIS is used for decision-making and in the formation of public health policies. If health authorities can model how diseases spread, they can decide on the best interventions and how to use them. For instance, GIS can be used to simulate potential outbreaks and evaluate the effectiveness of vaccination campaigns through spatial pattern-based distribution analysis (Baldock et al., 2025). Since surveillance is using more data, using GIS in public health is an essential step to help health systems be more ready and responsive. With the help of these systems, public health practitioners can have a more holistic approach to controlling infectious diseases, making responses oriented to the particular geographic and epidemiologic context of each outbreak (Figure 5.11).

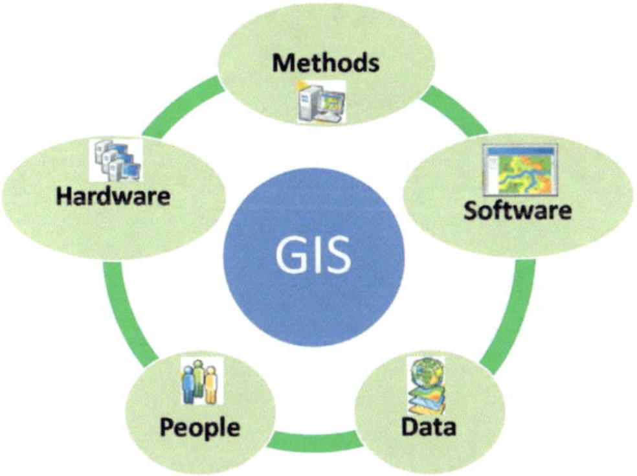

Figure 5.11. Geographic information systems (GIS).

Source: https://1.bp.blogspot.com/-TxfluLf0uy0/XOu75pEjtLI/AAAAAAAAAA8/k6TFC9n3Cc4xtF79zGvGkIJ6fYbpNTs_gCLcBGAs/s1600/introfig1.jpg.

5.3.3. Mobile Health Applications

The advent of mobile health apps has significantly transformed the landscape of infectious disease surveillance and tracking. Mobile health apps leverage the prevalence of smartphones to gather and analyze real-time health information, and thus allow for quick identification of disease outbreaks. By merging AI and data analytics, mobile health apps can track population health patterns, automate symptom monitoring, and provide early alerts for possible health threats. This forward thinking is a departure from previous methods of surveillance, which utilize slower systems of reporting that can have the potential to postpone public health responses. As such, the use of mobile health apps can enhance the capacity of authorities to respond promptly to infectious disease threats, which is crucial for controlling outbreaks before they escalate into larger public health emergencies (Olaboye et al., 2024). In places such as South Africa, the COVID-19 pandemic accelerated the use of innovative digital health interventions, further proving the effectiveness of mobile health technologies. As per current research, different digital technologies such as SMS-based interventions, telemedicine, and mobile applications were used to carry out screenings, track disease progression, and enhance communication during the pandemic (Mbunge et al., 2022). These applications provide crucial functionality like self-assessment of symptoms that enables one to track his or her state of health and minimize the workload on healthcare facilities. In addition, the inclusion of health applications in the monitoring of behavior and contact tracing has enabled transmission patterns to be identified, thereby making targeted interventions possible. This highlights the critical role of mobile health apps in strengthening public health interventions and guiding resource allocation during infectious disease outbreaks. As promising as mobile health apps are for disease surveillance, enormous challenges must be surmounted to make them effective and gain mainstream acceptance. Data privacy, security, and access are some of the concerns that limit the full potential of these technologies. Most people might be reluctant to provide personal health information because they fear surveillance or abuse, making data-driven responses less effective. Also, inequalities in access to the internet and digital skills have the potential to worsen health disparities, putting vulnerable groups at risk. To break these barriers, it is essential to have robust privacy legislation in place and to establish outreach channels that educate users about the benefits of mobile health apps. By overcoming these challenges, public health agencies can maximally utilize digital health technologies to enhance surveillance and monitoring of infectious diseases, ultimately improving health outcomes for all communities (Mbunge et al., 2022; Olaboye et al., 2024) (Figure 5.12).

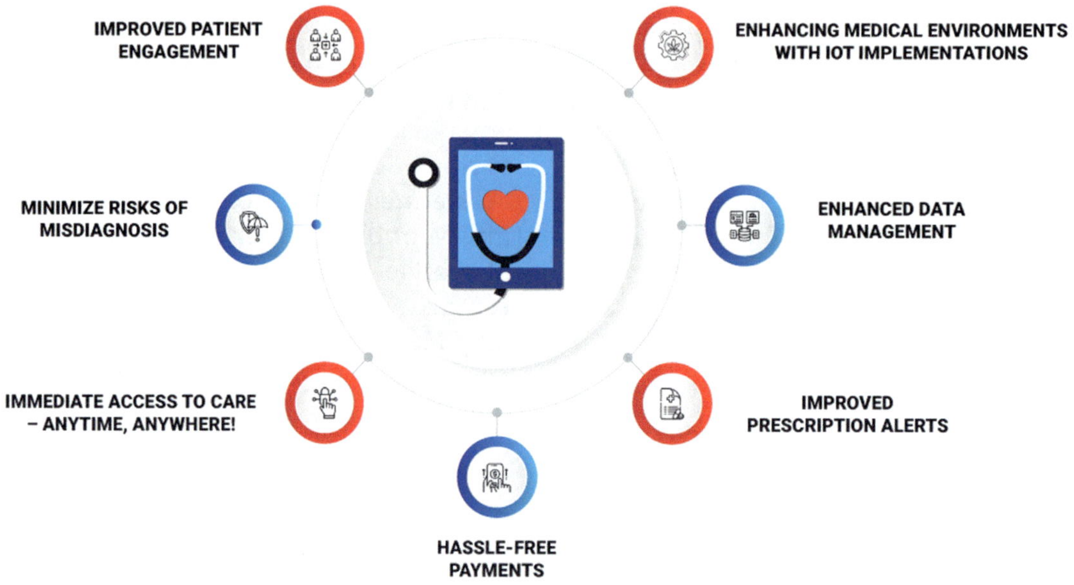

Figure 5.12. Mobile health applications.

Source: https://www.rishabhsoft.com/wp-content/uploads/2018/01/Benefits_Benefits-of-Mobile-Apps-for-Healthcare-Industry.jpg.

5.4. Role of Government and Public Health Organizations

Monitoring and surveillance of infectious diseases is primarily the responsibility of governments and public health agencies, which include gathering data and coordinating responses to emergencies. It is the duty of governments to establish effective monitoring systems that can detect and control outbreaks. This involves utilizing new technologies and health informatics, such as analyzing epidemiological trends in real-time. Additionally, public health agencies are responsible for helping different groups, such as local health departments, healthcare providers, and community agencies, coordinate to build a unified surveillance system. They help ensure that critical, essential data is adequately shared and promptly, which benefits decisions made in public health interventions. By concentrating efforts and resources, governments and public health agencies are better able to reduce the impact of infectious diseases on populations. The bioterrorism response also prompts serious questions about the systems that governments and public health agencies use. Surveillance systems need to address not only natural outbreaks but also be capable of dealing with possible biological threats, which tend to emulate infectious disease outbreaks. Integrating surveillance for both bioterrorism and emerging diseases is essential; as noted by Chyba (1998), differentiation between the two situations presents critical challenges to health authorities. Governments need to craft a communication strategy and protocols that maximize public awareness of possible threats. In the process, they can create an enlightened population more capable of participating in prevention activities and reporting suspicious cases promptly. Finally, a balanced strategy attends to both current infectious diseases and possible bioterrorist use, providing universal public health preparedness. Additionally, community involvement becomes a more critical factor in the quality of surveillance programs, especially when looking at the strength of community health workers (CHWs). Effective case management of diseases such as malaria demonstrates how local levels can enhance the sensitivity of surveillance systems. As highlighted in Buj et al. (2014), appropriately trained CHWs are capable of conducting diagnostic tests and delivering quality care, thus acting as essential bridging structures between the community and the formal health systems. If health systems provide CHWs with training and a sufficient budget, it will be easier to collect data and monitor diseases. This way of working enables the identification of infectious diseases and the observation of health patterns in various communities. Governments and public health authorities, through leveraging local knowledge and experience, can build a more resilient healthcare system that is adequately equipped to deal with public health challenges.

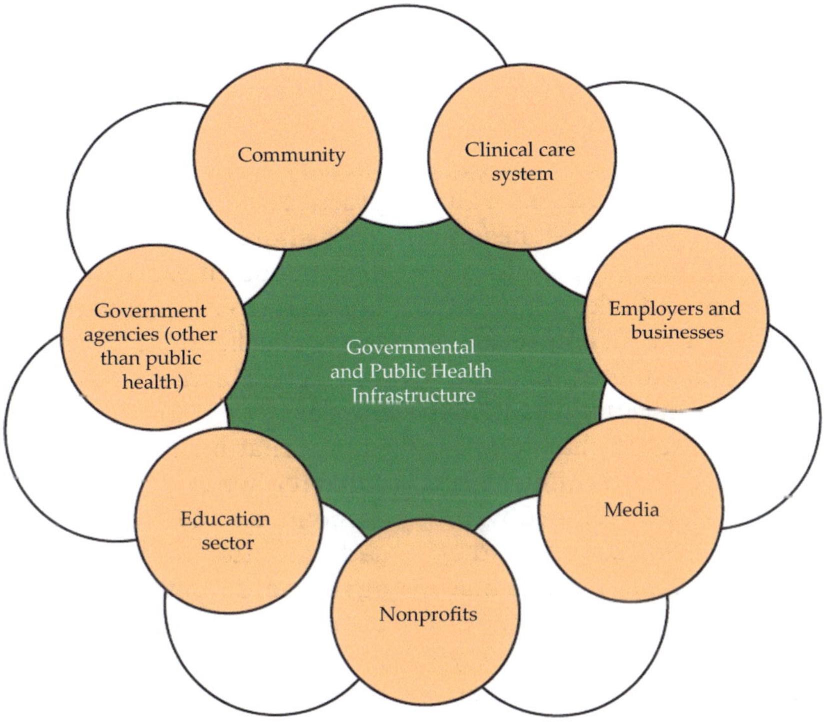

Figure 5.13. The role of government and public health organizations.

Source: https://nap.nationalacademies.org/openbook/23471/xhtml/images/img-213-1.jpg.

5.4.1. National Health Agencies and Their Responsibilities

National health agencies play a crucial role in public health infrastructure, monitoring and tracking infectious diseases within their respective areas. They do more than collect data; they carefully analyze and explain the information to follow the spread of diseases. Health agencies at the national level use complete frameworks to gather information on diseases, which requires cooperation from health care, government, and research organizations. Promoting integrated approaches enables national health authorities to design timely measures that prevent the spread of disease and keep the public safe. Efficient utilization and management of health data are fundamental to enhancing response strategies as well as ensuring that policies for health are evidence-based and responsive to such emerging issues as pandemics. Aside from their functions in data management, national health authorities also have the responsibility to respond to health emergencies that occur from natural epidemics and anthropogenic challenges, such as bioterrorism. The ability to detect and react in a timely manner to such incidents plays a vital role in reducing potential harm to populations. The review of earlier events suggests that it would be challenging to distinguish between bioterror attacks and natural epidemics. It is the job of national health organizations to build up their preparedness systems to spot these risks and take action to protect the public. This requirement emphasises the need for training, collaboration, and determining effective communication channels among different stakeholders so that health organisations can marshal resources effectively and respond promptly to health crises (Chyba, 1998). National health agencies also bear the responsibility to advocate for policy reforms that promote food safety and public health strategies in general. Comparing the impacts of food safety reforms across various countries and regions can provide valuable insights into enhancing data collection and analysis systems. Coordination across public health agencies is critical in developing harmonized surveillance activities that not only monitor infectious diseases but also emphasize prevention measures. National health agencies are therefore essential in responding to not only short-term health emergencies but also in developing long-term public health policies that encourage well-being and prevent disease outbreaks. Recommendations of U.S. programs, policies, and activities emphasize the necessity of ongoing improvement and responsiveness in national health approaches, ultimately supporting the stability and effectiveness of public health systems (N/A, 2010).

5.4.2. International Collaboration and Organizations

The role of global cooperation in monitoring and surveillance of infectious diseases has grown more crucial in today's globalized world. The WHO and similar organizations help coordinate international action on health problems, share important information, and unite how data is collected. When nations cooperate in this way, outbreaks are easier to find early, which helps reduce the risk of pandemics. Additionally, collaborating with other countries enables the sharing of resources, information, and best practices, which helps improve health systems. Joint efforts can significantly limit the impact of infectious disease outbreaks, as seen during the COVID-19 pandemic, when exceptional levels of collaboration were established to track and regulate the virus's transmission across borders. One of the significant challenges in international cooperation is the unequal capacity among countries to monitor and respond to infectious diseases. Low-resource settings often demonstrate limited access to advanced surveillance technologies and data collection systems. This disparity can lead to underreporting and inadequate response measures, ultimately compromising global health security. Organizations committed to international health should prioritize developing programs to increase laboratory capacity and enhance the collection of epidemiological data in these nations. With the correction of these imbalances, global collaborations can better prevent infectious disease spread and ensure all countries make stringent contributions to international surveillance efforts in global health. Such initiatives are necessary to address the ongoing challenge of AMR, which poses a significant threat to health and necessitates coordinated international action to enhance surveillance and prevention measures (Murray et al., 2022). Being open and sharing information is very important for successful cooperation in monitoring infectious diseases worldwide. Nations must implement standard reporting criteria and share information promptly to provide timely responses to new threats. Organizations like the Global Outbreak Alert and Response Network demonstrate such an attitude by unifying various stakeholders in a practice of keeping track of disease outbreaks in real-time. Furthermore, the involvement of non-state actors, including research centres and non-governmental organisations (NGOs), deepens the shared knowledge pool and incites creative solutions. The use of more surveillance systems worldwide makes it simpler to notice trends and apply interventions based on evidence, which boosts our ability to respond to future outbreaks. This predictive trend is particularly relevant when solving for the surge in noncommunicable diseases caused by infectious pathogens, where complete data can spur focused prevention efforts (Roth et al., 2020) (Figure 5.14).

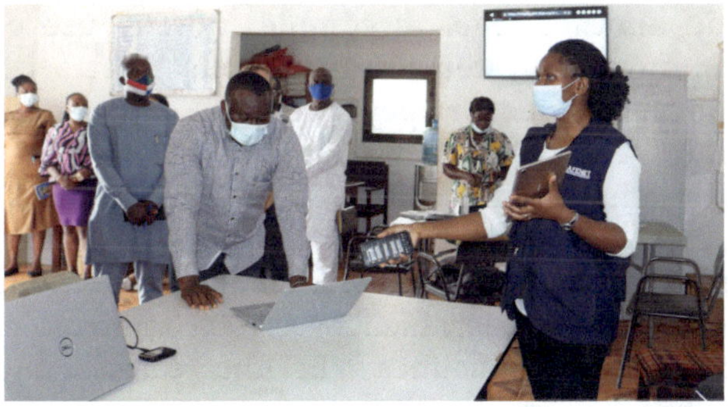

Figure 5.14. International collaboration and organizations.

Source: https://www.cdc.gov/global-health-protection/media/images/stories-from-the-field-old/Surveillance_Systems_Featured.jpg.

5.4.3. Policy-Making and Funding for Surveillance Programs

The success of infectious disease surveillance programs relies heavily on strong policies and effective funding mechanisms. Setting up systems for data collection and analysis should be a main priority for policymakers to monitor disease outbreaks. It means having laws as well as a commitment to teamwork with other fields, which is not limited to public health. The DSN Initiative makes it obvious that multi-sector cooperation is needed, as shown by the Rockefeller Foundation's findings in different areas. These studies demonstrate that having integrated disease surveillance systems enables communities to respond more promptly to emerging health threats, thereby strengthening their resistance to infectious diseases. Due to weak policies and inconsistent funding, these programs fail to reach their full potential, which in turn encourages people to demand more investment in healthcare. Besides making policies, ensuring sufficient funding for surveillance programs is also crucial for their success. Wealth facilitates the application of technology-based methods for the collection of data, training of personnel, and community mobilization efforts to raise public knowledge about infectious diseases. The assessment of current programs reveals that successful funding can significantly support the ability to monitor, and this ability can lead to improved health outcomes. In particular, reviews from initiatives such as the DSN provide insight into how strategic investment in connected networks can lead to more efficient disease identification and response approaches. For instance, evaluating the correlation between the level of funding and the surveillance results sheds light on how funding translates to actual public health outcomes. Policymakers must thus be aware of the key connection between the funding and the general sustainability of infectious disease surveillance activities. In addition, harmonizing funding mechanisms with holistic policy regulations is crucial for enhancing the strategic objectives of surveillance programs. Policymakers would do well to look to the incorporation of evidence-based advice from effective surveillance programs, including those in food safety. Reviewing the impact of such other reforms on data integration and prevention can give valuable lessons for enhancing infectious disease monitoring. Policy and funding mechanisms should be structured to maintain a unified approach that enables data sharing and inter-agency collaboration. By adopting these standard approaches, policymakers can design an environment that not only expands the scope of current surveillance programs but also lays a solid foundation for adapting to future public health emergencies. This overall strategy serves as the basis for the need for focused investment in health surveillance infrastructure to mitigate the impact of infectious diseases on global health systems.

5.5. Challenges in Surveillance and Monitoring

The successful monitoring and surveillance of infectious diseases are challenged by a myriad of issues that can severely erode the effectiveness of public health interventions. The most urgent requirement is for timely and accurate data collection, which is often hindered by the poor infrastructure in much of the country, particularly in rural or underdeveloped regions. Historical surveillance techniques, although essential, may not be sensitive enough or large-scale enough to capture outbreaks at their inception. More advanced technologies, such as digital epidemiology and data analysis, have been developed; however, their application is not consistent due to costs, technical, and human capacity constraints. Additionally, there needs to be someone accountable for gathering and interpreting such information, which calls for skilled personnel who are frequently in short supply or not adequately trained, especially in developing nations where infectious diseases have the most tremendous impact. Another significant challenge in communicable disease surveillance is integrating information from diverse sectors and fields. Efficient monitoring calls for coordination among health organisations, government agencies, and non-governmental organisations. Nonetheless, inconsistencies in communication, varying standards of data, and divergent goals among stakeholders may hamper effective sharing of robust data and cooperation. For example, healthcare systems may concentrate more on non-communicable diseases, thereby ignoring infectious disease preparedness and exposing themselves to acute outbreaks. As seen in the COVID-19 pandemic, the international community of health suffered from a cripplingly fragmented response to sharing data and information, creating an exacerbation of the health effects of the virus on global public health systems (Jackson et al., 2020). Without the streamlined integration of surveillance data, the capacity to respond to emerging threats is significantly reduced. Lastly, the ethical aspects of surveillance activities add another level of complexity. The use of monitoring systems is commonly met with concerns over privacy and data protection, which can result in public mistrust and non-adherence. For instance, the application of intrusive tracking technologies to track disease transmission may elicit fear among populations suspicious of government overreach or intrusion. In addition, inequalities in healthcare access and technology can lead to unequal surveillance practices, hence marginalized groups staying hidden in monitoring systems. Mitigating these ethical challenges is crucial for developing effective surveillance mechanisms that are accepted by the community. Using responsible and inclusive practices that are centered on transparency and citizen engagement will be critical for addressing such problems as well as increasing the surveillance of infectious diseases in future situations (Scheidwasser et al., 2025) (Figure 5.15).

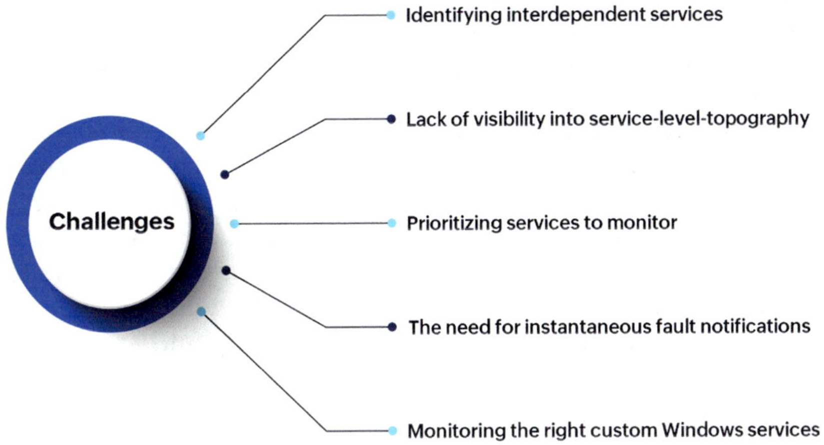

Figure 5.15. Challenges in surveillance and monitoring.

Source: https://www.manageengine.com/network-monitoring/images/windows-service-monitoring-challenges-1.jpg.

5.5.1. Data Privacy and Ethical Concerns

The expansion of digital surveillance and monitoring technologies for infectious diseases has raised significant concerns about data privacy and ethical considerations in their use. As more health authorities come to depend on geospatial analytics and artificial intelligence to tackle public health emergencies, problems such as consent, anonymisation, and data misuse have taken centre stage. For example, although the integration of different data sources can contribute to the improvement of disease surveillance, it also carries the risk of revealing personal information about subjects and thus violating their right to privacy. Ethical data handling is essential, as violations can result not only in a loss of public confidence in health organizations but also in unforeseen negative impacts on individuals under surveillance. So, it is critical to balance the importance of disease surveillance with the rights of individuals when planning future public health programs. The use of AI and mobile health data in infectious disease surveillance raises concerns that go beyond privacy alone. AI algorithms used in predictive modeling use data that can reflect past discrimination. This can lead to specific populations being identified incorrectly or overlooked, thereby increasing health inequalities rather than reducing them. Furthermore, as corporations amass and analyze enormous amounts of individual health information from mobile apps, the transparency of data practices is of primary importance. People need to be notified not only of how data will be utilized, but also of the possible consequences related to its gathering and analysis. The moral application of technology in this field requires strong frameworks with emphasis on fairness and accountability to guarantee that the advantages of surveillance are not at the expense of people's rights. Ultimately, the moral landscape of data privacy in the surveillance and monitoring of infectious diseases remains complex and nuanced. With every advancing innovation in technology, there is a challenge for health authorities to come up with clear policies and regulations that solve these challenges. The adoption of responsible data governance models is critical to curtail risks of data misuse and breaches. Additionally, collaborating with communities to foster greater understanding and acceptance of surveillance efforts can help establish trust, which is crucial in ensuring effective public health responses. By prioritizing ethics and privacy over technological development, health authorities can establish a surveillance model that balances public health with individual rights and social values. The debate that will continue to take place regarding the consequences of data use within epidemic control will be crucial to influence policies that conform to both public health objectives and to ethics (Figure 5.16).

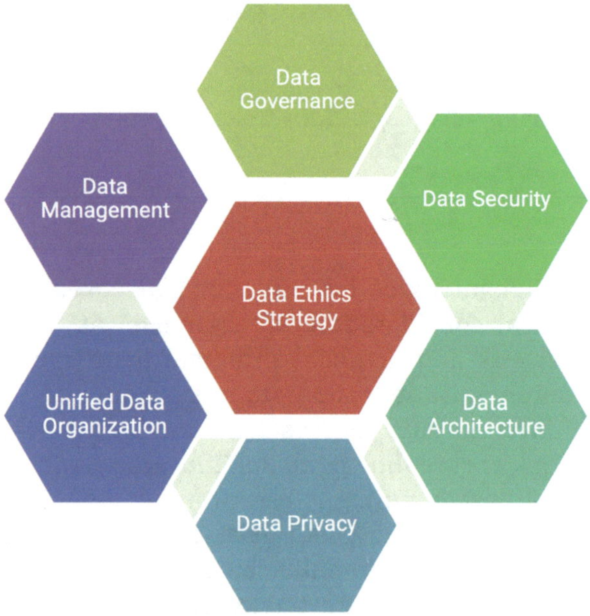

Figure 5.16. Data privacy and ethical concerns.

Source: https://www.informatica.com/content/dam/informatica-com/en/blogs/uploads/2021/blog-images/data-ethics-strategy.png.

5.5.2. Resource Limitations and Funding Issues

In infectious disease surveillance, resource shortages and funding constraints significantly impede effective response and monitoring efforts. Developing nations often face significant challenges in human resources, technology infrastructure, and funding, which can significantly hinder their ability to identify and respond to outbreaks. The Rockefeller Foundation's DSN Program was initiated to enhance human resources for disease surveillance in these areas so that national capacities for disease monitoring and reporting disease events would be improved. However, even with such programs, most countries fail to sustain these efforts in the long run due to ongoing financial constraints, which raise questions about the sustainability and effectiveness of surveillance systems within these vulnerable regions (Ancheta et al., 2010). The continuity of inadequate funding eventually prevents the construction of integrated networks that are required for quality disease monitoring and response. Furthermore, geographical disparities in funding distribution exacerbate existing gaps in disease surveillance capabilities. Capacity for early detection of outbreaks in many developing countries is still alarmingly low, primarily due to the fact that funding focuses on regions that already have strong health systems. This disparity hinders attempts to connect surveillance strategies for emerging and overlooked endemic zoonoses; areas that are most at risk frequently lack the available resources needed to apply effective surveillance measures (Bronsvoort et al., 2012). The multifaceted global regulatory landscape, coupled with inadequate communication between institutions and communities, hinders the integration of a unified response to infectious disease threats. The funding priorities need to be reevaluated with the focus on ensuring resources are reallocated to areas that are weakest in terms of surveillance. To overcome the constraints resulting from funding deficiencies and resource availability, new models of surveillance collaboration need to be explored, especially in vulnerable regions. Regional networks can be invested in to encourage countries with similar health concerns to collaborate, thereby maximising resource use. The DSN Initiatives model, with its focus on collaboration for disease surveillance, is a prime example of this potential through the creation of partnerships to build regional expertise and capacity. Through the creation of platforms for collaborative funding and strategic assistance, nations can strengthen not just their surveillance systems but also overall health infrastructure (Ancheta et al., 2010). Ultimately, assigning priority to funding for diseases that are endemic in developing countries and establishing sustainable systems to track both emerging and enduring threats is a pragmatic and fair means of enhancing global health security (Figure 5.17).

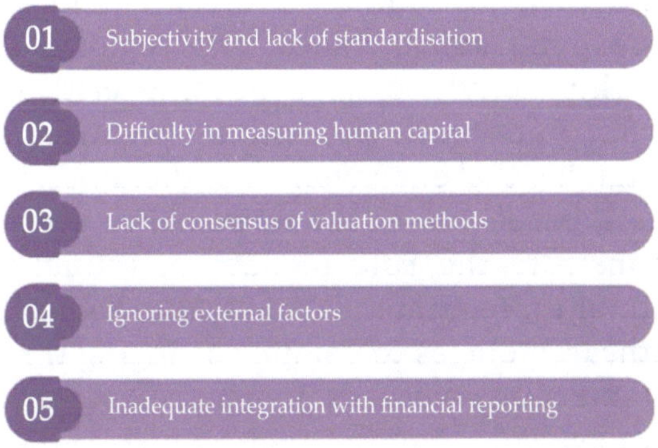

Figure 5.17. Resource limitations and funding issues.

Source: https://www.theknowledgeacademy.com/_files/images/Top_Limitations_of_Human_Resource_Accounting%282%29.png.

5.5.3. Variability in Reporting and Data Accuracy

There are often , significant differences in how reliable and accurate data is collected in different areas, which makes infectious disease surveillance more difficult. Inconsistency arises because various methods are employed to collect and report data, which can impact the accuracy and credibility of the information. If some healthcare facilities use technology differently, this can lead to unequal data transmission and analysis. When mixed with public and media perceptions, such inconsistency can alter the true picture of epidemiology. As emphasized by Chen et al. (2019), the re-emergence of infectious diseases presents considerable challenges in honestly evaluating and managing outbreaks. Hence, managing these inconsistencies in reporting becomes necessary to improve public health responses as well as sustain effective surveillance systems. The accuracy of data in infectious disease monitoring is essential, since errors have significant effects on public health interventions. Cases' detection variability usually stems from the disparate surveillance approaches used across different regions, as mentioned in Cliquet et al. (2019) raccoon rabies virus surveillance assessment. The research demonstrated that certain reporting methods, such as those involving unusual animal behaviour and deceased cases, had higher detection probabilities, underscoring the importance of method selection. In addition, the absence of standardized techniques supports the incidence of both under-reporting and over-reporting among diverse populations. Therefore, creating an integrated framework for surveillance that includes best practices from various approaches would be highly effective in offering improved accuracy in disease reporting and more credible information for decision-making. Apart from differences in methodology, demographic considerations can introduce significant variations in data accuracy and reporting. Groups with different access to healthcare and public health knowledge usually have quite different rates of infectious disease cases. Besides affecting the number of cases reported, this imbalance can also alter the perception of how many people are affected by the disease in a particular area. With the dynamics of online information during disease outbreaks, community responses can create panic and misinformation, further clouding the data landscape, as examined in Chen et al. (2019). Surveillance should also pay attention to these factors by analysing demographics to notice any trends in reporting locally. Only with an advanced method that handles data changes and the reasons behind them can effective surveillance systems be built to deal with the constant issues in infectious disease surveillance.

5.6. Case Studies of Successful Surveillance

Successful deployment of infectious disease surveillance systems is an essential component in public health responses. An example is the extensive analysis of AMR through recent large-scale analysis, where 4.95 million deaths linked to bacterial AMR were estimated in 2019 in 204 countries. The research employed a predictive statistical modeling method to assess data gathered from systematic reviews of literature and hospital surveillance, yielding substantial findings regarding the burden of AMR. By determining patterns in antibiotic resistance among several pathogens, this research effectively mobilized resources as well as informed health policy-making efforts targeted at reducing AMR's impact on global healthcare. Effective surveillance not only highlights key gaps in data—particularly in low-resource environments—but also underscores the need to scale up laboratory capacity to address this pressing concern (Murray et al., 2022). A notable second example of effective surveillance is the control of Helicobacter pylori infection, a cause of gastric cancer and peptic ulcers. The evolution from empirical trial-and-error treatments to an evidence-based therapy directed by antimicrobial stewardship principles defines a significant shift in the treatment of infectious diseases. Surveillance is now an essential component in the monitoring of treatment efficacy and resistance trends, enabling healthcare workers to tailor therapy according to local susceptibility data. This move underlines the importance of incorporating test of cure data into local stewardship initiatives. This integration guarantees best practices are shared with prescribers as well as public health practitioners, and ultimately contributes to improved patient care while minimizing the risk of resistance emergence. It is a graphic demonstration of the role that systematic surveillance plays in the effective management of chronic infections (Graham et al., 2021). The relationship between efficacious surveillance programs and public health impact is demonstrated through evidence-informed targeted interventions. For example, with the nation's AMRs growing alarmingly, numerous healthcare systems have implemented new surveillance strategies that enable them to monitor resistant pathogens and respond quickly. Local and regional data gathering activities have become critical to informing antibiotic prescribing practices and maintaining the' effectiveness of therapies. Such models, based on robust surveillance systems, demonstrate the role of data in influencing treatment recommendations and realigning healthcare policies to counter changing threats from infectious diseases. In a more data-driven health system, adopting real-time surveillance as part of routine practice will be critical in optimizing response and protecting community health (Murray et al., 2022).

5.6.1. The Ebola Outbreak and Response

The Ebola outbreak that occurred in 2014–2016 is a warning of how infectious diseases can significantly affect public health and the world as a whole. The epidemic, which originated in West Africa, demonstrated that countries and global health organizations were unprepared for such a crisis. Monitoring is crucial to the early detection and containment of infectious diseases. The Noguchi Memorial Institute for Medical Research (NMIMR) showcases how national research centers can fortify epidemic preparedness using strong surveillance systems. By upgrading laboratory capabilities and providing essential testing labs, NMIMR illustrated the value of localized resources in containing outbreaks. The institute's contribution to Ebola and other viral hemorrhagic fevers emphasised the need to bring together local and global efforts to realise comprehensive disease surveillance and response systems (Odoom et al., 2024). In addition, the building of a coordinated response to infectious disease outbreaks like Ebola requires that health systems emphasise systematic collection and analysis of data. Unfortunately, most outbreaks occur without essential data, making it difficult to appreciate their impact fully. The Ebola outbreak highlighted that restricted access to real-time information frequently impedes effective responses, leading to enhanced morbidity and mortality. The difficulties encountered were most forcefully felt in the arena of perinatal health, where higher risks of poor outcomes, including the death of the infant, mainly were unrecorded during the epidemic. This absence of systematic data collection not only hinders instantaneous response processes but also continues to maintain knowledge gaps on the effects of infectious disease outbreaks in vulnerable groups. As noted, the observation of perinatal health during epidemics should be given priority in expanded health surveillance systems (Malange et al., 2023). What was learned from the Ebola outbreak transcends immediate health effects to inform future public health policy. The integration of perinatal health monitoring into infectious disease surveillance can significantly enhance the understanding of community and health system resilience during epidemics. As an example, determining pregnancy outcomes within the Ebola framework is crucial for developing targeted interventions to protect mothers and infants. Data on total health must be gathered to inform the development of evidence-based response protocols, taking into consideration the special vulnerabilities of pregnant women. By integrating epidemiological studies with efficient health policies, public health workers can better prepare for and respond to future outbreaks. The integrated strategy of surveillance and monitoring, where not just the disease is considered but its larger implications on population health, will, in the long run, make the world better prepared against EIDs (Malange et al., 2023) (Figure 5.18).

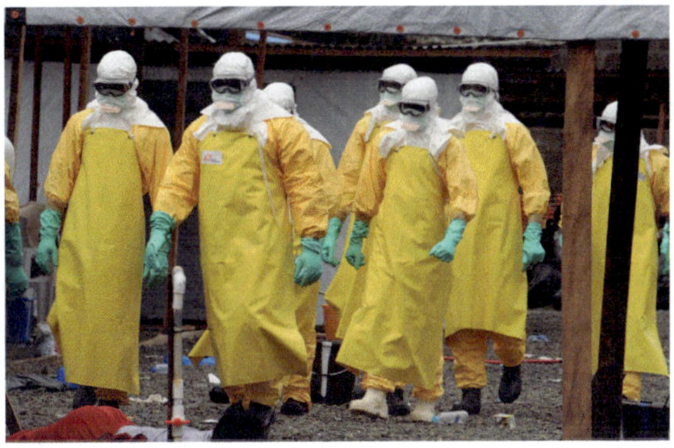

Figure 5.18. The Ebola outbreak and response.

Source: https://img.washingtonpost.com/rw/2010-2019/WashingtonPost/2014/08/31/Foreign/Images/Par7962517.jpg?uuid=yK80fjFeEeSPAgPGRLLX0A.

5.6.2. COVID-19 Tracking and Management

The COVID-19 pandemic highlighted the vital necessity of effective tracking and management systems in infectious disease surveillance and monitoring. Effective data collection and analysis helped in timely interventions, hotspot identification, and public health information dissemination. The GBD has played a key role in creating crucial health estimates, such as the effect of COVID-19 on global populations. The GBD 2021 data demonstrate a willingness to learn about disease burden by regularly improving and updating analytical techniques, which helps public health policymakers create evidence-informed interventions that are tailored to individual community needs. These strategies not only address immediate health threats but also support long-term health planning and policy-making to tackle infectious diseases in a comprehensive manner, extending beyond the ongoing pandemic (Ferrari et al., 2024). New variants of the SARS-CoV-2 virus added to the challenge in managing COVID-19, necessitating adaptive surveillance mechanisms. Due to the variation in infectivity and pathogenicity of such variants, monitoring their spread was an essential requirement. Wastewater surveillance (WWS) proved to be a critical tool in that case, enabling scientists to better monitor community-level infections compared to using conventional methods by themselves. Research has shown that WWS not only tracks the spread of SARS-CoV-2 but also provides information on new variants emerging in populations. The capability to identify these variants before their occurrence in clinical cases indicates the promise of WWS as an early warning system. Consequently, authorities can introduce timely interventions that reduce community transmission, ultimately protecting public health (Tiwari et al., 2023). The innovation of technology integration into surveillance activities has revolutionised the tracking and management of infectious diseases. Utilisation of geospatial information, mobile health technologies, and real-time monitoring systems has provided public health authorities with unmatched information regarding the dynamics of COVID-19 transmission. Through the convergence of conventional epidemiologic approaches with cutting-edge data collection methods, authorities can identify outbreaks more effectively and evaluate the effectiveness of actions taken. In addition, interdisciplinary collaboration between data science specialists, public health professionals, and environmental monitoring experts further contributes to these initiatives. As was apparent throughout the COVID-19 pandemic, detailed tracking and management initiatives will be critical to future infectious disease response, reiterating the need for flexible frameworks to handle the volatile nature of viral activity (Ferrari et al., 2024) (Figure 5.19).

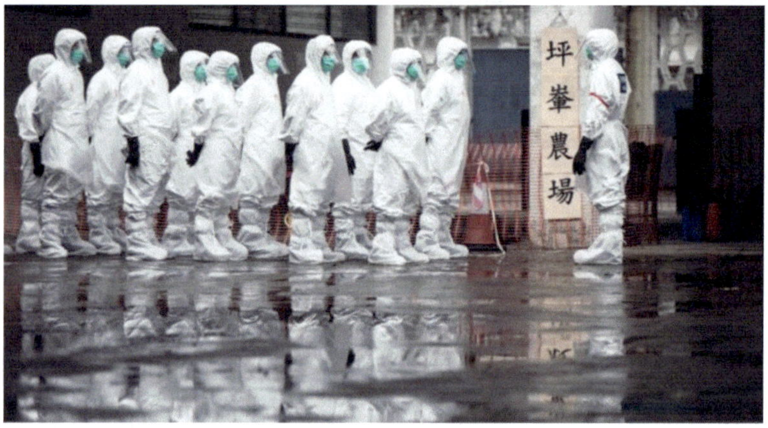

Figure 5.19. COVID-19 tracking and management.

Source: https://ichef.bbci.co.uk/news/640/cpsprodpb/87FF/production/_112751843_trackandtrace.jpg.

5.6.3. Lessons Learned from Past Surveillance Efforts

The historical background of surveillance activities in infectious disease control offers crucial lessons relevant to present-day strategies. Previous experiences have shown the value of constructing strong human capacities effective in disease surveillance. For instance, the Rockefeller Foundation introduced the DSN Initiative in 2007, which aimed to strengthen capacities in developing nations. The assessment of the DSN's role in the Mekong area emphasized the importance of regional networks that promote coordination between countries in surveillance and reporting outbreaks. Such coordinated platforms play an integral role in responding to cross-border health threats, demonstrating that global coordination can decisively enhance the responsiveness and agility of surveillance systems. By drawing on these lessons, public health responses today can prepare more effectively for emerging infectious disease threats by strategically investing in the establishment and maintenance of core capacities to limit vulnerability in global health responses (Ancheta et al., 2010). Further, the potential for successful community-level interventions has become an essential learning from experience in previous surveillance. A systematic review of literature on community case management (CCM) of malaria revealed that CHWs can provide quality care when trained and supervised accordingly. This highlights the importance of incorporating capacity building into surveillance mechanisms. Local health workers' participation strengthens both the quality of care provided and promotes community participation in disease surveillance. This frontline level engagement can also serve as an early warning system for health authorities, providing them with timely information that is vital in predicting outbreaks and responding to them in a timely manner. Successful surveillance must hence include integrated approaches strengthening the general health system so that CHWs are equipped with the tools and the desired support for effective implementation (Buj et al., 2014). Lastly, the shared experience of earlier surveillance programs puts in perspective the necessity of ongoing review and adaptation of strategies in light of actual outcomes. For example, results from the DSN Initiative revealed that stakeholder accountability is central to the sustainability of investments in surveillance. It is now clear that effective health surveillance is not a fixed entity, but rather one that requires continuous evaluation to innovate in response to new challenges. Incorporating lessons from previous experience, such as different health interventions and regular performance assessments, can contribute to an improved monitoring system that is potentially more resilient. In addition, recognising bottlenecks in referral processes within community health structures can inform improvements, thereby enhancing overall health service delivery. Sustained learning and adjustment form the foundation of proper surveillance, enabling public health organizations to react better to infectious disease risks in a changing environment (Ancheta et al., 2010; Buj et al., 2014).

SUMMARY

In summary, successful monitoring and surveillance of infectious diseases are essential for maintaining public health and mitigating the impact of outbreaks. The information gathered through systematic surveillance not only enables timely recognition of emerging pathogens but also assists in analyzing trends in disease transmission and the effectiveness of interventions. The growing burden of cardiovascular conditions underscores the need for comprehensive disease management processes, highlighting the crucial role of surveillance in addressing non-communicable diseases and their overlap with infectious threats, particularly in geographically heterogeneous environments (Roth et al., 2020). In the absence of strong monitoring structures, public health systems may struggle to deliver timely and required interventions to current and new diseases, ultimately compromising population health. In addition, the onset of new threats like the SARS-CoV-2 pandemic has highlighted the necessity for global surveillance networks. The rapid spread of the virus and its significant impact on global health systems lay bare the shortcomings in current monitoring measures. Improved surveillance not only facilitates the early detection of viral outbreaks but also provides insight into epidemiological patterns, which is vital for containment efforts (Singhal, 2020). Effective sharing of information between global health organisations and government agencies is critical to address world health emergencies effectively. Therefore, building these networks will be crucial in protecting public health and averting future pandemics. In conclusion, the convergence of high-tech surveillance methodologies with collaborative international efforts can significantly enhance our readiness and reaction to infectious disease threats. As we face persistent public health threats, both communicable and noncommunicable diseases require a holistic response that focuses on data-driven decision-making and resource distribution. Surveillance systems must evolve to address technological innovation and comprehensive data analysis, enabling health authorities to anticipate outbreaks and take proactive measures (Roth et al., 2020; Singhal, 2020). By continued dedication to such efforts, we can improve infectious disease resilience and thereby safeguard populations across the globe from future health threats.

Surveillance and monitoring of infectious diseases rely on complex strategies and mechanisms that aim to detect and control outbreaks effectively. One of the important initiatives is the DSN, initiated by the Rockefeller Foundation, which aims to strengthen human resources for disease surveillance in developing nations. This program seeks to and enhance national capacities in monitoring, reporting, and responding to outbreaks by way of improved coordination among regions and between global initiatives. The activities of DSNs, especially in areas frequently under-resourced and prone to vulnerability, highlight the necessity of establishing infrastructure for disease surveillance. This, in turn, will help develop a more sustainable disease management response to infectious diseases within various contexts, as pointed out by Ancheta et al. (2010). Aside from human capacity, breakthroughs in statistical methods are also vital for the successful monitoring of infectious diseases. For example, the Farrington algorithm and Poisson cumulative sum schemes have been pivotal in identifying aberrations within surveillance data. The statistical methods assist analysts in interpreting patterns of disease transmission and detecting outbreaks in a timely fashion, with adjustments for seasonality and spatial aggregation. By implementing these methodologies on field data, like evaluating rabies surveillance among Hessian foxes in Germany, scientists can develop insights that complement response measures. Not only do such technical measures enhance the reliability of data interpretation, but they also enable public health officials to make informed choices based on credible surveillance figures, as seen in Held et al. (2007). Ultimately, the main issues regarding infectious disease surveillance and monitoring reflect the linkage between human resource development and complex statistical approaches. Programs such as the DSN demonstrate the dedication to enhancing the detection and response capacity of diseases both regionally and globally. At the same time, the use of advanced statistical techniques enhances the validity of surveillance data, enabling more rapid responses to emerging health threats. As the global epidemiology of infectious diseases continues to evolve, these key components remain the cornerstone in informing successful public health strategies and policies that protect communities from epidemics and prepare for future challenges.

CLOSER LOOK:

WHOLE GENOME SEQUENCING (WGS):

Whole genome sequencing (WGS) has transformed modern biology by enabling scientists to examine the complete DNA blueprint of an organism with unprecedented detail. Taking a closer look at WGS reveals not only its scientific power but also its profound impact across medicine, research, agriculture, and public health. Unlike targeted sequencing methods that focus on specific genes or regions, WGS reads nearly every nucleotide in the genome, providing the most comprehensive view possible of genetic structure and variation. At its core, WGS involves breaking DNA into small fragments, reading these fragments through high-throughput sequencing technologies, and using computational tools to reconstruct the full genome. Advances in sequencing platforms have dramatically reduced both cost and time, making WGS accessible to a wide range of applications. This comprehensive approach is especially valuable for detecting genetic variants that might otherwise be missed, including single-nucleotide changes, small insertions or deletions, copy-number variations, and large structural rearrangements.

In clinical medicine, WGS is emerging as a powerful diagnostic tool. It can identify rare genetic mutations responsible for undiagnosed conditions, guide treatment decisions, and refine the understanding of inherited disease risk. Importantly, WGS allows clinicians to look beyond a predefined set of genes, which is crucial when symptoms do not point to a clear genetic cause. In oncology, sequencing tumor genomes helps uncover driver mutations, monitor evolution under therapy, and identify targeted treatment options.

WGS also plays a central role in infectious disease surveillance. Sequencing the genomes of bacteria, viruses, or parasites allows researchers to track outbreaks, map transmission pathways, monitor antimicrobial resistance, and detect emerging variants. The ability to compare whole genomes provides a level of resolution far beyond traditional typing methods, improving the speed and accuracy of public health responses. Beyond medicine, WGS is reshaping fields such as agriculture, where breeders use genomic information to enhance crop resilience, disease resistance, and yield. In conservation biology, sequencing endangered species helps inform protection strategies by revealing genetic diversity and population structure. In forensics, WGS offers high-precision identification and new tools for solving complex cases.

Despite its benefits, WGS also raises important considerations. Interpreting vast amounts of data requires significant expertise, and not all variants have clear clinical meaning. Ethical issues—such as privacy, data ownership, and incidental findings—must be addressed thoughtfully.

Ultimately, a closer look at whole genome sequencing reveals a technology that is both transformative and rapidly evolving, positioned to shape the future of science and medicine for decades to come.

REFERENCES

1. Adefemi, N. A., Ukpoju, N. E. A., Adekoya, N. O., Abatan, N. A., & Adegbite, N. a. O. (2023). Artificial intelligence in environmental health and public safety: A comprehensive review of USA strategies. *World Journal of Advanced Research and Reviews, 20*(3), 1420–1434. https://doi.org/10.30574/wjarr.2023.20.3.2591.
2. Alhumaid, N. K., Alajmi, A. M., Alosaimi, N. F., Alotaibi, M., Almangour, T. A., Nassar, M., Memish, Z. A., et al. (2024). Epidemiology of reportable bacterial infectious diseases in Saudi Arabia. *Infectious Diseases and Therapy, 13*, 667–684. https://www.semanticscholar.org/paper/80889fccfb88b0b038f64bee778a60893cc8bd70 (accessed on 30th May 2025).
3. Ancheta, C. A., Perez, E. S., Richter, K., Tempongko, M. S. B., Sunpuwan, M., Mendoza, O. M., Pachuen, O., et al. (2010). *Disease Surveillance Networks Initiative Asia: Final Evaluation*. https://core.ac.uk/download/86445039.pdf (accessed on 30th May 2025).
4. Anonymous, Baldock, C. (2025). *Understanding Animal Health in Southeast Asia: Advances in the Collection, Management and Use of Animal Health Information*. https://core.ac.uk/download/pdf/6377294.pdf (accessed on 30th May 2025).
5. Balmes, J., Ritz, B., & Tager, I. (2004). *Can Lessons from Public Health Disease Surveillance be Applied to Environmental Public Health Tracking?* https://core.ac.uk/download/pdf/3775836.pdf (accessed on 30th May 2025).
6. Bernstein, Ç. N., Eliakim, A. R., Fedail, S. S., Fried, M., Gearry, R. B., Goh, K. L., Hamid, S., et al. (2016). World Gastroenterology Organization global guidelines: Inflammatory bowel disease. *Journal of Clinical Gastroenterology, 50*, 803–818. https://doi.org/10.1097/mcg.0000000000000660.
7. Biu, P. W., Nwasike, C. N., Tula, O. A., Ezeigweneme, C. A., & Gidiagba, J. O. (2024). A review of GIS applications in public health surveillance. *World Journal of Advanced Research and Reviews, 21*, 030–039. https://doi.org/10.30574/wjarr.2024.21.1.2684.
8. Bronsvoort, B. M. de C., Cash, R. A., Daborn, C., Knobel, D., Auty, H., Handel, I., Institute of Medicine and National Research Council (U.S.) Committee on Achieving Sustainable Global Capacity for Surveillance and Response to Emerging Diseases of Zoonotic Origin, et al. (2012). *Bringing Together Emerging and Endemic Zoonoses Surveillance: Shared Challenges and a Common Solution*. https://core.ac.uk/download/9397884.pdf (accessed on 30th May 2025).
9. Budd, J., Miller, B. S., Manning, E., Lampos, V., Zhuang, M., Edelstein, M., Rees, G., et al. (2020). Digital technologies in the public-health response to COVID-19. *Nature Medicine, 26*, 1183–1192. https://doi.org/10.1038/s41591-020-1011-4.
10. Buj, V., Kedenge, S., Kim, J., Ngongo, N., et al. (2014). *Community Health Workers and Stand-Alone or Integrated Case Management of Malaria: A Systematic Literature Review*. https://core.ac.uk/download/19452714.pdf (accessed on 30th May 2025).
11. Carrasco, L. R., Cook, A. J. C., Moffitt, L. J., & Souza, M. D. M. S. (2025). *Economics of Robust Surveillance on Exotic Animal Diseases: The Case of Bluetongue*. https://core.ac.uk/download/pdf/6590971.pdf (accessed on 30th May 2025).
12. Casimiro-Soriguer, C., Pérez-Florido, J., Robles, E. A., Lara, M., Aguado, A., Rodríguez, I. M. A., Lepe, J. A., et al. (2024). The integrated genomic surveillance system of Andalusia (SIEGA) provides a One Health regional resource connected with the clinic. *Scientific Reports, 14*.

https://www.semanticscholar.org/paper/b91784b31077947d62fb818217c09086db8c8159 (accessed on 30th May 2025).

13. Chen, K., Shrivastava, U., & Tindol, B. (2019). The dynamics of real-time online information and disease progression: understanding spatial heterogeneity in the relationship. https://core.ac.uk/download/289123789.pdf (accessed on 30th May 2025).
14. Chyba, C. F. (1998). *Biological Terrorism, Emerging Diseases, and National Security*. https://core.ac.uk/download/71349580.pdf (accessed on 30th May 2025).
15. Clarke, K. C., McLafferty, S. L., & Tempalski, B. J. (1996). On epidemiology and geographic information systems: a review and discussion of future directions. *Emerg. Infect. Dis.* https://academicworks.cuny.edu/cgi/viewcontent.cgi?article=1230&context=hc_pubs (accessed on 30th May 2025).
16. Cleaveland, S., Halliday, J. E. B., Hampson, K., & Hanley, N. (2017). Driving improvements in emerging disease surveillance through locally-relevant capacity strengthening. *Science*. https://core.ac.uk/download/84148417.pdf (accessed on 30th May 2025).
17. Cliquet, F., Gelman, A., Glueck, T. F., Gruen, B., Homer, C., MacKenzie, D. I., Manning, S. E., et al. (2019). Not all surveillance data are created equal—A multi-method dynamic occupancy approach to determine rabies elimination from wildlife. *Journal of Applied Ecology*. https://core.ac.uk/download/288431474.pdf (accessed on 30th May 2025).
18. Ekirapa, A., Matthys, B., Zinsstag, J., Crump, L., Yatich, N., & Ettarh, R. (2011). *Disease Surveillance Networks Initiative Africa: Final Evaluation.* https://core.ac.uk/download/86445038.pdf (accessed on 30th May 2025).
19. Ferrari, A. J., Santomauro, D., Aali, A., Abate, Y. H., Abbafati, C., Abbastabar, H., Abd ElHafeez, S., et al. (2024). Global incidence, prevalence, years lived with disability (YLDs), disability-adjusted life-years (DALYs), and healthy life expectancy (HALE) for 371 diseases and injuries in 204 countries and territories and 811 subnational locations, 1990–2021: A systematic analysis for the Global Burden of Disease Study 2021. *The Lancet*, *403*, 2133–2161. https://doi.org/10.1016/s0140-6736(24)00757-8.
20. Forkuo, A. Y., Nihi, T. V., Ojo, O. O., Nwokedi, C. N., & Soyege, O. S. (2025). A conceptual model for geospatial analytics in disease surveillance and epidemiological forecasting. *International Medical Science Research Journal*. https://www.semanticscholar.org/paper/35172ca90ea76fde8df908d6f51e431966dcb53a (accessed on 30th May 2025).
21. Ghany, M. G., & Morgan, T. R. (2019). Hepatitis C guidance 2019 update: American Association for the Study of Liver Diseases–Infectious Diseases Society of America recommendations for testing, managing, and treating hepatitis C virus infection. *Hepatology*, *71*, 686–721. https://doi.org/10.1002/hep.31060.
22. Graham, D. Y., & Liou, J. M. (2021). Primer for development of guidelines for *Helicobacter pylori* therapy using antimicrobial stewardship. *Clinical Gastroenterology and Hepatology*, *20*, 973–983.e1. https://doi.org/10.1016/j.cgh.2021.03.026.
23. Habib, G., Lancellotti, P., Antunes, M. J., Bongiorni, M. G., Casalta, J. P., Del Zotti, F., Dulgheru, R., et al. (2015). 2015 ESC guidelines for the management of infective endocarditis. *European Heart Journal*, *36*, 3075–3128. https://doi.org/10.1093/eurheartj/ehv319.

24. Hausmann, J., Dörre, A., Katz, K., & Van, De. B. S. (2024). Lifting COVID-19-associated non-pharmaceutical interventions: Potential impact on notifications of infectious diseases transmitted from person to person in 2022 in Bavaria, Germany. *Frontiers in Public Health, 12*. https://www.semanticscholar.org/paper/c5f2b9b0cb48f1203d05da08f82b357c981fcfa5 (accessed on 30th May 2025).

25. Held, L., Höhle, M., & Paul, M. (2007). *Statistical Approaches to the Surveillance of Infectious Diseases for Veterinary Public Health*. https://core.ac.uk/download/12163041.pdf (accessed on 30th May 2025).

26. Jackson, D., Anders, R., Padula, W., Daly, J., & Davidson, P. (2020). Vulnerability of nurse and physicians with COVID-19: Monitoring and surveillance needed. *Journal of Clinical Nursing, 29*, 3584–3587. https://www.semanticscholar.org/paper/46d576dba3e00a947e279c8a0273a469fffa3620 (accessed on 30th May 2025).

27. Jancee, B. V., Lakshmi, B. S., Mohankumar, N., Nagarajan, M., & Murugan, R., et al. (2025). Deep learning for infectious disease surveillance integrating Internet of Things for rapid response. https://core.ac.uk/download/642896143.pdf (accessed on 30th May 2025).

28. Kimball, A. M., Gugerty, M. K., Abernethy, N., & Curran, S. (2011). *Disease Surveillance Networks Initiative Global: Final Evaluation*. https://core.ac.uk/download/86445037.pdf (accessed on 30th May 2025).

29. Kyu, H., Pinho, C., Wagner, J. A., Brown, J., Bertozzi-Villa, A., Charlson, F., Charlson, F., et al. (2016). Global and national burden of diseases and injuries among children and adolescents between 1990 and 2013: Findings from the Global Burden of Disease 2013 Study. *JAMA Pediatrics, 170*(3), 267–287. https://www.semanticscholar.org/paper/8d2b3b28c99d2b3265b24b9a903c3e33dfebdde0 (accessed on 30th May 2025).

30. Malange, V. N. E., Hedermann, G., Lausten-Thomsen, U., Hoffmann, S., Voldstedlund, M., Aabakke, A., Eltvedt, A., et al. (2023). The perinatal health challenges of emerging and re-emerging infectious diseases: A narrative review. *Frontiers in Public Health, 10*. https://www.semanticscholar.org/paper/515b3f86f7fad5714073d75c6396828d5e623532 (accessed on 30th May 2025).

31. Manyi-Loh, C. E., Mamphweli, S., Meyer, E. L., & Okoh, A. I. (2018). Antibiotic use in agriculture and its consequential resistance in environmental sources: Potential public health implications. *Molecules, 23*, 795. https://doi.org/10.3390/molecules23040795.

32. Mbunge, E., Batani, J., Gaobotse, G., & Muchemwa, B. (2022). Virtual healthcare services and digital health technologies deployed during coronavirus disease 2019 (COVID-19) pandemic in South Africa: A systematic review. *Global Health Journal, 6*, 102–113. https://doi.org/10.1016/j.glohj.2022.03.001.

33. Murray, C. J. L., Ikuta, K. S., Sharara, F., Swetschinski, L. R., Robles, A. G., Gray, A. P., Han, C., et al. (2022). Global burden of bacterial antimicrobial resistance in 2019: A systematic analysis. *The Lancet, 399*, 629–655. https://doi.org/10.1016/s0140-6736(21)02724-0.

34. N/A. (2010). Building the science foundation of a modern food safety system: Lessons from Denmark, the Netherlands, and the United Kingdom on creating a more coordinated and integrated approach to food safety information. https://core.ac.uk/download/71349712.pdf (accessed on 30th May 2025).

35. Newton, P. N., Bond, K. C., Abiola, V. O., Ade-Abolade, K., Adeyeye, M. C., et al. (2019). Global access to quality-assured medical products: The Oxford Statement and call to action. *The Lancet Global Health*, *7*, e1609–e1611. https://doi.org/10.1016/s2214-109x(19)30426-7.

36. Odoom, J. K., Lartey, B., Kyei-Baafour, E., Bonney, J. H. K., Kwadwo, K., Ofori, M., De Souza, D. K., et al. (2024). Seventh annual research meeting of the Noguchi Memorial Institute for Medical Research: Viral infections. *Ghana Medical Journal*. https://www.semanticscholar.org/paper/f865826c087e9b8c1246d51ec24fb4b57370f9c2 (accessed on 30th May 2025).

37. Olaboye, J. A., Maha, C. C., Kolawole, T. O., & Abdul, S. (2024). Innovations in real-time infectious disease surveillance using AI and mobile data. *International Medical Science Research Journal*, *4*, 647–667. https://www.semanticscholar.org/paper/2be4e00919fa943fe69e62e30c2e3e284c9c932f (accessed on 30th May 2025).

38. Roth, G. A., Mensah, G. A., Johnson, C. O., Addolorato, G., Ammirati, E., Baddour, L. M., Barengo, N. C., et al. (2020). Global burden of cardiovascular diseases and risk factors, 1990–2019. *Journal of the American College of Cardiology*, *76*, 2982–3021. https://doi.org/10.1016/j.jacc.2020.11.010.

39. Scheidwasser, N., Poulsen, L., Leow, P. R., Khurana, M., Iglesias-Carrasco, M., Laydon, D., Donnelly, C. A., et al. (2025). Deep learning from videography as a tool for measuring *E. coli* infection in poultry. *bioRxiv*. https://www.semanticscholar.org/paper/f4d39352ebe763870c72710f7251b943ea287798 (accessed on 30th May 2025).

40. Shi, B., Xia, S., Yang, G., Zheng, X., et al. (2021). Spatial patterns of *Plasmodium vivax* transmission explored by multivariate auto-regressive state-space modeling – A case study in Baoshan prefecture in southern China. https://core.ac.uk/download/551516519.pdf (accessed on 30th May 2025).

41. Singh, S., Sharma, P., Pal, N., Sarma, D., Tiwari, R., & Kumar, M. (2024). Holistic One Health Surveillance Framework: Synergizing environmental, animal, and human determinants for enhanced infectious disease management. *ACS Infectious Diseases*. https://www.semanticscholar.org/paper/6b9453e0c0a1c5682036d299f62a23f72ac170e8 (accessed on 30th May 2025).

42. Singhal, T. (2020). A review of coronavirus disease-2019 (COVID-19). *The Indian Journal of Pediatrics*, *87*, 281–286. https://doi.org/10.1007/s12098-020-03263-6.

43. Struelens, M. J., Ludden, C., Werner, G., Sintchenko, V., Jokelainen, P., & Ip, M. (2024). Real-time genomic surveillance for enhanced control of infectious diseases and antimicrobial resistance. *Frontiers in Science*. https://www.semanticscholar.org/paper/65d604db4663c0fe272f154ad588578efa1a306c (accessed on 30th May 2025).

44. Sumithra, S., Radhika, M., Venkatesh, G., Lakshmi, S., Jancee, B. V., Mohankumar, N., & Murugan, S. (2025). Deep learning for infectious disease surveillance integrating Internet of Things for rapid response. *International Journal of Electrical and Computer Engineering (IJECE)*. https://www.semanticscholar.org/paper/b384d0cef7e51cdcc43614dfb305ce03af9fbd50 (accessed on 30th May 2025).

45. Ternhag, A., Tegnell, A., Lesko, B., Skärlund, K., & Penttinen, P. (2004). Basic Surveillance Network, a European database for surveillance data on infectious diseases. *Euro Surveillance: Bulletin Européen sur les Maladies Transmissibles = European Communicable Disease Bulletin*, *9*(7), 1, 2. https://www.semanticscholar.org/paper/35e0185fdd0f26a6dc90ef84c906a1617857cc9f (accessed on 30th May 2025).

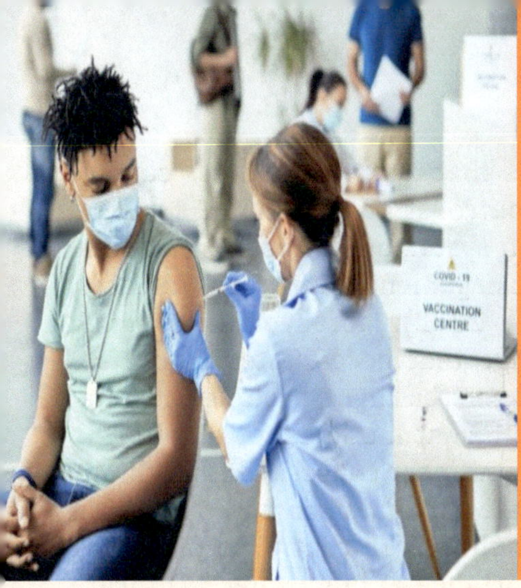

Chapter 6

INFECTIOUS DISEASE CONTROL STRATEGIES

Contents

Introduction

The importance of controlling infectious diseases has grown in recent years because of global health crises. Over the years, infectious diseases have been a significant danger to people, causing many cases of sickness and death. New medical techniques have given health systems access to many ways to prevent and treat illnesses, but issues such as AMR and new pathogens require them to update and adapt their practices constantly. The recent COVID-19 pandemic epitomises the urgency of deploying effective control measures, which not only include vaccination but also encompass public health policies and community behaviours that can mitigate disease spread (Tian et al., 2022). Since infectious diseases are constantly changing, these strategies are essential. Recently, scientists and technology have helped change how contagious diseases are handled. A significant breakthrough is the use of mRNA vaccines, which have proven to be very effective against COVID-19. As a result, scientists are now exploring the use of similar technologies for other infectious diseases, which could lead to significant changes in global vaccination practices. Examining these technologies reveals that we must address current outbreaks and prepare for future health emergencies. Therefore, control strategies should combine new research findings with practical use in public health. Through systematic utilization of these innovations, significant strides can be made in the prevention and management of infectious diseases, ultimately leading to more resilient healthcare systems (Tian et al., 2022). Moreover, the growing threat of antimicrobial resistance (AMR) poses a critical challenge that necessitates innovative strategies for controlling infectious diseases. AMR complicates patient treatment, prolongs hospital stays, and increases mortality. Therefore, it is crucial to develop efficient methods for monitoring and responding to it. A lot of research has shown that AMR is a significant concern, with millions of deaths each year due to bacterial resistance. For this reason, strategies that encompass infection control, responsible antibiotic use, and public health information should be central to managing infectious diseases. The use of data in AMR underscores the importance of enhancing healthcare facilities, both locally and globally, to address these threats. Only through a multifaceted approach that combines education, innovative technology, and robust health policies can societies effectively combat the rise of infectious diseases and safeguard public health (Figure 6.1).

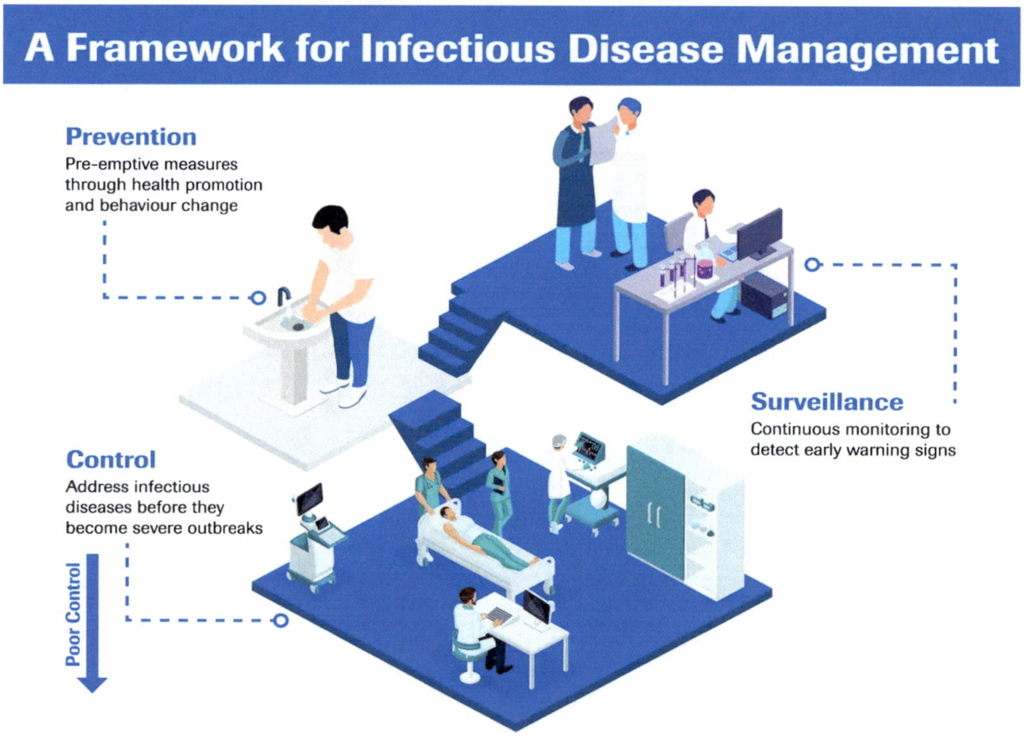

Figure 6.1. Infectious disease control strategies.

Source: https://rochediagram.com/wp-content/uploads/1.gif.

Definition of Infectious Diseases

Infectious diseases are a significant public health issue because bacteria, viruses, fungi and parasites cause them. They can spread within the host and lead to various health problems. Because they can be easily spread, infectious diseases can travel from one person to another, through insects or animals, or from the environment, which makes it difficult to prevent and manage them. In addition, the global spread of infectious diseases is made worse by AMR, changes in the environment and unequal social and economic conditions. This complexity underscores the importance of understanding infectious diseases from both biological and social perspectives, as illustrated by the annual mortality rates and health issues affecting diverse populations. They are essential in shaping effective ways to manage and control these diseases. In addition to harming health, infectious diseases impact the economy, social systems, and daily life. It is necessary to know the number of infectious diseases in a population to decide how to provide public health resources. It is clear from reviewing global health that millions of people lose their lives every year because of drug-resistant infections. In 2019 alone, approximately 4.95 million deaths were associated with bacterial AMR, highlighting the life-threatening implications of these diseases (Murray et al., 2022). Also, not having proper healthcare services and limited access to medicine make it more challenging to control infectious diseases. Therefore, we must develop robust approaches that encompass prevention, monitoring, and treatment to mitigate the far-reaching effects of these diseases on people worldwide. Infectious disease control works best when healthcare, public health, and social and political efforts are combined. Combining these approaches provides a clear understanding of how diseases are transmitted and how they can be prevented. Vaccination efforts have significantly helped in cutting down cases of preventable diseases, as is clear from programs that inoculate children against measles and polio. In parallel, ongoing research into the development of novel antibiotics and antiviral agents is essential in countering the threat of AMR (Roth et al., 2020). Also, public campaigns help communities learn about good hygiene habits and how to deal with health issues early. Ultimately, implementing these multifaceted strategies not only addresses the immediate threats posed by infectious diseases but also fosters resilience and preparedness for future outbreaks (Figure 6.2).

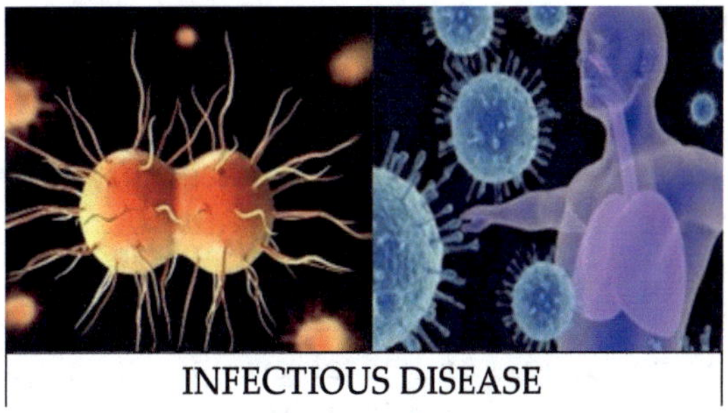

Figure 6.2. infectious diseases.

Source: https://www.dssimage.com/blog/wp-content/uploads/2022/09/Blog-Banner-2.png.

Importance of Controlling Infectious Diseases

Controlling infectious diseases helps protect public health and also maintains the stability of communities and their economies. Because infectious agents can spread fast, it is essential to manage their spread in an organized and planned way. By utilising vaccination, improved sanitation, and public health education, it is possible to mitigate the effects of disease outbreaks. Being able to react to EIDs quickly is essential, as shown by previous health crises. During major outbreaks, it becomes clear where healthcare systems are weak, which is why they should be regularly checked. For instance, a recent tabletop exercise conducted by the New York City Health + Hospitals focused on high-risk pathogens, indicating the necessity for robust communication protocols, staff education, and clear management procedures in the event of an outbreak (Dhagat et al., 2025). If these controls are absent, the consequences for public health can be severe, touching both personal well-being and economic growth. Additionally, continuous public health efforts are crucial for preparing people to respond to infectious diseases. The emergence of novel pathogens, as evidenced by the Zika outbreak in India, highlights the unpredictable nature of infectious threats (Chandra et al., 2024). By using advanced surveillance, it is easier to detect and follow disease transmission, which helps with early interventions. Additionally, utilising vector control, constructing better healthcare facilities, and effective communication with the public contribute to a community's strength. Efforts to contain outbreaks rely on teamwork among government organizations, partners from other countries, and local groups, so a quick response plan is ready. Having a wide range of strategies is crucial for preventing infectious diseases from causing serious harm and for enabling health systems to effectively manage any health emergency.

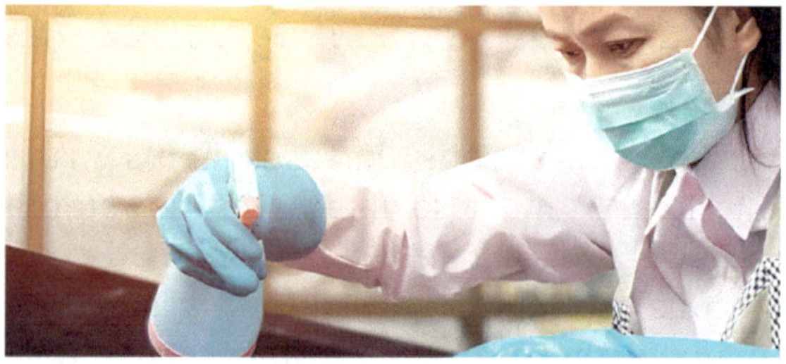

Figure 6.3. Controlling infectious diseases.

Source: https://learntastic.com/store/343024/images/infection-control-preventing-and-controlling-infectious-diseases-including-covid-19.png.

Managing infectious diseases is essential for health as well as for the overall social and economic situation. A stable environment with controlled infectious diseases helps economies, since widespread disease can cause problems for labor, healthcare and public services. When infectious disease control strategies are implemented, the public environment becomes safer, which helps social and economic activities flourish. Preventive actions help lower disease and death rates, resulting in less money spent on healthcare and fewer resources used in the future. Experiences from past outbreaks support better public health strategies and make communities safer from future risks. The continuous refinement of health strategies, informed by past experiences and emerging research, is paramount to safeguarding public health and ensuring that societies remain resilient in the face of infectious disease challenges (Chandra et al., 2024; Dhagat et al., 2025) (Figure 6.3).

Overview of Control Strategies

Strategies to control infectious diseases are designed to stop the spread and control any outbreaks. Some of the approaches are vaccination, treatment with antimicrobials, and public health actions. Vaccination is essential for disease control, as it plays a key role in preventing infectious bursal disease in poultry. The virus, which is genetically diverse, results in many young birds becoming ill and dying. Despite challenges posed by evolving virus strains, vaccination remains the primary strategy, leveraging both conventional and advanced vaccines, such as genetically engineered options, to bolster immunity and reduce disease incidence (Muneeb et al., 2024). Because vaccination strategies can be modified, they are crucial in addressing the evolving nature of infectious diseases. In addition, using chemicals and biological methods is essential for managing plant diseases. The management of bacterial canker in tomatoes highlights how careful balance is needed in farming. ways. Although copper-based chemicals are used in traditional strategies, the resistance and environmental issues they face suggest we should move toward more sustainable methods. New eco-friendly methods suggest combining both biological and non-biological substances with traditional techniques to enhance effectiveness and prevent both resistance and harm to plants. These innovative approaches exemplify a shift in thinking regarding disease control, underscoring the importance of sustainability in agricultural practices and disease management (Sedighian et al., 2025). If food production systems are not made environmentally friendly, they will not be sustainable in the long run. Infectious disease control strategies greatly benefit from community involvement and education. Making the public aware of how to prevent infectious diseases, such as by practising good hygiene and understanding the benefits of vaccines, can significantly reduce their occurrence. Public health campaigns aim to help people protect themselves and others, mainly in groups at high risk for transmission. Taking part in disease surveillance also helps communities notice outbreaks quickly and respond swiftly, which is essential for controlling the spread of infectious diseases. It is also necessary to focus on social and economic factors that cause health inequalities, so everyone can use preventive services and get healthcare. All these elements work together to make society stronger against infectious diseases, which leads to healthier communities.

6.1. Surveillance and Monitoring

Intense surveillance and monitoring are essential for controlling infectious diseases because they help find and respond to outbreaks in a timely way. Before, well-established disease surveillance systems helped public health organisations to collect, study, and share data in an organised way. The Centres for Disease Control and Prevention's initiative to develop a national environmental public health tracking (EPHT) network exemplifies this approach, linking environmental and chronic disease data to better understand public health dynamics.

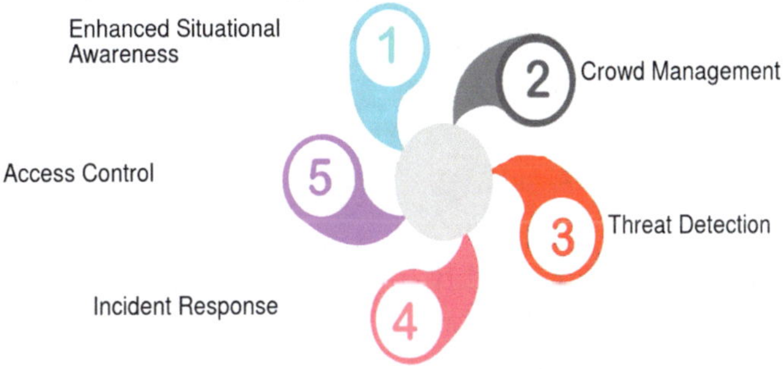

Figure 6.4. Surveillance and monitoring.

Source: https://fastercapital.co/i/Event-Security--How-to-Ensure-Your-Event-is-Safe-and-Secure--Surveillance-and-Monitoring-Systems.webp.

By continuously updating surveillance systems to integrate emerging technologies and data, public health entities can more accurately assess population-level exposure to various disease risk factors, creating a proactive stance against infectious disease threats (Balmes et al., 2004). It is essential for surveillance that countries cooperate at both the regional and global levels. Initiatives like the Disease Surveillance Network (DSN), launched by the Rockefeller Foundation, highlight the need to strengthen human resources and foster cooperation in developing countries. If countries can monitor and report outbreaks more effectively, these networks ensure a rapid response and limit the spread. Moreover, such collaborations make it possible to write detailed reviews that inform actions against diseases, mainly in areas that are prone to infectious diseases. The DSNs' focus on fostering connections between local and international efforts highlights the importance of a unified approach to disease surveillance, ultimately contributing to a more resilient global public health infrastructure (Ancheta et al., 2010). As we refine our methods of observation and monitoring, it is crucial to strike a balance between collecting information and taking action. The EPHT and similar systems not only connect data but also manage environmental issues that can cause chronic diseases, which can be exacerbated by infectious disease outbreaks. Ensuring that surveillance and intervention interact enables new and existing data to inform public health policies. However, after collecting data, it is necessary to continually monitor the surveillance systems to determine their effectiveness in preventing the spread of diseases. By maintaining an adaptive framework that regularly reviews and updates its strategies, public health agencies can enhance their responses to infectious disease challenges, thereby improving overall population health outcomes (Balmes et al., 2004) (Figure 6.4).

6.1.1. Role of Epidemiology in Disease Tracking

Epidemiology helps by monitoring and tracking the spread of diseases, providing vital information that is used to design strategies for controlling infections. They collect, study, and explain health data to see what patterns exist in the spread of diseases. The information helps manage outbreaks and can inform public health policy. For example, the tracking of AMR has illuminated the significant health burden it carries, estimating 4.95 million deaths associated with bacterial AMR globally in 2019, which highlights the urgent need for informed intervention strategies (Murray et al., 2022). Epidemiological information is used to respond quickly and plan long-term approaches to combat infectious diseases, ensuring resources are used efficiently. Interventions are directed where they are most effective. Real-time insights into diseases are evident in the way epidemiology helps manage emergent infectious diseases. In the COVID-19 pandemic, researchers applied epidemiology to find out how mental health was affected by the disease, proving that public health crises often go hand in hand. Findings indicated significant increases in the prevalence of major depressive and anxiety disorders due to pandemic-related disruptions, particularly among vulnerable populations (Santomauro et al., 2021). With such analysis, it is vital to monitor diseases by examining both the infectious agents and their effects on mental health and social factors. A comprehensive approach is necessary to develop strategies that address both the health issues and the impact of infectious diseases on society. Epidemiology is also crucial for guiding actions that help stop the spread of contagious diseases. Strong surveillance systems enable public health agencies to track the spread of diseases and identify associated risks, allowing them to take the necessary actions. If we know the levels of specific pathogens and how resistant they are to certain drugs, we can design better treatment and vaccination strategies. The assessment of AMR in specific locales reveals critical insights into tailored prevention initiatives, ensuring that resources are directed to areas with the greatest need (Murray et al., 2022). Also, regular epidemiological studies help to improve laboratory facilities and data collection, which is vital for keeping public health prepared for new threats.

6.1.2. Use of Technology in Surveillance Systems

Using technology in surveillance systems has changed the way infections are tracked and handled. Using mobile applications and big data analytics to collect detailed data allows for immediate tracking of how diseases are spreading. Because of this, public health officials can act quickly when new threats appear. For example, New Zealand and South Korea have effectively utilised technology to track and identify cases, which has helped reduce the spread of the virus. Collecting and examining a lot of data helps surveillance work better and leads to better decisions, which is in line with the main approaches used to contain COVID-19. Such technological interventions not only support immediate response efforts but also contribute to a more comprehensive understanding of disease dynamics, facilitating better preparedness for future outbreaks (Baker et al., 2020). Additionally, modern technology enables more accurate and faster diagnostic tests, which is crucial for effective surveillance. Rapid diagnostic tests and serological assays have made it easier to identify infected individuals, allowing for prompt interventions. They demonstrate that conducting extensive testing early can help prevent the spread of infections. In Singapore, by using serological analysis as well as traditional methods, health officials have learned about past infections and linked affected individuals which helps with containing the outbreak. This dual approach enables health authorities to implement targeted social distancing measures more effectively, demonstrating how technology transformation enhances public health strategies for controlling infectious diseases (Winter et al., 2020). Furthermore, the use of geospatial technology, such as Geographic Information Systems (GIS), has become indispensable in modern surveillance systems. GIS makes it easier to identify infection hotspots, which allows health officials to focus their efforts where they are most needed. With knowledge of disease patterns and demographics, authorities can identify who is most likely to get sick and establish effective interventions. Moreover, future advancements in artificial intelligence (AI) and ML hold significant potential to predict outbreaks before they escalate into widespread infections. As seen during the COVID-19 pandemic, effective surveillance systems reliant on technology not only improve the immediate response to health crises but also lay a robust foundation for ongoing public health efforts, thereby enhancing overall management of infectious diseases globally (Baker et al., 2020) (Figure 6.5).

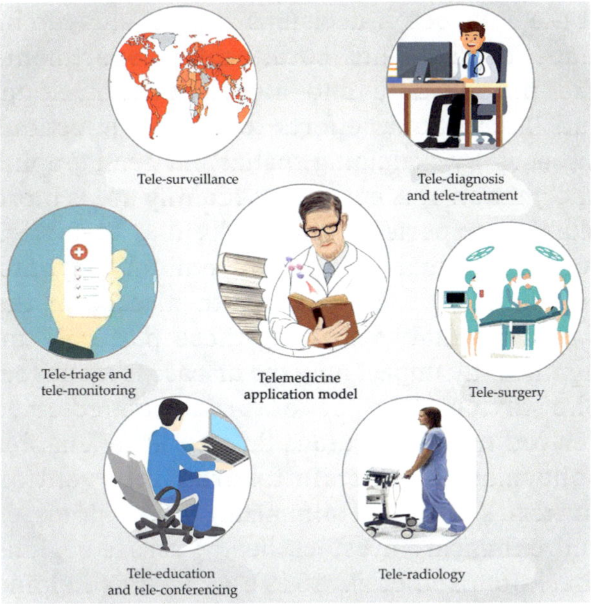

Figure 6.5. Use of technology in surveillance systems.

Source: https://images-provider.frontiersin.org/api/ipx/w=1200&f=png/https://www.frontiersin.org/files/Articles/646506/fmed-08-646506-HTML/image_m/fmed-08-646506-g001.jpg.

6.1.3. Importance of Data Collection and Analysis

Collecting and analyzing data is very important for controlling infectious diseases. way allows public health officials to watch for changes in diseases and how they spread, which helps them respond more quickly and effectively. Using real-time data from surveillance, it is possible to find out where and among whom outbreaks of infectious diseases are most likely to occur. Recent studies have suggested that combining mathematical models with routine surveillance can help us understand and project how diseases evolve. This multifaceted approach encourages the implementation of targeted strategies, optimizing resource allocation and increasing the chances of effective disease management (Bergquist et al., 2016). In addition, by looking at the data, better decisions and policies can be made. departments. Local health departments use proper data and also benefit national and international efforts to control infectious diseases. By examining spatial and demographic information, it is possible to identify areas more likely to experience outbreaks due to factors such as animal groups and building layouts. Simulations of foot-and-mouth disease in the U.S. show that identifying these patterns can significantly impact how the disease is managed. The articulation of outbreak trajectories derived from meticulous data scrutiny enables policymakers to craft tailored intervention strategies, therefore minimizing economic losses and enhancing livestock health across regions (Beck-Johnson et al., 2019). As well as helping with short-term measures, gathering and analyzing data is essential for defeating infectious diseases over time. Monitoring regularly allows for checking how well the strategies are working which helps with making management changes. Reviewing the process is essential to improving surveillance-response systems, as demonstrated by studies on eliminating tropical diseases. Studies that encompass various types of surveillance methods, both old and new, enable researchers to contribute to the critical understanding of how diseases spread. Such efforts demonstrate that through sustained data collection and meticulous analysis, we can enhance the efficacy of infectious disease control strategies significantly, moving closer to the goal of eradication (Bergquist et al., 2016).

6.2. Vaccination Programs

Infectious disease control plans rely on vaccination programs, which significantly decrease the number of communicable diseases. Because of strong immunisation efforts, there have been significant improvements in the health of children, as vaccines have reduced the number of deaths from diseases like measles, mumps, and rubella. Studies indicate that countries with high vaccination rates have seen at least a 90% drop in disease rates, demonstrating the effectiveness of vaccination programs. In contrast, places with low vaccination rates are still experiencing outbreaks of diseases that can be prevented by vaccines, highlighting the importance of stronger and more flexible vaccination programs to achieve global health goals. Sustained efforts to increase vaccine accessibility and education are essential, particularly in areas vulnerable to misinformation and healthcare inequities, ensuring the continued success of vaccination efforts in reducing disease prevalence and promoting community health overall (Karaut, 2024). In addition to improving public health, vaccination programs help build herd immunity within communities. If a large number of people are immune to a disease, it protects those who are unable to get vaccinated, such as those with medical issues. The concept of herd immunity highlights the importance of vaccination for many people, as it protects not just the individual but also the broader community. As people travel more and the world becomes more interconnected, infectious diseases can spread rapidly. Therefore, it is crucial for nations to collaborate on vaccination programs to control outbreaks and protect people worldwide. Still, some groups, such as the elderly and people with chronic health problems, might not react well to vaccines. This phenomenon highlights the complexity of achieving collective immunity and the need for targeted strategies to address these vulnerabilities while sustaining high coverage rates in the general population (Perfilyeva et al., 2024). It is tough to understand how vaccines influence the immune system. People who are always inflamed due to vulnerability may not react well to vaccination. Myeloid-derived suppressor cells (MDSCs) play a pivotal role in modulating immune responses, which may limit the effectiveness of vaccines in these populations. Understanding how MDSCs impact the immune system is crucial for enhancing vaccine efficacy in populations at higher risk of infection, including the elderly and individuals with chronic infections. Studying how to suppress MDSCs may lead to valuable findings and treatments to boost vaccine-induced immunity in these groups. Addressing the needs of these groups ensures that vaccination programs are inclusive and effective, ultimately advancing the goals of infectious disease control strategies (Perfilyeva et al., 2024) (Figure 6.6).

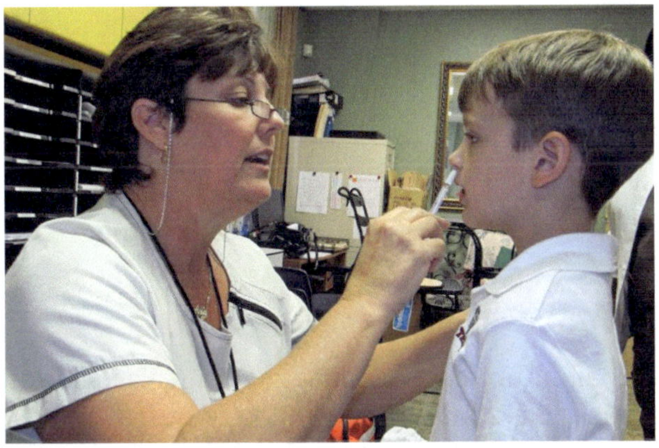

Figure 6.6. Vaccination programs.

Source: https://epi.ufl.edu/wordpress/files/2022/11/Article_Flu-vaccination-programs-have-potential-to-be-self-sustaining-in-florida_Image-1-1024x696.jpg.

6.2.1. Types of Vaccines and Their Effectiveness

Vaccination is now a key method for managing infectious diseases, and different vaccines are made to address specific pathogens. The main groups of vaccines are inactivated, live attenuated, subunit, and mRNA, and each works differently to protect the body. Inactivated vaccines are made from killed germs, which makes them safe, but usually requires several doses to build up strong immunity. On the other hand, live attenuated vaccines are made using weakened forms of the pathogen, which elicit strong immune responses, but they can be risky for individuals with weakened immune systems. The quick development and strong results of mRNA vaccines in the COVID-19 pandemic introduced a new area of vaccine technology. It is essential to be aware of different vaccines to develop effective ways to protect the public from infectious diseases. The way vaccines work depends largely on the characteristics of the pathogen and the immune system of the people to whom they are administered. In some cases, vaccines are administered first to individuals who are most likely to contract the disease or spread it, which is particularly effective for highly contagious diseases. This contrasts with morbidity-based approaches, which target those in high-prevalence areas, and are more beneficial for moderately transmissible strains (Pourbohloul et al., 2006). Vaccination delays can reduce the effectiveness of morbidity-based strategies, underscoring the importance of prompt vaccination. Considering such factors, public health officials can adjust their vaccination plans as the rate of virus transmission changes. This approach enables the design of vaccination strategies tailored to various situations. Among athletes and people at high risk, vaccination has played a significant role in controlling the spread of infections. Athlete health protocols now include vaccinations for influenza and pertussis to ensure athletes, their teams, and the community are protected. With infectious diseases being highly transmissible in competitive environments, taking proactive measures such as vaccinations is critical for maintaining the health of the population (d'Hemecourt et al., 2007). If athletes follow the recommended vaccinations and preventive measures, it raises herd immunity and helps control outbreaks during the sports season. Educating athletes on the importance of adhering to vaccination schedules presents a vital strategy in infectious disease control that extends beyond individual health, safeguarding broader community welfare (Figure 6.7).

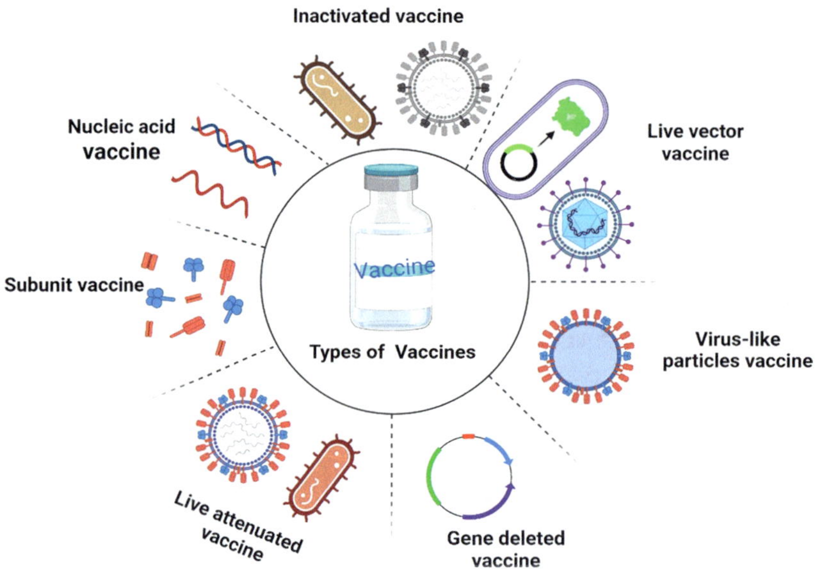

Figure 6.7. Types of vaccines and their effectiveness.

Source: https://images-provider.frontiersin.org/api/ipx/w=1200&f=png/https://www.frontiersin.org/files/Articles/1243835/fvets-10-1243835-HTML/image_m/fvets-10-1243835-g001.jpg.

6.2.2. Public Health Campaigns to Promote Vaccination

For infectious disease control, effective public health campaigns are essential to encourage vaccination and ensure that many people are immunised. They utilize social media, community outreach, and educational resources to connect with diverse individuals. By informing people about the benefits of vaccination, such campaigns can address hesitancy, fight false information, and encourage trust in health authorities. For example, using ethical guidelines in a campaign plan enables the identification and addressing of what people care about, making messages more effective for various demographic groups. Such an approach not only enhances public understanding of vaccinations' critical role in reducing disease transmission but also emphasizes the importance of collective responsibility in protecting public health and safety, as demonstrated by recent modeling studies that highlight equitable access to vaccines across communities (Zarebski et al., 2025). Additionally, the pharmaceutical industry significantly supports public health campaigns that encourage people to get vaccinated, as noted in recent literature. Along with making vaccines available, authorities take steps to inform the public about the value and safety of vaccination. They supply information and encourage people to make wise health decisions. Tackling AMR should involve public education on the correct use of antibiotics as well as efforts to promote vaccination. Suppose public health officials and pharmacists join forces. In that case, they can give accurate information and stress the preventive role of vaccines, which benefits the community. Innovative strategies, including the use of technology for monitoring vaccination trends, have the potential to enhance the efficiency and reach of these initiatives (Winata et al., 2024). The effectiveness of public health campaigns in encouraging vaccination is evaluated by their adaptability to new public opinions and health issues. It is essential to communicate openly and promptly during outbreaks to ensure people feel the need to get vaccinated. Involving community leaders in campaigns can help build trust and improve the credibility of the campaigns, which can address the reasons why some populations are not vaccinated. It allows people in the community get to know each other better and learn about health. When communities are more involved, they tend to get vaccinated more often, which helps control infectious diseases. By employing strategic communication and community involvement, public health campaigns can significantly contribute to sustaining public health initiatives and improving overall health resilience (Winata et al., 2024; Zarebski et al., 2025) (Figure 6.8).

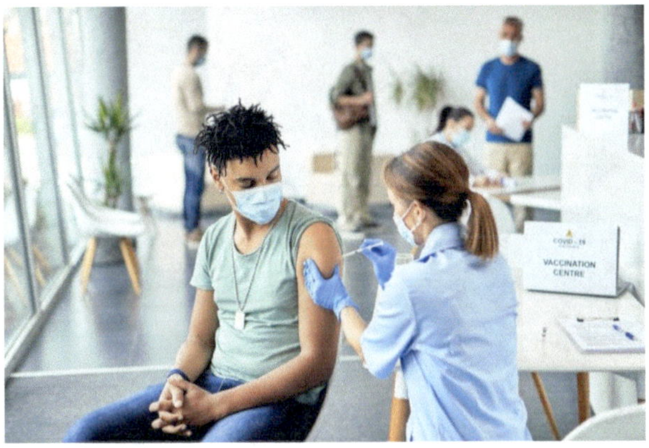

Figure 6.8. Public health campaigns to promote vaccination.

Source: https://publichealth.tulane.edu/wp-content/uploads/sites/3/2023/02/tulane-mph-blog-community-health-promotion-rural-areas.jpeg.

6.2.3. Challenges in Vaccine Distribution and Access

Getting vaccines to all regions is made more complicated by the logistical problems that can slow down and unevenly distribute the vaccines. If supply chains are not efficient, such as lacking sufficient cold storage, vaccines may spoil or be wasted, particularly in areas with limited resources. Additionally, vaccines are often administered first to people in cities, which exacerbates health disparities. According to studies on antibiotics, the same issues can happen with vaccines, where how well the healthcare system is built affects how widely they are distributed. Therefore, addressing these logistical issues is critical to ensuring that vaccines reach all populations promptly and effectively, thereby reducing the risk of disease outbreaks and improving overall public health outcomes (Murray et al., 2022). Another major problem in getting vaccines to people is that people may be hesitant or hear false information, which can discourage them from getting vaccinated. Many communities harbor doubts due to past wrongdoings or distrust in healthcare, potentially leading to lower vaccination rates. Informing the public about the safety and effectiveness of vaccines is crucial for building trust and gaining support. New methods of communication and specialised programs for vulnerable individuals can help more people get vaccinated. As evidenced by early experiences with SARS-CoV-2 vaccines, clarifying the rigorous testing and approval processes involved helps demystify the vaccination process and counter misinformation (Connors et al., 2021). Increasing public awareness through campaigns can greatly help overcome this challenge which will improve how vaccination programs work. The role of policies and governance in handling vaccine distribution is vital. To be effective, policies should be developed by different levels of government, private businesses, and international groups, ensuring that vaccines are accessible to all fairly. In many cases, political will is lacking, leading to disparities in distribution based on socioeconomic status (SES) or geographic location. Intellectual property rights and market monopolies can also hinder the production of affordable vaccines, which exacerbates the difficulties faced by people in developing countries. Reviewing these policies and guidelines enables stakeholders to develop a strategy that helps more people get vaccinated. Such systemic changes are vital for the success of infectious disease control strategies and the establishment of equitable healthcare systems (Connors et al., 2021) (Figure 6.9).

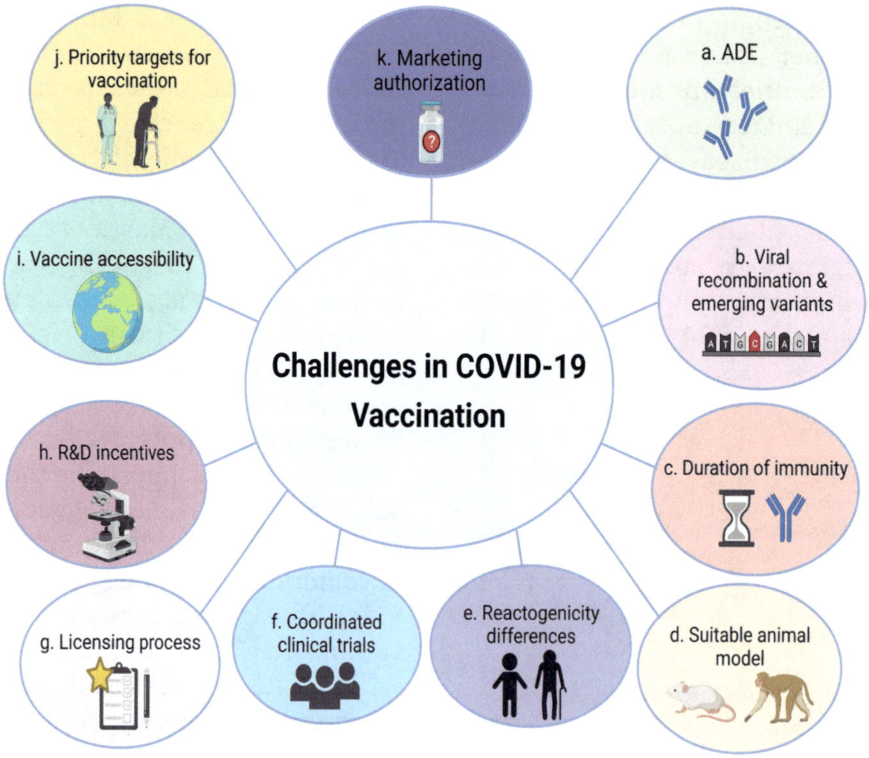

Figure 6.9. Challenges in vaccine distribution and access.

Source: https://www.mdpi.com/vaccines/vaccines-09-01474/article_deploy/html/images/vaccines-09-01474-g001.png.

6.3. Public Health Policies

Effective public health policies help guide the control of infectious diseases. Between 1850 and 1925, Chicago's urban population experienced a significant decrease in mortality rates, providing current health systems with practical lessons. The cause of the decline in the crude death rate was the reduction in deaths from infectious diseases and children, which occurred due to the introduction of public water and sewer systems. About 30 to 50 per cent of the decrease in mortality is linked to these investments, which demonstrates the significant impact clean water has on health. Such findings underscore the necessity of prioritising sound public health policies that target environmental health determinants and advocate for broader socioeconomic strategies to enhance community wellbeing (Ferrie et al., 2025). In recent years, emerging trends in infectious diseases, such as the increased incidence of hospital-acquired infections (HAIs), have prompted a reevaluation of existing public health policies in healthcare facilities. Due to rapid changes in infection control, nurses and infection control practitioners now have different roles. As infectious diseases evolve, these professionals must now adhere to new guidelines and focus more on data and teamwork. In addition, there is now a greater need for transparency in public health, so healthcare facilities must have robust systems to record and share infection rates. This shift not only reflects an evolving public health policy landscape but also highlights the importance of continuous training and adaptability in the healthcare workforce (Kaba et al., 2011). All in all, since public health policies and infectious disease control strategies are linked, different groups need to collaborate more closely. Those who make policies should recognize that addressing infectious diseases requires coordinated actions across healthcare, environmental, economic, and social sectors. Talking with local governments, community groups, and health professionals can lead to new ways to fight the causes of infectious diseases. When public health systems encourage partnerships and inclusive policies, they can better handle and prevent outbreaks, which helps protect the public health of many people. In this way, a synergistic approach positions public health policies not only as reactive measures but as proactive strategies essential for improving health outcomes and community resilience against future infectious disease threats (Figure 6.10).

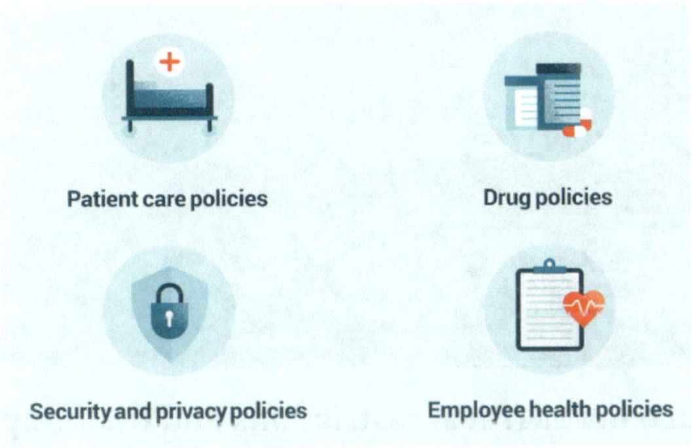

Figure 6.10. Public health policies.

Source: https://www.usa.edu/wp-content/uploads/2021/10/healthcare-policy-examples.png.

6.3.1. Implementation of Quarantine and Isolation Measures

Using quarantine and isolation is very important for controlling infectious diseases and forms an essential part of public health strategies. Quarantine is for people who might have been exposed to an infectious agent, but isolation is for people who have tested positive. All of these steps help lower the spread of disease during an outbreak by reducing the amount of contact between infected individuals and the general public. It was found that using quarantine and isolation, along with other non-pharmaceutical strategies, dramatically reduces the number of cases. The strategic implementation of these measures is particularly effective when diseases exhibit rapid transmission dynamics, ultimately serving as a safeguard to maintain public health and safety during crises such as pandemics or epidemics, as illustrated by the models' outcomes in Akter et al. (2024). Although quarantine and isolation are necessary, it is tough to put them into practice for vulnerable people. A case in point is the situation of displaced individuals in Burkina Faso during the COVID-19 pandemic, which shows the challenges brought by socioeconomic factors. When there are insufficient funds, inadequate housing, and poor communication, both the people affected and the humanitarian officials face greater challenges in addressing these issues. Even though people are aware of quarantine and isolation, many still misunderstand the differences between them, which can make it difficult to follow the rules. Humanitarian actors observed that societal and infrastructural limitations significantly impacted the implementation of public health strategies. Adapting the communication and implementation processes to address these barriers becomes critical, as evidenced by the experiences shared by IDPs in Kadio et al. (2024). Including community involvement in the use of quarantine and isolation helps ensure people follow the rules and that the measures are effective. Community members feel more responsible and involved when they are part of sharing and discussing public health information. When people from different backgrounds collaborate, it is easier to address cultural issues and get compliance. Additionally, designing plans that address the needs of IDPs and other specific groups enables authorities to manage quarantine and isolation more effectively. The successful integration of community feedback into the planning and execution phases of these measures not only improves public health outcomes but also empowers individuals, creating a more resilient and informed community as shown in various case studies (Akter et al., 2024; Kadio et al., 2024).

6.3.2. Travel Restrictions and Their Impact on Disease Spread

The implementation of travel restrictions in response to infectious disease outbreaks has emerged as a key strategy to mitigate the spread of pathogens across geographical boundaries. To prevent the spread of COVID-19, many countries closed their borders and banned travel, which helped contain the virus. By placing these restrictions, public health was protected by limiting the arrival of new cases from affected areas. Yet, these actions help control the disease, but they cause major economic problems. As indicated by the response to COVID-19, businesses faced temporary closures, significant job losses, and the need to restructure operations, underscoring the delicate balance public health officials must strike between safeguarding the population and maintaining economic stability (Phanphakdi et al., 2023). Information on how travel restrictions help control infectious diseases provides additional support for their use in managing outbreaks. In Hamadan, a study was conducted to investigate the effectiveness of various approaches, including travel restrictions, vaccination, social distancing, and mask-wearing, in reducing the spread of COVID-19. The study revealed that implementing these policies together could significantly reduce the number of infections. Specifically, travel restrictions were identified as a significant factor in reducing disease transmission, accounting for a more controlled spread of the virus (Soltanian et al., 2023). It proves that limiting travel during pandemics is essential and also helps control the spread of infectious diseases. However, it remains uncertain whether travel restrictions can be sustained in the long term to control contagious diseases. While the initial measures to halt the spread may be effective, maintaining these measures for an extended period can lead to fatigue, economic hardship, and dissatisfaction. Therefore, those making policies should understand that infectious disease transmission can change, and new variants could make earlier strategies less useful. As the global landscape adapts to new pathogens, a nuanced and flexible approach must be employed, one that combines travel restrictions with other public health initiatives, vaccination campaigns, and community engagement to foster a resilient societal response against future outbreaks (Phanphakdi et al., 2023; Soltanian et al., 2023) (Figure 6.11).

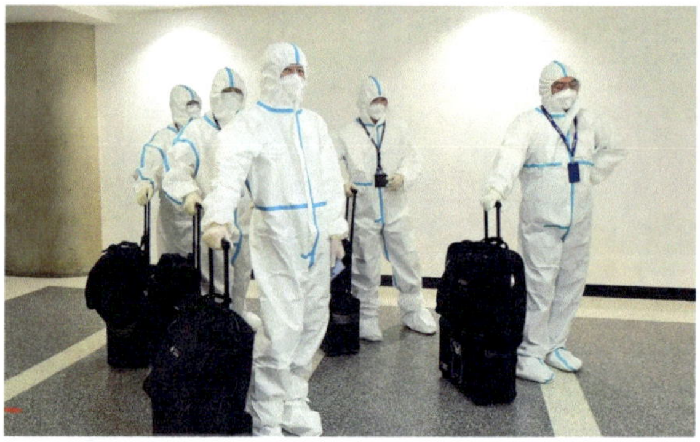

Figure 6.11. Travel restrictions and their impact on disease spread.

Source: https://i2-prod.mirror.co.uk/incoming/article28833180.ece/ALTERNATES/s1200d/0_FILES-US-HEALTH-VIRUS-CHINA-TRAVEL.jpg.

6.3.3. Legislation Supporting Infectious Disease Control

Infectious disease control strategies are significantly bolstered by robust legislation aimed at mitigating the spread of pathogens. Laws and regulations help public health by requiring the reporting of contagious diseases, which enhances the ability to monitor and respond to health threats. As an example, laws that require healthcare workers to inform public health about certain infectious diseases make it easier for officials to notice an outbreak and organize the right actions, such as vaccinations or quarantines. Being proactive in this way protects those who are at risk and also helps everyone in the community understand the importance of disease prevention. Therefore, good laws in this area form the base for organised efforts to address infectious diseases and help keep people safe from them. Also, laws that determine how money is distributed are essential for maintaining contagious disease control programs. Government policies provide the funds needed for research and new developments in diagnostics, treatments, and prevention. For example, the need for new herpes simplex virus vaccines underscores the importance of continuing to fund research to address serious health issues. As reported in the CDC/NIAID Joint Workshop, the lack of effective treatments and vaccines for genital herpes highlights the importance of legislative support in fostering research endeavors and expanding prevention strategies (Connolly et al., 2024). Such laws focus on quick health actions and also set up essential steps for future solutions that help the public. The COVID-19 pandemic illuminated the critical link between legislation and the training of healthcare professionals in infection prevention and control (IPC). Laws can help establish training programs for infectious disease doctors, equipping them with the skills to handle IPC tasks effectively. The recent evaluation of infection prevention training in infectious disease fellowship programs revealed significant gaps in standardized education regarding IPC practices (Winkler et al., 2024). It highlights the need for laws to establish training and certification standards for healthcare workers, thereby enhancing their skills in this area. Proper training prepares clinicians to handle infectious disease outbreaks and strengthens the healthcare system to face future public health issues.

6.4. Education and Awareness

Education and awareness play pivotal roles in controlling infectious diseases, providing communities with the necessary knowledge to make informed health decisions. When diseases like tuberculosis are prevalent, special education programs can educate people about how the disease is transmitted and how it can be treated. In India, for instance, increasing health literacy among community leaders has shown potential to address the high prevalence of multidrug-resistant tuberculosis (MDR-TB) by informing individuals of disease implications and the importance of adherence to treatment regimens. As indicated in recent studies, countries with robust public health initiatives that prioritise education generally report better outcomes in managing infectious diseases, emphasising the need for systematic educational interventions in high-burden regions (Gamon et al., 2013). Such actions help people and also encourage community members to work together, which is essential for dealing with public health crises. Getting the public informed and educated is often vital for the success of vaccination programs. For example, the Advisory Committee on Immunisation Practices (ACIP) has recognised that facilitating widespread knowledge about bacterial meningitis, particularly among adolescents and young adults, can significantly reduce infection rates through vaccination uptake. Making meningitis vaccines required for school attendance is an example of how laws can highlight the need for information about vaccines. In regions lacking such policies, community initiatives—like the Protect Alaska's Future campaign—demonstrate how grassroots awareness activities can stimulate dialogue, encouraging legislative support for critical public health measures (Hulstine et al., 2017). If communities value education, they will be better equipped to address infectious diseases and make vaccines more effective. Also, informing society about the effects of contagious diseases helps prevent them and strengthens the community. When people are well-informed, they are more likely to wash their hands, see a doctor when needed, and get vaccinated. Campaigns that correct misunderstandings about vaccines or how diseases are spread can help reduce vaccine hesitancy and boost the number of people vaccinated, which in turn decreases the number of diseases that can be prevented with vaccines. Various efforts, such as distributing educational materials to healthcare professionals, demonstrate the need for advocacy and awareness to sustain progress in disease prevention. By integrating education into public health initiatives, communities not only enhance their understanding of infectious diseases but also empower individuals to take proactive steps in safeguarding their health and that of others (Gamon et al., 2013; Hulstine et al., 2017) (Figure 6.12).

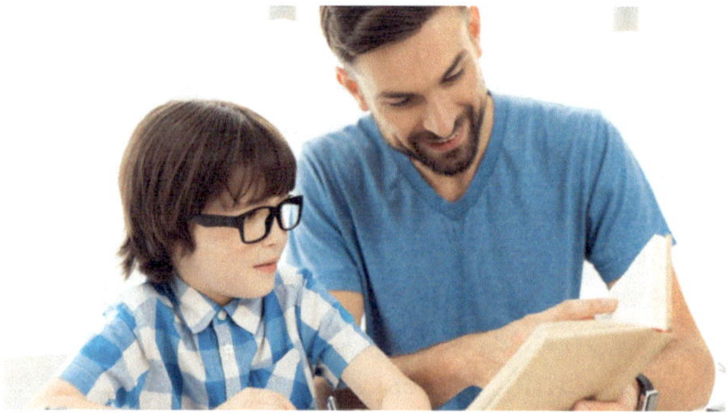

Figure 6.12. Education and awareness.

Source: https://stonesmentor.com/wp-content/uploads/2024/01/unnamed-1.webp.

6.4.1. Importance of Public Education on Hygiene Practices

Effective public education on hygiene practices is fundamental in the fight against infectious diseases, as it lays the groundwork for community awareness and behavior change. By disseminating information about hygiene, including regular hand washing, proper waste disposal, and maintaining clean living environments, communities can significantly reduce the transmission of pathogens. Educational programs about hygiene can help vulnerable populations stay healthier, as they may not have sufficient access to healthcare or detailed health information. By combining education with environmental awareness, communities can be empowered to engage more and develop a lasting culture of health. This approach is similar to infectious disease control, as it enables individuals to take care of their own health and hygiene, thereby reducing the spread of diseases. Such health education models highlight how using culturally relevant and engaging methods can encourage people to practice hygiene. According to research, involving local people, such as teachers and community leaders, in health interventions makes the interventions more effective for the target audience. This approach respects the participants' cultural background, encouraging them to trust the process and, in turn, remember and use hygiene practices. The literature points out that when programs are designed for local communities, they have helped people understand hygiene, sanitation, and how to detect diseases early. Due to a lack of access and awareness, many infectious diseases are prevalent in rural Indonesia. Community-based education helps people become stronger and take steps to prevent these diseases. They show that making education relevant to the community and culture is vital for controlling diseases. Teaching people about hygiene is essential for maintaining stable health over time and enabling them to fight off infectious diseases. In addition to promoting individual health, educating communities about hygiene can help society as a whole adopt healthier habits and attitudes. As an illustration, when hygiene education is combined with water and sanitation, it helps people understand that health is significant for both themselves and the community. For this reason, involving public education in infectious disease control is both valuable and necessary for lasting improvements in health. Future efforts must prioritize such educational initiatives, ensuring they are inclusive, accessible, and culturally relevant to sustain their impact over time, as emphasized by the findings regarding community engagement strategies in fostering effective hygiene practices and disease prevention (Gwadabe et al., 2025; Solehuddin, 2025) (Figure 6.13).

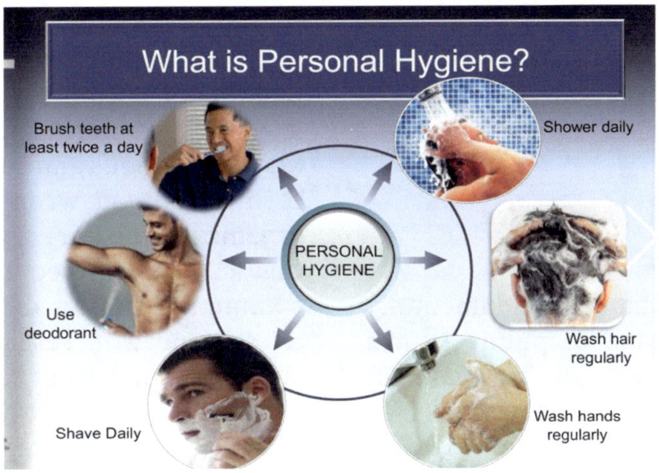

Figure 6.13. Importance of public education on hygiene practices.

Source:

6.4.2. Community Engagement in Disease Prevention

Community engagement serves as a pivotal strategy in the prevention and control of infectious diseases, particularly in low- and middle-income countries (LMICs). Involving community members helps health initiatives to be effective in meeting specific needs. By leveraging community resources, community-led approaches enable health interventions to reach and benefit a greater number of people. Actively taking part in disease control, such as through education and outreach, helps communities improve their health behaviours concerning HIV, malaria, and diarrheal diseases. This cooperative approach not only aligns with global health priorities but also supports the Sustainable Development Goals (SDGs) by fostering stronger health systems that prioritise community participation and empowerment (Indravudh et al., 2025). Also, the way communities engage can be quite different depending on their cultural traditions and economic situation. If participants trust and feel motivated, it becomes easier to carry out health interventions in the community. Still, there are obstacles, because community standards, a lack of resources, and biases within institutions can block the positive effects. Research suggests that when people feel they have control over health programs, they are more likely to continue participating and achieve better health outcomes. Therefore, understanding the contextual influences that dictate the success of these engagement strategies is crucial for designing effective disease prevention programs that resonate with community needs and values (Klingberg et al., 2024). Including community engagement in infectious disease control plans enhances program effectiveness and addresses ethical issues in health research and intervention. Since many now support participatory approaches, it is necessary to examine the possible challenges and biases they might introduce carefully. Sometimes, community engagement can lead to problems, including unrealistic expectations from the community or the community becoming financially dependent. So, even though encouraging people to participate in their communities is usually a good idea, it is necessary to analyse how these engagements take place. Fostering genuine collaboration while addressing harmful dynamics ensures that community engagement remains a viable and ethical strategy in the multifaceted landscape of infectious disease prevention (Klingberg et al., 2024).

6.4.3. Role of Social Media in Spreading Awareness

The advent of social media has fundamentally transformed the landscape of public health communication, particularly in the realm of infectious disease control. Platforms such as Twitter, Facebook, and Instagram provide invaluable channels for disseminating information quickly and widely, reaching audiences that traditional media may overlook. Given their expansive reach, these platforms have been pivotal in informing the public about EIDs, vaccination campaigns, and preventive health measures. By being able to post quickly and easily on social media, health organisations can help correct false information and clear up misunderstandings, especially when there is an emergency. Using these platforms for infectious disease awareness has been found to encourage more people to get involved and take care of their health, which helps prevent and control infectious disease outbreaks. It has been found that targeted social media campaigns can help shape people's opinions about vaccination and healthy living. For instance, mathematical modelling helps illustrate how social media can be used to disseminate information and encourage people to prioritise their health. In particular, campaigns that target specific groups can help health authorities tailor their messages to how groups perceive vaccines. Social media can also bring people together to take action for health; viral posts and shared experiences encourage individuals to get their networks involved in health initiatives. It is essential, as quick reactions by the public can lower the spread of diseases and improve how they are controlled. Additionally, social media enables health authorities to connect and interact with the public, not only for sharing information. Having feedback mechanisms means that health programs can communicate with the public and encourage them to be involved. It is important during health crises, as people may feel anxious and confused, which can cause them to spread wrong information. If health organisations share updates on social media, they can inform people and also help build a community during difficult health situations. As evidenced in research on optimal control strategies, awareness campaigns integrated into social media have proven effective in managing infectious diseases, highlighting the platform's vital role in shaping health behaviors that align with effective communicable disease control efforts (Basir et al., 2023; Ratra, 2023) (Figure 6.14).

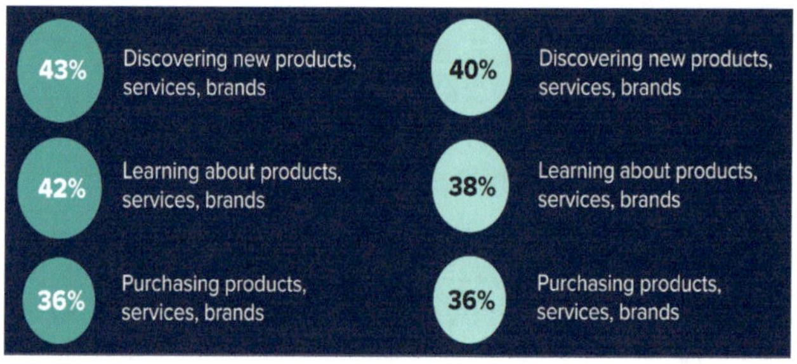

Figure 6.14. Role of social media in spreading awareness.

Source: https://media.sproutsocial.com/uploads/2021/06/harris-report-chart-6-1920x1080-1.png.

6.5. Treatment and Management

Effective treatment and management of infectious diseases require a multifaceted approach that integrates antiviral therapies, vaccination strategies, and public health policies. The introduction of antiviral medications, such as ribavirin for Crimean-Congo hemorrhagic fever (CCHF), has demonstrated promising results in managing specific viral infections. Since CCHF can be deadly, with a mortality rate ranging from 10% to 40% in those who get it, the success of these treatments is critical. For this reason, health systems should ensure that these treatments are available, particularly in areas where the risk of transmission is higher. Also, vaccination programs are effective in lowering the likelihood of disease outbreaks. When we use treatment and prevention simultaneously, we can mitigate the effects of infectious diseases and support improved public health. Recently, genomics has had a significant impact on the management and treatment of infectious diseases. Genomic technologies, particularly next-generation sequencing (NGS), allow for the rapid identification of infectious agents and real-time surveillance of pathogens. Because of this, health authorities can follow the spread of the disease and design appropriate interventions. Genomic epidemiology provides researchers with the means to study how pathogens evolve, enabling the development of more effective treatment strategies based on the genetic characteristics of each strain. In addition, understanding the genetic diversity of viruses like CCHFV is essential for developing effective vaccines and control strategies, highlighting the crucial role of genomics in managing infectious diseases today. It is essential for public health initiatives to handle the social factors that impact health to make the treatment and management of infectious diseases more effective. SES, the availability of healthcare, and education all play a significant role in determining who is likely to get infected and who can get prompt treatment. Therefore, strategies should address medical care as well as the health infrastructure and educate the community. An educational campaign can help people understand the early symptoms and seek medical care, which is very important for controlling diseases like CCHF that often cause death. By creating an environment that prioritizes equitable access to healthcare and disseminates knowledge about prevention and treatment, public health authorities can foster a resilient community better equipped to handle outbreaks and reduce their devastating effects (Figure 6.15).

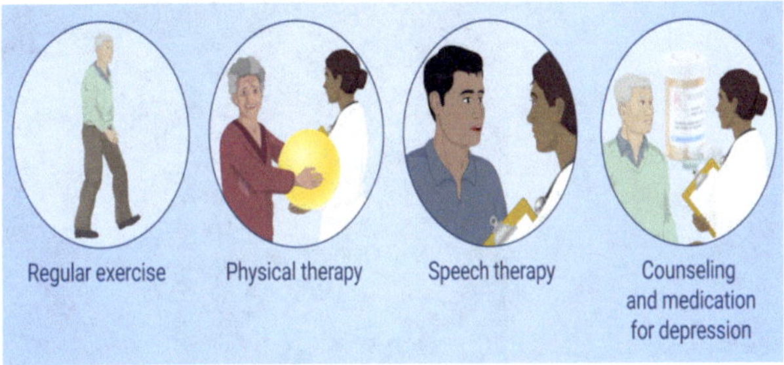

Figure 6.15. Treatment and management.

Source: https://external-content.duckduckgo.com/iu/?u=http%3A%2F%2Fwww.youandparkinsons.com%2Fen-pk%2Fslides%2Ftreatment-and-management-of-parkinsons-disease-complementary-and-supportive-therapies-for-parkinsons%2Fpk03-slides-m3_slide_17%24jpg&f=1&nofb=1&ipt=0d4aeaf44c05cf090475b322d780f9ea585762c2cad96cae3a4947a54f47b08d.

6.5.1. Advances in Medical Treatments for Infectious Diseases

The landscape of medical treatments for infectious diseases has witnessed substantial advancements due to the urgent need to tackle the escalating threat of antibiotic resistance. Antibiotics developed in the past are not working well against tough bacteria. For this reason, scientists have begun exploring new methods, particularly the development of novel antimicrobial agents. Metal nanomaterials have recently been considered a promising answer to this issue. Due to their unique properties, these nanoparticles can combat bacterial infections by disrupting bacterial cell walls and preventing the formation of biofilms. This burgeoning field of nanomedicine not only addresses the immediate challenge of drug resistance but also lays the groundwork for more effective treatment options, as highlighted in recent comprehensive reviews (Zhu et al., 2025). Utilising these new materials in treatment plans enables healthcare professionals to enhance their current efforts in controlling infectious diseases. There has been significant progress in using microbiome-based treatments, which are now being used more often in treatment plans. Given our understanding that the human microbiome influences health and disease, there is growing interest in utilizing microbiome modulation as a therapeutic approach for infectious diseases.

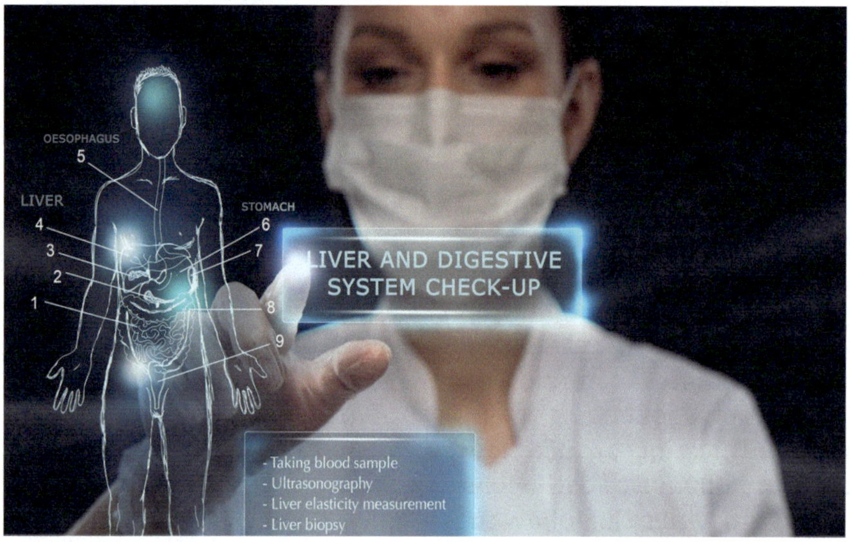

Figure 6.16. Advances in medical treatments for infectious diseases.

Source: https://i2.wp.com/www.lifeadvancer.com/wp-content/uploads/2016/09/Medical-Treatments-Future.jpg?fit=850%2C644&ssl=1.

Although most developments in this area have primarily benefited high-income countries, low- to middle-income countries also have considerable potential. By using targeted probiotics and live biotherapeutics, health crises related to maternal health, malnutrition, and infectious diseases can be addressed, which significantly benefits the health of people in these areas. Current efforts to characterize microbiomes from diverse populations aim to tailor strategies that effectively meet these specific health challenges, thus paving the way for more individualized treatment options that enhance overall efficacy (Gulliver et al., 2024). Besides these new methods, research and technological progress are necessary to keep improving treatments for infectious diseases. Teamwork among scientists, healthcare professionals, and policymakers is necessary to apply the study results and improve healthcare. As a result, people will be more likely to use nanomedicines and microbiome treatments, and this will also help address problems with healthcare access in less affluent areas. It is also crucial to strengthen public health efforts that focus on education, diagnosis, and prevention, as these are essential components of any comprehensive infectious disease control program. As we move forward, the amalgamation of novel treatment modalities and robust public health strategies will be crucial in effectively confronting the evolving challenges presented by infectious diseases (Figure 6.16).

6.5.2. Role of Healthcare Providers in Managing Outbreaks

In the realm of infectious disease control strategies, healthcare providers play a pivotal role in managing outbreaks and mitigating their impact on public health. Practitioners are the first to notice potential contagious diseases and take action. Because they pay close attention, have a strong clinical sense, and are aware of new diseases, they can detect unusual cases of illness early. When outbreaks are ongoing, healthcare providers must use effective methods to inform everyone about the risks and how to stay safe. Recognizing and reporting infectious cases early by healthcare professionals can significantly reduce the number of people who become infected, thereby slowing the spread of diseases. Their active participation in reporting not only facilitates local public health responses but also contributes to national and global efforts aimed at outbreak containment (Daskalakis et al., 2022). In addition, healthcare providers play a crucial role in developing and implementing vaccination and treatment plans during outbreaks. They have the role of administering vaccines, distributing medicines, and educating the public on the importance of vaccines for infection control. Besides their administrative duties, healthcare providers also assist individuals who face challenges accessing healthcare. They the community by providing information and collecting resources, which increases the number of people vaccinated and supports herd immunity. By partnering with public health agencies, these efforts can be better organised and made to include all people, ensuring they are based on evidence. The rapid deployment of resources and targeted vaccination initiatives, guided by the input of healthcare providers, can substantially reduce morbidity and mortality rates during an outbreak, as evidenced in various healthcare responses globally (Kuntz, 2020). Healthcare providers are involved in assessing how well outbreak control measures are working by gathering and analysing information about the situation. Using this feedback loop helps improve public health approaches, plan better for future emergencies, and strengthen healthcare systems against more outbreaks. After an outbreak, having healthcare providers participate in the analysis can help identify areas where the response plan needs improvement, which can guide the allocation of resources and training for the future. Drawing on their experiences, they can point out what works and what doesn't, which is vital for planning how to handle future outbreaks. By engaging in continuous education and professional development, healthcare providers remain equipped to adapt to evolving challenges posed by infectious disease outbreaks, reinforcing their essential role in safeguarding community health and improving response efficacy (Daskalakis et al., 2022) (Figure 6.17).

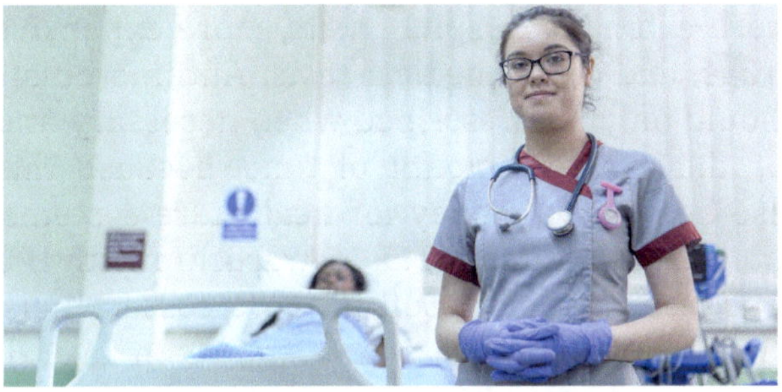

Figure 6.17. Role of healthcare providers in managing outbreaks.

Source: https://healthplan.co.uk/wp-content/uploads/2023/01/explaining-the-role-of-healthcare-professionals.jpg.

6.5.3. Importance of Antimicrobial Stewardship

The importance of antimicrobial stewardship cannot be overstated, particularly in today's world, where the prevalence of AMR continues to escalate. Antimicrobial stewardship involves using antimicrobials in the most effective manner possible, ensuring patient benefits and minimising the risk of antimicrobial resistance.

Strong stewardship programs can make a big difference in both patient health and public health by reducing the increasing rates of resistance. Worldwide, data reveal that 700,000 people die annually because of infections caused by resistant pathogens, which highlights the urgent need for strong stewardship efforts. The rise of AMR particularly threatens vulnerable populations in low-resource settings, emphasising the critical function of stewardship in reducing mortality and enhancing healthcare infrastructure, particularly in regions like sub-Saharan Africa with unique challenges (Kariuki et al., 2022). Apart from saving lives, antimicrobial stewardship is essential for the financial stability of health care systems. Using these programs helps control the high expenses associated with treating infections caused by resistant organisms. AMR-related expenses are estimated to be in the billions, mainly because they lead to more extended hospital visits, more expensive drugs, and extra medical tests. Antimicrobials should only be prescribed when necessary and for the correct amount of time, because this also helps save money for healthcare systems. Integrating antimicrobial stewardship with IPC practices can also result in more cost savings, which underscores its importance in overall infectious disease management. The convergence of effective stewardship and infection control is a crucial investment for health authorities aiming to tackle the multifaceted challenges of AMR (Murray et al., 2022). Also, teaching and training healthcare professionals is essential for antimicrobial stewardship programs to succeed. Providing prescribers with accurate information on antibiotic use helps the medical community respond to new cases of antibiotic resistance. This educational component fosters a culture where doctors recognize that certain infections do not require antibiotics. When healthcare systems update their training, it helps staff adhere to stewardship rules, which improves patient outcomes and reduces the likelihood of resistance. Having pharmacists, microbiologists, and infection control specialists on the team improves the stewardship framework by providing more effective ways to fight AMR. A concerted effort towards education, alongside policy implementation, will ensure that antimicrobial stewardship remains at the forefront of infectious disease control strategies globally, effectively addressing the existing gaps in combating both infections and resistance development within diverse settings (Kariuki et al., 2022).

6.6. Global Collaboration

Global collaboration stands as a cornerstone of effective infectious disease control strategies, especially in an increasingly interconnected world. The cooperative efforts of nations, organisations, and health entities are vital in creating a comprehensive and unified response to outbreaks. If countries use a variety of sources and experts, they can share information on diseases, findings from medical studies, and new ways to address them globally. They facilitate the spread of information, enabling public health actions to be supported by the latest and most accurate data. Collaboration has become increasingly important during global health emergencies, as demonstrated by the worldwide efforts during the COVID-19 pandemic. This approach emphasises that everyone has a responsibility to protect public health, as infectious diseases can affect people worldwide and necessitate a coordinated global response. In addition, effective infectious disease strategies depend on integrating health and environmental sustainability efforts, which underscores the importance of global cooperation. According to recent findings, the intersection of these fields presents unique opportunities to promote health outcomes while ensuring ecological integrity (Gwadabe et al., 2025).

For instance, integrated vector management

initiatives not only reduce the risks of vector-borne diseases but also contribute to the minimisation of pesticide resistance, showcasing the dual benefits of collaboration (Gwadabe et al., 2025). Mobile health apps and big data analysis are key in facilitating information sharing worldwide, allowing for close monitoring of disease outbreaks and the actions taken to address them. Because of this approach, governments, NGOs, and the private sector should join forces to help ensure sustainable practices that address health and environmental challenges, which strengthen global health security. Also, dealing with infectious diseases requires a lot of funding and resources, which emphasises the need for nations to cooperate globally. It has been found that the resources used for prevention and control have a significant effect on infectious disease outcomes. Allocating more funds to public health strategies is linked to lower mortality rates, highlighting the importance of countries pooling resources and sharing successful funding methods. Yet, providing more money alone, without a transparent team approach, could still leave public health emergencies unmanaged effectively. Because of this, it is essential to establish international partnerships and funding programs that ensure resources are shared fairly, allowing LMICs to enhance their control over infectious diseases. They create a strong global health system that can handle more outbreaks and protect people everywhere.

6.6.1. Role of International Organizations in Disease Control

International organisations play a pivotal role in the global strategy for controlling infectious diseases, acting as facilitators of dialogue, coordination, and resource allocation among nations. These organisations, such as the World Health Organisation (WHO) and various regional bodies, provide essential frameworks and guidelines that nations rely upon to strengthen their health systems. They encourage nations to cooperate, which allows them to exchange knowledge and skills needed to control and reduce the impact of outbreaks. Besides, these organisations often organise training programs to boost local health care skills, which helps countries handle sudden health emergencies better. Such collaborative frameworks are vital in establishing a cohesive global response to diseases that do not recognize borders, highlighting the necessity for international cooperation in health matters (N/A, 2009). Besides coordination, international organisations are essential for raising funds to help control diseases. They commonly oversee and share out money to fight public health threats, mainly in LMICs that do not have enough resources to deal with these issues themselves. As an example, when infectious diseases spread, these organisations set up ways to fund quick actions such as vaccination programs and emergency care. The help of international organisations provides immediate relief and supports long-term improvements in health systems, enabling countries to better prepare for future public health challenges. By advocating for and implementing sound financing mechanisms, they enhance global health security and would allow countries to prepare for and respond effectively to infectious diseases (Adu-Gyamfi et al., 2019). International organisations also play a role in preventing and responding early to infectious diseases, which is essential for controlling their spread. With the help of surveillance and epidemiological research, these organisations enable countries to monitor the onset and spread of diseases. Being vigilant is crucial in areas where outbreaks are likely, as it enables authorities to respond quickly and reduce the risk of transmission. They also make sure that health posts are set up at airports and borders, which helps with early identification and quarantine of those infected. This proactive approach not only aids individual countries but also contributes to global health stability, emphasizing the importance of preparedness and responsiveness in infectious disease control strategies (N/A, 2009) (Figure 6.18).

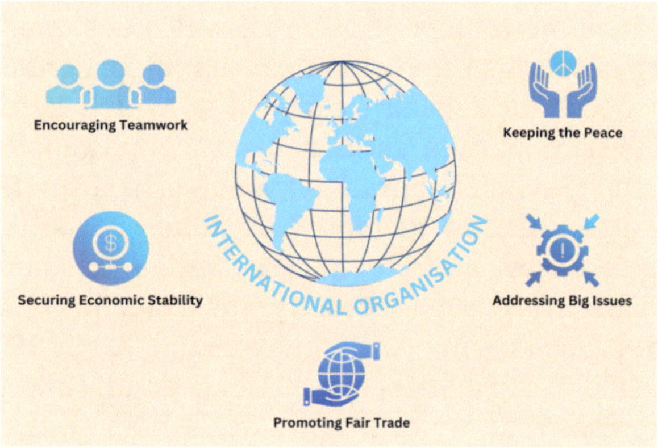

Figure 6.18. Role of international organizations in disease control.

Source: https://www.cheggindia.com/wp-content/uploads/2024/06/Importance-of-International-Organizations-1024x614.png.

6.6.2. Importance of Sharing Resources and Information

The sharing of resources and information is critical in the realm of infectious disease control strategies, as the collaborative effort between nations can enhance public health responses. Because diseases can affect any country, it is essential to collaborate for effective monitoring and control. The DSN helps to show how important this is by supporting better disease monitoring in developing countries. Such networks support collaboration among countries in a region, which is necessary for effective monitoring and response to diseases, helping nations respond quickly and collectively when outbreaks occur. By pooling resources and sharing data, countries can identify patterns and vulnerabilities shared across regions, making the response to infectious diseases faster and more coordinated, ultimately saving lives and reducing economic burden on healthcare systems (Ancheta et al., 2010). Reviews of projects such as the DSN Initiative further prove the success of collaborative networks. Rockefeller Foundation reports point out that strong collaboration between different fields improves disease monitoring and response. Participating in healthcare, environmental science, and emergency management helps create better plans for controlling infections. Because of this approach, nations can make better use of each other's strengths and new ideas to address both endemic and EIDs.

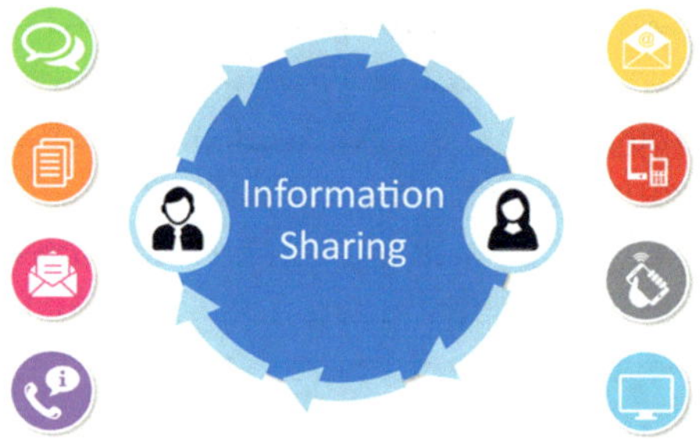

Figure 6.19. Importance of sharing resources and information.

Source: https://www.virtual-college.co.uk/-/media/vcwebsite2/images/ready-to-go-training/business-compliance/information-sharing-level-2/information-sharing_1.png?mw=750&hash=4E737E4DAF8945011CC61BAA82C9D40B48D427C5.

Furthermore, shared knowledge enriches the data pool, leading to better-informed decisions that can adapt to the evolving landscapes of infectious threats (Kimball et al., 2011). Making resources and information available to others ensures that the control of contagious diseases remains effective and trustworthy. These evaluations help review what has been done before and also help plan future actions in disease surveillance. This approach emphasises the importance of being open and flexible, allowing everyone to learn from both successes and failures. When information and resources are shared easily, organizations and countries can develop trust and strong public health systems. This interconnectedness is vital for tackling global health threats, reinforcing the idea that collaboration is not merely beneficial but imperative in the fight against infectious diseases (Kimball et al., 2011) (Figure 6.19).

6.6.3. Case Studies of Successful Global Initiatives

The global community has seen remarkable initiatives aimed at controlling infectious diseases, showcasing effective collaboration and innovative strategies. A prime example is the Global Polio Eradication Initiative (GPEI), launched in 1988, which brought together the WHO, UNICEF, and the Rotary Foundation. This initiative emphasised mass vaccination campaigns that significantly reduced polio incidence worldwide. By the early 2000s, the initiative had reduced polio cases by 99%, demonstrating how a worldwide effort could combat a long-standing health problem. Its success stems from adapting to each community's needs and leveraging technology to collect and deliver vaccines, an approach that has inspired other countries to emulate its approach to infectious diseases. Another significant case study is the Joint United Nations Program on HIV/AIDS (UNAIDS) and its 90-90-90 targets, aimed at ending the AIDS epidemic by 2030. In 2014, the initiative was started to diagnose, treat, and control the virus in people living with HIV. UNAIDS has encouraged cooperation among governments, non-governmental organisations, and the private sector, which has led to new ways of preventing and treating HIV. The program emphasised the importance of data in informing public health actions and enabling countries to track their progress and utilise resources effectively. In 2020, many nations had either achieved or were close to achieving the goals, showing that organized global actions can address health emergencies and guide future efforts against infectious diseases. The way the world dealt with COVID-19 has demonstrated the success of global health initiatives, primarily through collaboration on research and vaccine development.

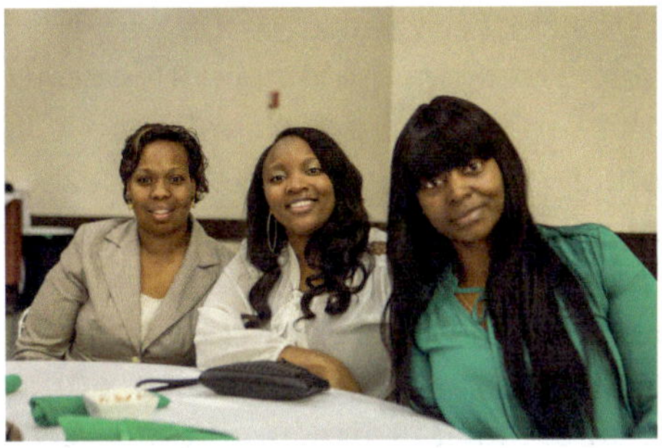

Figure 6.20. Case studies of successful global initiatives.

Source: https://infectiousdiseasesinitiative.org/images/galleries/2014/conference/18.jpg.

Organisations like the Coalition for Epidemic Preparedness Innovations (CEPI) played a pivotal role in mobilising resources for rapid vaccine research and development, facilitating partnerships among pharmaceutical companies and governments. The rapid development and distribution of vaccines are unlike anything seen before, demonstrating the collective commitment to addressing a global health issue. COVAX was also set up to help make vaccines available to everyone, especially in low- and middle-income countries, to address any differences in public health responses. Initiatives such as these underscore the importance of global cooperation, resource sharing, and strategic planning in infectious disease control, setting a precedent for future health emergencies (Kutikov et al., 2020; Tuite et al., 2020) (Figure 6.20).

SUMMARY

In concluding the examination of infectious disease control strategies, it is essential to emphasise the complex interplay between effective healthcare interventions and policy implementation. The increase in contagious diseases is linked to changes in global health, so a strong system for prevention and management is required. New approaches to treating diabetes, such as glucose-lowering therapies, demonstrate how advanced medical solutions can help prevent complications and enhance the health of populations. As illustrated in the context of Brazil, high-quality data can inform cost-effectiveness strategies that will enhance the prioritisation of healthcare resources, ultimately benefiting public health initiatives (Nogueira et al., 2023). The results of these studies can lower the number of sick people and also help ease the economic pressure on healthcare systems. Additionally, managing infectious diseases requires the use of both preventive strategies and medical treatments. The essential role of antimicrobial stewardship programs (ASPs) emerges as a critical component in optimising antimicrobial usage, thus combating the alarming rise of AMR that has claimed millions of lives (Echeverría-Esnal et al., 2023). Such stewardship initiatives strengthen public health measures and also enhance the ability of healthcare professionals, particularly clinical pharmacists, to implement effective interventions. When healthcare systems invest in learning and equipment, providers can use evidence-based methods that significantly lower the number of infectious diseases and their complications. In the end, controlling contagious diseases sustainably requires teams from different areas to cooperate beyond the usual healthcare settings. Managing these diseases effectively involves healthcare professionals, policymakers, and communities working together. When various stakeholders are involved and data is used, it becomes possible to design strategies that address new health challenges. More research is needed to develop new approaches that enhance the delivery of interventions and ensure equal access for all, particularly in underserved communities. Working together in this way will help build strong public health systems that can handle the challenges of infectious diseases in the 21st century.

To control infectious diseases, we must use a variety of techniques together. It was found that management of communicable diseases should be distinguished from the ways other resources are managed, for example, in fisheries and agriculture. By applying the lessons learned from these areas, public health can enhance its monitoring and response efforts. For example, using indicators and thresholds from integrated pest management can enhance the detection of diseases, improving both the speed and accuracy of disease detection. This transdisciplinary method not only fosters collaboration across different fields but also aids in tailoring strategies that are economically feasible and that clarify accountability among stakeholders, thus aligning diverse interests towards common public health objectives (Matsuda et al., 2024). It is also essential to use computational tools to assess and handle the daily risks of infectious diseases. Forecasting infection trends with ML algorithms has been very promising, especially when it comes to dealing with new variants like Omicron. Public health authorities can use spatiotemporal transmission intensity matrices to decide where to focus healthcare resources as infection rates change in different areas. Thanks to these approaches, it is easier to track and address outbreaks, which reduces the burden on healthcare services. In Hong Kong, for instance, the use of adaptive resource allocation strategies derived from empirical data resulted in substantial reductions in peak infection rates, underscoring the effectiveness of strategic, informed planning (Ren et al., 2022). Ultimately, integrating these separate approaches into a single plan enables swift action, flexibility, and ongoing benefits for public health. They suggest merging old public health methods with new technologies, including data analysis and flexible ways of managing problems. Insights from other management fields can add to current public health approaches and encourage more people to collaborate in governance. Sharing knowledge across different areas of science enhances public health and makes communities better equipped to respond to new outbreaks. Ultimately, establishing a culture of cooperation and innovation will be crucial in developing robust infectious disease control strategies that can effectively respond to emerging health threats (Matsuda et al., 2024).

CLOSER LOOK:

ADVISORY COMMITTEE ON IMMUNIZATION PRACTICES (ACIP):

The Advisory Committee on Immunization Practices (ACIP) plays a central role in shaping vaccine policy in the United States, functioning as an essential bridge between scientific evidence and public health action. Taking a closer look at ACIP reveals a structured, transparent, and highly collaborative process designed to ensure that immunization recommendations are grounded in rigorous data and aligned with the best interests of the population. ACIP is an independent panel of medical and public health experts convened by the Centers for Disease Control and Prevention (CDC). Its membership represents a wide range of specialties—including infectious diseases, pediatrics, internal medicine, nursing, pharmacy, and epidemiology—to ensure that multiple perspectives inform decision-making. In addition to voting members, ACIP includes non-voting liaisons from professional organizations and federal agencies, creating a forum for broad scientific collaboration. This multidisciplinary approach ensures that recommendations consider not only clinical evidence but also feasibility, equity, implementation, and public health impact.

One of ACIP's core responsibilities is evaluating new vaccines and determining how they should be used. This involves reviewing data on safety, efficacy, cost-effectiveness, disease burden, and real-world performance. The committee applies a structured evidence-assessment framework—commonly known as GRADE (Grading of Recommendations, Assessment, Development, and Evaluation)—to ensure consistency and transparency. Through public meetings and published documentation, ACIP provides insight into how scientific evidence translates into policy.

Once ACIP votes on a recommendation, it must be reviewed and approved by the CDC Director before becoming official U.S. immunization guidance. These recommendations influence the routine childhood and adult immunization schedules, insurance coverage mandates, and clinical practice nationwide. Because of this reach, ACIP plays a crucial role in promoting vaccine accessibility, preventing disease outbreaks, and maintaining high levels of community protection. ACIP's work is especially visible during public health emergencies. In times of emerging threats—such as novel respiratory viruses or sudden outbreaks—the committee rapidly evaluates data to guide vaccine prioritization, booster strategies, and risk-based recommendations. Its transparent process, which includes live-streamed meetings and publicly available reports, helps build public trust and enables clinicians to follow rapidly evolving guidance.

Ultimately, a closer look at the Advisory Committee on Immunization Practices reveals a model of evidence-based public health decision-making. By combining scientific rigor, open deliberation, and broad expertise, ACIP ensures that immunization policies remain responsive to new data and aligned with the goal of protecting population health.

REFERENCES

1. Aarøe, L., Petersen, M. B., & Arceneaux, K. (2017). The behavioral immune system shapes political intuitions: why and how individual differences in disgust sensitivity underlie opposition to immigration. *American Political Science Review, 111*(2), 277–294. https://doi.org/10.1017/s0003055416000770Adu-Gyamfi, S. (2019). *Ebola Hemorrhagic Fever in Africa: A Necessary Highlight.* https://core.ac.uk/download/480549437.pdf (accessed on 30th May 2025).
2. Akter, M., Nurunnahar, Ullah, M., Meetei, M. Z., Zaagan, A. A., & Mahnashi, A. M. (2024). An innovative fractional-order evolutionary game theoretical study of personal protection, quarantine, and isolation policies for combating epidemic diseases. *Scientific Reports, 14.* https://www.semanticscholar.org/paper/982b9e6dc77cf599133a114427472c0841a76f27 (accessed on 30th May 2025).
3. Ancheta, C. A., Perez, E. S., Richter, K., Tempongko, M. S. B., Sunpuwan, M., Mendoza, O. M., Pachuen, O., et al. (2010). *Disease Surveillance Networks Initiative Asia: Final Evaluation.* https://core.ac.uk/download/86445039.pdf (accessed on 30th May 2025).
4. Baker, M. G., Kvalsvig, A., & Verrall, A. J. (2020). New Zealand's COVID-19 elimination strategy. *The Medical Journal of Australia, 213*, 198–. https://doi.org/10.5694/mja2.50735.
5. Balmes, J., Ritz, B., & Tager, I. (2004). *Can Lessons from Public Health Disease Surveillance be Applied to Environmental Public Health Tracking?* https://core.ac.uk/download/pdf/3775836.pdf (accessed on 30th May 2025).
6. Basir, F. A., Rajak, B., Rahman, B., & Hattaf, K. (2023). Hopf bifurcation analysis and optimal control of an infectious disease with awareness campaign and treatment. *Axioms, 12*, 608. https://www.semanticscholar.org/paper/eb34ec901f7cda5518751947765f4eaa458e5f69 (accessed on 30th May 2025).
7. Beck-Johnson, L. M., Hallman, C., Lindström, T., Miller, R., et al. (2019). *Effects of Regional Differences and Demography in Modeling Foot-and-Mouth Disease in Cattle at the National Scale.* https://core.ac.uk/download/287606180.pdf (accessed on 30th May 2025).
8. Bergquist, R., Tanner, M., Utzinger, J., Yap, P., et al. (2016). Surveillance and response systems for elimination of tropical diseases: Summary of a thematic series in infectious diseases of poverty. *Infect. Dis. Poverty.* https://core.ac.uk/download/46605195.pdf (accessed on 30th May 2025).
9. Chandra, V., Gaidhane, A., & Choudhari, S. G. (2024). Public health strategies in the face of crisis: A comprehensive review of the Zika outbreak in India. *Cureus, 16.* https://www.semanticscholar.org/paper/46371d00ded47b5d1497227c5d2d2285e0d62771 (accessed on 30th May 2025).
10. Connolly, K. L., Bachmann, L., Hiltke, T., Kersh, E. N., Newman, L. M., Wilson, L., Mena, L., et al. (2024). Summary of the Centers for Disease Control and Prevention/National Institute of Allergy and Infectious Diseases Joint Workshop on Genital Herpes: 3–4 November 2022. *Open Forum Infectious Diseases, 11*(5), ofae230. https://www.semanticscholar.org/paper/5eec56195f3c1a8d19d853dabd16739eedae2c91 (accessed on 30th May 2025).

11. Connors, M., Graham, B. S., Lane, H. C., & Fauci, A. S. (2021). SARS-CoV-2 vaccines: Much accomplished, much to learn. *Annals of Internal Medicine, 174*, 687–690. https://doi.org/10.7326/m21-0111.

12. d'Hemecourt, P., & Luke, A. (2007). *Prevention of Infectious Diseases in Athletes.* https://core.ac.uk/download/323072758.pdf (accessed on 30th May 2025).

13. Da Gama, K. M., Romeiro, E. T., Da Silva, C. L., De Jesus, B. M. S., De Freitas, H. C., De Sousa, B. E., Dos Santos, V. S., et al. (2024). Strategies for control and prevention of emerging infectious diseases: Lessons learned and future directions. *Revista Ibero-Americana de Humanidades, Ciências e Educação.* https://www.semanticscholar.org/paper/360b6bb89cda4fe9ed2a82627c255169525048c2 (accessed on 30th May 2025).

14. Daskalakis, D., McClung, R. P., Mena, L., Mermin, J., McQuiston, J. H., Damon, I. K., Monroe, B., et al. (2022). Monkeypox: Avoiding the mistakes of past infectious disease epidemics. *Annals of Internal Medicine, 175*, 1177, 1178. https://doi.org/10.7326/m22-1748.

15. Dhagat, P., Coan, J., Ganguly, A., Puetz, C., Silvestri, D., & Madad, S. S. (2025). Enhancing healthcare preparedness: Lessons from a tabletop exercise on highly pathogenic avian influenza (HPAI). *Tropical Medicine and Infectious Disease, 10.* https://www.semanticscholar.org/paper/bcd1f3d4b20d0b9857c9c58ab8cd0f3d394f59f5 (accessed on 30th May 2025).

16. Echeverría-Esnal, D., Hernandez, S., Murgadella-Sancho, A., García-Paricio, R., Ortonobes, S., Barrantes-González, M., Padullés, A., et al. (2023). Cross-sectional survey on the current role of clinical pharmacists among antimicrobial stewardship programs in Catalonia: Much ado about nothing. *Antibiotics, 12.* https://www.semanticscholar.org/paper/08ec2c37bb1b5c77e2a2b935b33463c0c434a78e (accessed on 30th May 2025).

17. Ferrie, J. P., & Troesken, W. (2025). *Death and the City: Chicago's Mortality Transition, 1850–1925.* https://core.ac.uk/download/pdf/6606152.pdf (accessed on 30th May 2025).

18. Gamon, M. (2013). *Maribel Gamon – Multidrug-Resistant Tuberculosis in India: Solving a Problem by Reconstructing the Public Health Infrastructure.* https://core.ac.uk/download/67755957.pdf (accessed on 30th May 2025).

19. Gulliver, E., Di Simone, S. K., Chonwerawong, M., & Forster, S. C. (2024). Unlocking the potential for microbiome-based therapeutics to address the sustainable development goal of good health and wellbeing. *Microbial Biotechnology, 17.* https://www.semanticscholar.org/paper/aa6e9f35c0b283b76c0417d5c965d85a224fd009 (accessed on 30th May 2025).

20. Gwadabe, H. A., Elelu, S. A., Innocent, M. O., Ibrahim, G. O., Adekunle, I. J., & Abdulsalam, M. (2025). Exploring local-to-global win-win strategies for infectious disease control: Enhancing human health and sustainability. *Biological Sciences.* https://www.semanticscholar.org/paper/18c619905221b190ca54092850e62596841729c8 (accessed on 30th May 2025).

21. Hulstine, A. (2017). *Vaccine Implementation: Alaska 2017.* https://core.ac.uk/download/286607590.pdf (accessed on 30th May 2025).

22. Indravudh, P. P., McGee, K., Sibanda, E., Corbett, E. L., Fielding, K., & Terris-Prestholt, F. (2025). Community-led strategies for communicable disease prevention and management in low- and middle-income countries: A mixed-methods systematic review of health, social, and economic impact. *PLOS Global Public Health, 5.* https://www.semanticscholar.org/paper/0b37d67763a7423e336d6d4f456e4e0d7434ee47 (accessed on 30th May 2025).

23. Kaba, A. (2011). *The Changing Nature of Health Professionals' Work: The Impact of Infectious Disease.* https://core.ac.uk/download/639159949.pdf (accessed on 30th May 2025).
24. Kadio, K., Ly, A., Ouédraogo, A., Ag Ahmed, M. A., Yaya, S., & Gagnon, M. P. (2024). Implementation of lockdown, quarantine, and isolation measures in the context of COVID-19 among internally displaced persons in Burkina Faso: A qualitative study. *Conflict and Health, 18.* https://www.semanticscholar.org/paper/ed7fa356de90a46955f533909f3ae6cec7b05892 (accessed on 30th May 2025).
25. Karaut, T. S. (2024). Evaluating the effectiveness and coverage of vaccination programs in reducing the incidence of pediatric infectious diseases. *Asian Journal of Pediatric Research.* https://www.semanticscholar.org/paper/042260c9d1959d911f8737e15a55e4aa880e49fb (accessed on 30th May 2025).
26. Kariuki, S., Kering, K., Wairimu, C., Onsare, R., & Mbae, C. (2022). Antimicrobial resistance rates and surveillance in Sub-Saharan Africa: Where are we now? *Infection and Drug Resistance, 15,* 3589–3609. https://doi.org/10.2147/idr.s342753.
27. Kimball, A. M., Gugerty, M. K., Abernethy, N., & Curran, S. (2011). *Disease Surveillance Networks Initiative Global: Final Evaluation.* https://core.ac.uk/download/86445037.pdf (accessed on 30th May 2025).
28. Klingberg, S., Adhikari, B., Draper, C. E., Bosire, E. N., Nyirenda, D., Tiigah, P., & Mukumbang, F. C. (2024). Enhanced or hindered research benefits? A realist review of community engagement and participatory research practices for non-communicable disease prevention in low- and middle-income countries. *BMJ Global Health, 9.* https://www.semanticscholar.org/paper/0dcd625b8fda5cd5322abd39f8718b401a5ff5c3 (accessed on 30th May 2025).
29. Kuntz, J. (2020). Resilience in times of global pandemic: Steering recovery and thriving trajectories. *Applied Psychology, 70,* 188–215. https://doi.org/10.1111/apps.12296.
30. Kutikov, A., Weinberg, D. S., Edelman, M. J., Horwitz, E. M., Uzzo, R. G., & Fisher, R. I. (2020). A war on two fronts: Cancer care in the time of COVID-19. *Annals of Internal Medicine, 172,* 756–758. https://doi.org/10.7326/m20-1133.
31. Marangu, V. M., Kei, R. M., & Kithinji, D. K. (2024). Review of participatory epidemiology application in human health and nutrition and future directions. *African Journal of Science, Technology and Social Sciences.* https://www.semanticscholar.org/paper/1c411ab3d70d6810c6151abbdf244ffc2f352676 (accessed on 30th May 2025).
32. Matsuda, H., & Watanabe, A. (2024). A comparative study of population management approaches in infectious disease control, population management of fisheries and wildlife, and integrated pest management in agriculture. *Population Ecology.* https://www.semanticscholar.org/paper/17aaa41e9ad3ec7d1bb56bfd26aa0e6813dee3d0 (accessed on 30th May 2025).
33. McCloskey, B., Dar, O., Zumla, A., & Heymann, D. (2014). Emerging infectious diseases and pandemic potential: Status quo and reducing risk of global spread. *The Lancet Infectious Diseases, 14,* 1001–1010. https://doi.org/10.1016/s1473-3099(14)70846-1.
34. Muneeb, J. M., Pawaskar, D. K., Muteeb-Ullah-Rafiqui, Siddiqui, R., Shabir, N., Pawaskar, N. K., & Rasool, A. (2024). A comprehensive overview of infectious bursal disease, a major threat to poultry health and production. *International Journal of Advanced Biochemistry Research.* https://www.semanticscholar.org/paper/e7b68f8ee6839c70fdeaee185034f726f110eda3 (accessed on 30th May 2025).

35. Murray, C. J. L., Ikuta, K. S., Sharara, F., Swetschinski, L. R., Robles, A. G., Gray, A. P., Han, C., et al. (2022). Global burden of bacterial antimicrobial resistance in 2019: A systematic analysis. *The Lancet, 399*, 629–655. https://doi.org/10.1016/s0140-6736(21)02724-0.

36. N/A. (2009). *The U.S. Government's Global Health Policy Architecture: Structure, Programs and Funding*. https://core.ac.uk/download/71348672.pdf (accessed on 30th May 2025).

37. Nogueira, A., Barreto, J., Moura, F., Luchiari, B., Abuhab, A., Bonilha, I., Nadruz, W., et al. (2023). Comparative effectiveness and cost-effectiveness of cardioprotective glucose-lowering therapies for type 2 diabetes in Brazil: A Bayesian network model. *Health Economics Review, 13*. https://www.semanticscholar.org/paper/8138a95537f0a26b76453f162fc32aab4bb16b9f (accessed on 30th May 2025).

38. Nyiramana, M. P. (2024). The role of genomics in infectious disease control. *Research Invention Journal of Public Health and Pharmacy*. https://www.semanticscholar.org/paper/789b946d9579ac4e4b96a072b56ff2cc1b335481 (accessed on 30th May 2025).

39. Perfilyeva, Y., Aquino, A., Borodin, M. A., Kali, A., Abdolla, N., Ostapchuk, Y., Tleulieva, R., et al. (2024). Can interventions targeting MDSCs improve the outcome of vaccination in vulnerable populations? *International Reviews of Immunology*. https://www.semanticscholar.org/paper/3bb077458a8703a30485a7f2f28fc0315243183f (accessed on 30th May 2025).

40. Phanphakdi, W. (2023). Managing strategy and organizational policy for growth and sustainability after COVID-19 crisis: Case study of large-sized listed companies. In *15th Global Conference on Business and Social Sciences on 14–15 September 2023, Novotel Bangkok Platinum Pratunam, Thailand*. https://www.semanticscholar.org/paper/c375e3825d08215211c29dd8b51d4a23fe42b3e3 (accessed on 30th May 2025).

41. Pourbohloul, B., Brandriss, B., Grenfell, B., Cauchemez, S., Dauer, C., Dezso, Z., et al. (2006). *A Comparative Analysis of Influenza Vaccination Programs*. https://core.ac.uk/download/pdf/4063374.pdf (accessed on 30th May 2025).

42. Ratra, N. (2023). Mathematical modeling for infectious disease control and vaccination strategies: Insights from India. *International Journal of Science and Research (IJSR)*. https://www.semanticscholar.org/paper/7dff416ad1eb06538d430a108434412447d1e1a8 (accessed on 30th May 2025).

43. Ren, J., Liu, M., Liu, Y., & Liu, J. (2022). Optimal resource allocation with spatiotemporal transmission discovery for effective disease control. *Infectious Diseases of Poverty, 11*. https://www.semanticscholar.org/paper/4b04a5944c1390e1bafb46b0ce5160869a466fec (accessed on 30th May 2025).

44. Roth, G. A., Mensah, G. A., Johnson, C. O., Addolorato, G., Ammirati, E., Baddour, L. M., Barengo, N. C., et al. (2020). Global burden of cardiovascular diseases and risk factors, 1990–2019. *Journal of the American College of Cardiology, 76*, 2982–3021. https://doi.org/10.1016/j.jacc.2020.11.010.

45. Santomauro, D., Mantilla, H. A. M., Shadid, J., Zheng, P., Ashbaugh, C., Pigott, D. M., Abbafati, C., et al. (2021). Global prevalence and burden of depressive and anxiety disorders in 204 countries and territories in 2020 due to the COVID-19 pandemic. *The Lancet, 398*, 1700–1712. https://doi.org/10.1016/s0140-6736(21)02143-7.

46. Sedighian, N., Guineheux, A., van der Wolf, J. M., & Déziel, E. (2025). Ecofriendly control

strategies against *Clavibacter michiganensis*, the causal agent of bacterial canker of tomato. *Plant Disease*. https://www.semanticscholar.org/paper/8bd4e3337c1c9e8eb49fbdf625ebd2cf5518598f (accessed on 30th May 2025).

47. Solehuddin, M. (2025). Community-based health education for infectious disease prevention in Ulu Bawang Barat District. *Pengabdian: Jurnal Abdimas*. https://www.semanticscholar.org/paper/02c1e0f0dc589870abff0a4d4c9228be7b585fe9 (accessed on 30th May 2025).

48. Soltanian, A., Ahmaddoost-Razdari, R., Mahjub, H., & Poorolajal, J. (2023). Impact of COVID-19 Disease Control Committee (CDCC) policies on prevention of the disease using Bayes network inference in west of Iran. *BMC Public Health, 23*. https://www.semanticscholar.org/paper/4df67383fe9f686dea81d385c4011067567a6b24 (accessed on 30th May 2025).

49. Srivastava, S., Kumar, S., Sharma, P. K., Rustagi, S., Mohanty, A., Donovan, S., Henao-Martínez, A., et al. (2024). Control strategies for emerging infectious diseases: Crimean-Congo hemorrhagic fever management. *Health Science Reports, 7*. https://www.semanticscholar.org/paper/0070505be9f28cb5bfef53d331b24da065a5ce2c (accessed on 30th May 2025).

50. Tian, Y., Deng, Z., & Yang, P. (2022). mRNA vaccines: A novel weapon to control infectious diseases. *Frontiers in Microbiology, 13*. https://doi.org/10.3389/fmicb.2022.1008684.

51. Tuite, A. R., Bogoch, I. I., Sherbo, R., Watts, A., Fisman, D. N., & Khan, K. (2020). Estimation of Coronavirus Disease 2019 (COVID-19) burden and potential for international dissemination of infection from Iran. *Annals of Internal Medicine, 172*, 699–701. https://doi.org/10.7326/m20-0696.

52. Winata, N., Hasyim, D. M., & Primulyanto, B. A. (2024). Pharmaceutical involvement in infectious disease control: Strategies, challenge and solutions. *Journal of Pharmacopoeia*. https://www.semanticscholar.org/paper/6d4a88c6d5c2c4b236078cbbb6abec8f42b3c6d3 (accessed on 30th May 2025).

53. Winkler, M. L., Paras, M. L., Wright, S. B., & Shenoy, E. S. (2024). National survey of infectious disease fellowship program directors: A call for subspecialized training in infection prevention and control and healthcare epidemiology. *Infection Control & Hospital Epidemiology, 45*, 562–566. https://www.semanticscholar.org/paper/f91f7f4c0b558cfd8bfbd70e260a239fedbcba0e (accessed on 30th May 2025).

54. Winter, A. K., & Hegde, S. T. (2020). The important role of serology for COVID-19 control. *The Lancet Infectious Diseases, 20*, 758, 759. https://doi.org/10.1016/s1473-3099(20)30322-4.

55. Zarebski, A., Tellioglu, N., Stockdale, J. E., Spencer, J. A., KhudaBukhsh, W. R., Miller, J. C., & Zachreson, C. (2025). *Including Frameworks of Public Health Ethics in Computational Modeling of Infectious Disease Interventions*. ArXiv, abs/2502.00071. https://www.semanticscholar.org/paper/7f7ba7440a5fb46f45853c29125b49d627411362 (accessed on 30th May 2025).

56. Zhang, Z. (2025). Analysis report on trends in public infectious disease control in China. *Frontiers in Public Health, 12*. https://www.semanticscholar.org/paper/4ba1cea3b1fc7cdf85387969e53c95573d70dd43 (accessed on 30th May 2025).

57. Zhu, C., Diao, Z., Yang, Y., Liao, J., Wang, C., Li, Y., Liang, Z., et al. (2025). Recent advances and challenges in metal-based antimicrobial materials: A review of strategies to combat antibiotic resistance. *Journal of Nanobiotechnology, 23*. https://www.semanticscholar.org/paper/b1e04af99aa63f6766174eceb99e39c21b4fc7e4 (accessed on 30th May 2025).

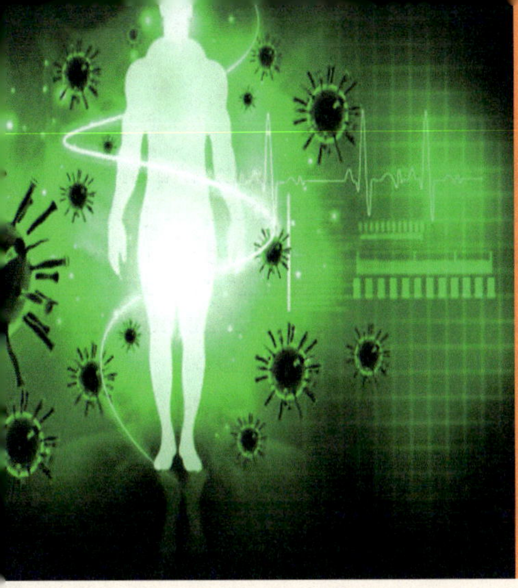

Chapter 7

EMERGING AND REEMERGING INFECTIOUS DISEASES

Contents

Introduction

Understanding the scope of emerging and reemerging infectious diseases (EIDs) necessitates a comprehensive overview of the dynamics that influence their spread and impact on global health. The term emerging infectious diseases (EIDs) refers to newly identified pathogens or previously recognized pathogens that have significantly increased in incidence or geographic range. In contrast, some contagious diseases that were once less common are resurfacing due to changes in society, the environment, and human activities. It demonstrates how contagious diseases interact with the environment and human well-being, which calls for us to be watchful and adapt to new challenges. The interaction between people and the environment, mainly due to urbanisation and globalisation, is a significant reason infectious diseases appear. Mosquitoes, which can carry arboviruses such as those from *Ae. aegypti* and *Ae. albopictus*, are now more likely to occur in cities. Due to modern transportation, diseases can spread rapidly across the globe and reach new areas quickly. The presence of these vectors in cities indicates that disease transmission has evolved, utilising human and urban resources alongside natural sources. This change necessitates an urgent reassessment of public health strategies to combat the challenges posed by these emerging threats effectively (Lwande et al., 2019). Besides ecological and environmental factors, how society and politics respond to infectious diseases is very important. During the COVID-19 pandemic, it was clear that political views and social settings affected how likely people were to get vaccinated. In places where most people vote Republican, fewer people are vaccinated, and this leads to higher rates of both infection and death, showing how political views can hinder public health measures. Trust in health professionals and science needs to be restored, and communication plans should be made that are not influenced by political views. Addressing the social determinants of health is essential to ensure better preparedness and response to EIDs, ultimately fostering a unified approach to safeguard global health (Albrecht, 2022) (Figure 7.1).

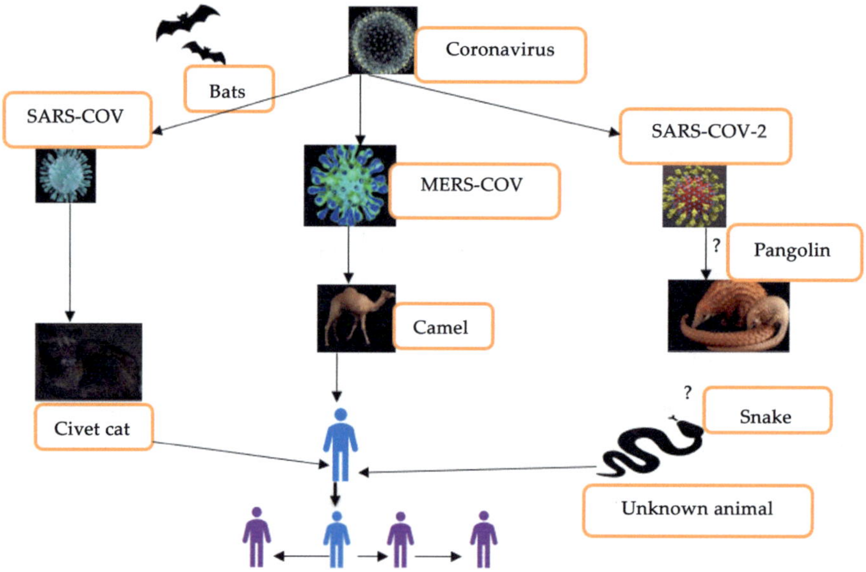

Figure 7.1. Emerging and reemerging infectious diseases.

Source: https://www.clinmedjournals.org/articles/ijva/ijva-7-067-004.jpg.

Definition of Emerging Infectious Diseases

EIDs represent a critical category within the field of epidemiology, encompassing newly recognised infections or those that have recently increased in incidence or geographic range. These diseases often arise from complex interactions among human populations, pathogens, and environmental factors, leading to significant public health challenges. EIDs may be defined as including zoonotic infections that can spread from animals to humans, highlighting the close proximity of wildlife ecosystems to human health. As these diseases become increasingly common, including those caused by novel coronaviruses, it is clear that we need better surveillance and health services everywhere. Since EIDs are unprecedented, it is necessary to study their causes, how they spread, and their effects on people's health in a complete way. Also, knowing what EIDs are requires considering the reasons why they emerge. Changes in the environment, land use, and climate help cause EIDs by allowing humans to interact more with wild animals, which can result in diseases spreading from animals to humans. Deforestation can destroy the habitats of many species, leading animals to move closer to people, which increases the risk of zoonotic diseases. Due to this combination of social and environmental changes, it is increasingly challenging to predict and control outbreaks. For this reason, defining EIDs requires understanding both the pathogens and the larger ecological and social contexts that enable these diseases to spread, as these aspects significantly influence public health strategies. Also, identifying diseases as emerging or reemerging is crucial for preparing and responding to health issues. Since reemerging infectious diseases are back due to reasons such as antibiotic resistance, fewer vaccinations or changes in society, they need different management approaches than newly emerging diseases. In some regions, tuberculosis and malaria are reappearing, which shows how reemergence can be challenging and calls for ongoing attention and updated public health measures. It is important to join forces in veterinary health, environmental science, and global health when trying to tackle EIDs. A multifaceted approach that incorporates surveillance data, research on pathogen behavior, and coordinated public health responses is essential to mitigate the impact of both emerging and reemerging infectious diseases (EIDs) (Baker et al., 2020; Verity et al., 2020) (Figure 7.2).

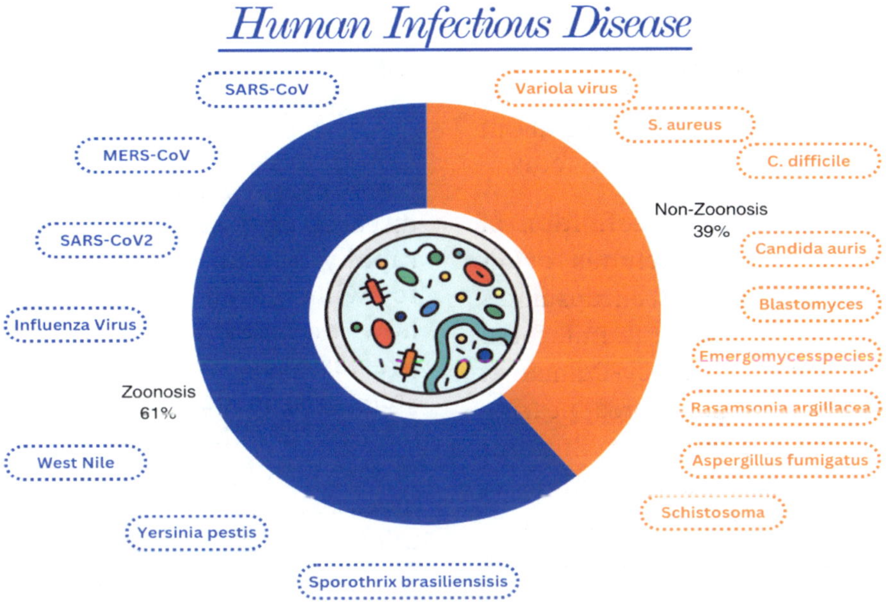

Figure 7.2. Emerging infectious diseases.

Source: https://www.mdpi.com/genes/genes-15-00908/article_deploy/html/images/genes-15-00908-g003.png.

Definition of Reemerging Infectious Diseases

The classification of reemerging infectious diseases plays a vital role in understanding their impact on public health. These diseases are called reemerging because they have increased in numbers after a period when they were less common, primarily due to changes in the environment, microbial adaptation, and societal development. It highlights the strong connections between human actions, environmental changes, and health threats, underscoring the need for public health to be adaptable and responsive. In Canada, Lyme disease is being noticed more often because Ixodes scapularis, the vector, is moving northward. The convergence of urban development and climate change has had significant implications for the spread and risk associated with such diseases, thereby emphasizing the importance of socio-ecological factors in the epidemiology of reemerging infections (Logan et al., 2023). Because reemerging diseases are constantly changing, it is important to keep researching and staying alert to infectious diseases. Although established infections are known to be dangerous, reappearing diseases, which are often perceived as new threats, require special attention. For instance, in the case of the Zika virus (ZIKV), its classification as an emerging infection was solidified following its rapid spread in Brazil, leading to a surge in congenital anomalies such as microcephaly. Realizing that pregnant women can get both well-known and novel infections has led to new worries about the health of both the mother and the fetus.

The Institute of Medicine's definition of emerging infections, which includes drug-resistant and reemerging diseases, encapsulates this complexity by recognizing the multifaceted nature of infectious threats (Meaney-Delman et al., 2017). Fighting diseases that are reappearing requires using surveillance, carrying out research, and taking immediate action. It involves studying the societal and natural factors that contribute to outbreaks and examining the relationships between human activities and diseases. Additionally, diseases that recur can exploit gaps in vaccination and the public health system. Because urban areas with Lyme disease are affected by environmental conditions and the human population, public health strategies should be adjusted to prevent risks. Ultimately, fostering interdisciplinary collaborations and enhancing community awareness can be instrumental in effectively tackling the evolving landscape of infectious diseases (Logan et al., 2023) (Figure 7.3).

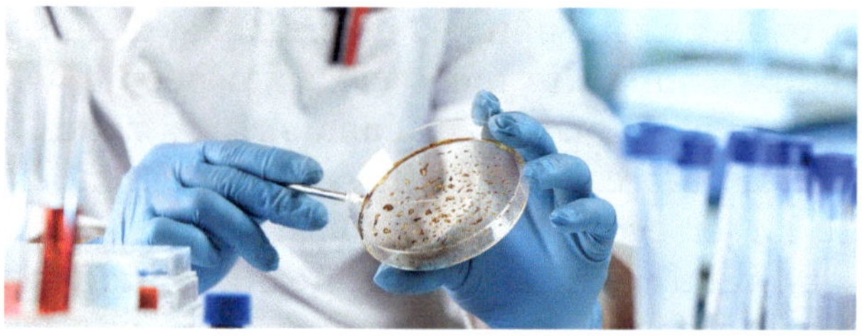

Figure 7.3. The classification of reemerging infectious diseases.

Source: https://www.hopkinsmedicine.org/-/media/images/health/1_-conditions/infectious-diseases/researcher-checking-a-petri-dish-hero.jpg?h=500&iar=0&mh=500&mw=1300&w=1297&hash=5C43F6C5C319BC7F9BA84A175B54E47A.

Importance of Studying These Diseases

The study of EIDs is paramount not only for public health but also for global security. These diseases pose substantial threats, as they can rapidly spread across populations, leading to widespread outbreaks. Understanding how diseases are transmitted, healthcare professionals can take effective preventive steps and manage outbreaks effectively. The CDC and similar agencies play a crucial role in this task by guiding efforts to identify and investigate major infectious diseases. Their initiatives include conducting applied research and maintaining surveillance systems that detect and mitigate risks associated with these pathogens. Being proactive in this way helps to create vaccines and other solutions that strengthen public health against future dangers. It is also essential to understand the economic impact of these diseases. Economies may suffer, health systems may be disrupted and infectious diseases may overload healthcare resources. When outbreaks occur, healthcare expenses increase, and productivity at work drops due to illness. When infectious diseases are studied first, countries can use their resources to predict and handle potential outbreaks. When new pathogens are studied, they become known threats, which makes it easier to control them. As noted, rapid mobilization of research capabilities to address knowledge gaps is crucial for managing risks associated with emerging pathogens (Buchanan et al., 1997). Therefore, focusing on these diseases helps protect both health systems and the economy in a world where countries are becoming more connected. Additionally, understanding how infectious diseases spread enables the development of effective public health policies. They can rely on research to develop policies that help improve people's vulnerability and resilience. Efforts to prevent diseases, such as vaccination and public education, rely on data collected from continuous research. Because of globalization and climate change, such initiatives are crucial since they help prevent and control infectious diseases. Working together, researchers, healthcare providers, and policymakers create a strategy that improves how response efforts are carried out. Consequently, the importance of studying these diseases transcends mere scientific inquiry; it is a cornerstone of enhancing societal health, economic vitality, and global preparedness.

7.1. Historical Context

Throughout history, the emergence and reemergence of infectious diseases have often coincided with significant socio-political and environmental transformations. It is clear from the relationship between human actions and disease spread that changes in land use, urban life, and globalisation can make it easier for infectious agents to spread. The Black Death in the 14th century and the 1918 flu pandemic demonstrate that changes in human mobility and living patterns can facilitate the rapid spread of pathogens. When people move into new areas, the chance of getting zoonotic diseases rises. Because of this, what we have learned from previous epidemics helps us understand what might cause future outbreaks, especially as human-wildlife contacts and changes in climate continue to disrupt the natural balance in nature. In the context of blood safety, historical approaches to managing infectious agents have laid the groundwork for current pathogen reduction technologies (PRTs). Screening techniques have advanced significantly over the last century, providing a deeper understanding of the risks associated with blood-borne pathogens. In the 1940s, blood donations were checked for syphilis and other infectious diseases, and over time, testing for viruses such as hepatitis B and HIV was added. Because of the ongoing risk of EIDs, new laboratory methods and PRTs were needed to ensure blood transfusions were safe. The establishment of rigorous protocols during workshops convened by organisations such as the FDA illustrates a proactive approach that builds on historical responses to HIV and hepatitis outbreaks, ultimately guiding contemporary efforts to bolster blood safety amid evolving disease threats (Atreya et al., 2019). Furthermore, how people have responded to EIDs over the years has been affected by both new medical knowledge and changes in society. How public health organisations respond to new threats shows the influence of broader social and political trends. For example, the recent emergence of the Zika and Ebola viruses has necessitated a review of public health's response and resource utilisation, highlighting the need for flexible strategies in combating infectious diseases. Such outbreaks have highlighted the weaknesses in health systems worldwide and encouraged countries to collaborate on surveillance and response. Learning from past experiences, combined with new technology, underscores the need for robust and adaptable strategies to address EIDs. Adapting to these challenges requires an unwavering commitment to research, public policy reform, and global cooperation in a landscape characterised by unpredictable health threats (Cameron et al., 2019).

7.1.1. Overview of Past Pandemics and Outbreaks

Throughout history, pandemics and outbreaks have emerged as significant public health challenges, reshaping societies and economies on a global scale. In the 14th century, the Black Death, a form of bubonic plague, significantly reduced Europe's population and brought about substantial changes to society and the economy. In the same way, the 1918 influenza pandemic killed millions and changed health care systems, resulting in new medical research. The recent cases of ZIKV and Ebola virus disease show that people are still at risk from EIDs. All of these events have helped us realize that surveillance, quick action, and better medical practices are key to managing major health issues. The emergence and recurrence of infectious diseases are strongly influenced by ecological, biological, and human factors. With vector-borne diseases, the warming climate helps pathogens and their carriers, such as *Aedes albopictus*, to spread and also move to new regions because of globalization and people traveling. To address these problems, public health authorities are recommended to use early warning systems and integrated surveillance, according to studies that look at cross-border cooperation. By understanding past pandemics and their causes, public health efforts can be enhanced to better handle future outbreaks. This holistic approach is necessary to enhance resilience against infectious diseases in the face of an ever-evolving threat landscape (Jenkins et al., 2024). Another dimension to consider in understanding past outbreaks is the impact of antimicrobial resistance (AMR) on disease management. Due to the rise in drug-resistant infections, it is becoming increasingly clear that some current treatment protocols are less effective than they once were, as evidenced by *Staphylococcus aureus* strains that resist standard antibiotics. This problem has become even clearer after COVID, highlighting the need to find new ways to overcome resistance patterns that threaten good care. Advancements in genomics and machine learning (ML) provide promising avenues for rapid diagnosis and understanding the genetic underpinnings of resistance. Considering past pandemics, it is essential to utilise advanced technology to develop new treatments and enhance our methods for addressing emerging threats. By studying resistance over the past decade and deploying new strategies, we can make a more robust health infrastructure ready to confront future public health crises (Gopikrishnan et al., 2024) (Figure 7.4).

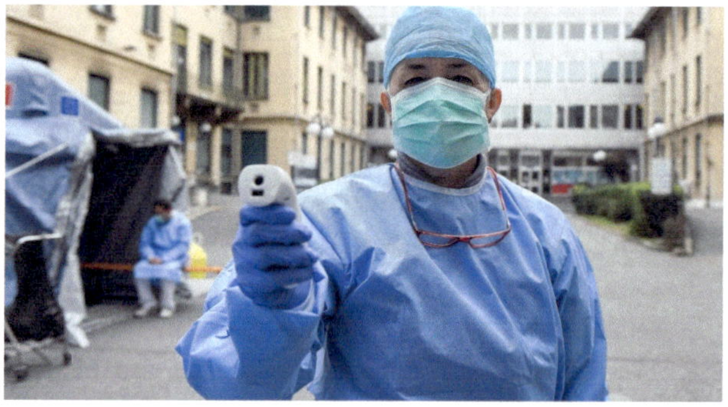

Figure 7.4. Overview of past pandemics and outbreaks.

Source: https://cf-images.us-east-1.prod.boltdns.net/v1/static/694940094001/d85da6ca-a19a-4fac-ba85-2c9c616a62ca/02179336-d530-4cd5-87bb-38ac8c602ba1/1280x720/match/image.jpg.

7.1.2. Factors Contributing to the Emergence of Diseases

The emergence of infectious diseases is often attributed to a complex interplay of various factors, including environmental, sociological, and technological changes. A significant reason is the way people's behaviours and lifestyles are changing because of urbanisation and globalisation. When people migrate and live in crowded areas, diseases have more chances to be transmitted. Modern transportation methods, such as airplanes, enable people to travel quickly across the globe, which in turn helps pathogens spread more rapidly. Changes in the climate have also influenced where vectors live, which has helped infectious agents that were previously controlled to increase. As a result, it is essential to understand how human actions contribute to the rise of diseases for successful public health efforts. Zoonotic transmission is another crucial reason why infectious diseases appear. Many of the major EIDs originate from animals, highlighting the connection between animal and human health, known as One Health. For instance, when people modify their farming practices and expand into areas where wildlife resides, it disrupts the natural balance and increases the likelihood of humans contracting zoonotic diseases. Furthermore, the emergence of more virulent strains complicates matters. The introduction of new ways to diagnose infections has helped us realise that many bacteria thought not to be serious are now recognised as major health threats. As highlighted in various studies, comprehensive monitoring of animal health and the ecosystems they inhabit is essential to mitigate the risks associated with zoonoses (Greub et al., 2015). The breakdown of public health infrastructure is a significant reason why infectious diseases appear. Thanks to medical progress, infectious diseases are now less common; unfortunately, recent studies show that public health resources are not improving. It has been pointed out in several studies that the loss of this infrastructure interferes with effective disease monitoring, quick responses, and full public health measures. A lack of funds prevents organizations from identifying pathogens and managing diseases, which weakens their ability to deal with disease outbreaks. Strategic plans from the CDC encourage government and private groups to join forces and strengthen the public health system. Innovations in laboratory-based surveillance and improved communication networks are foundational steps toward addressing the challenges posed by emerging microbial threats (Satcher et al., 1995) (Figure 7.5).

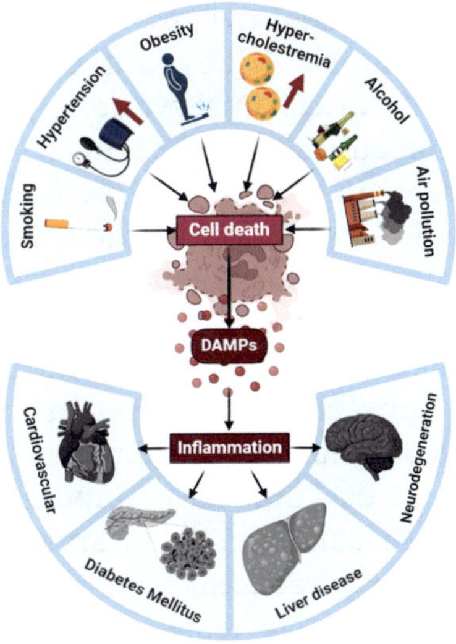

Figure 7.5. Factors contributing to the emergence of diseases.

Source: https://media.springernature.com/lw685/springer-static/image/art%3A10.1038%2Fs41419-025-07563-7/MediaObjects/41419_2025_7563_Figa_HTML.png.

7.1.3. Lessons Learned from Historical Events

Lessons learned from historical events surrounding infectious diseases have provided critical insights into the management of emerging and reemerging health crises. A notable example is the management of hospitals during the COVID-19 pandemic, which highlighted the importance of having effective incident command systems. Hospitals in Iran found that screening, separating patients by need, and having call centers were important for handling the rising needs for care. Strategies such as managing staff and offering education helped healthcare centers be better prepared for the outbreak. This experience illustrates not only the significance of immediate response strategies but also underscores the need for continuous improvement in health systems to prepare for future pandemics, ensuring they are resilient and adaptive to unexpected surges in patient numbers (Seyedin et al., 2022). Moreover, historical observations reveal that non-pharmaceutical interventions (NPIs) are essential tools in controlling infectious disease outbreaks. Studies reviewing the use of NPIs in crises show that how well and effectively they are received depends on the situation. For example, environmental cleaning and WASH services are often appreciated and can be effectively carried out in informal settlements, which are typically crowded and have limited access to healthcare. In some cases, interventions that restrict personal freedoms have been opposed, even though they have helped to stop the spread of disease. Understanding these nuances can inform the design and implementation of NPIs during emergent health threats, ensuring they align with the community's needs and context (Polonsky et al., 2022). Teaching about history in public health today helps prevent outbreaks and encourages people to be more involved in health care. The importance of community engagement for public health interventions is highlighted by history, since it helps people affected by the interventions to follow and respond better. When knowledge gaps are identified in past responses, future research should aim to develop targeted interventions that address the unique needs and circumstances of individuals. When healthcare systems gather and record evidence and past experiences, they become more ready for future challenges and support the health of the community. Using this approach, which is based on past experiences, will be essential for dealing with the various difficulties of EIDs.

7.2. Mechanisms of Disease Emergence

The understanding of disease emergence is fundamentally linked to the dynamic interplay between pathogens and their hosts, significantly characterised by zoonotic transmission. Many EIDs occur when pathogens move from animals to humans, often facilitated by changes in the environment and human activities. Deforestation and urbanisation have led to closer contact between animals and humans, increasing the risk of SARS-CoV-2 and other zoonotic diseases spreading. Mosquitoes can spread to new areas due to climate change, which alters the habitats that enable them to infect people who were not previously at risk. This complex interaction highlights the necessity of a comprehensive approach in monitoring zoonotic infections, as the evolution of pathogens often closely tracks alterations in environmental conditions and human encroachment into wildlife habitats (Choi, 2021). Along with ecological changes, how people live and the number of people in a population also play a significant role in causing diseases. Due to urbanization, cities become crowded, allowing infectious diseases to spread quickly in places where healthcare services are insufficient. Travel and trade around the world help people and animals move quickly from one country to another, which can spread diseases. The rise in antimicrobial use has led to the development of resistance in microbes, making it increasingly difficult to treat certain infections. Clinical studies have shown that flu strains are constantly evolving, which means public health systems must remain prepared for unexpected outbreaks. Particularly, the emergence of influenza strains accentuates the urgent need for robust surveillance and innovative therapeutic strategies to mitigate the impact of both EIDs (Degu et al., 2020). The process by which pathogens escape the host's immune system is also critical in understanding disease emergence. Coronaviruses and influenza viruses have developed special ways to get past the first defense system in the body. For example, some viruses can delay the activation of the immune system, allowing the virus to replicate quickly and cause a more severe disease. As a result of this reaction, the virus is transmitted and can also cause hyperinflammation in the host, as seen in COVID-19 patients with high levels of inflammatory markers. Therefore, discoveries about these processes help significantly in making better vaccines and treatments. By comprehensively addressing these various mechanisms of disease emergence, public health initiatives can more effectively prepare for and respond to the challenges posed by EIDs (Choi, 2021) (Figure 7.6).

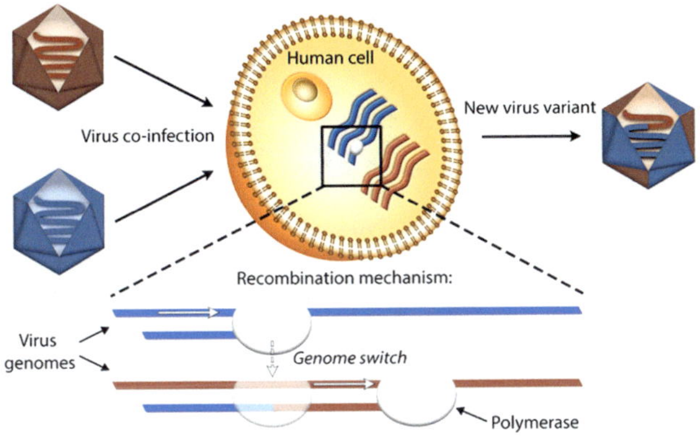

Figure 7.6. Mechanisms of disease emergence.

Source: https://scx1.b-cdn.net/csz/news/800a/2021/mechanism-underlying-t.jpg.

7.2.1. Environmental Changes and Their Impact

Environmental changes, particularly those stemming from human activities such as urbanization and deforestation, have significant repercussions on the emergence and spread of infectious diseases. Land-use and land cover (LULC) changes can create new habitats for pathogens and vectors, thereby amplifying the risk of exposure to EIDs. For example, some research suggests that altering land use can alter the local environment, which may increase the likelihood of mycobacterial infections infecting humans. This discourse lacks studies on the significant land use changes that happen in tropical parts of Meso- and South America and Southeast Asia. Addressing the health implications of LULC alterations is crucial, as these changes can simultaneously affect both human and animal health, highlighting the need for a multidisciplinary approach in future studies (Guégan et al., 2025). Due to climate change, infectious diseases are increasing in frequency and becoming more prevalent, presenting new challenges for public health. When the climate changes, it can affect where and how many disease vectors are present, which can alter the spread of diseases. For example, floods, changes in temperature and variations in humidity can directly change the habitats of organisms that carry diseases. Such environmental changes can intensify the relationship between hosts and pathogens which may cause diseases to be transferred between species. In addition, when air quality is poor and precipitation patterns change, it can weaken the immune systems of hosts, potentially exacerbating EIDs. Consequently, understanding the interplay between climate change and disease emergence is essential for developing effective surveillance and intervention strategies (Liao et al., 2024). To deal with the link between environmental changes and EIDs, the world needs to take action through global monitoring and research. Because climate change can increase the chances and impact of outbreaks, new ideas for disease control and tracking are needed. It will be necessary for experts from different fields to collaborate in designing systems that can monitor the interactions between pathogens and hosts as the environment changes. Technologies leveraging artificial intelligence (AI) can further enhance these efforts by providing timely data on disease trends and potential outbreak threats. As we move forward, public health entities must adopt a holistic approach that integrates environmental health, veterinary science, and epidemiology to build resilience against the inevitable challenges posed by EIDs (Liao et al., 2024).

7.2.2. Human Behavior and Urbanization

The rapid pace of urbanisation has significant implications for human behaviour, particularly concerning public health. As cities grow due to migration, people often live in crowded areas with insufficient resources and infrastructure. Such conditions in this environment encourage the spread of infectious diseases due to overcrowding, poor sanitation, and inadequate access to healthcare. Also, people in cities often interact with animals, which can result in more zoonotic diseases, as happened with COVID-19. Public health can better address EIDs by understanding the social and cultural aspects of city living and encouraging preventive actions. Considering these factors is necessary for designing urban planning strategies that focus on health and well-being as cities continue to grow. Human behavior becomes even more critical as cities change because of globalization and new technologies.

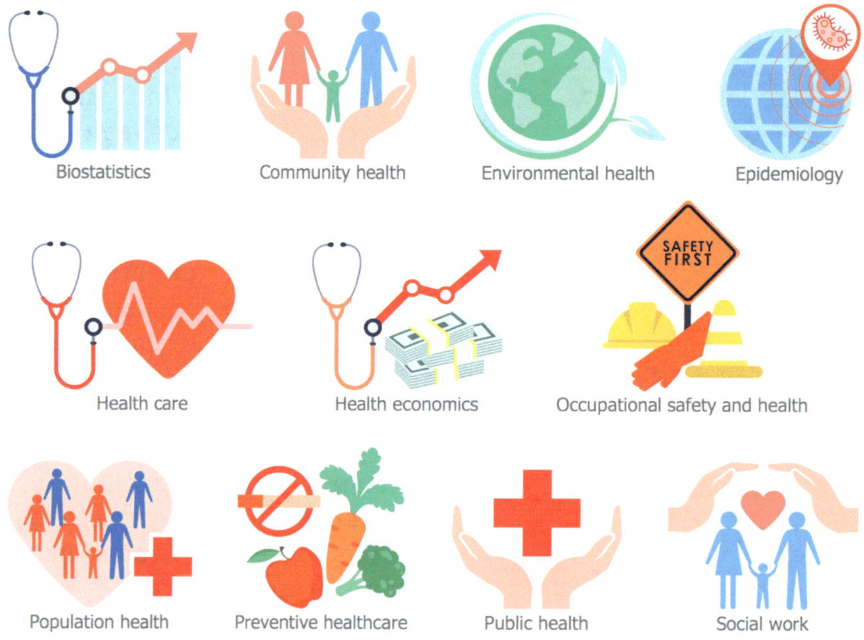

Figure 7.7. Human behavior and urbanization particularly concerning public health.

Source: http://conceptdraw.com/How-To-Guide/picture/public-health/Health-Sciences-Design-Elements-Public-Health.png.

Changes in lifestyle due to urban growth can facilitate the emergence and recurrence of infectious diseases. For example, more travel and trade since the pandemic has allowed pathogens to move quickly from one country to another. Research has shown that living in cities can alter what people eat, their housing, and their ability to move, which may all affect the spread of diseases. Additionally, the use of digital technology for communication may decrease people's interaction with their communities, potentially making it more challenging to address public health issues collectively. When cities change, it is essential to study the behaviors of their populations to guide disease prevention and health improvement so that public health systems can be ready for future infectious disease challenges. Studying how human actions are affected by urbanisation requires knowledge from public health, sociology and urban planning. As cities continue to grow, we must support initiatives that promote good health and help prevent disease outbreaks. Community involvement, better education and better access to healthcare can help people resist EIDs. Having green spaces in cities improves mental health and encourages people to exercise, which allows them lead healthier lives. Additionally, utilising technologies that support disease monitoring and promote preventive health actions can significantly enhance public health. The collaboration between policymakers, urban planners, and public health officials is crucial in developing comprehensive strategies to address the challenges posed by urbanization and ensure that human behavior is aligned with health-promoting practices, paving the way for a more resilient urban populace, thereby addressing the vulnerabilities associated with urban densification and growth (Figure 7.7).

7.2.3. Globalization and Travel

Globalization has significantly transformed the way individuals travel, ultimately influencing the spread of EIDs. Due to increased international travel, cities have become very crowded, making it easier for diseases to spread. Modern methods of transportation, such as air travel, enable viruses and bacteria to travel from one place to another in a remarkably short time. Because people travel across the globe, an infectious disease outbreak in one place can rapidly become a worldwide pandemic, as has happened in many health crises over the last two decades. Understanding the implications of such widespread connectivity is essential for public health authorities tasked with monitoring, controlling, and preventing the spread of diseases that may arise due to increasing travel activity in a globalized world (Sims et al., 2020). The COVID-19 pandemic vividly illustrates how infectious diseases can spread rapidly in our global society. The virus was first found in Wuhan, China and it quickly spread to other countries, proving that modern travel helps diseases spread faster than ever before. Besides travel, cities are growing and the creation of wet markets has made it easier for pathogens to move from animals to humans. Tourists and business travellers who visit these markets help create the conditions for diseases to appear. Additionally, the high volume of travellers can strain healthcare systems, making it more challenging to quickly identify and isolate those infected with diseases. Consequently, an analysis of globalization and travel reveals critical insights into the dynamics of disease proliferation, underpinning the need for effective surveillance and response mechanisms to safeguard public health (Malta et al., 2020). Strategies for globalisation, travel, and infectious diseases should put the highest priority on early detection and control. Strong screening at airports and land borders is necessary to identify and separate infected individuals before they can help the virus spread further. Governments should also cooperate on international health projects to establish standard rules that lead to more effective responses to emerging health threats. WBE helps authorities monitor diseases in populations and identify any changes in public health. Because lifestyles are becoming more global, public health strategies must adjust accordingly. With the inevitability of future outbreaks, it is crucial for global health frameworks to adapt and evolve, fostering an interconnected approach for safeguarding populations worldwide while maintaining the benefits of globalization and travel (Sims et al., 2020).

7.3. Case Studies of Emerging Diseases

Investigating emerging diseases is crucial for understanding the dynamics of public health crises. The COVID-19 pandemic, which started with SARS-CoV-2, demonstrated the interconnectedness of human actions, healthcare access, and pathogen transmission. Healthcare workers, who are in the frontline against this disease, showed differing levels of understanding and feeling about preventing it. A study conducted in Nepal assessed the knowledge of community health workers regarding COVID-19, revealing that a significant percentage believed proper use of personal protective equipment (PPE) significantly mitigated transmission risks. However, this case study also highlighted areas of concern, such as the lack of availability of essential medical supplies and a need for ongoing educational initiatives to improve knowledge and attitudes among healthcare personnel, ultimately affecting health outcomes and containment measures during the pandemic (Shrestha et al., 2021). EIDs are also interesting because they elucidate the molecular processes that enable viruses to infect the body. The case study highlighted the study of SARS-CoV-2's spike protein, which reveals essential points about managing and treating the disease. Assays were created to study the virus's ability to fuse cells, and it was found that SARS-CoV-2 was more effective at cell fusion than previous viruses such as SARS-CoV. Based on this insight into how viruses are constructed, scientists were able to develop effective inhibitors, such as EK1C4, which proved effective against SARS-CoV-2 and other coronaviruses. The innovation represented by such targeted therapeutic development underscores the importance of research in combating emerging diseases. It highlights the critical need for ongoing investigations into viral interactions and responses, particularly as new variants emerge (Xia et al., 2020). Examining case studies of new diseases helps scientists and supports better public health strategies all over the world. The COVID-19 pandemic has shown that infectious diseases can seriously affect societies and economies, which requires a combined effort that uses epidemiology, public health, and global cooperation. The results from different case studies provide helpful advice for being ready for future outbreaks. It is clear from the studies on healthcare workers and new treatments that all aspects of education, resources, and research should be given priority. By doing so, it will enhance readiness to address current and future health emergencies, ensuring that lessons learned from case studies inform proactive strategies and ultimately reduce the impact of EIDs on global health (Xia et al., 2020; Shrestha et al., 2021).

7.3.1. Zika Virus (ZIKV) Outbreak

The emergence of the ZIKV has been notably influenced by various environmental and socioeconomic factors, highlighting the critical linkage between human health and ecological conditions. Recent outbreaks, particularly in Brazil, have highlighted the complexities of co-circulating ZIKV with other arboviruses, such as dengue virus (DENV) and chikungunya virus (CHIKV), which complicates disease management and vector control strategies. Between 2023 and 2024, an ecological study found that dengue cases increased by 322% and Oropouche fever cases by 300%, indicating that arboviral diseases are becoming more prevalent in Brazil's various regions. As conditions become favorable for vector proliferation, it becomes essential for public health interventions to adapt dynamically to the intricate interactions among these viruses and their respective vectors, paving the way for context-specific control measures (Daudt-Lemos et al., 2025). Climate is now recognised as a key factor influencing the spread of ZIKV, which is further affected by changes in land use and economic conditions. Studies in northeastern Brazil have found a link between changes in land cover, increased fires, and a rise in ZIKA infections. The wide temperature range that Aedes mosquitoes can tolerate allows for more outbreaks in urban areas. More research has shown that bigger cities with a poorer quality of life are more likely to experience arboviral infections. Understanding these relationships is indispensable for developing targeted public health strategies and effectively mitigating the risk of future Zika outbreaks (Lopes et al., 2024). ZIKV outbreaks can result in problems for the economy and public health systems, aside from just the health issues they cause. When the 2015–2016 outbreak occurred, it became clear that ZIKV was linked to more cases of microcephaly and other birth defects, which created immediate public health concerns. Women who could have children were very concerned about their reproductive health, which caused more tension in society. As the number of cases continued to rise, it became clear that health systems required more integrated disease monitoring and greater community involvement. Educating the public about how to prevent ZIKV, along with better control of infected insects, is essential for facing the existing and future problems caused by ZIKV and similar viruses. This holistic approach is necessary for safeguarding communities against the looming threats of EIDs (Lopes et al., 2024; Daudt-Lemos et al., 2025) (Figure 7.8).

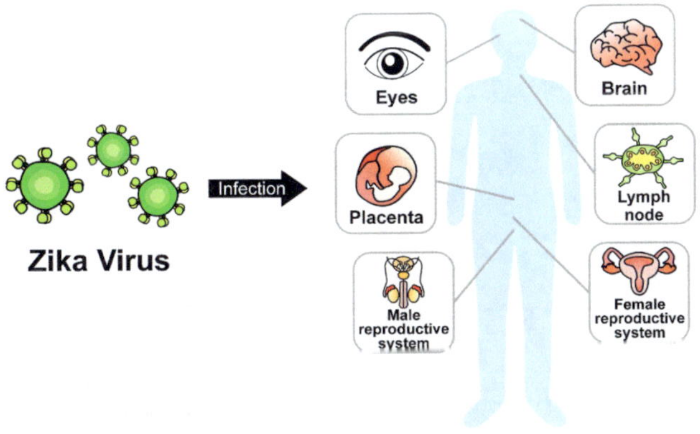

Figure 7.8. Zika virus outbreak.

Source: https://www.mdpi.com/vaccines/vaccines-10-01517/article_deploy/html/images/vaccines-10-01517-g001.png.

7.3.2. Ebola Virus Resurgence

The resurgence of the Ebola virus in recent years is emblematic of the broader phenomenon of EIDs that continue to challenge global health systems. The outbreaks of Ebola in West Africa have pointed out weaknesses in public health systems, monitoring, and ways to respond. Ecological changes, like deforestation and climate change, make it easier for wildlife to come into contact with humans, which helps Ebola reappear. In addition, the rise of globalisation and urbanisation causes more people to move, which allows pathogens to spread quickly around the world. As noted in the context of malaria, understanding and improving the interplay between local health dynamics and global threats is essential for combating these reemerging diseases within their respective frameworks (Greenspan et al., 2007).

Dealing with the renewed Ebola virus outbreak requires a plan that stresses the importance of national public health institutes and global teamwork. According to Greenspan et al. (2007), these institutions are critical for implementing revised International Health Regulations that encourage collaborative surveillance and information sharing about infectious disease outbreaks. They help find and respond to Ebola cases quickly and also support the ability to deal with different EIDs. To implement effectively, it is essential to stop outbreaks and investigate the reasons behind disease transmission and spread in society. Paying attention to these aspects, public health narratives may shift from simply reacting to zoonotic infections like Ebola to taking steps to prevent them. What we have learned from earlier Ebola outbreaks emphasises the need for increased awareness and preparedness for future cases. For example, helping people in the community and educating them about health is crucial for preventing the spread of Ebola when it returns. Local communities should be informed about the signs, risks, and ways to avoid Ebola, so that wrong information does not spread. It is also essential to prioritise more research on vaccines and treatment guidelines in the global health agenda, so healthcare systems can respond effectively to outbreaks. The concerted efforts to enhance local and international health systems will be instrumental in ensuring that the resurgence of Ebola and other infectious diseases does not lead to devastating public health crises (Ali et al., 2022).

7.3.3. COVID-19 Pandemic

The COVID-19 pandemic, which is an EID, has demonstrated the close connection between global health and social responses. As the virus spread globally, it revealed that countries were less protected than people thought, challenging the notion that Western governments were leaving infectious diseases behind. Because of this, people started to reconsider how diseases first appeared, which led to a significant change in public health stories. Many experts have studied the effects of pandemics and the emergence of EIDs in the early 1990s. The phenomenon of COVID-19 has not only catalyzed scientific inquiry. Still, it has also spurred interdisciplinary dialogues among humanities and social science scholars, revealing the multifaceted nature of health crises in contemporary society (Silva et al., 2023). The effects of the COVID-19 pandemic have varied significantly around the world, highlighting that local factors play a substantial role in shaping the development of viral infections and public health responses. In Mozambique, COVID-19 has combined with arboviruses and malaria to cause a more serious health situation. Studies have found that viral infections are common in this setting and that arboviruses and malaria can be present together in febrile patients, which makes it harder to diagnose and treat them. From March 2020 to September 2021, Mozambique experienced three distinct COVID-19 waves, with the number of cases rising sharply in each. This scenario reflects broader trends observed in various countries, where health systems have had to adapt to the emergent realities posed by the pandemic, necessitating proactive surveillance and enhanced public health strategies to address multiple co-occurring infectious diseases (Ali et al., 2022). The pandemic has, therefore, made it clear that there are significant problems in healthcare and disease monitoring in places with limited resources. The simultaneous appearance of multiple infectious diseases in Mozambique highlights the need for a comprehensive public health approach that considers environmental, social, and economic factors. The pandemic has also encouraged a new way of thinking about and handling EIDs around the world. By combining work from different fields and integrating historical insights with modern epidemiology, health experts can develop more effective strategies to prevent and control diseases. This integrative approach is vital, especially as EIDs continue to threaten global health security and as humanity faces an era characterized by increased zoonotic spillover events and changing ecological conditions exacerbated by climate change (Silva et al., 2023) (Figure 7.9).

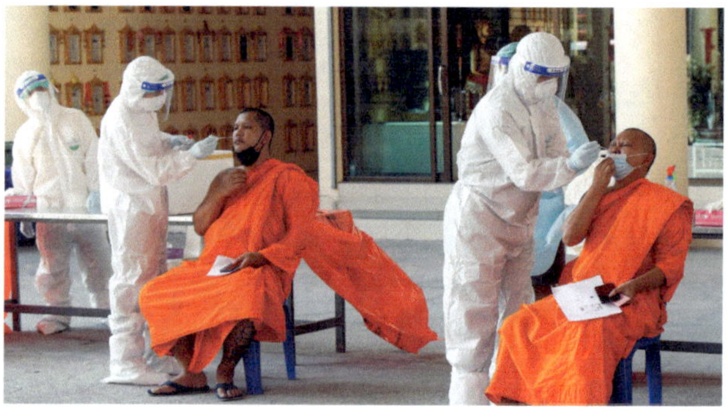

Figure 7.9. COVID-19 pandemic.

Source: https://static01.nyt.com/images/2021/05/10/world/10virus-briefing-plateau-sub/10virus-briefing-plateau-sub-videoSixteenByNine3000-v2.jpg.

7.4. Reemerging Infectious Diseases

The landscape of reemerging infectious diseases is shaped significantly by sociopolitical and environmental factors that influence the transmission dynamics of pathogens. A good example is the worldwide problem of vaccine-preventable diseases, which affects high-risk groups such as people in correctional facilities. Because it is often hard for prisoners to get medical care, vaccination rates are usually low, which increases the risk of disease outbreaks within and outside prisons. Research indicates that vaccination rates for diseases like COVID-19 and the hepatitis B virus (HBV) are starkly inadequate in many institutions, which raises immediate public health concerns. As highlighted in recent studies, improving vaccine uptake in prisons can have far-reaching implications, yielding community-wide benefits by mitigating the overall risk of transmission and contributing to pandemic preparedness efforts across the broader population (Moazen et al., 2024). The reason pathogens return is due to the interaction between microbial agents, human actions, and environmental changes, highlighting the need for a combined public health approach. For example, tuberculosis and malaria are returning, and they are now resistant to the usual ways they are treated. Human activities, such as urban expansion and climate change, contribute to altering the patterns of these diseases. Because pathogens continually evolve, it is essential to continually improve and update diagnostic techniques. New technologies in bioinformatics and ML help quickly recognize and describe infectious agents. By harnessing these technologies, public health officials can quickly respond to outbreaks and make informed decisions regarding interventions to curb the spread of reemerging contagious diseases (Ristori et al., 2024). Tackling reemerging infectious diseases requires strategies that combine science with community involvement. It is essential to bring together healthcare providers, researchers, and policymakers to strengthen systems that watch for changes in disease patterns. This way of thinking is also used in public health education to explain why vaccinations are necessary and what risks come from being hesitant about them. When vaccination is not available to everyone, especially those who need it most, the virus can continue to return and disrupt global health security. Ultimately, a concerted focus on both the scientific and social dimensions of reemerging infectious diseases is imperative to prevent their resurgence and protect community health at large (Moazen et al., 2024).

7.4.1. Definition and Examples

Emerging infections are illnesses that either show up in a population recently or have existed but are becoming more common or found in more places. Such diseases often occur due to interactions between environmental changes, technological advancements, and human actions. The ZIKV, which attracted worldwide attention in the early 2010s, was mainly caused by urban growth, changes in the climate, and increased travel. They both facilitate the virus's spread, making it more difficult to stop and control the disease. When people are more connected globally, there is a greater chance for emerging diseases to spread, which makes it harder for public health officials to manage and use resources. Unlike new infectious diseases, reemerging diseases were once contained but have appeared again, usually more dangerous. The rise of infectious diseases is attributed to the failure of public health measures, the increasing resistance of bacteria to antibiotics, and environmental changes. A pertinent example of this is the resurgence of tuberculosis (TB) worldwide, linked closely to the rise of multidrug-resistant strains. The rise of infectious diseases like TB is also linked to poverty and lack of healthcare, which makes it harder to manage infections. It is essential to understand this dynamic when planning strategies to address new and recurring health threats. EIDs affect more than public health, also impacting the economy and social life. SARS-CoV, which emerged in 2002–2003, significantly impacted international health systems and disrupted trade and travel, highlighting the interconnection between health and economics. The SARS-CoV-2 pandemic, which has just occurred, has demonstrated how infectious diseases can quickly impact the world's economies and health systems, resulting in significant changes in social behavior and policies. As outlined in recent research, most RNA viruses affecting humans originate from zoonotic sources and highlight the need for increased surveillance and preventative measures to mitigate future outbreaks (Sperk et al., 2020). The problem is to grasp how diseases develop and to find new methods to tackle them as they change in reaction to changes in humans and their surroundings.

7.4.2. Factors Leading to Reemergence

The resurgence of infectious diseases such as whooping cough (*Bordetella pertussis*) highlights the multifaceted factors that contribute to reemergence, particularly in highly immunized populations. Immunity is decreasing, as evidenced by the rise in pertussis cases among adolescents and adults, despite most of them having received vaccinations. Because acellular vaccines lose their effectiveness, more people in these populations are getting infected. In the last three decades, these changes in epidemiology have caused concern in public health, mainly because unvaccinated infants are still at high risk of severe illness.

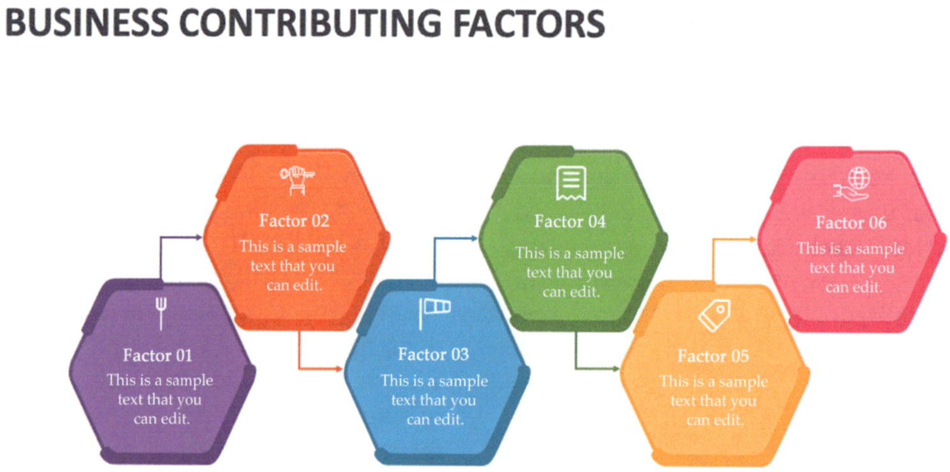

Figure 7.10. Factors leading to reemergence.

Source: https://www.collidu.com/media/catalog/product/img/a/b/abda0145ed9ef4c5ec3da83f10db08b79819e132dc96e016b60a6161a42bc491/business-contributing-factors-slide5.png.

This complicated interplay between vaccine-related immunity and disease prevalence indicates the importance of ongoing surveillance and evaluation of immunisation programs to adapt and respond effectively to emerging patterns of infectious diseases, as emphasised in numerous studies over the past decade (Philip et al., 2014). Changes in the genes of pathogens are also a reason why infectious diseases are coming back. Changes in bacteria can help them become more harmful or immune to vaccines and drugs that are currently used. The evolution of *Bordetella pertussis* has been observed to render vaccines less effective, making it harder to maintain herd immunity. Because of antibiotic-resistant strains, people who are infected have fewer treatment choices, which leads to more cases and greater health risks. To manage this situation, we must understand how these mutations occur, which can be achieved through further research and monitoring of genomic data.

By identifying drifts in pathogen genetics, public health officials can update vaccination strategies and mitigate outbreaks before they escalate, stressing the importance of integrating scientific advancements into public health planning (Philip et al., 2014). Finally, changes in the environment, primarily climate change, make it easier for infectious diseases to resurface and warrant close observation. Climate changes affect disease patterns by altering habitats and enabling disease vectors and pathogens to reach new areas. Higher temperatures and greater humidity help mosquitoes multiply, and these insects can carry diseases like malaria and dengue. Also, climate change helps AMR by making it easier for pathogens to live and change. For this reason, using a One Health method that joins efforts for human, animal, and environmental health is very important to handle the connections between these factors. Enhancing education and awareness among healthcare providers and the general public will serve to reduce the burden of emerging infections in the context of a changing environment, ultimately contributing to improved public health outcomes (Figure 7.10).

7.4.3. Public Health Implications

When infectious diseases emerge or reemerge, they pose significant public health challenges that necessitate a range of responses. As outlined in Greub et al. (2015), emerging pathogens are increasingly recognized as formidable threats to microbiological public health. Better tools for diagnosis and environmental changes make it easier for people to contract pathogens. The effects of urbanization, climate change, and other social and cultural factors make diseases harder to control and lead to a rise in their incidence. So, improve surveillance, research, and education for communities to address these risks and respond to new dangers. Zoonotic and waterborne diseases are also a key concern because they have resurfaced due to environmental and population changes. Greub et al. (2015) highlight the significant number of emerging bacterial infections that typically originate from animal sources or contaminated water, posing unique challenges for health authorities. People who are immunocompromised are more likely to get seriously ill and are therefore a primary concern in public health. To address these public health issues, we need to employ strategies that encompass environmental health, veterinary public health, and active policy development. Working together across different sectors and adopting a One Health approach will be necessary to prevent outbreaks and enhance disease control. The social and political environment can make it harder to deal with EIDs, as is happening in Venezuela now. As per, the country is dealing with several epidemics and poor health, which has resulted in infectious diseases coming back as a result of social and economic problems. This exemplifies how public health crises can hinder global health advancements and impede the attainment of Sustainable Development Goals (SDGs). Because health systems, migration crises, and diseases are linked, it is essential for both national and international efforts to manage public health well. Therefore, prioritizing emerging health issues through collaborative global efforts is crucial for safeguarding public health in affected regions and ensuring continued progress towards global health equity (Figure 7.11).

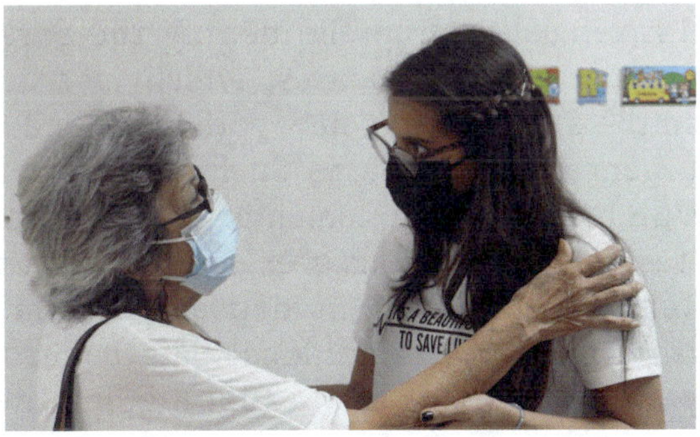

Figure 7.11. Public health implications.

Source: https://internationalmedicalcorps.org/wp-content/uploads/2022/04/VEZ_A-senior-adult-thanks-an-International-Medical-Corps-volunteer-e1651277047588.png.

7.5. Role of Technology in Disease Surveillance

The use of technology has significantly improved the monitoring of diseases, particularly for emerging infectious diseases. New tools are now used to speed up and improve the accuracy of collecting information about disease outbreaks. For example, digital health tools such as apps and online systems facilitate real-time monitoring of disease prevalence and its geographic distribution. It allows for quicker detection of outbreaks and stronger control, which helps cut down the effects of infectious diseases on public health. Furthermore, the integration of AI and ML algorithms into surveillance systems has improved predictive modeling, allowing for more informed decision-making and resource allocation during potential epidemics (Sims et al., 2020). They highlight the need to use technology to improve how public health deals with new health threats. Technology is also important in WBE, which offers a different way to monitor public health. WBE examines wastewater samples to identify pathogens and monitor changes in community health, which helps track the spread of infectious diseases. It helps to monitor health better and also alerts communities early when outbreaks are detected. Studying pooled wastewater enables health officials to rapidly identify the spread and resistance of diseases, which is crucial given the emergence of new pathogens and the resurgence of old diseases. Such advancements in WBE present a complementary approach that addresses the limitations of existing surveillance systems, particularly in densely populated urban areas where traditional data collection may fall short (Sims et al., 2020). Using these technologies represents a significant step toward being more proactive in public health. Using PRTs demonstrates how technology and disease monitoring join forces to ensure blood safety. Workshops organised by health agencies such as the FDA have shown a strong effort to improve blood safety by including PRTs in blood banks. They can remove known and unknown pathogens from blood, which decreases the risk of getting infections from transfusions, especially those caused by EIDs. Research findings are used to create and implement effective screening and mitigation measures, which in turn influence the management of blood safety. Also, it is essential to consider how PRT adoption affects the economy, which shows that prioritizing patient safety and cost-effectiveness is necessary. Overall, the collaborative efforts in developing and implementing these technologies reflect a broader commitment to enhancing disease surveillance and response mechanisms in an ever-evolving public health landscape (Figure 7.12).

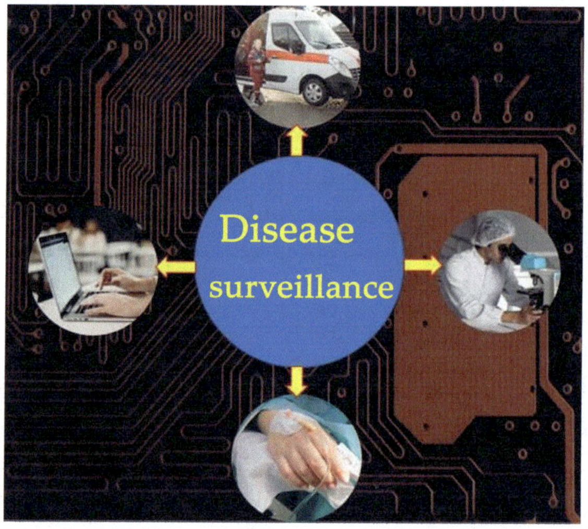

Figure 7.12. Role of technology in disease surveillance.

Source: https://blogger.googleusercontent.com/img/b/R29vZ2xl/AV vXsEgQdL6zDBEpp KYQQMYkAkRkK0u QXLsVuuO cc3rATl3wm66b86fK 20MeHkJ3mpG9gDyCN xpLQZeBFylA7l NP0002p mSR2oagY9n_ vKaYgcMDPNtIo Vxc6DWatyYSkFuG ccupi MJG1e TuED7E_lrhKCxiIVzQH- VMvWxS8XkDm-s2TcPloO0e0wrS 2hkog/s548/12.jpg.

7.5.1. Advances in Diagnostic Tools

Because infectious diseases continue to emerge and recur, new and improved diagnostic tools are necessary to detect them promptly and accurately. CRISPR and other technologies have recently made a significant impact on molecular diagnostics by providing new ways to detect and monitor pathogens and diseases. New technologies enable the conduct of detailed and sensitive tests in various locations, including remote areas. CRISPR-based diagnostics utilise the targeting capabilities of Cas12 and Cas13 to rapidly identify infectious agents.

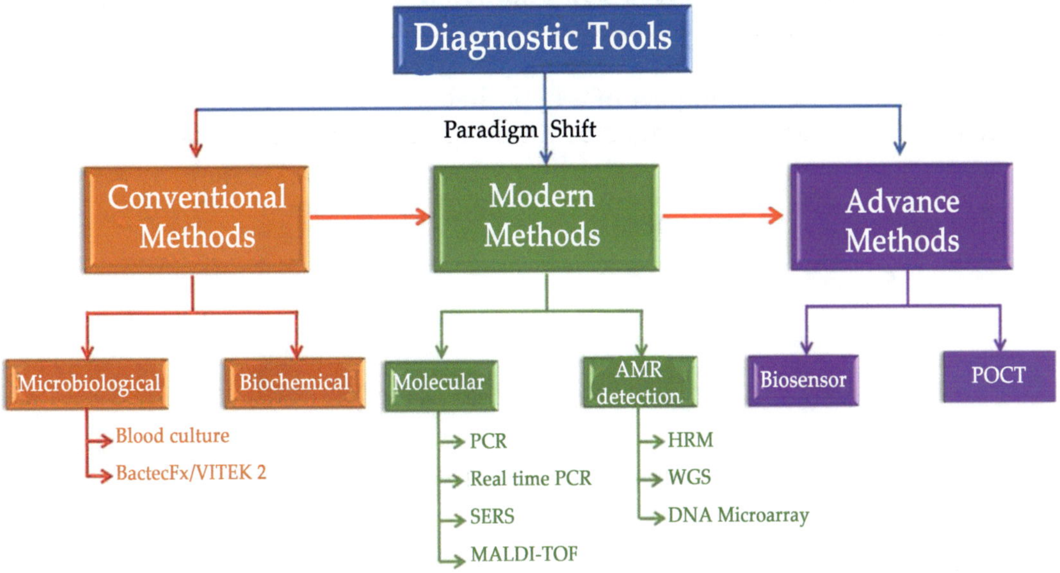

Figure 7.13. Advances in diagnostic tools.

Source: https://www.mdpi.com/diagnostics/diagnostics-13-00277/article_deploy/html/images/diagnostics-13-00277-g001.png.

Through multiplex detection methodologies, healthcare providers can simultaneously identify multiple pathogens, thereby enhancing the diagnostic capabilities necessary to manage complex disease outbreaks effectively (Lahari et al., 2025). Moreover, point-of-care testing (POCT) tools have gained traction, particularly in low-resource settings where access to traditional laboratory facilities is limited. The main goal of recent developments is to make affordable and portable POCT devices that can help with poverty-related infectious diseases in sub-Saharan Africa. They provide quick results that help doctors make informed decisions about treatment, and they also address issues such as access and reliability. With digital technology included in these platforms, it becomes possible to share and manage data more easily, which should make the diagnostic process more efficient. By emphasising the development and implementation of POCT tools tailored to local epidemiological contexts, public health initiatives can address critical gaps in the detection and management of EIDs (Ofori et al., 2024). As new diagnostic tools are developed, we must continue to address both the technical and contextual challenges associated with their use. Problems like misdiagnosis, which can have severe health impacts, underscore the importance of using reliable and robust testing methods. People are now realizing that a mix of education, training, community involvement, and new technology is essential. If stakeholders work together and set up stable supply lines for diagnostic materials, they can make sure that new diagnostic tools benefit people who need them most. Collectively, these efforts are essential for building resilient health systems capable of responding effectively to the dynamic landscape of EIDs (Ofori et al., 2024) (Figure 7.13).

7.5.2. Use of Data Analytics and Modeling

Using data analytics and modeling helps experts understand how infections are transmitted and what might cause an outbreak. Advanced computational models, such as the SEIR (Susceptible-Exposed-Infectious-Recovered) framework, enable researchers and public health officials to simulate the spread of diseases under various intervention scenarios. For instance, researchers conducted a simulation to project the potential impact of a hypothetical Ebola virus outbreak in India; without intervention, it was estimated that millions could be affected within two years (Sau, 2017).

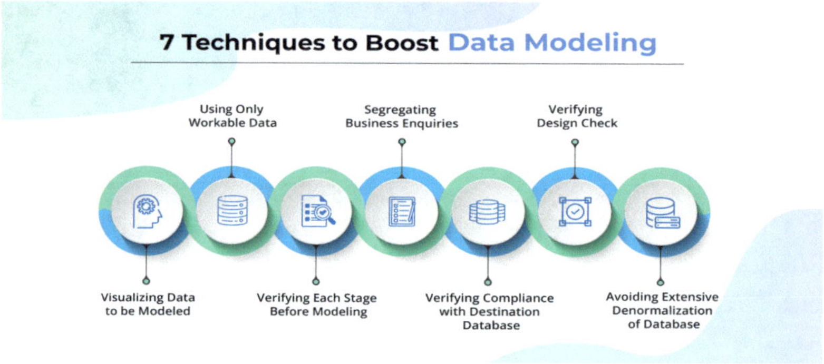

Figure 7.14. Analytics and modeling.

Source: https://www.techment.com/wp-content/uploads/2023/05/Data-Modelling-02-2048x1065.png.

These models show that acting promptly to infectious diseases depends on having timely data. Additionally, utilising data analytics in public health facilitates the integration of diverse data types, which is essential for accurate epidemiological analysis. Global Burden of Disease (GBD) studies exemplify this use of analytics by evaluating the impact of risk factors and diseases across different demographics worldwide (Adebola et al., 2024). They utilize vast data to determine the prevalence of diseases and the number of deaths from them, which aids in planning and resource distribution in public health. Even so, there are still problems, mainly in middle- and low-income countries, where insufficient data makes it difficult to estimate accurately. By using advanced data analytics such as ML and big data analytics, the ability to gather and study data improves, which helps public health efforts against infectious diseases. Working together, data scientists, public health experts, and policymakers will help enhance and apply precision public health strategies based on strong data analysis. Relying on advanced models enables quick actions against EIDs, ensuring health systems can effectively handle potential outbreaks. As evidenced by previous models predicting the spread of the Ebola virus, these analytical frameworks can guide preventive measures to contain outbreaks effectively (Sau, 2017). GBD studies also help by pointing out where diseases are more common, which is key in forming health policies and choosing what to focus on. In this ever-evolving landscape of infectious diseases, the synergy between data analytics and public health practices will be essential in achieving sustainable health outcomes and safeguarding communities worldwide (Figure 7.14).

7.5.3. Global Health Networks and Collaboration

Working together across borders is very important for dealing with EIDs. Since these diseases are constantly evolving, the world needs to respond collectively and coordinate its actions. When countries and different sectors join forces, they share essential information and resources. Additionally, the One Health approach, which emphasises the interconnectedness of human, animal, and environmental health, has gained popularity among interdisciplinary teams. By integrating expertise from fields such as veterinary medicine and public health, organizations can develop comprehensive strategies for disease prevention and control, as demonstrated through research collaborations across regional and international platforms (Rantam et al., 2017). Also, the worldwide impact of infectious diseases shows that different stakeholders such as governments, non-governmental organizations, and academic institutions should join forces. Because health problems such as HIV/AIDS and malaria are so complex, there is a need for countries to cooperate and share knowledge about surveillance, prevention, and treatment. Effective health planning requires paying attention to the various factors that contribute to diseases, including social and economic issues and health inequities. Engaging diverse disciplines, such as nutrition and environmental science, further bolsters the groundwork necessary to tackle these pressing global health issues (Flores et al., 2025). Apart from preventing diseases, global health networks help set up a lasting structure for future health security. When guidelines and policies are designed to emphasise teamwork between different sectors, global health initiatives are more prepared to handle new risks. Being part of these networks helps health professionals get the knowledge and skills needed to address outbreaks. Ultimately, the ongoing commitment to global health networks facilitates not just reactive measures but also proactive strategies aimed at anticipating future challenges posed by infectious diseases, thereby enhancing overall public health security across nations (Rantam et al., 2017).

7.6. Public Health Strategies

Public health strategies play a significant role in controlling the effects of EIDs. Surveillance helps medical authorities spot health threats early on. By leveraging existing resources, a national network can facilitate the identification of pathogens and inform strategies to reduce the impact of these diseases. As advanced molecular methods are now required, federal agencies are exploring how to perform pathogen-agnostic testing on human samples. By developing interconnected networks among clinicians, laboratory scientists, and bioinformaticians, the United States can strengthen its public health infrastructure and better respond to infectious disease outbreaks, as noted in research on existing pathogen surveillance capacities (Downie et al., 2024). Public health education and awareness campaigns are essential for any strategy to fight EIDs. Awareness changes the way individuals and communities act, which can have a big effect on how diseases are transmitted. It was found in a recent study that many people in Guangzhou are unaware of how to prevent or avoid diseases like MERS and Zika. It is clear from the findings that education and income play a key role in knowledge, so special health information strategies should be designed for vulnerable groups. Such initiatives are vital in ensuring that communities are well-informed, thereby enhancing their capacity to engage in preventive behaviours that lower disease risk (Ma et al., 2022). In addition, public health strategies should involve the cooperation of government bodies, healthcare workers, and community-based organisations. To handle EIDs, it is necessary to join efforts from epidemiology, health information sharing, and community involvement. Public health agencies should promote partnerships that leverage the strengths of different groups to effectively respond to health threats as a cohesive team. Improving the way agencies communicate can lead to prompt sharing of information on outbreaks and how to prevent diseases. Moreover, the role of technology in improving data collection and analysis cannot be understated, as it enables health officials to monitor disease trends in real time and implement strategic responses effectively, ultimately strengthening the overall public health response (Downie et al., 2024).

7.6.1. Vaccination and Immunisation Programs

EIDs can be controlled and prevented mainly through vaccination and immunisation programs. In the past, these programs have helped lower the number of cases of measles, polio, and smallpox, showing that vaccinating many people is effective. New pathogens are emerging, and some previously controlled infectious diseases are reappearing. The National Academy of Sciences' Institute of Medicine warns that the erosion of public health infrastructure significantly contributes to these challenges, necessitating robust vaccination strategies to mitigate the risks posed by infectious agents (Satcher et al., 1995). Vaccines protect each person and also help reduce the number of infections and stop outbreaks in the community. As a result, maintaining and enhancing immunization efforts is crucial for controlling EIDs. Effective vaccination programs can only be achieved when there is more public awareness and when healthcare services are made more accessible. If communities improve adult health care and encourage people to know more about health, they will grasp the role of vaccines in stopping the spread of diseases. Research indicates that improved health awareness and community participation lead to higher vaccination rates, ultimately contributing to healthier populations (Andrus et al., 2004). Moreover, when decisions are made locally, communities can design vaccination programs that suit them, which leads to more people getting involved. Removing barriers to vaccination will strengthen our ability to address new threats, which is vital for public health in combating infectious diseases. Besides community involvement, using advanced technologies and monitoring diseases is necessary for vaccination programs to succeed. Using surveillance systems, public health officials can quickly identify and address outbreaks, which helps determine vaccination plans. Laboratory-based surveillance and enhanced communication networks facilitate the identification of new immunisation needs, particularly in response to the emergence of novel pathogens (Satcher et al., 1995).

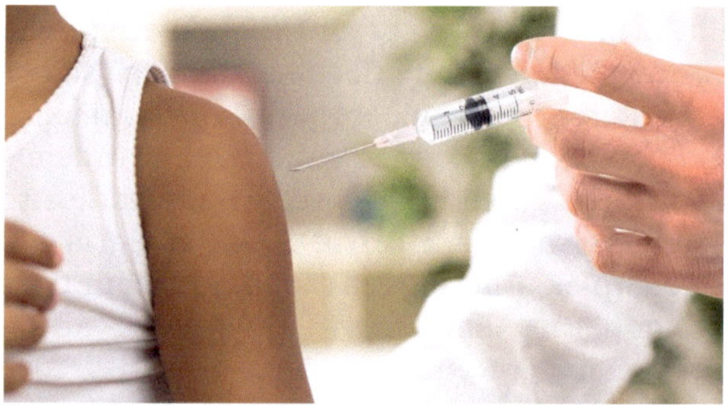

Figure 7.15. Vaccination and immunization programs.

Source: https://ichef.bbci.co.uk/news/1024/cpsprodpb/F6AF/production/_97815136_child-vaccination_150917_gt.jpg.

In addition, collaboration among government offices, medical professionals, and international teams helps to respond to EIDs in a coordinated manner. The continual adaptation and evaluation of vaccination programs, coupled with epidemiological insights, will be pivotal in safeguarding populations and minimizing the impact of infectious diseases on public health (Figure 7.15).

7.6.2. Education and Awareness Campaigns

Educating and informing people is very important in fighting EIDs, as it helps communities respond better to public health problems. Their primary purpose is to share essential details about diseases and encourage people to adopt healthy habits. Public health officials can utilise social media, organise community workshops, and distribute pamphlets to effectively connect with diverse populations. Having community leaders involved is key, since they can raise the level of trust and encourage more people to be involved, especially where healthcare resources are scarce. If people become better at understanding health information, they are more likely to recognise symptoms and seek medical advice, which helps prevent diseases from spreading. In certain circumstances, targeted education can significantly enhance the public's understanding of health problems. For instance, in countries grappling with high rates of tuberculosis, including multidrug-resistant tuberculosis (MDR-TB), tailored strategies are required to address unique socio-cultural factors. They should use messages that are meaningful to local people and align with their traditions and health-related ideas. Workshops can be organized to teach people about the importance of taking medicine as directed and also about the broader effects of infections and drug resistance. Such proactive approaches can build a robust framework for compliance with treatment protocols, ultimately reducing the prevalence of diseases like TB, which is critical given the alarming statistics circulating its effectiveness in diverse settings, as highlighted by Gamon et al. (2013). Also, for education and awareness campaigns to work well everywhere, it is important to keep evaluating and updating them. It is essential to know the local situation such as current healthcare services and how involved the community is, when planning a campaign. By teaming up with healthcare providers, policymakers, and public health organizations, we can address the special needs and problems of every community. Therefore, using evidence-based approaches is crucial, as it enables the distribution of resources more effectively and enhances the success of interventions, particularly in low- and middle-income countries. Research on AMR highlights the importance of adopting a One Health approach and carefully reviewing policies to make educational messages effective across various health sectors. Education and awareness campaigns are instrumental in shaping behaviors and perceptions regarding infectious diseases, ultimately leading to a more informed public capable of combating health threats effectively (Aarestrup et al., 2015) (Figure 7.16).

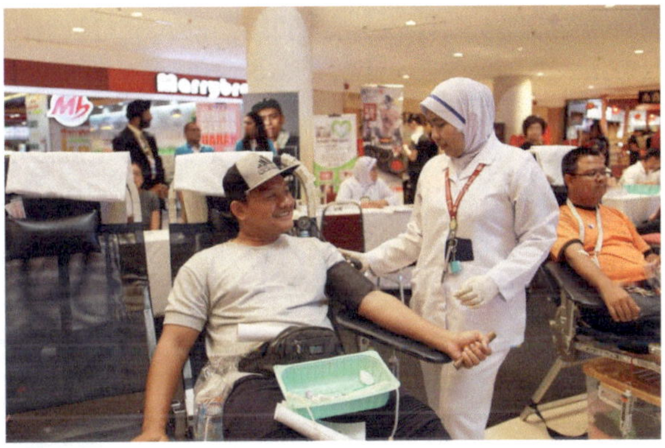

Figure 7.16. Education and awareness campaigns.

Source: https://qiu.edu.my/wp-content/uploads/2018/09/Public-Health-Campaign-2018-3.jpg.

7.6.3. Policy and Regulatory Measures

The emergence and re-emergence of infectious diseases demonstrate the need for robust policies and regulations worldwide. Because people and goods cross borders daily, it is easy for pathogens to be carried from one region to another. Thus, governments should have complete surveillance systems to detect and manage infectious disease risks quickly. Governments, health organizations, and researchers must team up to find strategies that support public health and still allow for effective disease control. By fostering international cooperation, nations can share vital information on disease outbreaks, thereby improving the overall preparedness and response to emerging infectious challenges, as the nature of these diseases transcends national boundaries and requires a coordinated global approach to address them effectively (Bettcher et al., 1997). Emphasising communication and swift action in regulations is crucial for combating infectious diseases. Centres for Disease Control and Prevention (CDC)-like entities play a vital role in this regard as they direct national programs aimed at enhancing the identification, investigation, and control of infectious diseases. They have detailed systems in place to track the number of cases, investigate disease spread, and assess the effectiveness of their public health actions. Additionally, the development and distribution of vaccines and biological reagents are crucial for controlling infectious diseases. Such public health regulations ensure that local health departments receive the necessary support and resources to manage potential outbreaks effectively, underscoring the need for a strong regulatory backbone in any nation's health policy framework to safeguard public health. Also, the rise of new infectious diseases means policies must be flexible to handle the challenges caused by globalisation and urbanisation. Preventive measures, vaccination and good hygiene should be promoted through public health education campaigns. Encouraging health literacy among people allows governments to support communities in stopping the spread of diseases. It is essential that these policies address current problems and plan for future risks by investing in research and strategic planning. As the global interconnectedness of economies and societies grows, so too does the imperative for dynamic policy responses that reflect the complex and evolving landscape of infectious diseases, ensuring that public health priorities remain at the forefront of governmental agendas (Bettcher et al., 1997).

SUMMARY

Infectious diseases are constantly changing, which creates significant difficulties for public health systems everywhere. The examination concludes by emphasising the need for immediate and active action to address EIDs. As we have seen, these diseases have spread across the world due to increased travel, climate change, and the rise of social and economic factors. Because of these conditions, public health authorities should give priority to new surveillance approaches such as WBE, which allows for flexible monitoring of diseases. Analysing wastewater data in real time helps health officials be more prepared for outbreaks and protect people from risks. The need for such advancements has never been greater, given the vulnerabilities exacerbated by rapid population growth and environmental shifts (Sims et al., 2020). Additionally, having well-organised plans and responses is essential to effectively handle the challenges of EIDs. Based on the analysis, cooperation among public health, environmental science, and economic policy is required for a complete approach to managing diseases. Getting different sectors involved increases the reach of actions and strengthens society's ability to resist health threats. Since EIDs are systemic, an inclusive approach is required that sees how all parts of society are connected. More resources and support should be provided to institutions to ensure they can collaborate effectively and quickly in the event of an outbreak. A failure to address these interconnected elements may lead to inadequate responses, further exacerbating the impact of infectious diseases on human health and safety (AlMossawi et al., 2019). All things considered, overcoming the problems of EIDs requires combining innovative methods of surveillance, collaboration across different sectors, and robust institutional structures. They are essential for a public health system to effectively address the challenges of infectious diseases. Since EIDs can be unpredictable, constant focus, financial support, and flexible solutions are needed to prevent and control them. The effects of these strategies are essential for the economy and society as well as for health. Thus, mobilising efforts across diverse sectors and leveraging new technologies will be crucial in safeguarding communities and ensuring a proactive stance against the rise of infectious diseases in an increasingly interconnected world (AlMossawi et al., 2019; Sims et al., 2020).

EIDs are still a significant problem for public health everywhere. A major part of this issue is that organisations must have the resources necessary to handle these risks. Essential steps should focus on bringing healthcare, environmental management, and economic planning together to work collaboratively. In these areas, investment is necessary to improve the response to infectious diseases. By analysing relevant literature on epidemic preparedness interventions, researchers have identified that a collaborative ethos—alongside fiscal and social commitments—bolsters national capacity to respond to EIDs effectively (Almossawi et al., 2019). Improving these networks enables countries to respond quickly during outbreaks, thereby supporting public health worldwide. Understanding the complexity of emerging pathogens enables us to design more effective strategies for prevention and control. The danger posed by these pathogens is a major point, as their virulence can vary significantly and impact public health in various ways. New studies using ML techniques have found that some aspects of the environment can help predict how severe human-infectious RNA viruses are. Traits such as transmissibility, the ability to infect multiple organ systems, and transmission routes are crucial in assessing the potential impact of emerging viruses (Brierley et al., 2019). By studying viruses in detail, scientists can determine what factors contribute to more severe disease outcomes. It enables better planning and directs actions to mitigate the risks of newly emerging infectious diseases. It is crucial to identify key points and methods for addressing the issues caused by EIDs. A good response plan should be able to adapt to the unique features of each new disease, considering how it spreads and its severity. Because preparedness activities are based on different situations, the responses can be adjusted to match the needs of each community. It is essential to implement interventions that address weaknesses in the existing response framework while emphasising the need for multisectoral engagement (Almossawi et al., 2019). Emphasising these important aspects allows public health efforts to handle new threats and support better health outcomes for everyone in the community.

CLOSER LOOK

VETERINARY PUBLIC HEALTH:

Veterinary Public Health (VPH) is a crucial field that bridges the gap between animal health, human health, and the environment. It focuses on the prevention, control, and monitoring of diseases that can be transmitted between animals and humans, known as zoonoses. With over 60% of human infectious diseases originating from animals, VPH plays an essential role in safeguarding public health.

At its core, Veterinary Public Health emphasizes disease surveillance, food safety, and environmental protection. Veterinary professionals work to identify and manage animal-borne pathogens such as Salmonella, Brucella, and rabies, which have significant implications for human populations. This includes monitoring livestock, wildlife, and companion animals, as well as implementing measures to reduce disease transmission. For example, vaccination campaigns, quarantine regulations, and vector control programs are essential tools in reducing outbreaks.

Food safety is another vital aspect of VPH. Veterinary experts ensure that animal-derived products, including meat, milk, and eggs, are safe for human consumption. They monitor production processes, inspect slaughterhouses, and test for microbial contamination or chemical residues. By enforcing hygienic practices along the food chain, VPH minimizes risks of foodborne illnesses and promotes public confidence in animal products.

Environmental health is increasingly recognized as part of VPH. Livestock management practices, waste disposal, and the use of antimicrobials in animals all have environmental implications. Improper handling can lead to water contamination, antimicrobial resistance, and ecological imbalances. Veterinary public health initiatives aim to promote sustainable farming practices, responsible drug use, and ecological stewardship, integrating animal, human, and environmental health—a concept now widely known as "One Health."

The significance of Veterinary Public Health has been highlighted by global health emergencies, such as avian influenza, Ebola, and the COVID-19 pandemic, all of which have links to animal hosts. Through research, policy development, and education, VPH professionals help prevent disease emergence, reduce transmission risks, and strengthen public health systems.

In conclusion, Veterinary Public Health is a dynamic and interdisciplinary field that protects both human and animal populations. By combining veterinary science, epidemiology, food safety, and environmental management, VPH professionals play a pivotal role in maintaining a healthy, safe, and sustainable world. As human populations grow and interactions with animals increase, the relevance of Veterinary Public Health continues to expand, emphasizing its critical contribution to global health security.

REFERENCES

1. Dar, O. A., Hasan, R., Schlundt, J., Harbarth, S., Caleo, G., Dar, F. K., Littmann, J., Rweyemamu, M., Buckley, E. J., Shahid, M., Kock, R., Li, H. L., Giha, H., Khan, M., So, A. D., Bindayna, K. M., Kessel, A., Pedersen, H. B., Permanand, G., . . . Heymann, D. L. (2015c). Exploring the evidence base for national and regional policy interventions to combat resistance. *The Lancet, 387*(10015), 285–295. https://doi.org/10.1016/s0140-6736(15)00520-6Albrecht, D. E. (2022). Vaccination, politics and COVID-19 impacts. *BMC Public Health, 22*. https://doi.org/10.1186/s12889-021-12432-x.
2. Ali, S. (2022). *Epidemiological Analysis of Emerging and Re-emerging Virus Infections in Mozambique*. https://core.ac.uk/download/591918950.pdf (accessed on 30th May 2025).
3. AlMossawi, H. J., Longacre, C., Kak, N., & Joshi, S. (2019). Key strategies to address emerging and reemerging infectious diseases: A systematic analysis. *Research Square*. https://doi.org/10.21203/rs.2.14861/v1.
4. Almossawi, H., Longacre, C., Kak, N., & Joshi, S. (2019). *Key Strategies to Address Emerging and Reemerging Infectious Diseases: A Systematic Analysis [Preprint]*. https://www.semanticscholar.org/paper/5326a2399aafc5cdc8c73402d3fa3b8727b28b3c (accessed on 30th May 2025).
5. Alonso, A., Fauci, A. S., Bisht, K., Borovsky, P., Bukreyev, A., Butcher, B., Earl, P., et al. (2005). Emerging infectious diseases: A 10-year perspective from the National Institute of Allergy and Infectious Diseases. https://core.ac.uk/download/pdf/8706962.pdf (accessed on 30th May 2025).
6. Alvarado-Socarras, J., Barbella-Aponte, R. A., Bello, R. J., Bonilla-Aldana, D. K., et al. (2019). Infectious diseases, social, economic and political crises, anthropogenic disasters and beyond: Venezuela 2019 – Implications for public health and travel medicine. https://core.ac.uk/download/299842880.pdf (accessed on 30th May 2025).
7. Andrus, J. K., & Castillo-Solórzano, C. (2004). *Rubella Elimination and Improving Health Care for Women*. https://core.ac.uk/download/pdf/8712033.pdf (accessed on 30th May 2025).
8. Atreya, C. D., Glynn, S. A., Busch, M. P., Kleinman, S., Snyder, E. L., Rutter, S., AuBuchon, J. P., et al. (2019). Proceedings of the Food and Drug Administration public workshop on pathogen reduction technologies for blood safety 2018 (Commentary, p. 3026). *Transfusion, 59*, 3002–3025. https://doi.org/10.1111/trf.15344.
9. Baker, M. G., Kvalsvig, A., & Verrall, A. J. (2020). New Zealand's COVID-19 elimination strategy. *The Medical Journal of Australia, 213*, 198. https://doi.org/10.5694/mja2.50735 (accessed on 30th May 2025).
10. Bettcher, D. W., Käferstein, F. K., & Motarjemi, Y. (1997). *Foodborne Disease Control: A Transnational Challenge*. https://core.ac.uk/download/pdf/8257395.pdf (accessed on 30th May 2025).
11. Bloch, E. M., Sullivan, D., Casadevall, A., Shoham, S., Tobian, A., & Gebo, K. A. (2024). Applying lessons of COVID-19 and other emerging infectious diseases to future outbreaks. *mBio, 15*. https://www.semanticscholar.org/paper/5548e164316c9d7717be2dc8bd5d83858a501c46 (accessed on 30th May 2025).
12. Brierley, L., Pedersen, A. B., & Woolhouse, M. (2019). Tissue tropism and transmission ecology predict virulence of human RNA viruses. *PLOS Biology, 17*. https://www.semanticscholar.org/paper/3fb87cfef0c6409f46ade73c46bcf196179f2752 (accessed on 30th May 2025).

13. Buchanan, R. L. (1997). *Identifying and Controlling Emerging Foodborne Pathogens: Research Needs*. https://core.ac.uk/download/pdf/8257375.pdf (accessed on 30th May 2025).

14. Cameron, S. A., & Sadd, B. M. (2019). Global trends in bumble bee health. *Annual Review of Entomology, 65*, 209–232. https://doi.org/10.1146/annurev-ento-011118-111847.

15. Choi, Y. (2021). Emerging and re-emerging fatal viral diseases. *Experimental & Molecular Medicine, 53*, 711, 712. https://www.semanticscholar.org/paper/15b9bcd000ca6a021085a64f3e00d73333ef3c09 (accessed on 30th May 2025).

16. Da Silva, M. A. D., & Skotnes-Brown, J. (2023). *Emerging Infectious Diseases and Disease Emergence: Critical, Ontological and Epistemological Approaches*. https://core.ac.uk/download/587387815.pdf (accessed on 30th May 2025).

17. Daudt-Lemos, M., Ramos-Silva, A., Faustino, R., de Noronha, T. G., Vianna, R. A. O., Cabral-Castro, M., Cardoso, C. A. A., et al. (2025). Rising incidence and spatiotemporal dynamics of emerging and reemerging arboviruses in Brazil. *Viruses, 17*. https://www.semanticscholar.org/paper/b47f0c8cc1386a30c5f815053e869958b5768f68 (accessed on 30th May 2025).

18. Degu, S., Gemeda, N., Abebe, A., Berihun, A., Debebe, E., Sisay, B., Gemeda, H., et al. (2020). In vitro antifungal activity, phytochemical screening and thin layer chromatography profiling of *Impatiens tinctoria* A. Rich root extracts. *Annals of Microbiology and Infectious Diseases*. https://www.semanticscholar.org/paper/6dd741076b501867d6a4fd01ea86dffb17285edf (accessed on 30th May 2025).

19. Downie, D. L., Rao, P., David-Ferdon, C., Courtney, S., Lee, J. S., Quiner, C., MacDonald, P. D. M., et al. (2024). Surveillance for emerging and reemerging pathogens using pathogen-agnostic metagenomic sequencing in the United States: A critical role for federal government agencies. *Health Security, 22*, 85–92. https://www.semanticscholar.org/paper/e2ccd070a016a9a8c23ca6cc7f0cc9effbabacc6 (accessed on 30th May 2025).

20. Fidler, D. P. (1996). *Globalization, International Law, and Emerging Infectious Diseases*. https://core.ac.uk/download/pdf/8257124.pdf (accessed on 30th May 2025).

21. Flores, R., & Gillespie, S. (2025). *Health and Nutrition: Emerging and Reemerging Issues in Developing Countries*. https://core.ac.uk/download/pdf/6288820.pdf (accessed on 30th May 2025).

22. Frölich, L., Flier, W., Gustavsson, A., Rossini, P., & Holzapfel, D. (2022). Response to the letter titled "The conundrum of the AD continuum." *Alzheimer's & Dementia, 19*. https://www.semanticscholar.org/paper/3f6ecece927fd5e6a05e846e5eb02d2e7b813398 (accessed on 30th May 2025).

23. Gamon, M. (2013). *Maribel Gamon – Multidrug-Resistant Tuberculosis in India: Solving a Problem by Reconstructing the Public Health Infrastructure*. https://core.ac.uk/download/67755957.pdf (accessed on 30th May 2025).

24. Gopikrishnan, M., & Haryini, S. G. C. (2024). Emerging strategies and therapeutic innovations for combating drug resistance in *Staphylococcus aureus* strains: A comprehensive review. *Journal of Basic Microbiology, 64*. https://www.semanticscholar.org/paper/aa557e66e847b52d7b34373d4cb119b2a91c70cf (accessed on 30th May 2025).

25. Greenspan, A. L., Andrus, J. K., Baker, M., Centers for Disease Control and Prevention, Heymann, D. L., Rodier, G., et al. (2007). *Global Public Health Security*. https://core.ac.uk/download/pdf/8397494.pdf (accessed on 30th May 2025).

26. Greub, G., & Vouga, M. (2015). *Emerging Bacterial Pathogens: The Past and Beyond.* https://core.ac.uk/download/77149050.pdf (accessed on 30th May 2025).

27. Gudipati, S., Herc, E., & Zervos, M. J. (2020). Can the One Health approach save us from the emergence and reemergence of infectious pathogens in the era of climate change: Implications for antimicrobial resistance? https://core.ac.uk/download/352938764.pdf (accessed on 30th May 2025).

28. Guégan, J. F., Vargas, C. C. E., Chevillon, C., Sylla, A., Dogbe, M., Fast, K. M., Pechal, J. L., et al. (2025). Land use and land-cover changes and emerging non-tuberculous and tuberculous infectious diseases in human and animals: A mixed-methods review of research findings from global and spatio-temporal perspectives. *Environmental Research: Health.* https://www.semanticscholar.org/paper/274d1f4a8e563f7ed669027ae444741b328fe30f (accessed on 30th May 2025).

29. Jenkins, C., Levin-Zamir, D., Le, C., Mazzilli, S., von Schreeb, S., & Denmark. (2024). 5.C. Scientific session: Strengthen resilience against emerging vector-borne diseases through the ECDC Fellowship Programs. *The European Journal of Public Health, 34.* https://www.semanticscholar.org/paper/5a50c005c66356d5027eeec2387cfb50e9cab4e6 (accessed on 30th May 2025).

30. Lahari, S., Sneha, Y., Sathwika, C., Tharun, M., & Rao, T. (2025). Innovations and implementations of clustered regularly interspaced short palindromic repeats in next-generation diagnostic tools: A review of current and emerging techniques. *Journal of Clinical Sciences.* https://www.semanticscholar.org/paper/b9630519667be2b3e0833dc3c3324741f51e71d2 (accessed on 30th May 2025).

31. Lee, W. K., & Shin, S. R. (2024). Development of Emerging Infectious Diseases Preventive Health Behavior (EID-PHB) Scale and validation of the complex models. *Journal of Multidisciplinary Healthcare, 17,* 445–460. https://www.semanticscholar.org/paper/1c4f255219132e39fc6cce07ae2db07e22b2bac8 (accessed on 30th May 2025).

32. Liao, H., Lyon, C. J., Ying, B., & Hu, T. Y. (2024). Climate change, its impact on emerging infectious diseases and new technologies to combat the challenge. *Emerging Microbes & Infections, 13.* https://www.semanticscholar.org/paper/44b2ef0c91804a3c1099427c3060b9ab9df2ef48 (accessed on 30th May 2025).

33. Logan, J. J., Hoi, A. G., Sawada, M., Knudby, A., Ramsay, T., Blanford, J., Ogden, N., et al. (2023). Risk factors for Lyme disease resulting from residential exposure amidst emerging *Ixodes scapularis* populations: A neighborhood-level analysis of Ottawa, Ontario. *PLOS ONE, 18.* https://www.semanticscholar.org/paper/f307d4f877a3d89ab6a58fe5ff09241a8e5c43d6 (accessed on 30th May 2025).

34. Lopes, E. D., Nuvoloni, F. M., & Moreno, G. S. (2024). *Environmental Influence on Arboviruses Emerging and Reemerging Infectious. G*eography Department, University of São Paulo. https://www.semanticscholar.org/paper/d740a37f8bba9f95c59d0c0aee91b334163a8171 (accessed on 30th May 2025).

35. Lwande, O. W., Obanda, V., Lindström, A., Ahlm, C., Evander, M., Näslund, J., & Bucht, G. (2019). Globe-trotting *Aedes aegypti* and *Aedes albopictus*: Risk factors for arbovirus pandemics. *Vector-Borne and Zoonotic Diseases, 20,* 71–81. https://doi.org/10.1089/vbz.2019.2486.

36. Ma, X., Lu, J. X., & Liu, W. (2022). Knowledge of emerging and reemerging infectious diseases

in the public of Guangzhou, Southern China. *Frontiers in Public Health, 10*. https://www.semanticscholar.org/paper/51b8709e97ccc3dc7f2bd0b011c89654de0605e3 (accessed on 30th May 2025).

37. Malta, M., Rimoin, A. W., & Strathdee, S. A. (2020). The coronavirus 2019-nCoV epidemic: Is hindsight 20/20? *EClinicalMedicine, 20*, 100289. https://doi.org/10.1016/j.eclinm.2020.100289.

38. Mangen, J. F. (2024). Vaccines in the era of emerging infectious diseases: Immune mechanisms and innovations. *Newport International Journal of Public Health and Pharmacy*. https://www.semanticscholar.org/paper/b15f181b5777a59a0cf99634de5eabfeb07f9b7b (accessed on 30th May 2025).

39. Meaney-Delman, D., Jamieson, D., & Rasmussen, S. (2017). Addressing the effects of established and emerging infections during pregnancy. *Birth Defects Research, 109*, 307–310. https://www.semanticscholar.org/paper/11da6540b5a398df7f2f7e5ce05b4d27f190ac25 (accessed on 30th May 2025).

40. Moazen, B., Ismail, N., Agbaria, N., Mazzilli, S., Petri, D., Amaya, A., D'Arcy, J., et al. (2024). Vaccination against emerging and reemerging infectious diseases in places of detention: A global multistage scoping review. *Frontiers in Public Health, 12*. https://www.semanticscholar.org/paper/47b9e4acb15674a0d1e6e23bc3d17324c863f4a9 (accessed on 30th May 2025).

41. N/A. (2025). *National Center for Infectious Diseases (CVC)*. https://core.ac.uk/download/144186063.pdf (accessed on 30th May 2025).

42. Ofori, B., Twum, S., Yeboah, S. N., Ansah, F., & Sarpong, K. A. N. (2024). Towards the development of cost-effective point-of-care diagnostic tools for poverty-related infectious diseases in sub-Saharan Africa. *PeerJ, 12*. https://www.semanticscholar.org/paper/f3ace656f0266d5f2d80c3bbaeb39793f6d32cd3 (accessed on 30th May 2025).

43. Onifade, A., Adefunmilola, A., Auta, H. S., Daniel, E. O., Emmanuel, E., et al. (2024). *Review of Global Burden of Disease Studies: Trends, Challenges, and Future Directions*. https://core.ac.uk/download/618286874.pdf (accessed on 30th May 2025).

44. Philip, L. (2014). A systematic review on the risk factors associated with the resurgence of pertussis in highly immunized countries within the last ten years (2004 2014). https://core.ac.uk/download/71425255.pdf (accessed on 30th May 2025).

45. Polonsky, J., Bhatia, S., Fraser, K., Hamlet, A., Skarp, J., Stopard, I., Hugonnet, S., et al. (2022). Feasibility, acceptability, and effectiveness of non-pharmaceutical interventions against infectious diseases among crisis-affected populations: A scoping review. *Infectious Diseases of Poverty, 11*. https://www.semanticscholar.org/paper/b16884c00a790ff7c1bddef93a9136d6182b787f (accessed on 30th May 2025).

46. Rantam, F. A., Mufasirin, Srianto, P., & Suwarno. (2017). *The Role of Human, Animal, Environment to Maintain Ecosystem as Global Food Security*. https://core.ac.uk/download/pdf/304643100.pdf (accessed on 30th May 2025).

47. Ristori, M. V., Guarrasi, V., Soda, P., Petrosillo, N., Gurrieri, F., Longo, U., Ciccozzi, M., et al. (2024). Emerging microorganisms and infectious diseases: One Health approach for health shared vision. *Genes, 15*. https://www.semanticscholar.org/paper/7c7c97d1a79459ce06be4f48b48c8fc298d73a8a (accessed on 30th May 2025).

48. Satcher, D. (1995). *Emerging Infections: Getting Ahead of the Curve*. https://core.ac.uk/download/pdf/8248073.pdf (accessed on 30th May 2025).

49. Sau, A. (2017). A simulation study on hypothetical Ebola virus transmission in India using Spatiotemporal Epidemiological Modeler (STEM): A way towards precision public health. https://core.ac.uk/download/206133132.pdf (accessed on 30th May 2025).

50. Seyedin, H., Bagherzadeh, R., & Dowlati, M. (2022). Hospital management in infectious disease outbreak: Lessons learned from COVID-19 epidemic. *Health in Emergencies & Disasters Quarterly*. https://www.semanticscholar.org/paper/2b5c97f1b46471d88a1de599cbce3f88e1934327 (accessed on 30th May 2025).

51. Shrestha, A., Thapa, T. B., Giri, M., Kumar, S., Dhobi, S., Thapa, H., Dhami, P. P., et al. (2021). Knowledge and attitude on prevention of COVID-19 among community health workers in Nepal—a cross-sectional study. *BMC Public Health, 21*. https://doi.org/10.1186/s12889-021-11400-9.

52. Sims, N., & Kasprzyk-Hordern, B. (2020). Future perspectives of wastewater-based epidemiology: Monitoring infectious disease spread and resistance to the community level. *Environment International, 139*, 105689. https://doi.org/10.1016/j.envint.2020.105689.

53. Sperk, M., van Domselaar, R., Rodriguez, J., Mikaeloff, F., Sá Vinhas, B., Saccon, E., Sönnerborg, A., et al. (2020). Utility of proteomics in emerging and re-emerging infectious diseases caused by RNA viruses. *Journal of Proteome Research, 19*, 4259–4274. https://www.semanticscholar.org/paper/6db52ada64a4a8a4af368875535727ff879aae5b (accessed on 30th May 2025).

54. Verity, R., Okell, L., Dorigatti, I., Winskill, P., Whittaker, C., Imai, N., Cuomo-Dannenburg, G., et al. (2020). Estimates of the severity of coronavirus disease 2019: A model-based analysis. *The Lancet Infectious Diseases, 20*, 669–677. https://doi.org/10.1016/s1473-3099(20)30243-7.

55. Wang, S., Li, W., Wang, Z., Yang, W., Li, E., Xia, X., Yan, F., et al. (2024). Emerging and reemerging infectious diseases: Global trends and new strategies for their prevention and control. *Signal Transduction and Targeted Therapy, 9*. https://www.semanticscholar.org/paper/d020161ba5918186fd2e8744bd9dfeec9a36869f (accessed on 30th May 2025).

56. Xia, S., Liu, M., Wang, C., Xu, W., Lan, Q., Feng, S., Qi, F., et al. (2020). Inhibition of SARS-CoV-2 (previously 2019-nCoV) infection by a highly potent pan-coronavirus fusion inhibitor targeting its spike protein that harbors a high capacity to mediate membrane fusion. *Cell Research, 30*, 343–355. https://doi.org/10.1038/s41422-020-0305-x.

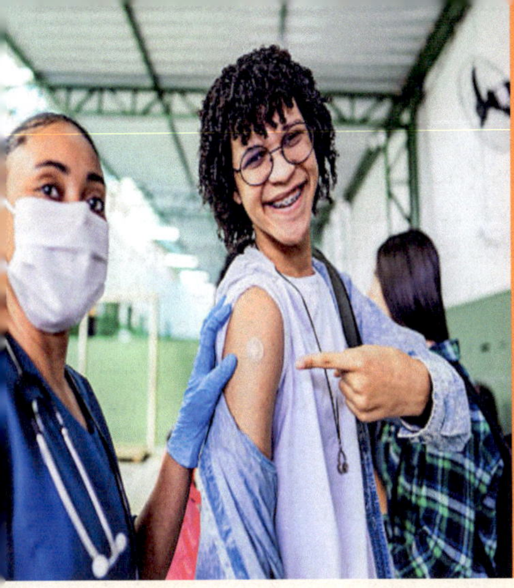

Chapter 8

EPIDEMIOLOGY OF COMMON INFECTIOUS DISEASES

Contents

Introduction

A foundational understanding of epidemiology is critical for addressing infectious diseases, which continue to pose significant public health challenges worldwide. Epidemiology reveals how diseases spread and affect different groups of people, providing us with essential knowledge about health conditions. It includes various techniques for collecting and studying data on infections, which helps locate people at risk and review ways to manage these diseases. Lately, social epidemiology has gained importance by looking at the ways social factors impact health. Research has shown that economic disparities, stress, and institutional inefficiencies can exacerbate disease transmission, highlighting the necessity of a multi-faceted approach in understanding infectious disease dynamics (Plotnikov et al., 2025). Therefore, learning epidemiology is crucial for comprehending the challenges in public health efforts aimed at controlling infectious diseases. Using systematic research methods adds more to our understanding of common infectious diseases. For instance, research protocols such as those developed for acute undifferentiated febrile illnesses (AUFIs) illustrate the breadth of epidemiological studies aimed at pathogen identification in diverse settings. Such studies are typically conducted in collaboration with various international groups to establish a comprehensive database on infectious diseases in regions with diverse health systems. By employing rigorous data collection methods, including laboratory testing for viral, bacterial, and parasitic agents, researchers can discern patterns of disease outbreaks and risk factors prevalent within specific populations (Cabada et al., 2024). The combination of clinical and epidemiological data helps explain how diseases develop and spread, which guides better public health actions. Besides helping us understand how diseases are spread, epidemiology also plays a major role in forming health policies and prevention plans. officials. Public health officials use epidemiological findings to design proper responses, direct resources, and choose the best ways to help populations at risk for infectious diseases. Additionally, epidemiology's use of concepts from sociology, economics, and psychology helps provide a broader perspective on health. Epidemiological information enables policymakers to tackle the root causes of health issues, including poverty and inadequate education, thereby reducing the risk of infectious diseases. As the landscape of infectious diseases evolves, especially in the context of emerging pathogens and changing societal dynamics, a well-rounded introduction to epidemiology remains indispensable for developing comprehensive strategies to enhance population health and effectively combat infectious diseases (Plotnikov et al., 2025).

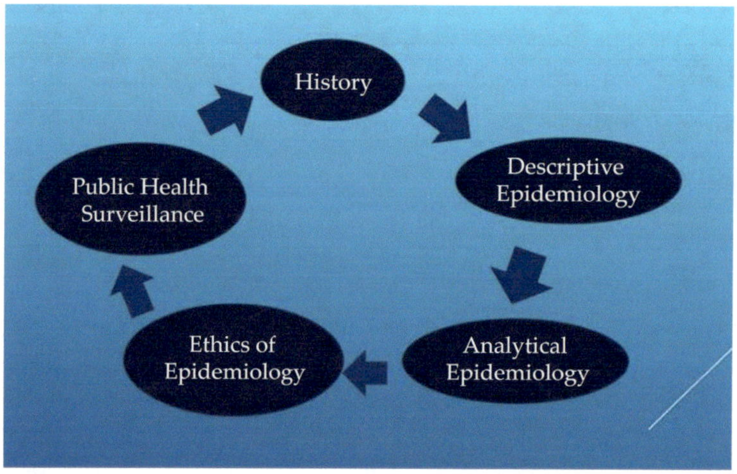

Figure 8.1. Epidemiology.

Source: https://slideplayer.com/slide/14023366/86/images/2/Approaching+Epidemiology.jpg.

Definition and Scope of Epidemiology

Epidemiology is a branch of science that examines how health-related conditions are spread and what factors influence them in specific populations. It is an essential method for studying how diseases are spread, how often they occur in different groups, and what affects health results. Epidemiology focuses on infectious diseases, chronic illnesses, injuries, and also on environmental health. Epidemiology encompasses more than just data collection; it employs advanced methods and theories to develop effective public health strategies. Observational studies and controlled trials enable epidemiologists to identify risk factors and patterns, which in turn help them develop policies to control diseases and underscore the importance of epidemiology in public health. Because public health issues are complex, mainly due to EIDs and global pandemics, epidemiology is constantly evolving. Due to the COVID-19 pandemic, researchers have had to adopt new methods for studying epidemiology to better understand the virus and develop effective responses.

The realities of post-infectious complications, such as Multi-System Inflammatory Syndrome in Children (MIS-C) and Post-Acute Sequelae of SARS-CoV-2 infection (PASC), highlight the importance of a comprehensive epidemiological approach that goes beyond acute disease transmission. As noted, although pediatric patients typically showed resilience against severe acute COVID-19 infection, the substantial morbidity associated with such sequelae underscores the critical need for ongoing research into the long-term effects of infectious diseases on health outcomes, emphasising the vital role of epidemiology in contemporary health management (Parzen-Johnson et al., 2024). As well as monitoring diseases, epidemiology plays a crucial role in ensuring the safety of medical procedures, such as blood transfusions. The creation of hemovigilance systems, which started in Japan and France in the 1990s, demonstrates how epidemiology supports better patient safety and quality in health care. They are designed to detect and prevent adverse outcomes from transfusions, illustrating how epidemiology can help prevent diseases by ensuring safe medical procedures. Although the United States has made strides, its hemovigilance system remains incomplete, showing that further integration of epidemiological insights is necessary for broader health safety efforts (Whitaker et al., 2019). This multifaceted application of epidemiology not only addresses immediate health crises but also contributes to building resilient health systems capable of adapting to shifting disease trends (Figure 8.2).

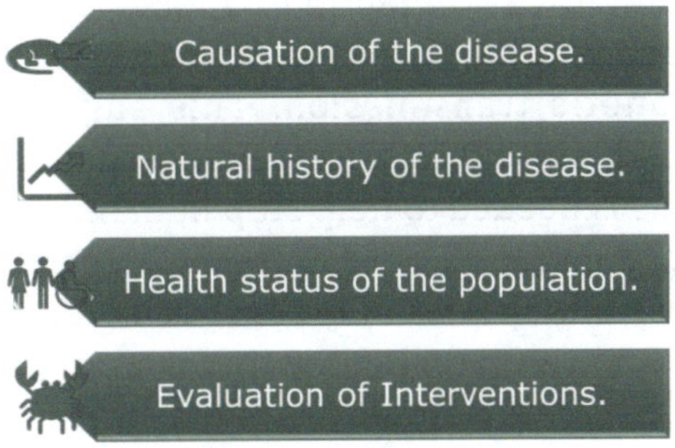

Figure 8.2. Scope of epidemiology.

Source: https://image6.slideserve.com/12044525/scope-of-epidemiology-l.jpg.

Importance of Studying Infectious Diseases

Public health and epidemiology rely on the study of infectious diseases to understand the factors that cause diseases to spread and persist. Examining how pathogens are spread within different groups enables epidemiologists to identify factors that increase the likelihood of infectious disease outbreaks. For example, a cross-sectional study on *Camel brucellosis* highlights the importance of conducting thorough epidemiological research to determine the prevalence of the disease and identify associated social and environmental factors. The study demonstrated a 4.8% overall seroprevalence of Brucella in a specific region, revealing district variations and significant risk factors related to herd management, highlighting the need for targeted interventions to enhance public health strategies and reduce disease transmission among both livestock and humans, as suggested by the findings of this critical analysis (Mohomed et al., 2024). It is also important to recognise how wildlife, domestic animals, and human health are all connected when studying infectious diseases. This concept, commonly known as the One Health approach, underscores the importance of studying diseases that can be transmitted from animals to humans and impact epidemiology. Research in Brazil on rodents has shown that infectious agents are shared between wildlife and homes, potentially leading to zoonotic transmission. This suggests that thorough surveillance of wildlife and domestic animals is needed to help stop human infections. The interactions across different habitats reveal that various species may serve as reservoirs for diseases, underscoring the importance of multi-species epidemiological studies in mitigating risks effectively and informing public health policies (Marinho-Júnior et al., 2023). As well as protecting public health, studying infectious diseases helps create new medicines and vaccines. Learning about the epidemiology of diseases allows researchers to find out how diseases are spread and where to intervene, which can be transformed into medical solutions that protect people. An example is Leishmaniasis, where studying both the insects and the animals they infect helps us create better ways to control the disease. Scientists can develop better vaccines and treatment approaches by identifying the ways diseases are transmitted and the environments where they thrive. Thus, the investigation of infectious diseases is not just a matter of interest; it is a necessary commitment that underpins global health security and offers invaluable insights into emerging infectious trends that threaten human populations (Marinho-Júnior et al., 2023) (Figure 8.3).

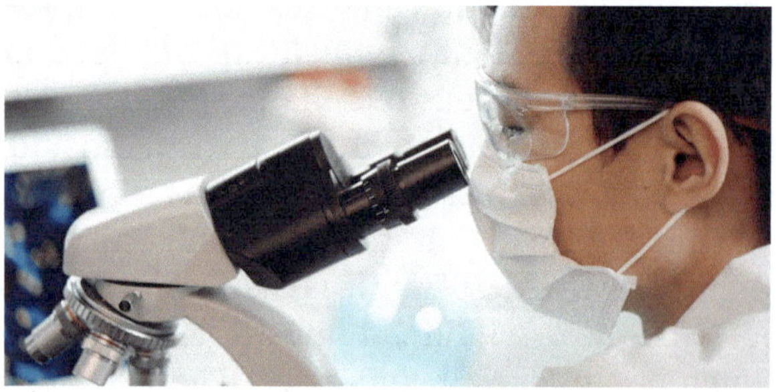

Figure 8.3. Studying infectious diseases.

Source: https://nanocellect.com/wp-content/uploads/2020/06/12.png.

Historical Context and Evolution of Epidemiological Methods

Essential developments in epidemiology throughout history have helped in understanding and managing infectious diseases. It was the Greeks and Romans who started the field of epidemiology by monitoring diseases and developing basic public health policies. It was in the 19th century that epidemiology began to develop as a formal science, largely due to the efforts of individuals like John Snow. By researching cholera cases in London, he made people realise the value of mapping diseases and using data to find patterns, which became important in modern epidemiology. Because of this evolution, health policies now focus on using data to enhance hygiene and sanitation and also recognise the role of social factors in determining health for different groups. As new technologies appeared and data were collected, epidemiology continued to develop during the 20th century. Thanks to statistical methods such as cohort and case-control studies, researchers could better link what people are exposed to with their health. These techniques made it possible to identify what causes infectious diseases, which helped create effective public health measures. Furthermore, the establishment of organisations such as the Centres for Disease Control and Prevention (CDC) underscored the importance of collaborative efforts in epidemiological research. Now, the use of molecular epidemiology and systems biology combines genetic, environmental, and social factors to give a better understanding of how diseases develop. It is clear from this progress that epidemiology has to change to address the more complex issues created by new infectious diseases. The recent cases have shown that understanding history is essential for dealing with new contagious diseases. For example, the emergence of SARS-CoV-2 highlighted the importance of studying zoonotic spillovers, and SARS and MERS had previously demonstrated the need for such research. Both Gorbalenya et al. (2020a) and Gorbalenya et al. (2020b) emphasise the necessity of studying viruses at the species level, which directly influences public health preparedness and response strategies. Having this historical knowledge enables us to gain a deeper understanding of virus-host interactions and predict future outbreaks. So, changes in epidemiology over time highlight the relationship between past events and current issues, showing why the discipline is essential for tackling infectious diseases worldwide.

8.1. Types of Infectious Diseases

Among infectious diseases, there is a wide variety, and they can mainly be grouped into bacterial, viral, fungal, and parasitic types. Pneumonia and strep throat, which are bacterial infections, are known for their rapid reproduction and the inflammation they cause in specific areas. A delay in diagnosing and treating these microorganisms can lead to significant health complications. Unlike bacteria, viral infections such as influenza and HIV use cells in the body to reproduce, which can result in several health issues and possible long-term problems. Both bacterial and viral diseases are essential in epidemiology because they affect many people and harm public health, so it is necessary to keep monitoring them and find new ways to prevent and control them. Although fungal infections are not as common as bacterial or viral infections, they are now recognised as a significant health risk, particularly for individuals with weakened immune systems. If candidiasis and aspergillosis are missed and handled promptly, they can result in a lot of sickness and deaths. Studying these infections highlights the need for precise diagnosis and the importance of monitoring antifungal use in hospitals. Because antifungal resistance is on the rise, health care systems should strengthen their surveillance strategies. It is, therefore, essential to be aware of fungal infections to prevent their negative impact on individuals who are more susceptible in hospitals and long-term care facilities. Protozoa, helminths, and ectoparasites are the main causes of parasitic infections, which are also critical infectious diseases. Malaria is an example caused by *Plasmodium* species, and giardiasis is the result of *Giardia lamblia*. The occurrence of these diseases varies by location, influenced by environmental and socio-economic conditions. For example, malaria is most common in tropical and subtropical areas, which results in a lot of sickness and death. As parasitic diseases are on the rise, it is essential to employ targeted public health measures, including vector control and improved sanitation. Also, knowing how parasites develop and spread is essential to create good prevention methods. All infectious diseases bring different problems and require a combined effort in public health.

8.1.1. Bacterial Infections

Bacterial infections are a significant part of the worldwide epidemiology of common infectious diseases. Among these, urinary tract infections (UTIs) are the most prevalent, affecting millions each year, particularly women. Most of the pathogenic bacteria are found in the gastrointestinal tract, which shows that the microbiology of the body is an essential part of infection. Research has shown that having multiple UTIs can significantly impact patients' quality of life, making it crucial to develop effective preventive strategies. For these issues, clinics that bring together infectious disease specialists and urologists have become very important. Such structures enable the categorisation of patients into complicated or uncomplicated cases, leading to tailored treatments that mitigate both recurrence and antibiotic resistance (Kling et al., 2025). It is essential to understand what causes bacterial infections to keep happening. Antibiotic-resistant bacteria are now a problem for public health, as they make it harder to treat infections caused by bacteria. As a result of the COVID-19 pandemic, more people are travelling and less surveillance, making people more concerned about multidrug-resistant organisms. Because of this, the world must pay close attention to respiratory infections among travellers. Infections like MERS-CoV and Henipavirus demonstrate the importance of monitoring the spread of diseases that can be transmitted by people traveling globally. They demonstrate that robust public health measures and international cooperation are essential to prevent outbreaks and facilitate a swift response. Vulnerable populations, including immunocompromised travelers, are especially at risk and require targeted strategies to minimize their exposure to potentially life-threatening infections (Norman et al., 2024). Because bacterial infections are changing, health authorities need to keep strong preventive strategies in place. The presence of non-infectious syndromes alongside bacterial infections highlights the wide range of challenges in the epidemiology of infectious diseases. It has been found through research that a large number of people sent for UTI management actually have asymptomatic bacteriuria or other non-infectious diseases. Because of this mistake, patients may receive unnecessary antibiotics, which adds to the bigger problem of AMR. Interdisciplinary clinics are effective in identifying the main health problems, which helps manage them well and decreases the risk of misusing drugs. Applying several treatments, such as vaginal estrogen and methenamine monotherapy, has shown that it is possible to treat recurrent UTIs and lower the risk of resistance. Consequently, recognising the nuanced landscape of bacterial infections is crucial for advancing treatment modalities and optimising patient outcomes (Kling et al., 2025). Through continued research and interdisciplinary collaboration, the epidemiology of bacterial infections can be better understood and effectively addressed within the larger context of infectious diseases (Figure 8.4).

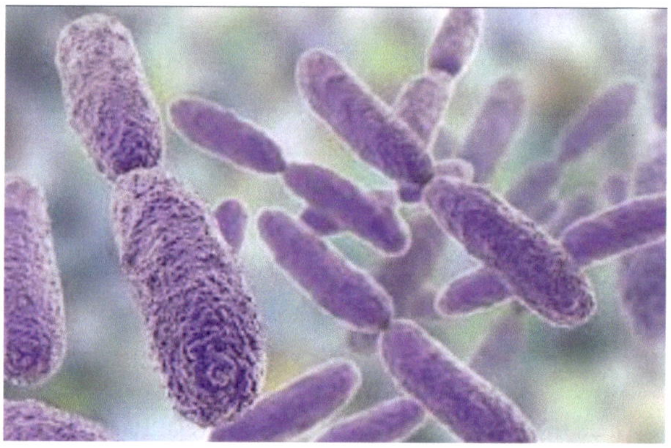

Figure 8.4. Bacterial infections.

Source: https://encrypted-tbn0.gstatic.com/images?q=tbn:ANd9GcTyCPBa7UkhLFDVVHTekGIzNdDKgI040wSi2A&s.

8.1.2. Viral Infections

Public health relies heavily on understanding viral infections through their epidemiology, particularly in terms of how they spread and the number of people affected in different populations. Many cases of hepatitis B, hepatitis C, and influenza have been reported due to their high numbers and the significant effect they have on healthcare systems. A study encompassing data from the Ministry of Health in Saudi Arabia reveals that males exhibit a higher susceptibility to these viral infections compared to females, indicating potential biological or behavioural factors influencing infection rates (Aleyeydi et al., 2024). The findings over four years highlight the need for well-targeted public health actions to reduce the spread, particularly among groups that may not have sufficient access to vaccines or information on how to prevent the virus. Also, the way viral infections interact with social and environmental factors should not be ignored. For example, diseases like dengue fever and measles are in medicine, but their occurrence varies depending on the weather and location. The data from Saudi Arabia shows that viral cases were much lower during the COVID-19 pandemic, which suggests that strict public health measures can significantly reduce infections. This observation compels further examination of how behavioural changes during pandemics can effectuate long-lasting shifts in the epidemiological landscape of viral diseases (Aleyeydi et al., 2024). It is essential to understand these factors to design good strategies and change health policies if the pandemic returns. In reviewing less common yet significant viral infections, one must consider the agricultural impact, particularly in livestock and poultry industries affected by diseases such as Infectious Bursal Disease (IBD). There is a very high seropositivity rate of 95.7% for IBD in backyard chickens in Ethiopia. As a result, this illustrates how viral infections impact human health, as well as the food supply and economy in farming communities. Since risk factors include immunity and how well biosecurity is practised, it is essential to use thorough vaccination and educational efforts to address these viral infections. Such investigations into host-specific viral diseases reveal the pressing necessity for a multifaceted approach that encompasses human, animal, and environmental health in tackling the challenges posed by viral infections in various contexts (Figure 8.5).

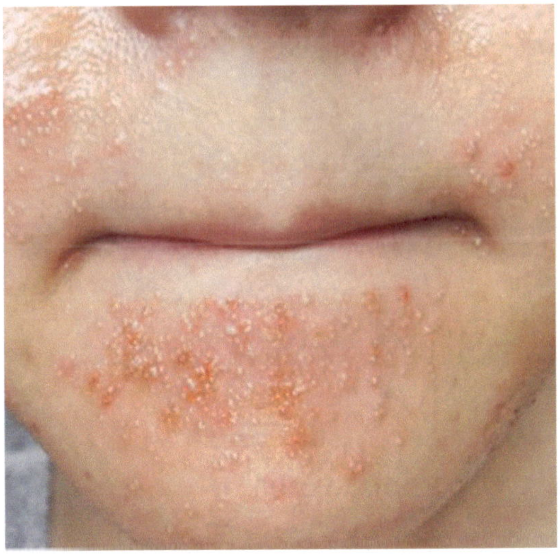

Figure 8.5. Viral infections.

Source: https://trueclinic.com.my/wp-content/uploads/2020/03/bacterial-infection-1.jpg.

8.1.3. Fungal and Parasitic Infections

Fungal and parasitic infections add a lot to the global problem of infectious diseases, mainly impacting infants and livestock. In Uttarakhand, infectious and parasitic infestations accounted for 26.92% of the dermatologic conditions observed in infants. Fungal infections accounted for 49% of all infections, which points to the need for more attention and quick treatment to prevent the complications they can cause. The findings emphasise that while non-infectious dermatological conditions predominate, the substantial presence of fungal infections necessitates further research into their epidemiology and management in pediatric settings (Bist et al., 2017). These infections also cause significant problems in both people and animals. A study in southern Morocco on skin diseases in dromedary camels revealed that dermatophytes were responsible for 30% of the cases. This highlights that both humans and animals can fall ill from fungal and parasitic pathogens, with the primary reasons being environmental factors, inadequate animal care, and improper treatment. The interplay of these factors signifies the importance of implementing preventive measures and effective treatment protocols to control these infections in both human and animal populations (Bengoumi et al., 2019). Epidemiological studies of fungal and parasitic infections suggest that a range of factors, including environmental, human-related, and biological aspects, play a role. The immune systems of young infants and animals are not fully developed, so they may be more likely to get these pathogens. The studies mentioned above have found that controlling the disease mainly depends on improving hygiene and teaching people about it. Due to increased travel and climate changes, these infections may spread more, necessitating continued research and public health efforts. Consequently, a multidisciplinary approach is essential to address the challenges posed by fungal and parasitic infections, ultimately aiming to reduce their incidence and improve health outcomes across various populations (Figure 8.6).

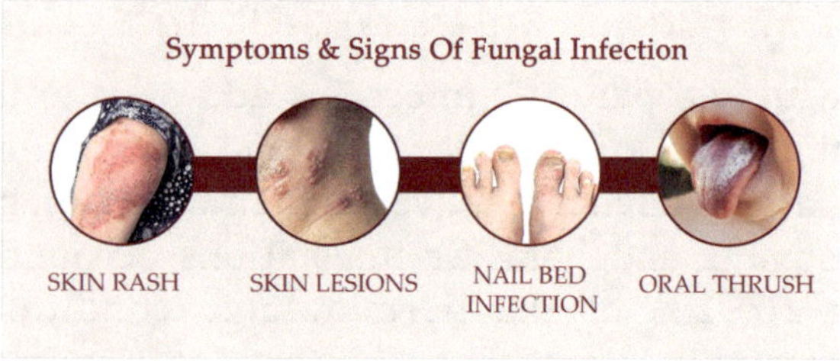

Figure 8.6. Fungal and parasitic infections.

Source: https://www.medindia.net/images/common/patientinfo/950_400/symptoms-and-signs-of-fungal-infection.jpg.

8.2. Transmission Dynamics

Understanding transmission dynamics is essential in epidemiology because they reveal how diseases can be transmitted within populations. The interaction between infectious agents and their hosts is crucial in shaping the course of an outbreak. Using mathematical models, scientists can imitate these processes and discover what affects the rate of transmission, such as the number of hosts, how they interact, and the environment. As an example, studies on polymorphic viral populations have found that some strains are more virulent than others, which influences how the virus spreads and evolves. A study found that when the population of susceptible bacterial cells was large, a variant with a higher propensity to lyse these cells became favoured, highlighting the intricate balance of selection pressure in epidemiological dynamics (Benhamou et al., 2024). Additionally, the link between wildlife and livestock is crucial for understanding how zoonotic diseases are transmitted. The example of African swine fever (ASF) and *Salmonella choleraesuis* illustrates how contact between wild and domestic animals can facilitate the spread of infections. In Sweden, surveys have shown that wild boars are often seen near pig farms, increasing concerns about disease transmission. Notably, the epidemiological similarities between ASF and *S. choleraesuis* underscore the importance of recognizing shared traits across diverse pathogens when conducting surveillance and implementing biosecurity measures (Ernholm, 2024). It points out that we should study both the direct ways diseases are passed and the environmental factors that might affect disease spread. It also points out how people's behavior influences the spread of infectious diseases. The way movement, social habits, and farming practices occur in a community can impact the spread of diseases. The way people act, such as hunting and managing farms, significantly influences how different species interact at the wildlife-livestock boundary. When local hunters are involved and good reporting methods are used, surveillance efforts can be significantly improved. They make it easier to understand how diseases are spreading locally and help develop stronger ways to control EIDs. The integration of theoretical, experimental, and observational data is essential in developing comprehensive strategies that address the complexities of disease transmission in various environments (Figure 8.7).

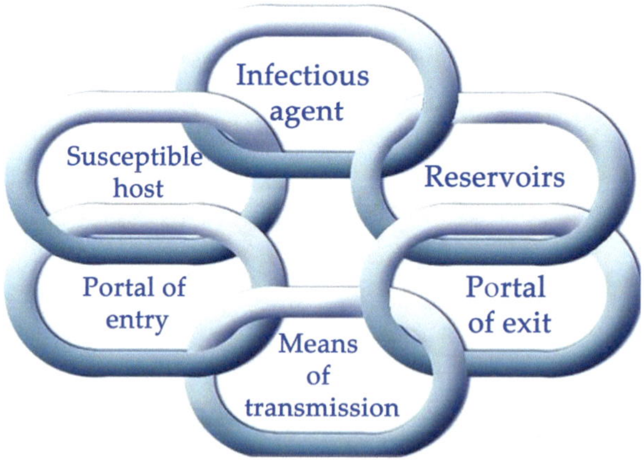

Figure 8.7. Transmission dynamics.

Source: https://image.slidesharecdn.com/dynamicsofdiseasetransmission-131123005720-phpapp02/95/dynamics-of-disease-transmission-2-638.jpg?cb=1385168646.

8.2.1. Modes of Transmission (Direct and Indirect)

Epidemiology of infectious diseases typically highlights that transmission can occur directly or indirectly. An infection occurs through direct transmission when the agent passes from one infected person to another susceptible person by touching, breathing, or swapping bodily fluids. Leptospirosis is a typical example, and people can get it by touching the urine of infected animals, which is often found in areas with animal waste. This zoonotic disease exemplifies how direct transmission mechanisms can particularly impact public health in regions where sanitation is inadequate, accentuating the need for effective surveillance and control measures (Pal et al., 2017). In indirect transmission, pathogens are transmitted by coming in contact with contaminated objects or the environment. Using the same personal items, for instance, toothbrushes, has been found to increase the risk of passing on hepatitis B and C viruses. The fact that some pathogens spread indirectly rather than directly prompts us to consider how pathogens are transmitted. Notably, incidents where indirect contact might facilitate a higher viral load associated with transmission underscore the complexity of understanding these transmission dynamics, particularly in clinical guidelines (Lin et al., 2016). The situation is further complicated by premastication, which may not seem important but has been shown to lead to more HBV infections in children. It is still essential to tell direct from indirect transmission when studying infectious diseases. Recognising how different pathogens spread through various means helps public health officials plan effective steps to reduce the number of cases. Avoiding contact with polluted water can help prevent leptospirosis, and good hygiene habits can stop hepatitis from spreading. Understanding these modes of transmission encourages a robust public health response, as it empowers communities to adopt preventive measures tailored explicitly to the pathogens that threaten them (Lin et al., 2016; Pal et al., 2017). By addressing both direct and indirect routes holistically, we can foster healthier environments and effectively combat the spread of infectious diseases (Figure 8.8).

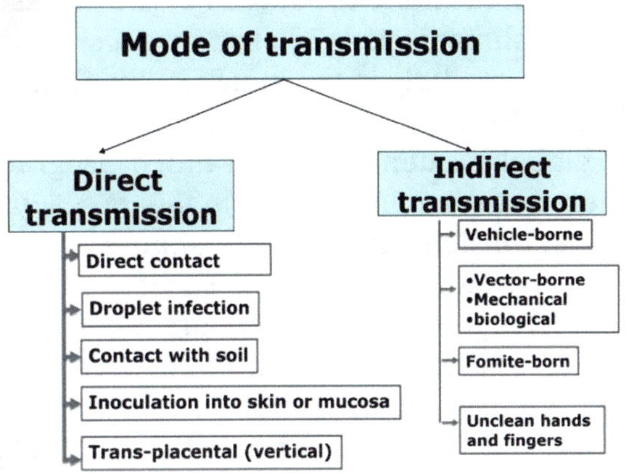

Figure 8.8. Modes of transmission (direct and indirect).

Source: https://hi-static.z-dn.net/files/dea/8c3e2b444be87a0bd72bb58641485daf.jpg.

8.2.2. Role of Vectors in Disease Spread

In epidemiology and public health, the way vectors spread infectious diseases is significant. Mosquitoes, ticks, and sandflies carry pathogens and help them move from one organism to another. Malaria, dengue fever, and leishmaniasis primarily use these insects to spread, highlighting the importance of understanding their biology and habitat. Since vectors and their hosts rely on each other, the spread of diseases becomes complicated, so it is essential to study what affects vector populations. Also, the rise in diseases spread by vectors highlights the need for specific actions to prevent their effects on public health, especially considering global climate change and urban growth, which may impact both vector habitats and human contact. Vector-borne diseases (VBDs) significantly contribute to worldwide morbidity and mortality, emerging as major public health concerns. WHO points out that more than 700,000 deaths each year are linked to these diseases, mostly in areas where the vectors live. Epidemiology of leishmaniasis requires examining how vectors, pathogens, and the environment facilitate the spread of the disease. Visceral leishmaniasis (VL) serves as a striking example, particularly in the Indian subcontinent, which has historically accounted for the majority of the global burden. Although much progress has been made in fighting *Leishmania donovani*, there are still significant gaps in understanding where and how the disease is spread. Having this knowledge helps develop practical ways to reduce vector populations and break the cycle of disease transmission, which can result in better public health and disease control. Improvements in how we study vectors should be used to learn more about how diseases are transmitted. New developments, for example, xenodiagnosis, help us to understand how vectors and infected hosts interact, which affects the risk of disease transmission. By studying how hosts infect their vectors, researchers can learn about the way specific diseases, such as VL, spread. Even though these approaches have great potential, implementing them is difficult because of logistical and ethical issues, mainly when using human subjects. Having modern research centres is very important, mainly in regions where VBDs are common. Addressing these challenges will be key for generating the requisite knowledge needed for effective vector control, particularly in light of increasing AMR attributed to vector-borne pathogens, as highlighted by the urgent need for innovative public health strategies in the context of AMR (Singh et al., 2020; Murray et al., 2022).

8.2.3. Environmental Factors Influencing Transmission

Infectious diseases are spread by various environmental factors, including weather, soil, and human activities. Temperature changes can strongly affect the life cycles of pathogens and the insects that carry them. For example, a temperature rise can cause mosquitoes to reproduce more, which increases the risk of diseases like malaria and dengue fever. Additionally, the environment, including the presence of wetlands or cities nearby, can alter the number and variety of these insects. It is essential to understand how climate affects disease vectors to predict outbreaks and take effective actions. Therefore, it is essential to investigate how environmental conditions influence the spread of common infectious diseases to better prepare for public health emergencies. The transmission of contagious diseases largely depends on the quality and pollution level of the air. Research has shown that as air pollution increases, people's immune systems become weaker, making them more susceptible to infections. Research on airborne viruses, for instance, avian influenza, found that air pollution in the environment played a significant role in making these viruses present in the air. Specifically, a study conducted in the Aogu Wetland in Taiwan analysed 357 ambient air samples to evaluate the concentration of airborne avian influenza viruses, finding correlations between air quality and virus transmission (Zhang et al., 2022). It shows that keeping an eye on the environment and controlling pollution is essential to managing infectious disease outbreaks. Additionally, when socioeconomic issues are combined with environmental issues, the spread of infectious diseases can worsen. Due to the high population and activity in cities, the risk of disease increases because of crowding and increased interaction among people. For instance, a study examining hand, foot, and mouth disease (HFMD) in Xinjiang, China, highlighted that urbanization, along with climatic factors such as rising temperatures and precipitation, significantly influenced HFMD incidence (Huang et al., 2021). In these areas, the number of cases was usually lower because there is more agriculture. These findings illustrate how understanding the connection between socio-environmental factors and infectious disease transmission can guide targeted interventions and public health strategies aimed at controlling disease spread in different communities (Figure 8.9).

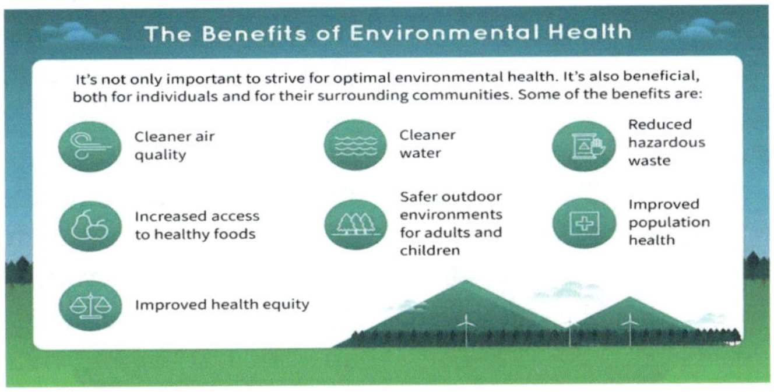

Figure 8.9. Environmental factors influencing transmission.

Source: https://s3.amazonaws.com/utep-uploads/wp-content/uploads/online-regis-college/2020/11/16062934/RC-MPH-2020-Q3-Skyscraper-8-Environmental-Factors-That-Affect-Health-miniIg1-v2-1000x613.jpg.

8.3. Epidemiological Surveillance

Infectious diseases are better controlled and managed with the help of epidemiological surveillance. When health officials collect, study, and analyse health data, they can identify outbreaks, monitor changes in diseases, and take action to prevent them. Different methods, such as passive and active surveillance, are used to collect detailed data from many other populations. For instance, the decline in incidence rates of HFMD following rigorous monitoring has underscored the value of surveillance in not only tracking disease prevalence but also understanding epidemiological patterns in specific regions, such as the Jiashan area in China from 2016 to 2022 (Yuan et al., 2024). Better data collection enables practitioners to refine their approaches, thereby reducing the impact of infectious diseases on community health. It is critical to have effective epidemiological surveillance when dealing with EIDs that can lead to acute meningitis and encephalitis. Identifying the diseases and their causes allows health authorities to assess how many people are affected and what actions are most important to take. The results from recent studies in Kazakhstan exemplify the importance of integrating comprehensive laboratory diagnostics with epidemiological data (Zhakipbayeva et al., 2023). In addition, recognising that enteroviruses cause many of these illnesses underscores the importance of implementing vaccination programs, which can help reduce both the incidence of sickness and mortality rates. Frequent and careful observation by the public health community allows them to prevent epidemics before they happen. Additionally, epidemiological surveillance is most effective when healthcare providers, laboratories, and governmental agencies collaborate. The use of different levels in data collection ensures that the data is accurate and can be shared easily among all parties involved. For instance, the sharing of longitudinal surveillance data regarding HFMD and acute meningitis has facilitated a deeper understanding of disease dynamics and spurred coordinated responses in affected areas (Zhakipbayeva et al., 2023; Yuan et al., 2024). Better surveillance and data analysis tools allow public health organisations to predict outbreaks better and organise resources. As such, the ongoing commitment to enhancing epidemiological surveillance is crucial for developing evidence-based policies that bolster public health resilience against common infectious diseases (Figure 8.10).

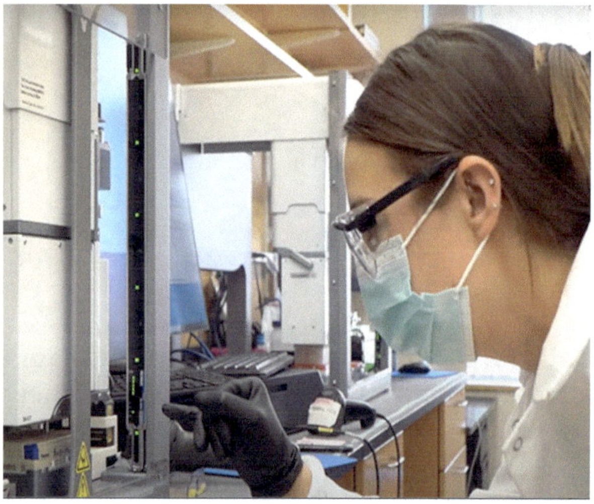

Figure 8.10. Epidemiological surveillance.

Source: https://www.broadinstitute.org/files/news/images/2022/GPviralsequencing-box.png.

8.3.1. Definition and Purpose of Surveillance

In public health and epidemiology, surveillance involves the regular collection, examination, and interpretation of health data to track disease prevalence and trends. to understand the patterns and spread of infectious diseases, which keep changing due to factors like changes in location, environment, and people's habits. Surveillance extends beyond simply collecting data; it necessitates ongoing review to support informed public health actions and decisions. Surveillance mainly aims to respond quickly to outbreaks and guide the creation of strategies to prevent them. Collecting and acting on data enables health officials to address new health issues and manage resources effectively, ultimately reducing the impact of infectious diseases on the population. Surveillance is primarily used to detect and monitor outbreaks of infectious diseases, which can range from small to large and be very serious. With effective surveillance, early warning signs of an epidemic can be found, which helps stop the disease from spreading further. During the COVID-19 pandemic, real-time monitoring data enabled experts to track the virus's spread and evaluate the effectiveness of various public health measures. Surveillance helps us identify and study the ways AMR happens, which makes it essential for controlling infections that are hard to treat. By correlating resistance patterns with specific pathogens, health authorities can tailor their strategies to combat the growing threat of AMR, thus demonstrating how surveillance shapes broader public health initiatives (Murray et al., 2022).

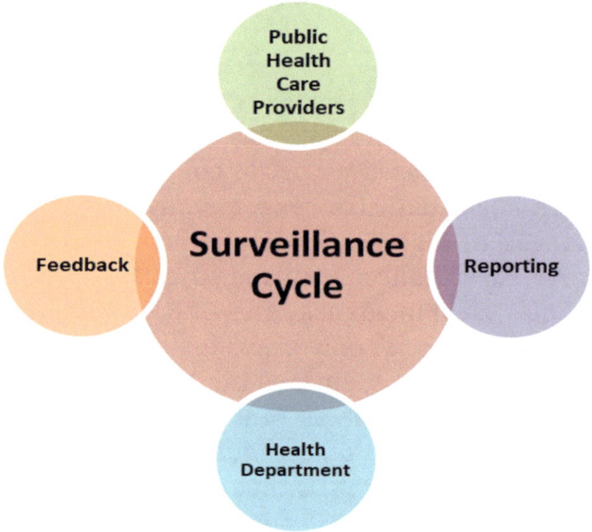

Figure 8.11. Surveillance, in the context of public health and epidemiology.

Source: https://www.researchgate.net/publication/368866999/figure/fig1/AS:11431281123372915@1677701227221/Surveillance-Cycle-approach-is-used-gather-process-and-share-public-health-related-data.png.

Additionally, surveillance is significant for its influence on the establishment of laws and allocation of resources. Surveillance information usually directs health officials to focus their funds and resources on regions and diseases that are most concerning. For instance, utilising information from surveillance systems can lead to more efficient allocation of laboratory resources and targeted public health activities in areas where infectious diseases are most prevalent. By combining surveillance, laboratory data, and healthcare records, we can gain a more thorough understanding of infectious diseases. By utilising data from multiple sources, including faecal samples and respiratory tests, public health officials can make informed decisions regarding patient management and isolation protocols, as illustrated in studies of COVID-19 that emphasise the need for varied sampling methods to gauge infection spread accurately (Chen et al., 2020) (Figure 8.11).

8.3.2. Types of Surveillance Systems (Active Versus Passive)

Surveillance systems are essential for epidemiology of common infectious diseases because they collect data that helps direct public health actions. There are two main types of surveillance systems: active and passive. In active surveillance, information about diseases is often collected by reaching out to healthcare providers and laboratories. This approach is beneficial in identifying EIDs, as it ensures that information is collected promptly and accurately. For example, in the context of bovine tuberculosis (BTB) management in Sweden, a detailed control program based on thorough tuberculin testing was implemented, highlighting how active surveillance enhances disease detection and monitoring efforts (Wahlström et al., 2004). Though active surveillance is expensive, it usually gives a clear picture of the disease and its trends, which can guide effective prevention measures. In comparison, passive surveillance depends on health professionals and laboratories to send in disease data without any extra encouragement. Because healthcare professionals report cases as they work, this system is faster and covers more people. Even though this approach works well for known infectious diseases, it could fail to detect cases of new or less common diseases due to the limitations of current reporting systems. For instance, the Royal Australian & New Zealand College of Obstetricians & Gynecologists (RANZCOG) recommends specific testing for sexually transmissible infections (STI) and blood-borne viruses (BBV), capturing data that reflects adherence to guidelines (Combs et al., 2008). So, although passive surveillance provides valuable insights into disease trends, it may not be as fast or precise as active surveillance. Choosing between active and passive surveillance methods can significantly impact public health and resource utilisation. Active surveillance generally provides better data, but it is expensive and requires a lot of staff, making it impractical in places with limited healthcare support. Alternatively, passive surveillance is a low-cost method for monitoring diseases in large populations, although it may not provide comprehensive details. When these systems are used together, health authorities can better handle outbreaks of infectious diseases. Using both types of surveillance, public health officials can combine their strengths to set up reliable systems that guide fast actions and improve the health of people affected by infectious diseases.

8.3.3. Importance of Data Collection and Analysis

Understanding and handling common infectious diseases in epidemiology depends greatly on data collection and analysis. Good data helps public health officials notice patterns, detect outbreaks and measure how well their efforts work. The relationship between robust data systems and public health outcomes is evident in regions plagued by severe acute respiratory illness (SARI), particularly in sub-Saharan Africa. Although SARI has a significant impact on children's health, many countries in this region have lacked proper surveillance systems in the past. The considerable gaps in data collection have led to underestimated mortality rates and ineffective responses to the disease's prevalence (Gessner, 2015). Therefore, having reliable and regular data monitoring is necessary to prevent outbreaks and look after vulnerable people. Additionally, examining epidemiological data enables researchers to identify factors that increase the risk of infectious diseases, which helps them plan effective prevention measures. For example, the study of salmonellosis and campylobacteriosis cases in Slovakia has revealed that detailed data have shown changes in how diseases are transmitted over the past decade. The findings demonstrate that while salmonellosis cases initially surged, there has been a statistically significant decline in incidence across the European Union (Zeleňáková et al., 2012). These findings play a key role in setting up and improving health-related policies. In this way, collecting epidemiological data continuously is essential for tracking the spread of diseases and for updating public health plans to address foodborne and infectious diseases. As well as helping us understand contagious diseases, collecting and analyzing data encourages public health bodies worldwide to cooperate and communicate. The WHO and national health authorities utilise teamwork in sharing data to identify patterns and address ongoing health issues. For instance, the effort to consolidate influenza surveillance data across several sub-Saharan African nations has helped to illuminate the regional burden of influenza-related morbidity and mortality (Gessner, 2015). By working together and sharing data, countries can learn from each other, which helps them respond together to infectious disease outbreaks. Ultimately, the prioritization of systematic data collection and analysis is indispensable for advancing public health responses and safeguarding communities from the threat of infectious diseases (Figure 8.12).

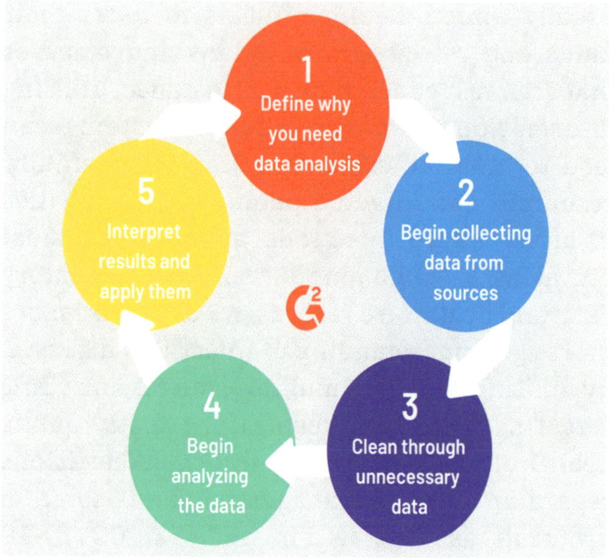

Figure 8.12. Importance of data collection and analysis.

Source: https://learn.g2.com/hs-fs/hubfs/data-analysis-process.png?width=1625&name=data-analysis-process.png.

8.4. Risk Factors for Infectious Diseases

Gaining knowledge about the factors that cause infectious diseases is very important for preventing and managing them. One significant category of risk factors includes demographic variables, such as age, sex, and socioeconomic status (SES). Children and the elderly are usually more likely to get infections because their immune systems are either not fully developed or are weakening. People with fewer resources often struggle to get needed healthcare, which can make infections more common and serious. Such differences underscore the importance of addressing social factors that contribute to infectious diseases, ensuring that those at risk receive the necessary support. The environment is critical in the spread of infectious diseases. The ways pathogens spread can be affected by climate change, urban growth, and sanitation.

As temperatures rise, mosquitoes can inhabit more areas, leading to increased cases of malaria and dengue fever. Additionally, poor sanitation facilitates the spread of waterborne diseases, particularly in densely populated urban areas where germs can proliferate. Therefore, it is crucial to integrate public health, environmental science, and urban planning to address these ecological risks and enhance communities' capacity to combat infectious diseases. Healthcare-associated infections (HAIs) present a unique set of risk factors within clinical settings, warranting focused research and intervention. Research shows that invasive devices such as catheters and ventilators significantly increase the risk of HAIs, with odds ratios showing that the risk is over four times higher. Sedation is also linked to more infections, probably because some anesthetic procedures weaken the immune system. Since HAIs are very common in intensive care units, it is crucial to prioritise infection control and the proper use of antibiotics in hospitals. Ongoing surveillance and understanding of these risk factors, such as those identified in Shrestha et al. (2022), are essential for developing targeted strategies to reduce the incidence of HAIs and protect patient safety.

8.4.1. Socioeconomic Factors

Socioeconomic factors play a significant role in the spread and number of infectious diseases. In places where SES is low, it is often more difficult for people to get healthcare, which makes infectious diseases more severe. Because of poor healthcare services, a lack of education, and poverty, people in vulnerable groups often experience more cases of hepatitis C. A study conducted in Afghanistan noted that a staggering 80.71% of hepatitis C cases occurred in married individuals with low education levels, highlighting how socioeconomic determinants correlate with health outcomes (Danish et al., 2025). Because of these differences, it is essential to target public health actions that consider both medical issues and the social factors that influence health, in order to prevent and control infectious diseases. Also, environmental elements such as sanitation and housing play a significant role in how contagious diseases spread in society.

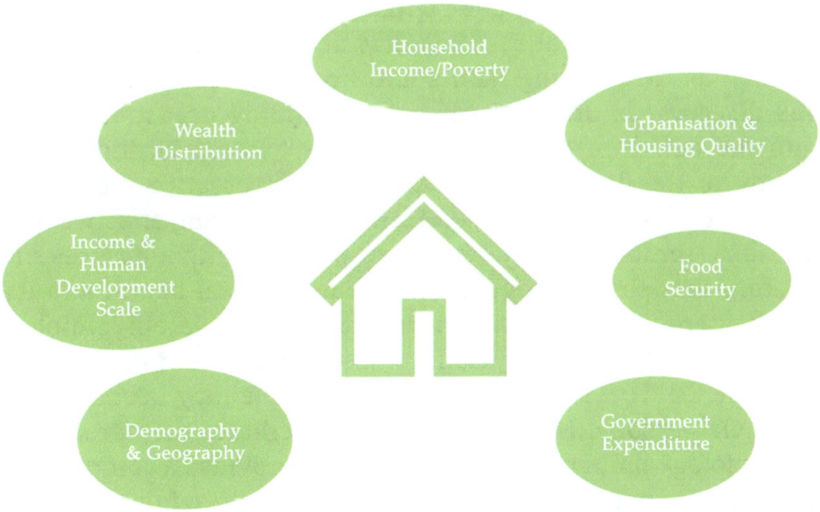

Figure 8.13. Socioeconomic factors.

Source: https://thinkpacific.com/app/uploads/2020/06/Socio-economic-factors.png.

When cities are crowded and their infrastructure is insufficient, it can be harmful to public health. A comprehensive analysis in Bangladesh revealed that poor hygiene practices and limited availability of healthcare exacerbate the prevalence of infectious diseases, such as conjunctivitis and other eye disorders (Chowdhury et al., 2024). Because of how SES and environment are related, those in lower SES groups often live in places with a greater risk of exposure to infectious agents. Thus, addressing these environmental causes is essential in the broader effort to prevent infectious diseases. Education is vital for influencing actions that can stop the spread of infectious diseases. Individuals with lower levels of education are often unaware of how to prevent infections, resulting in a higher incidence of infections. In the case of hepatitis C in Afghanistan, lower education levels among those infected underscore the need for comprehensive health education programs tailored to these communities (Danish et al., 2025). Additionally, as evidenced in Bangladesh, strategies to combat eye diseases are hampered by a lack of awareness regarding proper hygiene and health practices, which further intensifies the incidence of ailments (Chowdhury et al., 2024). Therefore, enhancing educational outreach and ensuring that vulnerable populations receive knowledge on hygiene, prevention, and available health services is paramount in mitigating the impact of infectious diseases within these communities (Figure 8.13).

8.4.2. Behavioral Factors (e.g., Hygiene Practices)

Studying how hygiene habits affect the spread of common infectious diseases is very important. How people behave can significantly influence both how many people get infected and the spread of diseases. Properly washing your hands is a significant way to prevent the spread of infectious agents. Washing your hands often, especially after touching dirty things or before you eat, can significantly decrease the chances of getting respiratory infections or stomach problems. Studies emphasise the need for public health campaigns that reinforce these hygiene practices, ultimately aiming to enhance community awareness regarding the importance of cleanliness as a primary defence against infections (Aprillia et al., 2024). Also, behavioural factors affect not only personal hygiene but also the social and cultural customs that determine the health of the community. The way people behave, such as their eating habits and how they seek medical care, can impact the number of infectious diseases. In other words, understanding breastfeeding culture can provide valuable insights into the health of mothers and children. Research indicates that breastfeeding contributes significantly to the health of infants, offering protective measures against infections during early development, underscoring the importance of promoting effective nutritional behaviours across diverse populations (Ibrahim, 2023). Therefore, public health measures should cover hygiene, nutrition, and the factors that shape people's behaviours. Mental health and its relationship with behaviour must be considered when looking at infectious disease epidemiology. Worrying about health can cause people to neglect their hygiene, which makes them more likely to get sick. When a health crisis, such as the COVID-19 pandemic, occurs, people may become more anxious and less likely to take care of their personal hygiene, which can facilitate the spread of the illness. Hence, understanding how psychology influences health behaviors provides a comprehensive understanding of disease prevention. Helping people improve their mental well-being and hygiene awareness may encourage them to follow preventive measures and thus lower the number of infectious diseases in communities. Emphasizing this intersection of mental health and hygiene is essential for effective epidemic control and fostering resilient populations (Figure 8.14).

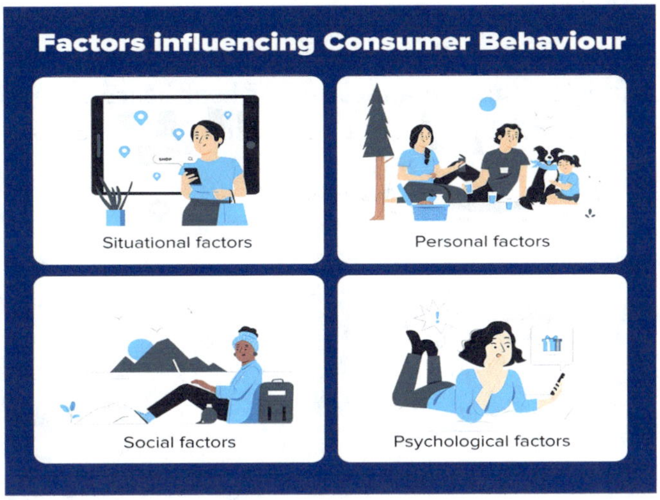

Figure 8.14. Behavioral factors (e.g., hygiene practices).

Source: https://wpswings.com/wp-content/uploads/2022/10/factors.jpg.

8.4.3. Biological Factors (e.g., Age, Immunity)

The role of biological factors in the epidemiology of common infectious diseases is profound, particularly in relation to age and passive immunity. Because their immune systems are not fully developed, infants and adolescents are more likely to get infections. As an illustration, children are more likely to get IBD, which is most common in chicks between three and six weeks, and is a major issue in poultry farming everywhere. In Ethiopia, seropositivity rates for IBDV in backyard chickens reached 95.7%, underscoring the importance of age as a critical biological factor in infection dynamics (Beshah et al., 2024). Because maternal antibodies provide temporary protection, young individuals are more likely to get infected with infectious diseases as the immunity fades. Immunity plays a crucial role in determining the likelihood of contracting infectious diseases. If people have pre-existing immunity from earlier infections or vaccinations, the chance of contracting the disease may be significantly lower in some populations. In the context of autoimmune diseases, such as rheumatoid arthritis (RA), patients exhibit compromised immune responses, resulting in increased vulnerability to infections.

Patients may experience even more immunosuppression when they receive immunomodulatory treatments, which could lead to more co-infections. In a cohort study, it was reported that 70% of RA patients had at least one cardiovascular risk factor, highlighting the complex interplay between immune status, age, and the risk of concurrent infectious diseases (Yano et al., 2023). Therefore, public health strategies should be tailored to take into account people's immunity when handling contagious disease epidemiology. Apart from age and the immune system, genes, the environment, and nutrition all play a role in determining how likely someone is to get an infectious disease. For example, people with certain genetic traits might have different immune responses, which can influence how severe and what the result of an infection will be. Besides, when there are too many people in an area and sanitation is poor, it can make infectious diseases more likely to spread, especially among those who are most at risk, such as the elderly or people with weak immune systems. To deal with the epidemiology of these conditions, we need to look at the biological factors as a group. Understanding the varying degrees of immunity across different demographic groups can inform vaccination strategies and the allocation of healthcare resources, ultimately aiding in the control and prevention of common infectious diseases (Figure 8.15).

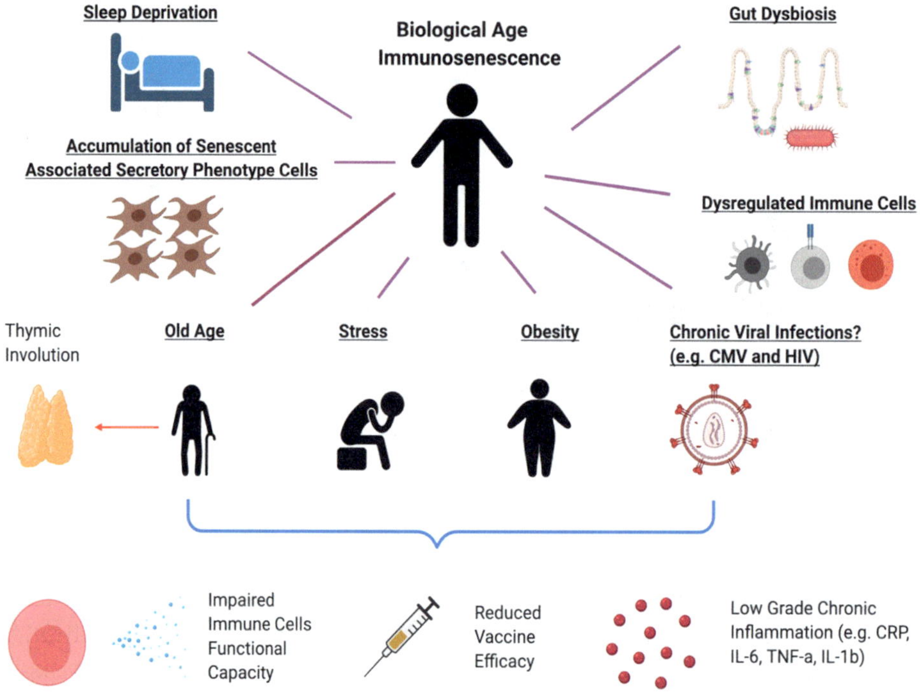

Figure 8.15. Biological factors (e.g., age, immunity).

Source: https://www.researchgate.net/publication/346528029/figure/fig3/AS:963914393210886@1606826508944/Various-external-stressors-that-results-in-biological-age-related-immunosenescence.png.

8.5. Impact of Infectious Diseases

The impact of infectious diseases extends far beyond individual health, influencing global economic stability and societal structures. One example is AMR, which has become a major issue due to giving antibiotics too often and not having proper infection control. About 4.95 million people died in 2019 due to bacterial AMR, demonstrating that it is a significant cause of death globally. Most of these deaths were caused by lower respiratory infections, which stresses the need for strong public health measures to address AMR and manage infectious diseases. It is essential to understand the extent to which AMR affects low-resource areas with numerous endemic diseases, in order to inform policies that improve healthcare and provide effective treatments. Such comprehensive approaches are vital as they can significantly mitigate the health and economic burdens posed by infectious diseases in affected populations (Murray et al., 2022). Infectious diseases are more common in marginalised regions, which worsens health inequalities and slows down development. The SARS-CoV-2 pandemic has shown that public health systems are weak everywhere, including in Africa, and that international health cooperation is not as strong as it should be. Africa needs a robust public health system to manage both new and existing diseases. The health of the continents is also challenged by the rise of non-communicable diseases and the ongoing problem of AMR, which makes it harder to manage health care. Thus, managing these issues well requires a complete public health strategy with local health goods production, trained staff, and strong relationships with other countries that consider local needs. These strategies are crucial for building resilient health systems that can effectively combat the threats posed by infectious diseases (Nkengasong et al., 2020). Infectious diseases cause huge economic damage by reducing productivity and straining healthcare systems. According to the WHO, infectious diseases lead to about 227 million years of healthy life lost in Africa each year, which is equivalent to a productivity loss of over $800 billion. Since many infectious diseases are a major problem, they hold back the economies of affected regions, resulting in more poverty and fewer health services for people. Tackling the reasons for infectious disease transmission, making healthcare accessible, and investing in local health help promote lasting economic growth. As we strive for comprehensive solutions, it is crucial to recognise the interdependence of health, financial stability, and social well-being across all societies, particularly in regions most affected by infectious diseases (Murray et al., 2022) (Figure 8.16).

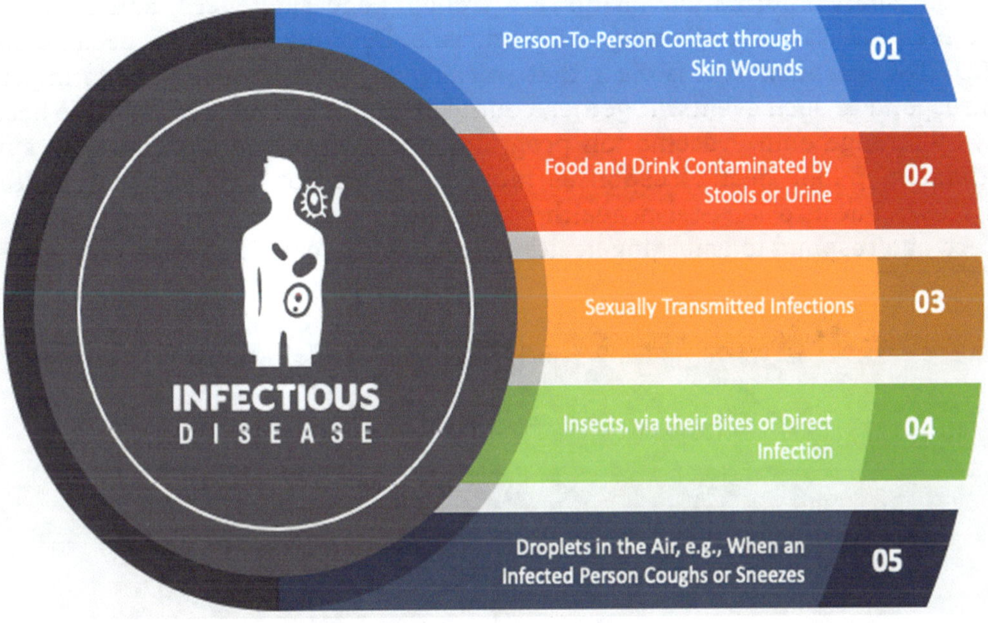

Figure 8.16. Impact of infectious diseases.

Source: http://cdn.sketchbubble.com/pub/media/catalog/product/optimized1/0/3/035e7be3332 91c8e7f62bf733a35f7eef63d9770c8a0a9f1d746997c3a2c6348/infectious-disease-mc-slide3.png.

8.5.1. Public Health Implications

The emergence of infectious diseases, particularly those resulting from novel pathogens such as SARS-CoV-2, raises significant public health implications that extend beyond immediate clinical concerns. The rapid global transmission of COVID-19 highlights the interconnectedness of today's world and the urgent need for swift action to halt outbreaks. To be effective, public health needs systems that can quickly identify and isolate cases so that transmission does not spread. Recent studies have found that people may still release the virus through their respiratory and intestinal secretions even after their symptoms subside, which could impact the guidelines for isolating them. The implications here necessitate reevaluation of existing public health guidelines to incorporate comprehensive testing and the assessment of multiple specimen types to ensure containment strategies are robust and effective in reducing transmission risk (Chen et al., 2020). Along with taking action to prevent and respond to outbreaks, the COVID-19 pandemic has highlighted the need for public health systems to address disparities in healthcare access. Many vulnerable people have difficulties accessing testing, treatment, and prevention, which makes infectious diseases more severe in these communities. Due to this difference, there is a pressing need for equitable healthcare policies that facilitate access to vaccinations and promote health awareness. In addition, pandemics have greatly affected mental health and the economy, which highlights the many different aspects of public health challenges. Addressing these issues requires a holistic approach that integrates social determinants of health into public health frameworks, thereby strengthening community resilience and response capabilities in the face of future outbreaks (Zhāng et al., 2020). Nations need to cooperate to deal with the public health problems linked to infectious disease outbreaks. Countries should share information on disease trends, gene sequences, and how interventions work so that everyone can address new health threats. Because the world became so connected during the COVID-19 pandemic, it is clear that working together is necessary to improve how we prepare and respond to such events. Together, countries can develop more effective health policies, for example, by strengthening vaccination programs and addressing diseases that spread across borders. Ultimately, public health responses must prioritise not only the immediate control of infectious diseases but also long-term health system strengthening, enhancing global capacity to prevent, detect, and respond to emerging health threats effectively (Chen et al., 2020) (Figure 8.17).

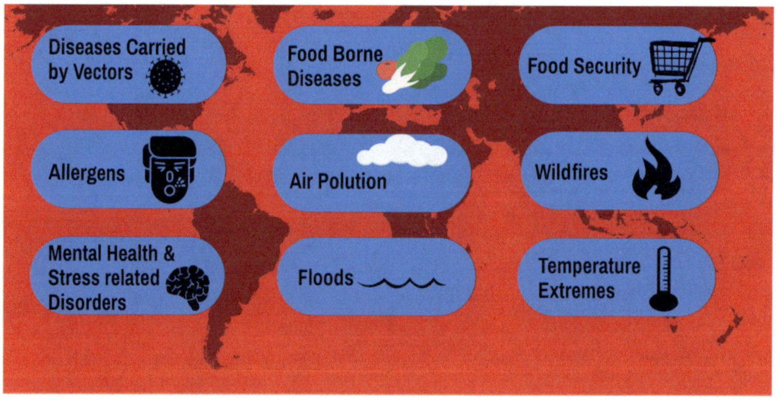

Figure 8.17. Public health implications.

Source: https://www.mphonline.org/wp-content/uploads/2020/06/mph-9-climate-effects-768x512.png.

8.5.2. Economic Consequences

The economic consequences of common infectious diseases exert a profound impact on public health systems and national economies. The costs of treatment and managing the disease are a significant issue. For example, acute infectious gastroenteritis (AGE) in the United States results in substantial healthcare resource utilisation, costing an average of $1,338 per outpatient visit, translating to an overwhelming total of $333,060,182 for the entire population studied (Wieters et al., 2024). Besides healthcare, these financial problems can also be seen in households that lose income, have medical bills, and suffer from less productivity because of illness. Therefore, being aware of the economic impacts of such diseases is crucial for developing effective public health policies. Along with the costs of treating illnesses, infectious diseases put pressure on the workforce and reduce productivity. Infectious diseases often cause many workers to miss work, which can reduce productivity and the economy's output. Increased healthcare claims and insurance premiums usually result from infectious diseases, which adds to the problems faced by both employers and employees. The economic impact is most noticeable in developing regions because of the higher rates of infectious diseases, which prevent them from growing economically. By analyzing data on antibiotic use and resistance strategies in sub-Saharan Africa, it becomes evident that these health-related economic repercussions necessitate targeted interventions to mitigate their effects (Wieters et al., 2024). Above that, infectious diseases can cause lasting economic problems that might be hard to notice in the beginning. Infectious diseases can cause conditions that recur, leading to long-term health problems that impact the productivity of individuals and communities. As a result, the demand for healthcare services increases, placing additional pressure on the system. In areas where tourism or trade plays a big role, outbreaks can cause a major drop in visitors and economic activity which can threaten the stability of the community. Thus, the economic consequences of infectious diseases present a multifaceted challenge that requires comprehensive strategies, not only aimed at immediate health interventions but also at fostering long-term economic resilience and recovery (Moon et al., 2023).

8.5.3. Social and Psychological Effects

The intersection of social and psychological effects arising from common infectious diseases plays a critical role in understanding their broader epidemiological impact. Infectious diseases can cause people in the community to feel more fearful and anxious, as was the case during the COVID-19 pandemic, when there was a considerable rise in major depressive disorder and anxiety disorders. Because of the lockdowns, social distancing, and constant media updates, many people experienced more uncertainty, which made their mental health problems worse and caused new cases to appear. According to research, daily SARS-CoV-2 infection rates and reduced human mobility were directly correlated with increased prevalence rates of these disorders, underlining the profound link between societal response to disease outbreaks and mental health outcomes (Santomauro et al., 2021). It shows that health crises are not only about medicine but also have a substantial impact on people's mental health. Pandemics often cause changes in social life, which can have a big effect on people's mental health. When people are unable to interact socially and lose their social networks, they may feel isolated and helpless, particularly those who are more vulnerable. The breakdown of society can make mental health issues worse for people affected by the infectious disease. It was found that females and younger people were more affected by the pandemic, which makes it necessary to create targeted actions to reduce these differences. Epidemiological data from various locations reveal that regions most severely impacted by the pandemic reported the highest increases in mental health disorders, indicating a strong relationship between disease prevalence and social well-being (Johnson et al., 2020). Therefore, understanding the impact of infectious diseases on society is crucial for developing public health strategies that address both physical and mental health. Infectious diseases affect people mentally and emotionally, so public health strategies should always include mental health support. COVID-19 showed clearly that mental health systems around the world need to be improved. Both controlling the spread of the infection and supporting the mental health of those affected should be essential parts of any mitigation strategy. Some helpful actions are to encourage support groups in the community and create policies that work to decrease the stigma around mental health problems. By acknowledging the interplay between infectious diseases and mental health, health authorities can create responsive, inclusive strategies that minimize the psychological toll of outbreaks while simultaneously addressing the epidemiological aspects (Santomauro et al., 2021). Ultimately, prioritizing mental health in the context of epidemiology is not merely beneficial but essential for the resilience and recovery of communities facing infectious diseases (Figure 8.18).

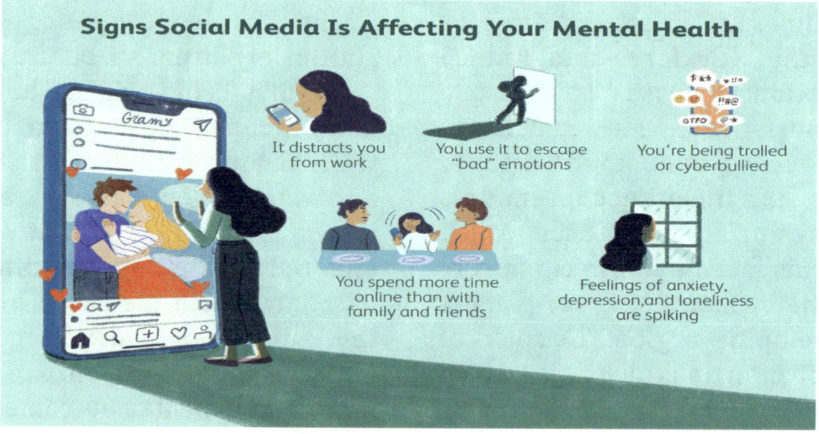

Figure 8.18. Social and psychological effects.

Source: https://www.verywellmind.com/thmb/ioxfQrLyAo5cwLXzRhlVELUFIgY=/1500x0/filters:no_upscale():max_bytes(150000):strip_icc()/link-between-social-media-and-mental-health-5089347-color-withtext-54a445186bb44974b059ac7b6494bcdf.gif.

8.6. Prevention and Control Strategies

In addressing the prevention and control strategies for common infectious diseases, a multifaceted approach is crucial. Early identification and action are crucial for managing risks, particularly in areas where outbreaks frequently occur, such as communities and schools. For instance, the study of HFMD and herpangina (HA) outbreaks in Zhejiang Province from 2021 to 2023 highlights the importance of timely reporting and management of cases. Nearly all outbreaks occurred in childcare settings, indicating that they are significant sources of disease transmission. Separating students and stopping classes can help prevent many infections, as delays cause more cases to appear. Thus, early detection coupled with strategic intervention can considerably alter the course of an outbreak, leading to better public health outcomes (Chen et al., 2025). Additionally, public health education helps prevent outbreaks from occurring. Educational programs should teach parents, caregivers, and teachers about the signs and symptoms of infectious diseases, for example, HFMD and HA.

Such programs can help communities notice early signs and prompt them to report these to the appropriate health officials. Also, encouraging students and staff to wash their hands and keep shared spaces clean can significantly lower the spread of diseases in these places. The effectiveness of these strategies is demonstrated by the correlation between the speed of outbreak management and the number of cases, indicating that informed communities can have a significant impact on infections. Enhanced education not only equips individuals with the necessary tools to combat these diseases but also fosters a culture of proactive health management within populations (Chen et al., 2025). In the case of sexually transmitted infections (STIs) like genital herpes, prevention strategies require a different set of approaches. Since there is no cure and diagnostics are still not perfect, it is essential to stress preventive actions such as teaching about sexual health and organising outreach programs. Public health initiatives should aim to provide comprehensive information regarding herpes simplex virus types 1 and 2 (HSV-1 and HSV-2), promoting safe sexual practices and awareness of transmission methods. Additionally, investigating new vaccines and treatments remains very important, as the CDC/NIAID workshop on genital herpes demonstrated. Such collaborative efforts can lead to innovative strategies for controlling STIs and establishing measures that reduce their incidence and impact on public health, thereby enhancing the overall effectiveness of prevention and control initiatives (Figure 8.19).

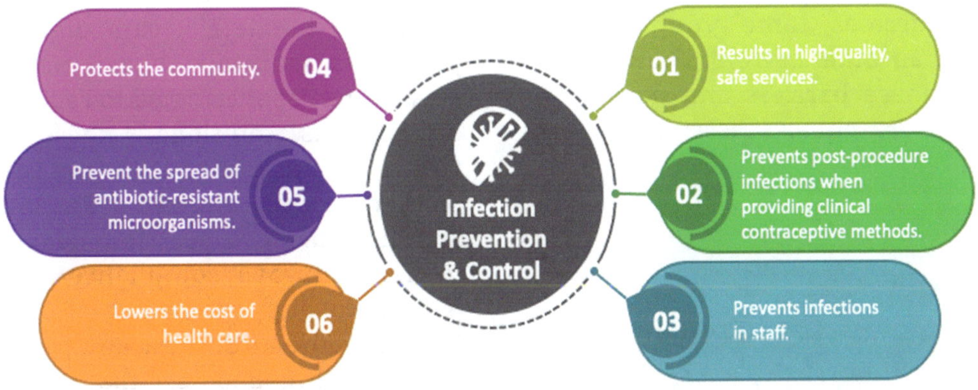

Figure 8.19. Prevention and control strategies.

Source: https://cdn.sketchbubble.com/pub/media/catalog/product/optimized1/1/f/1f7d0441caa9d0e4cee43466188a98f54ae491b354e8d992892dceb6f182016b/infection-prevention-and-control-mc-slide5.png.

8.6.1. Vaccination Programs

Vaccination programs play a crucial role in controlling infectious diseases, making a significant contribution to public health through the prevention of outbreaks and the reduction of morbidity and mortality rates. Vaccines stimulate a strong immune response, enabling people to resist certain diseases and support community immunity, which in turn helps protect those who cannot be vaccinated. As a result of vaccination, polio and measles have almost disappeared in many places across the globe. Nonetheless, these achievements depend on maintaining high vaccination rates to prevent the return of these diseases, which underscores the need for ongoing efforts to address people's fears and doubts about vaccines. Comprehensive vaccination programs have also been linked to a significant drop in the number of infectious diseases. Screening people along with vaccination can make public health even better. For example, in Catalonia, the integration of sickle cell disease (SCD) screening with standard-care treatments, including anti-pneumococcal vaccination, has exemplified how vaccination can not only prevent infections but also support the management of specific health conditions. Clinical results from patients who were screened and those who were not revealed that early vaccination significantly reduced SCD-related problems, proving that vaccination is linked to other healthcare strategies. It highlights the need for public health measures that support vaccination and early screening. The success of vaccination programs depends on several social and cultural factors, so these should be considered when planning and carrying out public health measures. If not everyone can get or accept vaccines, some groups may be more at risk than others. Work should focus on identifying these barriers and developing solutions to ensure equal access to vaccines for everyone.

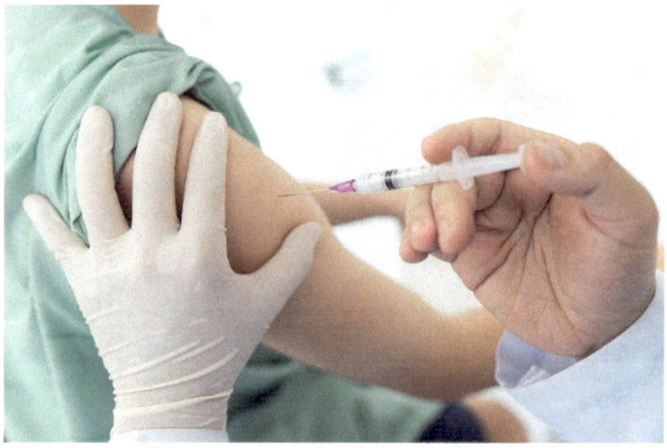

Figure 8.20. Vaccination programs.

Source: https://www.westtorrens.sa.gov.au/files/assets/public/v/1/services/health/immunisation.jpg?w=1080.

Research on chronic diseases, such as psoriasis, reveals significant gaps in healthcare for affected individuals, which may also be reflected in vaccination programs. Addressing these disparities not only enhances the efficacy of vaccination efforts but also aligns with global health goals aimed at achieving comprehensive health coverage for all individuals, thereby mitigating the impact of common infectious diseases on society (Torres et al., 2023; de Aledo-Castillo et al., 2024) (Figure 8.20).

8.6.2. Public Health Campaigns and Education

Public health campaigns are essential tools in the fight against infectious diseases, serving to inform and educate the public about health risks and prevention strategies. These campaigns often leverage a variety of communication methods, including social media, traditional advertising, and community outreach, to reach diverse populations. For example, during the COVID-19 pandemic, campaigns encouraged people to maintain social distancing, wear masks, and get vaccinated to reduce the number of infections. Additionally, these efforts aim to reduce the number of cases and educate people on how the disease can be prevented. Interesting stories and messages that people can relate to help improve compliance and encourage people to support health initiatives, which leads to more awareness and proactive actions about health. Besides, the impact of public health campaigns is greatly increased when strong educational programs about particular infectious diseases support them. By targeting educational efforts, such as those regarding Shiga toxin-producing *Escherichia coli* (STEC), public health officials can raise awareness about transmission routes and risk factors associated with these pathogens. Emphasising hygiene and safe food handling in schools can significantly reduce the number of cases and stop outbreaks. In particular, teaching parents and caregivers to recognize the signs and symptoms of STEC infections matters a lot, as children are more likely to suffer from severe outcomes. So, when people are informed about health issues, they can respond better, which results in better health and less disease pressure on healthcare systems, as observed in many regions using epidemiological data to change their strategies. Incorporating cultural and behavioral concepts into public health campaigns helps the messages reach and influence the people intended. When campaigns consider and address the impact of culture and society on health, they encourage more people in the community to take part. For example, the lockdown during the COVID-19 pandemic significantly impacted smoking behaviors in various populations, demonstrating how external factors could influence public health trends (Sabbah et al., 2022). Additionally, data show that educational levels impacted smoking rates during this period, indicating the need for tailored campaigns that consider demographic variables (Sabbah et al., 2022). As seen in the context of STEC infections, targeted and culturally sensitive education can improve surveillance and response, ultimately fostering a resilient public health framework that can adapt to emerging infectious disease threats (Figure 8.21).

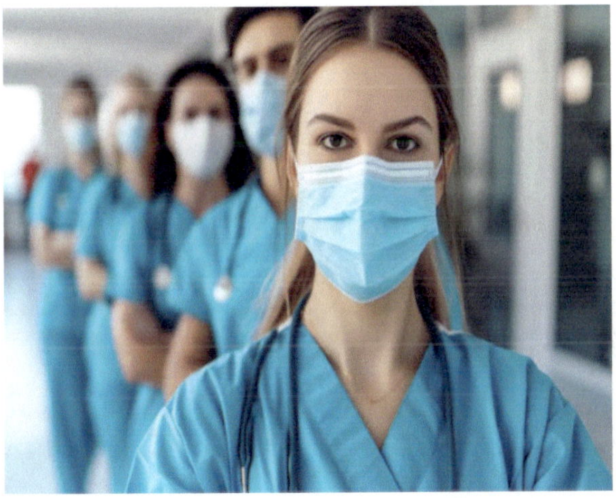

Figure 8.21. Public health campaigns and education.

Source: https://img.freepik.com/premium-photo/public-health-campaigns-healthcare-professionals-leading-public-health-initiatives_765582-10555.jpg.

8.6.3. Role of Healthcare Systems in Disease Management

The role of healthcare systems in disease management is pivotal in mitigating the impacts of infectious diseases. Well-equipped healthcare systems enable people to receive quick diagnoses, treatment, and prevention, all of which are crucial for controlling outbreaks. Effective disease management involves integrating healthcare services, including monitoring, vaccination, and treatment design for specific pathogens. For example, a well-organised healthcare effort can help reduce the effects of AMR, which has caused many cases of serious illness and death around the world. A recent study estimated that approximately 4.95 million deaths were associated with bacterial AMR in 2019 alone, underlining the urgent need for comprehensive healthcare strategies that address this challenge (Murray et al., 2022). As healthcare systems improve, the use of evidence-based approaches and public health actions will play a larger role in controlling common infectious diseases. Due to the SARS-CoV-2 pandemic, it is now evident that healthcare systems in resource-poor regions require improvement. Because of the pandemic, it has become clear that health infrastructure needs to be stronger and more adaptable to health emergencies. Creating a new public health order involves upgrading disease monitoring and response, as well as supporting the local production of vaccines and tests. This approach aims to reduce dependency on external sources and fortifies healthcare systems against future outbreaks (Nkengasong et al., 2020). Increasing healthcare infrastructure allows countries to identify better, handle and control outbreaks, which lowers the impact of infectious diseases and supports public health. In addition, healthcare systems help educate people and involve them in the community, which is essential for stopping diseases. Discussing how diseases are transmitted, how to prevent them, and the role of vaccination can significantly impact public health. Targeted educational programs can help individuals at risk understand how to manage their health effectively. Also, when the community is involved in healthcare efforts, people become more trusting and cooperative, which results in better compliance with health recommendations. Community involvement has proven crucial in enhancing the effectiveness of healthcare interventions during previous infectious disease outbreaks. The integration of health systems with public education and community collaboration not only enhances disease management but also ensures a more sustainable approach to addressing the ongoing challenges posed by infectious diseases (Nkengasong et al., 2020; Murray et al., 2022) (Figure 8.22).

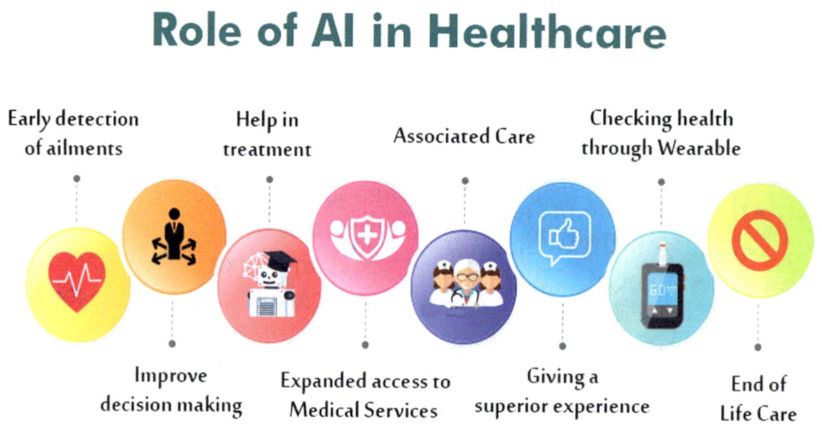

Figure 8.22. Role of healthcare systems in disease management.

Source: https://www.tutorsindia.com/academy/wp-content/uploads/2021/04/Role-of-AI-in-Healthcare.jpg.

SUMMARY

In concluding our exploration of the epidemiology of common infectious diseases, it is imperative to emphasise the dynamic nature of infectious disease patterns and the factors influencing their transmission. The data collected in various studies indicate that in regions such as Saudi Arabia, both brucellosis and tuberculosis remain prevalent. Due to the decline in COVID-19 infections, public health officials now face both challenges and new opportunities, as the findings indicate a decrease in many bacterial infections. Understanding these evolving patterns is therefore crucial for developing targeted interventions aimed at reducing disease burden and improving community health outcomes, thereby laying the foundation for future disease control strategies (Alhumaid et al., 2024). It is also essential to examine how antibiotic use affects AMR as we address problems with infectious diseases. Antibiotic use in sub-Saharan Africa is high, especially for Watch group antibiotics, which leads to more cases of AMR. Many patients said they used antibiotics without the required supervision from a doctor which highlights the risk of a public health crisis due to unchecked antibiotic prescriptions. Addressing these issues is crucial for implementing effective antimicrobial stewardship programs that strike a balance between the need for treatment and the imperative to curb resistance, as highlighted in the assessment of antibiotic use patterns across multiple healthcare facilities (Wieters et al., 2024). To have a complete approach to infectious disease epidemiology, it is crucial for health authorities, researchers and the public to cooperate. Results from disease surveillance and antibiotic use indicate that improved data collection and monitoring can lead to more effective public health actions. Future studies should include more variables such as socioeconomic conditions, travel experiences, and death rates, to better understand the factors that spread infectious diseases. By prioritising these areas, public health officials can better allocate resources, inform policy decisions, and ultimately safeguard community health against the ever-evolving threats posed by infectious diseases (Alhumaid et al., 2024; Wieters et al., 2024).

When studying the epidemiology of common infectious diseases, several important aspects are revealed that demonstrate the complexity of this field. Observational research is fundamental because it provides the basis for much of what we know in clinical and public health. It is crucial to study the causes, mechanisms of disease development, and factors determining their distribution among people. Observational studies, which are not as controlled as randomized trials, still give important insights due to the larger and more varied groups they often involve. The STROBE Statement emphasises the need for rigour in reporting these studies, guiding researchers to present their methods and findings in a detailed manner to enhance transparency and reproducibility in public health research (Vandenbroucke et al., 2007). Recognising these critical factors is essential for a comprehensive study of infectious diseases. Investigations into infectious diseases by epidemiologists mainly focus on discovering and understanding what increases the chances of the disease being transmitted and experienced. The environment, the social and economic situation, and the healthcare system all have a big impact on epidemiology. In many cases, outbreaks occur because people lack proper sanitation, are unvaccinated, or cannot access healthcare. Because these factors interact, it becomes challenging to control diseases and demands that public health uses several methods. In addition, it is essential to review new risk factors; although traditional indicators are still helpful, discussing climate change and its effects on infectious diseases is also crucial. This holistic perspective is critical for developing effective prevention strategies and ultimately reducing disease burden (Berkwits et al., 2007). It is also essential in infectious disease epidemiology that public health officials, researchers and the community work together. Good communication and sharing of information help data from observational studies affect policy decisions and healthcare strategies. This approach enables the incorporation of new knowledge into existing protocols, thereby enhancing the prevention and control of infectious diseases. It is also essential for epidemiology to use new technologies and approaches, such as digital health and analytics, to remain strong. By leveraging these partnerships and new ideas, the public health community can tackle both current and future challenges posed by infectious diseases. Understanding these dynamics highlights the importance of a comprehensive epidemiological approach in addressing the ongoing global health concerns associated with infectious diseases (Vandenbroucke et al., 2007).

CLOSER LOOK

PRE-EXISTING IMMUNITY:

Pre-existing immunity refers to the immune system's prior readiness to recognize and respond to a pathogen due to previous exposure or vaccination. This phenomenon significantly influences the body's ability to fight infections, the effectiveness of vaccines, and the progression of infectious diseases. Understanding pre-existing immunity is vital for immunologists, epidemiologists, and public health professionals, as it shapes strategies for disease prevention and outbreak control. At the core of pre-existing immunity is the adaptive immune system, which relies on memory B cells and T cells. When an individual is exposed to a pathogen—either through natural infection or vaccination—the immune system generates specific antibodies and memory lymphocytes targeted against that pathogen. On subsequent exposures, these memory cells allow for a faster and more robust immune response. For example, individuals previously infected with certain strains of influenza often mount quicker antibody responses upon re-exposure, sometimes mitigating symptoms or preventing reinfection altogether.

Pre-existing immunity can be both beneficial and challenging. On the positive side, it enhances protection against pathogens and can reduce the severity of disease. This is a key principle behind booster vaccinations, which aim to strengthen or refresh the immune memory. In populations with widespread pre-existing immunity, outbreaks of diseases such as measles or polio are often limited, highlighting the community-level impact of immune memory.

However, pre-existing immunity can also complicate responses to infections and vaccines. In some cases, prior exposure to related but distinct strains of a virus can lead to an altered immune response, a phenomenon known as "original antigenic sin." This can result in suboptimal protection or even heightened disease severity, as seen in certain dengue virus infections. Additionally, pre-existing immunity may interfere with the efficacy of new vaccines, particularly for rapidly mutating pathogens like influenza or coronaviruses, necessitating careful vaccine design and strain selection.

Research into pre-existing immunity has expanded with advances in immunology and genomics. Scientists now explore how cross-reactive immune responses—where immunity against one pathogen affects responses to another—impact disease dynamics and vaccine strategies. Understanding these interactions helps guide public health policies, including vaccination campaigns and pandemic preparedness plans.

In conclusion, pre-existing immunity is a central component of the human immune response, shaping susceptibility, disease outcomes, and vaccine effectiveness. While it provides valuable protection against previously encountered pathogens, it also presents challenges in managing evolving infectious diseases. Continued research into the mechanisms and implications of pre-existing immunity is essential for optimizing public health interventions and improving global disease control.

REFERENCES

1. Sabbah, H. A., Assaf, E., Taha, Z., Qasrawi, R., Ismail, L. C., Dhaheri, A. A., Hoteit, M., Al-Jawaldeh, A., Tayyem, R., Bawadi, H., AlKhalaf, M., Bookari, K., Kamel, I., Dashti, S., Allehdan, S., Waly, M., Al-Halawa, D. A., Mansour, R., Ibrahim, M., . . . Group, O. B. O. T. R. C. C. S. (2022). Impact of COVID-19 lockdown on smoking (waterpipe and cigarette) and participants' BMI across various sociodemographic groups in Arab countries in the Mediterranean Region. *Tobacco Induced Diseases, 20*(November), 1–16. https://doi.org/10.18332/tid/155007Aleyiydi, M. S., Alshiban, N. M., Alajmi, A. M., Alosaimi, N. F., Alotaibi, M., Nassar, M. S., Alhumaid, N. K., et al. (2024). Epidemiology of viral infectious diseases reported in Saudi Arabia. *Infectious Diseases and Therapy, 13*, 1893–1905. https://www.semanticscholar.org/paper/e26ec01893069a935532dd6ed81b602e559280f6 (accessed on 30th May 2025).
2. Alhumaid, N. K., Alajmi, A. M., Alosaimi, N. F., Alotaibi, M., Almangour, T. A., Nassar, M., Memish, Z. A., et al. (2024). Epidemiology of reportable bacterial infectious diseases in Saudi Arabia. *Infectious Diseases and Therapy, 13*, 667–684. https://www.semanticscholar.org/paper/80889fccfb88b0b038f64bee778a60893cc8bd70 (accessed on 30th May 2025).
3. Aprillia, Y. T., Adawiyah, A. R., Ambarwati, K., & Tenrilemba, F. (2024). Factors associated with breastfeeding self-efficacy and COVID-19 pandemic anxiety in post-partum mothers. *Jurnal Kesehatan Masyarakat*. https://www.semanticscholar.org/paper/485f425f53595c6aef0af183b65940b8645b1e25 (accessed on 30th May 2025).
4. Bengoumi, M., Faye, B., Kamili, A., Tligui, A., et al. (2019). Invited review: Camel skin diseases survey in Morocco. *Journal of Camelid Science*. https://core.ac.uk/download/288641826.pdf (accessed on 30th May 2025).
5. Benhamou, W., Blanquart, F., Choisy, M., Berngruber, T. W., Choquet, R., & Gandon, S. (2024). Evolution of virulence in emerging epidemics: From theory to experimental evolution and back. *Virus Evolution, 10*. https://www.semanticscholar.org/paper/d0a32a584805efba4855dd8ae57fdb79cfdffbbf (accessed on 30th May 2025).
6. Berkwits, M., & Guallar, E. (2007). Risk factors, risk prediction, and the apolipoprotein B–apolipoprotein A-I ratio. *Annals of Internal Medicine, 146*, 677–679. https://www.semanticscholar.org/paper/3d596fc645c70616059ff677bf86370cbc9aa81f (accessed on 30th May 2025).
7. Beshah, A., Ahmed, A., & Dandecha, M. (2024). Epidemiology and risk factors of infectious bursal disease: A review. *Journal of Bacteriology and Mycology*. https://www.semanticscholar.org/paper/fd0edafe0f7fee295d72e3743f473e81da29b0d1 (accessed on 30th May 2025).
8. Bist, J. S., Kumari, N., Mehta, A. K., Rana, R., et al. (2017). Prevalence of skin diseases among infants in a tertiary medical facility in Uttarakhand. *International Journal of Research in Medical Sciences*. https://core.ac.uk/download/539910210.pdf (accessed on 30th May 2025).
9. Cabada, M., Aguilar, P. V., Rodas, J. D., Hidalgo, M., Mozo, K., Gonzalez-Diaz, E. S., Jiménez-Coello, M., et al. (2024). Establishment of a multisite umbrella cohort study protocol to describe the epidemiology and aetiologies of acute undifferentiated febrile illness in Latin America. *BMJ Open, 14*. https://www.semanticscholar.org/paper/b604da63c38f95e7b9e98ffa47be6a6862093398 (accessed on 30th May 2025).
10. Casabonne, D., Almeida, J., Nieto, W. G., Romero, A., Fernández-Navarro, P., Rodríguez-Caballero, A., Muñoz-Criado, S., et al. (2012). Common infectious agents and monoclonal

B-cell lymphocytosis: A cross-sectional epidemiological study among healthy adults. *PLoS ONE, 7.* https://www.semanticscholar.org/paper/91a0009a5983097c8e1d7f025ebe67945d762a88 (accessed on 30th May 2025).

11. Chen, C., Gao, G., Xu, Y., Pu, L., Wang, Q., Wang, L., Wang, W., et al. (2020). SARS-CoV-2–positive sputum and feces after conversion of pharyngeal samples in patients with COVID-19. *Annals of Internal Medicine, 172*, 832–834. https://doi.org/10.7326/m20-0991.
12. Chen, Y., Sun, W., Ren, X., Gu, X., Song, K., Wang, P., Cao, Y., et al. (2025). Characteristics and timeliness of intervention in 47 school-based enterovirus outbreaks in Zhejiang Province, China. *Frontiers in Public Health, 13.* https://www.semanticscholar.org/paper/04e4200e736e964943959ba4277b3a4fcabae88a (accessed on 30th May 2025).
13. Chowdhury, I. H., Hasan, M. M., Hamid, S. A. T., & Abdulmajeed, S. M. (2024). Epidemiology of eye diseases in Bangladesh. *IP International Journal of Ocular Oncology and Oculoplasty.* https://www.semanticscholar.org/paper/145b2a104230efe14184edb0e2aea873bed2f003 (accessed on 30th May 2025).
14. Combs, B. G., Giele, C. M., Kwan, K. S. H., Mak, A., et al. (2008). Audit of antenatal testing of sexually transmissible infections and blood borne viruses at Western Australian hospitals. https://core.ac.uk/download/61303469.pdf (accessed on 30th May 2025).
15. Connolly, K. L., Bachmann, L., Hiltke, T., Kersh, E. N., Newman, L. M., Wilson, L., Mena, L., et al. (2024). Summary of the Centers for Disease Control and Prevention/National Institute of Allergy and Infectious Diseases Joint Workshop on Genital Herpes: 3–4 November 2022. *Open Forum Infectious Diseases, 11*(5), ofae230. https://www.semanticscholar.org/paper/5eec56195f3c1a8d19d853dabd16739eedae2c91 (accessed on 30th May 2025).
16. Danish, S. M., Asghari, S. J., Hashimi, S. A., Furmoli, M. E., Zamani, M. U., & Amiri, S. H. (2025). The prevalence and associated demographic factors of hepatitis C infections among patients referred to Hospital of Infectious Diseases in Kabul, Afghanistan: A cross-sectional study. *Afghanistan Journal of Basic Medical Science.* https://www.semanticscholar.org/paper/afcdc5fa1c4ba4fb740dbd885c9d81629d9c453f (accessed on 30th May 2025).
17. de-la-Torre, A., Mejía-Salgado, G., Cifuentes-González, C., Rojas-Carabali, W., Cuevas, M., García, S., Rangel, C. M., et al. (2024). Epidemiology, clinical features, and classification of 3,404 patients with uveitis: Colombian Uveitis Multicenter Study (COL-UVEA). *Graefe's Archive for Clinical and Experimental Ophthalmology, 262*, 2601–2615. https://www.semanticscholar.org/paper/b028ac766610c315b297c224533c9d9244e407b5 (accessed on 30th May 2025).
18. Ernholm, L. (2024). Wild boar at the farm gate: Infectious diseases and epidemiology at the wildlife-livestock interface. *Acta Universitatis Agriculturae Sueciae.* https://www.semanticscholar.org/paper/842bd7e92a4657f41e8f98f27b8661cbf46d633c (accessed on 30th May 2025).
19. Gessner, B. (2015). Severe acute respiratory illness in Sub-Saharan Africa. *The Journal of Infectious Diseases, 212*(6), 843, 844. https://www.semanticscholar.org/paper/78d588cc35a8b297763ff968fa6ca6258fe97de3 (accessed on 30th May 2025).
20. González de Aledo-Castillo, J. M., Argudo-Ramírez, A., Benéitez-Pastor, D., Collado-Gimbert, A., Almazán Castro, F., Roig-Bosch, S., Andrés-Masó, A., et al. (2024). Newborn screening for sickle cell disease in Catalonia between 2015 and 2022—Epidemiology and impact on clinical events. *International Journal of Neonatal Screening, 10.* https://www.semanticscholar.org/paper/42954009dc23677c245e9f07cfe2d531e5d39e9a (accessed on 30th May 2025).

21. Gorbalenya, A. E., Baker, S. C., Baric, R. S., de Groot, R. J., Drosten, C., Gulyaeva, A., Haagmans, B. L., et al. (2020a). The species severe acute respiratory syndrome-related coronavirus: Classifying 2019-nCoV and naming it SARS-CoV-2. *Nature Microbiology, 5*, 536–544. https://doi.org/10.1038/s41564-020-0695-z.
22. Gorbalenya, A. E., Baker, S. C., Baric, R. S., de Groot, R. J., Drosten, C., Gulyaeva, A., Haagmans, B. L., et al. (2020b). Severe acute respiratory syndrome-related coronavirus: The species and its viruses – a statement of the Coronavirus Study Group. *bioRxiv (Cold Spring Harbor Laboratory)*. https://doi.org/10.1101/2020.02.07.937862.
23. Hong, J., Zhao, Z., Su, Q., Huang, J., Chen, X., Le, J., Liu, X. L., et al. (2022). [Research advances in transmission dynamic models on hand, foot, and mouth disease]. *Zhonghua Liu Xing Bing Xue za Zhi = Zhonghua Liuxingbingxue Zazhi, 43*(6), 966–973. https://www.semanticscholar.org/paper/86eece148266c16aa30ce6d5844090969c809b02 (accessed on 30th May 2025).
24. Huang, R., Wei, J., Li, Z. W., Gao, Z., Mahe, M., & Cao, W. (2021). Spatial-temporal mapping and risk factors for hand foot and mouth disease in northwestern inland China. *PLOS Neglected Tropical Diseases, 15*. https://www.semanticscholar.org/paper/7980fad961ecfd6c1115d5d6c2281e7a9db0bc4b (accessed on 30th May 2025).
25. Ibrahim, M. E. (2023). Epidemiology, pathogenicity, risk factors, and management of *Helicobacter pylori* infection in Saudi Arabia. *Biomolecules and Biomedicine, 24*, 440–453. https://www.semanticscholar.org/paper/a4b64abd21f75f568e11a61e6a86b8c257f2d4e4 (accessed on 30th May 2025).
26. Johnson, D. E., Burtness, B., Leemans, C. R., Lui, V. W. Y., Bauman, J. E., & Grandis, J. R. (2020). Head and neck squamous cell carcinoma. *Nature Reviews Disease Primers, 6*. https://doi.org/10.1038/s41572-020-00224-3.
27. Kling, K., Zembower, T., Moore, W. J., Colbert, S., Schaeffer, A., & Williams, J. (2025). P-1562. Epidemiology, management, and outcomes of a novel complex urologic infections interdisciplinary clinic. *Open Forum Infectious Diseases, 12*. https://www.semanticscholar.org/paper/69d820c7d7a87f073d3a5445ee2026683db0cba7 (accessed on 30th May 2025).
28. Kokkinaki, K. G., Saridomichelakis, M., Mylonakis, M., Leontides, L., & Xenoulis, P. (2023). Seroprevalence of and risk factors for feline coronavirus infection in cats from Greece. *Comparative Immunology, Microbiology and Infectious Diseases, 94*, 101962. https://www.semanticscholar.org/paper/1a7a1b6164b29a8962a1cb76432037b751ff5f16 (accessed on 30th May 2025).
29. Lin, J., & He, J. (2016). Clinical guideline inconsistency regarding the prevention of hepatitis B and C virus transmission. *Infection Control & Hospital Epidemiology, 37*, 744, 745. https://www.semanticscholar.org/paper/fe7a1a79b92c2e1b7a64aaadbfe0de7cbf7df4c3 (accessed on 30th May 2025).
30. Loconsole, D., Giordano, M., Centrone, F., Accogli, M., Casulli, D., De Robertis, A. D., Morea, A., et al. (2020). Epidemiology of Shiga toxin-producing *Escherichia coli* infections in Southern Italy after implementation of symptom-based surveillance of bloody diarrhea in the pediatric population. *International Journal of Environmental Research and Public Health, 17*. https://www.semanticscholar.org/paper/3870e1640ee7611566042b0f280b07dd99ba1765 (accessed on 30th May 2025).

31. Mackay, I. M., & Arden, K. E. (2015). MERS coronavirus: Diagnostics, epidemiology and transmission. *Virology Journal, 12*. https://doi.org/10.1186/s12985-015-0439-5.

32. Marinho-Júnior, J. F., Monteiro, J. F. C. L. S., de Carvalho, A. W. S., de Carvalho, F. G., Cavalcanti, M. P., Shaw, J., Courtenay, O., et al. (2023). High levels of infectiousness of asymptomatic *Leishmania (Viannia) braziliensis* infections in wild rodents highlights their importance in the epidemiology of American Tegumentary Leishmaniasis in Brazil. *PLOS Neglected Tropical Diseases, 17*. https://www.semanticscholar.org/paper/05990c3ea2b54105ae27cafc6cb4268 4242c7c25 (accessed on 30th May 2025).

33. Mohomed, A. A., Ahmed, Z., Jabi, A. A., Salad, A. A., Mohamed, M. O. S., Mio, J. B., & Jimale, S. A. (2024). Sero epidemiology of *Camel brucellosis* and its public health significances at three selected districts in Erer Zone, Somali Region. *American Journal of Aquaculture and Animal Science*. https://www.semanticscholar.org/paper/d8a33270ba9c4c6a52225c9bc58d6570f36eb58e (accessed on 30th May 2025).

34. Moon, R., Bleak, T. C., Rosenthal, N., Couturier, B., Hemmert, R. B., Timbrook, T., Brown, H., et al. (2023). Epidemiology and economic burden of acute infectious gastroenteritis among adults treated in outpatient settings in US health systems. *The American Journal of Gastroenterology, 118*, 1069–1079. https://www.semanticscholar.org/paper/9b6e0c2202d4 16b2924a31fd6c76c8a3828ec6c0 (accessed on 30th May 2025).

35. Murray, C. J. L., Ikuta, K. S., Sharara, F., Swetschinski, L. R., Robles, A. G., Gray, A. P., Han, C., et al. (2022). Global burden of bacterial antimicrobial resistance in 2019: A systematic analysis. *The Lancet, 399*, 629–655. https://doi.org/10.1016/s0140-6736(21)02724-0.

36. Nkengasong, J. N., & Tessema, S. K. (2020). Africa needs a new public health order to tackle infectious disease threats. *Cell, 183*, 296–300. https://doi.org/10.1016/j.cell.2020.09.041.

37. Norman, F. F., & González-Sanz, M. (2024). Pulmonary infections in the returning traveler. *Current Opinion in Pulmonary Medicine, 30*, 243–251. https://www.semanticscholar.org/paper/dc0cd0a5e22873ffb6e04cd273cbb3ba78f3c31c (accessed on 30th May 2025).

38. Pal, M., & Hadush, A. (2017). *Leptospirosis: An Infectious Emerging Waterborne Zoonosis of Global Significance, 2017*, 1–4. https://www.semanticscholar.org/paper/796b950a94875fe4 1f0032d670b4566b2da734df (accessed on 30th May 2025).

39. Parzen-Johnson, S. L., & Katz, B. Z. (2024). Navigating the spectrum of two pediatric COVID-19 complications: Multi-system inflammatory syndrome in children and post-acute sequelae of SARS-CoV-2 infection. *Journal of Clinical Medicine, 13*. https://www.semanticscholar.org/pa per/5fd60e27ac5b577a12117af5751d7e45dbcea691 (accessed on 30th May 2025).

40. Plotnikov, A. A., Zaykova, O., Rusakova, E. V., & Grebennikova, T. V. (2025). Social epidemiology: Relevance, approaches, main directions and development trends. *ЗДОРОВЬЕ НАСЕЛЕНИЯ И СРЕДА ОБИТАНИЯ – ЗНиСО / Public Health and Life Environment*. https://www.semanticscholar.org/paper/722d8a5471ce3c823118176450981daaa3286134 (accessed on 30th May 2025).

41. Santomauro, D., Mantilla, H., A. M., Shadid, J., Zheng, P., Ashbaugh, C., Pigott, D. M., Abbafati, C., et al. (2021). Global prevalence and burden of depressive and anxiety disorders in 204 countries and territories in 2020 due to the COVID-19 pandemic. *The Lancet, 398*, 1700–1712. https://doi.org/10.1016/s0140-6736(21)02143-7.

42. Shrestha, S., Trotter, A., & Shrestha, P. (2022). Epidemiology and risk factors of healthcare-associated infections in critically ill patients in a tertiary care teaching hospital in Nepal: A

prospective cohort study. *Infectious Diseases, 15.* https://www.semanticscholar.org/paper/a309acdb54e5c6acfcd38b98230764cd930a6676 (accessed on 30th May 2025).

43. Singh, O. P., Hasker, E., Boelaert, M., Sacks, D. L., & Sundar, S. (2020). Xenodiagnosis to address key questions in visceral leishmaniasis control and elimination. *PLOS Neglected Tropical Diseases, 14*, e0008363–e0008363. https://doi.org/10.1371/journal.pntd.0008363.
44. Smiyan, O., Taramak, L., Smiian, K., Vasilyeva, O., Loboda, A., Petrashenko, V., Moshchych, O., et al. (2023). Modern view from Ukraine on etiology, pathogenesis and clinical-diagnostic aspects of community-acquired pneumonia in children. *Eastern Ukrainian Medical Journal.* https://www.semanticscholar.org/paper/e0553743e87b650e272876936edcd67d1e98dbcc (accessed on 30th May 2025).
45. Torres, T., Filipe, P., Menezes, B. F., Figueiredo, A., Pinto, S. A., Sousa, B. A., Rebelo, C., et al. (2023). Epidemiology of psoriasis in Portugal: A population-based study. *Acta Medica Portuguesa.* https://www.semanticscholar.org/paper/2212b929e6450009dba9de42612fb8b74f852eb1 (accessed on 30th May 2025).
46. Vandenbroucke, J., Von Elm, E., Altman, D., Gøtzsche, P., Mulrow, C., Pocock, S., Poole, C., et al. (2007). Strengthening the reporting of observational studies in epidemiology (STROBE): Explanation and elaboration. *PLoS Medicine, 4.* https://www.semanticscholar.org/paper/401d9f8e12297ac2d79a2ad75e7b7486ea7ca894 (accessed on 30th May 2025).
47. Wahlström, H. (2004). *Bovine Tuberculosis in Swedish Farmed Deer.* https://core.ac.uk/download/11694788.pdf (accessed on 30th May 2025).
48. Wen, C. P., Chang, C. H., Tsai, M. K., Lee, J. H., Lu, P. J., Tsai, S. P., Wen, C., et al. (2017). Diabetes with early kidney involvement may shorten life expectancy by 16 years. *Kidney International, 92*, 388–396. https://doi.org/10.1016/j.kint.2017.01.030.
49. Whitaker, B., Belov, A., & Anderson, S. (2019). Progress in US hemovigilance: Can we still learn from others? *Transfusion, 59.* https://www.semanticscholar.org/paper/40c30551ff19df784137e136de6bb8d9856e7897 (accessed on 30th May 2025).
50. Wieters, I., Johnstone, S., Makiala-Mandanda, S., Poda, A., Akoua-Koffi, C., Abu Sin, M., Eckmanns, T., et al. (2024). Reported antibiotic use among patients in the multicenter ANDEMIA infectious diseases surveillance study in sub-Saharan Africa. *Antimicrobial Resistance and Infection Control, 13.* https://www.semanticscholar.org/paper/36b70b627f625a1ae3a1de23df011db4b4fd4046 (accessed on 30th May 2025).
51. Yano, M., & Salido, E. (2023). AB0385 Risk factors and cardiovascular diseases among patients with rheumatoid arthritis in a tertiary government hospital in the Philippines. *Annals of the Rheumatic Diseases.* https://www.semanticscholar.org/paper/0e97ff555585ffbeec404687b0f455148fc295af (accessed on 30th May 2025).
52. Yuan, Y., Chen, Y., Huang, J., Bao, X., Shen, W., Sun, Y., Mao, H. (2024). Epidemiological and etiological investigations of hand, foot, and mouth disease in Jiashan, northeastern Zhejiang Province, China, during 2016 to 2022. *Frontiers in Public Health, 12.* https://www.semanticscholar.org/paper/55849113f24814544480105dcd7a9a687545ec55 (accessed on 30th May 2025).
53. Zeleňáková, L., Žiarovská, J., Kráčmar, S., Mura, L., Kozelová, D., Lopašovský, Ľ., Kunová, S., et al. (2012). Application of epidemiological information system (EPIS) in the Slovak Republic within the surveillance of salmonellosis and campylobacteriosis outbreaks in the European Union

(2001–2010). *Acta Universitatis Agriculturae et Silviculturae Mendelianae Brunensis, 60*, 189–200. https://www.semanticscholar.org/paper/a847bc29e05e42d5d0539b6bfc12339597185ea0 (accessed on 30th May 2025).

54. Zhakipbayeva, B. T., Berezovskiy, D. V., Bumburidi, Y., Berdiyarova, N., Kulzhanova, K. D., Agabayev, M. A., Whistler, T., et al. (2023). 1335. Etiological and epidemiological features of acute meningitis and encephalitis in hospitalized patients, Kazakhstan, 2019–2020. *Open Forum Infectious Diseases, 10*. https://www.semanticscholar.org/paper/97c656f0a88f08d1b7613c715804a5b13e09b57b (accessed on 30th May 2025).

55. Zhang, J. L., Chen, Z. Y., Lin, S. L., King, C., Chen, C. C., & Chen, P. S. (2022). Airborne avian influenza virus in ambient air in the winter habitats of migratory birds. *Environmental Science & Technology*. https://www.semanticscholar.org/paper/4cd85efdd7c85db274f5fc273389802c5b53be70 (accessed on 30th May 2025).

56. Zhāng, Y. Z., & Holmes, E. C. (2020). A genomic perspective on the origin and emergence of SARS-CoV-2. *Cell, 181*, 223–227. https://doi.org/10.1016/j.cell.2020.03.035.

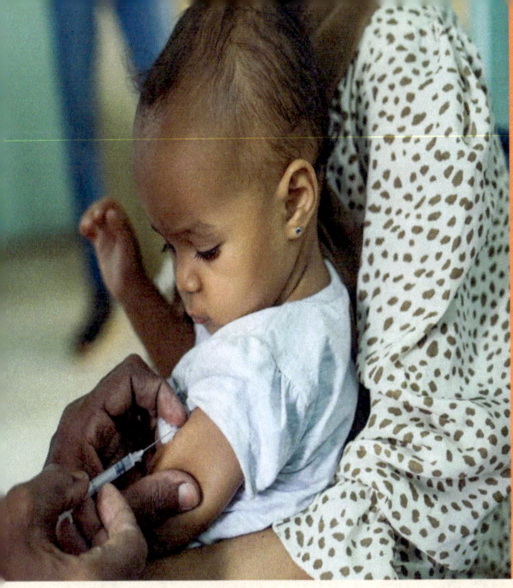

Chapter 9

VACCINES AND IMMUNIZATION PROGRAMS

Contents

Introduction

The profound impact of vaccines on public health cannot be overstated, serving as a cornerstone in controlling infectious diseases and reducing mortality rates globally. Due to vaccination programs, diseases such as smallpox are nearly eradicated, and polio and measles have become significantly less common. They are essential for reaching herd immunity. which safeguards people who cannot be vaccinated because of medical issues. When new vaccines are introduced, such as those developed rapidly for COVID-19, it is essential to understand how vaccines have been used in the past. Recent developments in maternal immunity highlight the need for targeted vaccination efforts, especially as pregnant women are at increased risk for severe influenza complications, necessitating robust immunization policies to protect both mothers and infants (Regan et al., 2021). The rapid development of new vaccines during the COVID-19 pandemic underscores the difficulty and importance of immunization programs today. The quick progress of these vaccines was possible because global health agencies, researchers, and pharmaceutical companies worked together, demonstrating the strength of science during emergencies. Even so, carrying out mass vaccination campaigns calls for attention to safety and accessibility, especially in different economic and social settings. It is clear from evaluations of vaccines that robust clinical trials are necessary to confirm their safety and effectiveness, ensuring that people continue to trust vaccination programs. A systematic review of existing data on COVID-19 vaccines reveals gaps in knowledge regarding long-term safety profiles and immunogenicity, warranting a cautious and informed approach to mass immunization (Sathian et al., 2021). Teaching people about the importance of vaccines is a key part of successful vaccine distribution. Even though vaccines have been proven to stop diseases from coming back, false information about them can quickly cause people to hesitate to get vaccinated. It demonstrates that healthcare workers should engage with communities, address their concerns, and emphasise the importance of group immunity. Also, public health policies should be updated to guarantee that vaccines are accessible to people in underserved and marginalized communities. While continuing with vaccinations, we must ensure transparency, provide information, and include everyone, which helps create a setting that encourages more people to be vaccinated. Ultimately, the establishment of effective vaccines and immunization programs relies on not just scientific advances but also social commitment to health equity and the common good (Figure 9.1).

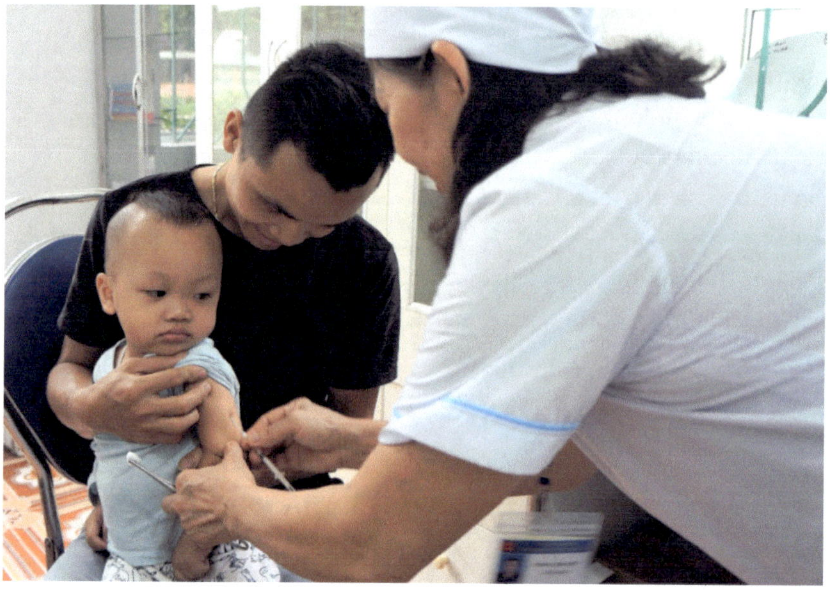

Figure 9.1. Vaccines and immunization programs.

Source: https://www.who.int/images/default-source/wpro/countries/viet-nam/news/2020/immunization-week.tmb-1920v.jpg?Culture=en&sfvrsn=be10e92e_2.

Definition of Vaccines

A vaccine is a substance that helps the immune system of a person develop resistance to a certain infectious disease. Vaccines typically contain an agent that resembles a disease-causing microorganism, which is composed of either weakened or inactivated versions of the microbe, its toxins, or its surface proteins. Vaccines work by imitating an infection, which causes the body to respond with the production of antibodies. Acquired immunity after vaccination can prevent more infections, which lowers the number and severity of diseases. Therefore, vaccines are crucial for public health as they protect both individuals and the community through herd immunity. This concept is essential in public health because it ensures that a sufficient number of people in a group are immune to an infectious disease, thereby making it less likely to spread. It is essential to carry out vaccine campaigns well so that public health benefits are maximized, especially in immunization programs. Countries worldwide have established national immunisation programs (NIPs) that outline the schedules for various vaccines to be administered at key stages of childhood and beyond. They rely on data from epidemiology and are designed to handle or eliminate infections that are a significant health concern. Healthcare professionals, including paediatricians, play a pivotal role in these programs, as evidenced by a study in Turkey highlighting the necessity for enhanced physician education on vaccine efficacy and the importance of routine immunisations, especially for vulnerable populations such as children (Dinleyici et al., 2018). The orderly use of vaccines in these programs has helped reduce polio and measles, proving how vital vaccines are for protecting the public. Although vaccination is very beneficial, it is still challenging to get many people to accept and follow the recommended vaccine schedule. Due to misinformation, cultural beliefs, and a lack of trust in medical systems, people are less willing to get vaccinated, which is a significant problem for immunisation efforts everywhere. As illustrated by various studies, including one focusing on the perceptions of healthcare professionals regarding meningitis vaccines in Turkey, a comprehensive understanding of the scientific basis of vaccines can help address these concerns (N/A, 2016). Public health should focus on educating people and being clear about the safety and effectiveness of vaccines to fight misinformation and encourage more people to get vaccinated. When communities are engaged and trust is built, hesitancy is reduced, which helps immunisation programs achieve their goal of protecting people's health.

Importance of Immunisation Programs

Immunisation programs serve as a critical frontier in public health, safeguarding populations against infectious diseases that could otherwise lead to significant morbidity and mortality. Vaccination helps each person resist disease and also adds to the protection of the entire community. This idea is particularly important for diseases that spread easily, as it requires a sufficient number of people to be vaccinated to prevent outbreaks. Because of global vaccination, smallpox has been completely eradicated, and the number of measles and polio cases has dropped significantly. Strong immunization programs can help address the financial problems linked to healthcare, missing work, and lasting disability, which supports the well-being of communities. The persistence of vaccine-preventable diseases (VPD) emphasises the need for sustained and well-coordinated immunisation efforts. Digital health technologies are making it possible to improve immunisation programs significantly. Using mobile health applications and electronic health records, health authorities can make vaccination easier, increase the number of people vaccinated, and monitor campaigns as they happen. They have been successful in addressing challenges such as vaccine hesitancy and logistical issues, particularly during public health emergencies like the COVID-19 pandemic. A detailed review of case studies shows that digital approaches support better communication and education of the public, which results in more people getting vaccinated. Because of these changes, it is essential to keep updating immunisation strategies to benefit from new technologies that improve public health. While evolving immunisation programs, a strong digital system should also address ethical and privacy matters. The role of immunisation programs is essential for both people's health and the agriculture sector. For instance, effective vaccination schemes in livestock management have proven to mitigate the impact of outbreaks caused by diseases such as Newcastle disease virus (NDV). Trials have shown that combining live attenuated and inactivated vaccines effectively protects poultry populations, thereby reducing economic losses for farmers. They demonstrate that human health and agriculture are closely linked, and that immunization has effects in other areas as well. The integration of comprehensive vaccination programs in both human and veterinary health is not only essential for disease prevention but also for sustaining livelihoods, ultimately reinforcing the intrinsic value that these programs hold in promoting public health security and economic stability (Figure 9.2).

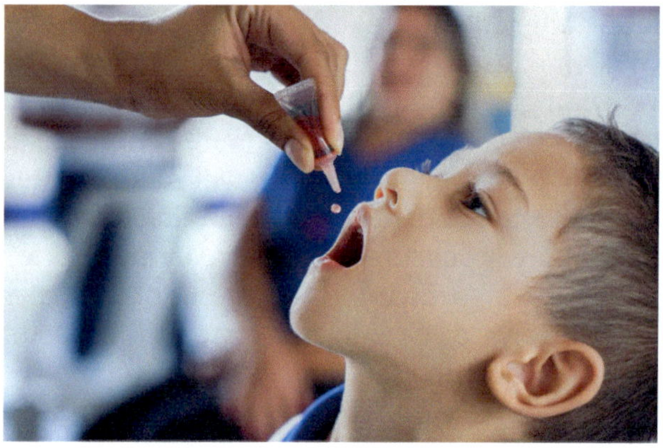

Figure 9.2. Immunization programs.

Source: https://www.unicef.org/sites/default/files/styles/media_large_image/public/UNI408835.jpg.webp?itok=gqrnI2qJ.

9.1. History of Vaccination

The history of vaccination is a cornerstone in the development of public health and disease prevention techniques. In the late 18th century, Edward Jenner proposed using cowpox to help people avoid getting smallpox. This vital discovery made it possible to eradicate smallpox, demonstrating that vaccines can eliminate diseases. After Jenner's early experiments, there was a rise in vaccination in the 19th and 20th centuries, and scientists began making vaccines for rabies, diphtheria, and tuberculosis. Because of these first vaccines, it became possible to develop and distribute vaccines on a large scale to protect people from infectious diseases. Because vaccines were recognised as essential for health, the 20th century witnessed many improvements in vaccine technology and the creation of organised immunisation programs.

The invention of the polio vaccine by Jonas Salk in the 1950s significantly changed how viral diseases were prevented. Many countries organised mass immunisation programs, which significantly reduced polio and proved that vaccinating many people at once works. Furthermore, these campaigns laid the groundwork for global health initiatives, such as the Expanded Program on Immunisation (EPI) created by the WHO in 1974, which aimed to increase vaccine coverage for children in various countries. At this time, governments made it a priority to include immunisation as a central part of health care for everyone. Lately, new developments in vaccine research have kept changing the way immunisation programs work. The rapid development of COVID-19 vaccines using mRNA technology has underscored the importance of new methods in vaccine production. They are effective against EIDs and also show how science can react quickly to worldwide health emergencies. Research studies examining the antibody response to vaccines, including those focused on healthcare workers and the effectiveness of booster doses, illustrate the ongoing evolution of vaccination strategies in the face of changing disease threats (Otoguro et al., 2025). As demonstrated, contemporary vaccination efforts seek to ensure widespread immunity and response effectiveness, reinforcing the necessity of vaccines within public health frameworks (Kaabi et al., 2023) (Figure 9.3).

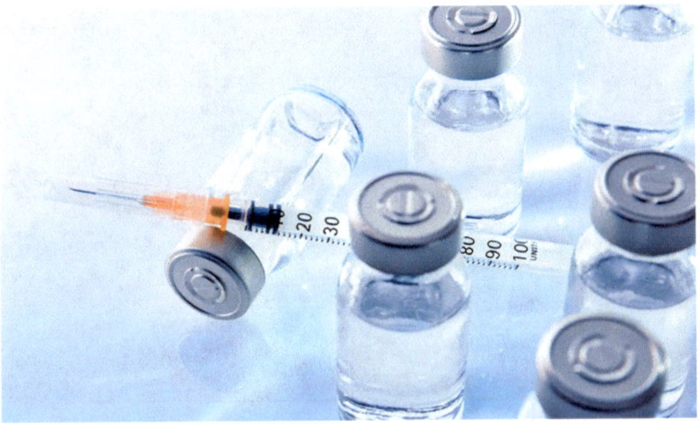

Figure 9.3. History of vaccination.

Source: https://a57.foxnews.com/a57.foxnews.com/static.foxnews.com/foxnews.com/content/uploads/2019/03/640/320/1862/1048/iStock-vaccine.jpg?ve=1&tl=1?ve=1&tl=1.

9.1.1. Early Methods of Immunization

The early methods of immunisation date back centuries and laid the foundation for contemporary vaccination practices. Variolation was the primary method of preventing smallpox in the 18th century. People were given material from the sores of those who had mild smallpox, which would protect them from the more dangerous form. While variolation helped lower the number of smallpox deaths, it was unsafe and sometimes made the recipient sick or caused death. The exercise showed that controlled exposure to the disease could help build immunity, which became a key idea in the development and use of vaccines in public health. The move from variolation to vaccination brought about a significant change in immunisation, leading to the development of organised vaccination programs based on immunological research. Edward Jenner, in the late 18th century, made immunisation possible by finding that cowpox material could protect people from smallpox. Jenner showed that inoculating a boy with cowpox could guard against smallpox infection. It was not only a single achievement but also the beginning of the organised development of vaccines everywhere. Because of Jenner's work, it became clear that a weakened or similar pathogen could be used to stimulate the immune system without causing the disease. As more microorganisms were studied, vaccination became more common, leading to the development of vaccines for rabies and anthrax. These initial attempts showed that vaccination could play a significant role in stopping diseases. During the 19th and early 20th centuries, as microbiology and immunology advanced, the way immunisation was understood kept changing. Louis Pasteur and Robert Koch built on Jenner's achievements by studying and isolating pathogens, which led to the creation of vaccines for rabies and cholera. Because of Pasteur's discovery that pathogens could be weakened, vaccine development became safer and more effective. The influence of science on public health became very clear during this period. With the success of vaccines understood, nations initiated mass vaccination campaigns to protect their populations and achieve herd immunity. Alongside these developments, public health campaigns emerged to promote trust in vaccines, which is essential for their acceptance and integration into routine healthcare practices, as highlighted by discussions on public trust in healthcare systems and vaccine efficacy in contemporary studies (Tebruegge et al., 2015; Larson et al., 2018).

9.1.2. Development of the Smallpox Vaccine

The development of the smallpox vaccine in the late 18th century marks a pivotal moment in the history of medicine and public health. In 1796, Edward Jenner demonstrated that contracting cowpox could help prevent smallpox, which helped establish vaccination as a means to prevent diseases. Jenner's technique was to inject cowpox material into people, which triggered their immune system and protected them from the serious effects of smallpox. The discovery saved lives and also challenged standard medical practices, making vaccination an accepted scientific method for fighting infectious diseases. Jenner's work showed how vaccinations could help, which encouraged scientists to develop more vaccines and set up immunization programs worldwide. In the years that followed, the vaccine was improved and standardised, which made it safer and more effective. In the late 1800s, governments and health organisations began to promote vaccination in many countries, recognising the significant harm smallpox caused to people. Making vaccination against smallpox mandatory in many countries greatly reduced the number of smallpox cases. Still, even with all the advantages, some communities began to resist vaccination because of their cultural beliefs, false information, and doubts about medical treatments. This hesitance evokes contemporary discussions around vaccine skepticism, illustrating that even successful vaccines like that for smallpox were not universally embraced, highlighting the complex interplay between public health initiatives and societal attitudes towards medical practices (Bird et al., 2023). As a result of the smallpox vaccination program, the WHO announced in 1980 that smallpox had been eradicated, which was a significant achievement for global health. As a result, it was demonstrated that public health strategies and vaccines could eradicate a disease, encouraging people to believe in vaccinations. After this, countries started to introduce other vaccination programs for polio and measles, motivated by the successful removal of smallpox. However, as noted in studies of vaccine hesitancy, the remnants of doubt regarding vaccines persist, suggesting that some of the challenges faced in the smallpox campaign are still relevant today (Johnston et al., 2020). Thus, the legacy of the smallpox vaccine is not only its success in controlling a notorious disease but also a case study in the ongoing battle against misinformation and skepticism within public health (Figure 9.4).

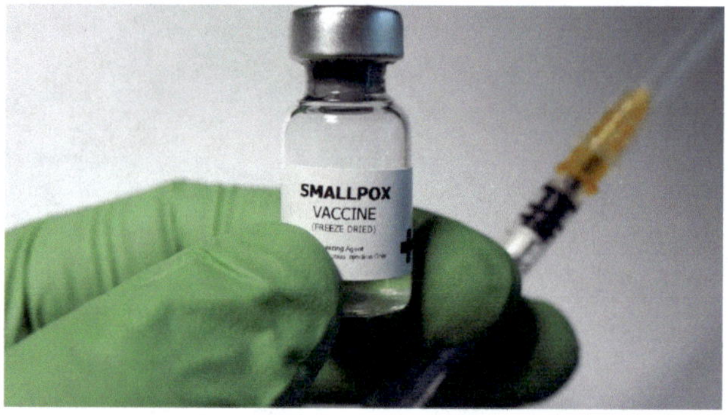

Figure 9.4. Development of the smallpox vaccine.

Source: https://www.usatoday.com/gcdn/media/2020/05/19/USATODAY/usatsports/247WallSt.com-247WS-707866-imageForEntry1-b4H.jpg?crop=1365,768,x0,y0&width=1365&height=768&format=pjpg&auto=webp.

9.1.3. Milestones in Vaccine Discovery

The journey of vaccine discovery has witnessed pivotal milestones that significantly shaped public health. Following Edward Jenner's introduction of smallpox vaccination in 1796, which involved using a living virus, the field has continued to evolve. Jenner's experiments demonstrated that using weakened forms of pathogens can stimulate the immune system, a finding that later proved crucial in the development of vaccines. This idea led to the invention of vaccines for rabies and tetanus in the late 19th century, which began the use of a planned approach to immunization. Thanks to vaccines, the number of sicknesses and deaths from infectious diseases decreased, and people began to value preventive healthcare, making immunisation a main priority for public health. The development of vaccines has typically progressed in tandem with advancements in science and technology. In the 20th century, Jonas Salk and Albert Sabin developed inactivated and attenuated vaccines for polio, which showed the link between vaccines and disease control. Salk's inactivated polio vaccine (IPV) was a critical advancement, paving the way for the eventual near-eradication of polio in many parts of the world. Sabin's oral polio vaccine (OPV) further demonstrated the feasibility of mass immunisation campaigns, allowing for easier distribution in low-resource settings. They were part of a broader movement in public health, including the establishment of international vaccination programs. As a consequence, coordinated efforts, such as the Global Polio Eradication Initiative (GPEI), arose to combat what was once a prevalent and debilitating disease. In recent years, researchers have focused on developing effective vaccines due to EIDs, which present both challenges and opportunities for progress. The ongoing pursuit of a human immunodeficiency virus (HIV) vaccine remains a critical milestone that underscores the complexities inherent in vaccine development. Even with extensive research and clinical trials, the genetic diversity of HIV makes it challenging to induce broadly neutralizing antibodies through vaccination, as recent studies on germline-targeting methods have demonstrated. Such approaches in vaccine science use modern genetic techniques and immunogen designs to boost the immune system against specific pathogens. As the landscape of infectious diseases evolves, so too must vaccination strategies and programs, underscoring the importance of innovation in the field (Bulcha et al., 2021; Sun et al., 2023).

9.2. Types of Vaccines

Vaccines are primarily categorised into various types, all designed to stimulate the immune system against specific diseases. Live attenuated vaccines are considered very effective because they use weakened versions of viruses or bacteria. They act much like real infections, so the body's immune response is strong and lasts a considerable amount of time. Examples include the measles, mumps, and rubella (MMR) vaccine, which has significantly reduced the incidence of these diseases worldwide. Even so, live vaccines are not recommended for individuals with weakened immune systems, highlighting the need for alternative vaccine options. With inactive vaccines, dead pathogens are used, which cannot infect you, but they still help your body build up immunity, much like the polio vaccine. The different vaccines are made for other groups and health situations, showing why it is important to have customised vaccination plans. Another major group includes vaccines made with parts of pathogens instead of the whole organism, such as subunit, recombinant, and conjugate vaccines. They are designed to stimulate the immune system using specific antigens, which reduces the chance of causing disease. For example, the hepatitis B vaccine utilises a protein from the virus to stimulate both T-cells and B-cells, resulting in successful immunisation. Similarly, conjugate vaccines link polysaccharides from bacterial capsules to proteins, as seen in the *Haemophilus influenzae* type b (Hib) vaccine. This way of thinking boosts our personal immunity and may also lower the number of people who spread the disease. The strategic deployment of these vaccines within immunisation programs is essential, particularly in populations vulnerable to severe bacterial infections (Friedman et al., 2025). Thanks to mRNA vaccines, especially those developed for COVID-19, the possibilities in vaccination have expanded significantly. Instead of using the old method, mRNA vaccines use genetic instructions to make cells produce antigens that trigger the immune system. It has many benefits, for example, it allows for quick production and can be adjusted to new EIDs. Additionally, the mRNA approach has demonstrated success against various pathogens and shown promising results in clinical trials. Still, the special storage and distribution needed for mRNA vaccines make it hard for them to be widely used, so a strong infrastructure and public awareness are necessary. As vaccination programs evolve to incorporate new technologies, it is crucial to understand the various types of vaccines available, ensuring equitable access and informed decision-making to enhance public health protections across communities (Goishi-Bessey et al., 2016) (Figure 9.5).

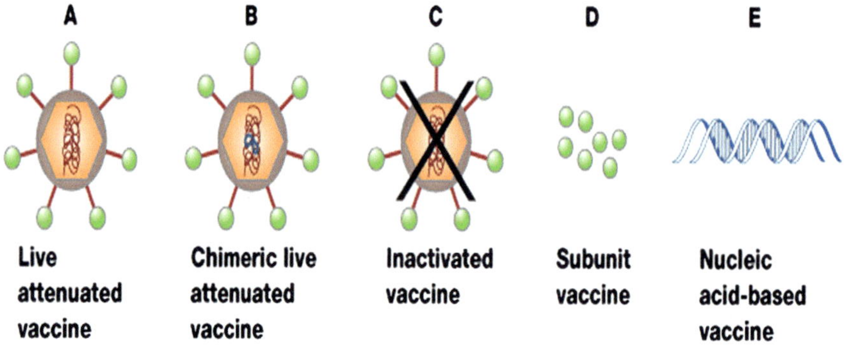

Figure 9.5. Types of vaccines.

Source: https://www.nature.com/scitable/content/ne0000/ne0000/ne0000/ne0000/22405302/1_2.jpg.

9.2.1. Live Attenuated Vaccines

Live attenuated vaccines are crucial components in the realm of immunisation programs due to their ability to provide robust and long-lasting immunity against various infectious diseases. These vaccines contain live pathogens that have been weakened or attenuated, rendering them incapable of causing disease while still eliciting an immune response. The immune system sees the weakened pathogens as the original ones, so it produces antibodies and starts other immune cells. Because live attenuated vaccines work like natural infections, they a stronger and longer-lasting immune response than inactivated vaccines, which only stimulate one part of the immune system. Their ability to prevent diseases like MMR shows why they are given to people in most countries. Live attenuated vaccines are also effective in animals, demonstrating their versatility and applicability in various settings beyond human medicine. As an example, in evaluating a combined live vaccine for bovine respiratory disease, researchers used *Mycoplasma bovis* and bovine herpesvirus type 1 to create a marker vaccine. This study found that the live attenuated vaccine increased the number of CD4+, CD8+, and CD19+ cells in cattle, which are essential for their immune system. As a result of vaccination, the immune system produced more IL-4 and IFN-γ, which are necessary for a good immune response. The use of this vaccine demonstrates that live attenuated vaccines can both stop disease and support animal health and productivity, which is positive for the agricultural sector. Additionally, live attenuated vaccines have played a crucial role in reducing disease outbreaks among livestock, underscoring their importance in public health. Following a camelpox outbreak in Kazakhstan, the country considered both live and inactivated vaccines to protect its camel herds. According to the field trials, camels vaccinated with the live attenuated camelpox vaccine produced antibodies quickly, and 99% of them showed antibodies by day 28. Unlike the live vaccine, the inactivated vaccine took longer to stimulate the immune system. Clinical disease was prevented in vaccinated camels, but unvaccinated camels all displayed severe symptoms. This situation highlights the importance of using live attenuated vaccines effectively to prevent disease spread and maintain animal health, which in turn helps secure food and jobs in affected areas.

9.2.2. Inactivated Vaccines

Inactivated vaccines, which consist of pathogens that have been killed or inactivated through various methods, play a crucial role in immunisation programs worldwide. Because inactivated vaccines do not replicate, they are often safer for people with weak immune systems than live attenuated vaccines. Since these vaccines elicit a weaker immune response, people typically require multiple doses to achieve the desired level of immunity. Still, boosters can strengthen the immune system, which helps inactive vaccines control and prevent infectious diseases. Vaccines such as the inactivated poliovirus vaccine (IPV) exemplify the potential of inactivated formulations in contributing to public health goals, particularly in the fight against poliovirus transmission. Inactivated vaccines are essential for developing new ways to immunise people, especially for fighting poliovirus. IPV, while historically recognised for its inability to induce robust mucosal immunity on its own, has shown remarkable promise in conjunction with oral poliovirus vaccines (OPV). Research indicates that IPV can strengthen the intestinal immune system in those who have received OPV, which is a significant improvement in efforts to stop poliovirus transmission. As populations begin to use only inactivated vaccines, the synergy between IPV and OPV could be beneficial. The enhancement of mucosal immunity could accelerate efforts toward global polio eradication by providing more comprehensive protection across various age groups, particularly older children, who are more likely to exhibit stronger immunity following an IPV booster than from OPV alone (Anis et al., 2015). Giving IPV in regular and extra immunisation programs can greatly help public health efforts. Adding IPV to immunisation programs is necessary to reduce health gaps in various communities. It is also crucial to apply our knowledge of inactivated vaccines in practice to sustain immunity and achieve global vaccination goals. It is clear from epidemiological and vaccination data that the extensive use of inactivated vaccines can lead to significant reductions in disease, as seen in the near eradication of polio in many areas. Continued support and education regarding the importance of inactivated vaccines ensure that healthcare professionals are well-equipped to promote their benefits and address potential hesitancy among the population (N/A, 2012). Thus, inactivated vaccines are pivotal in the ongoing efforts to enhance immunisation programs and protect communities from infectious diseases (Figure 9.6).

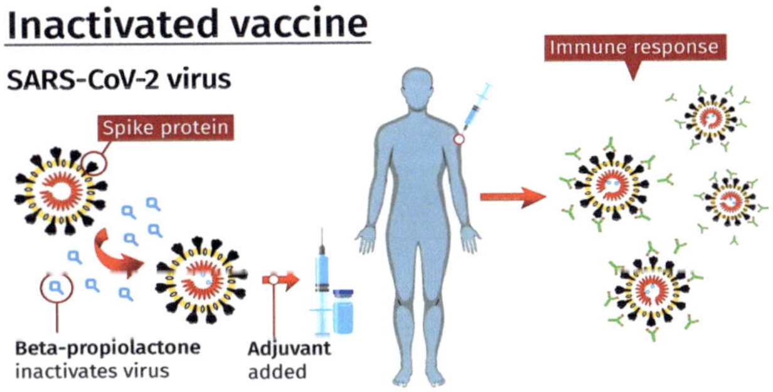

Figure 9.6. Inactivated vaccines.

Source: https://i.cbc.ca/1.6012349.1620074119!/fileImage/httpImage/image.jpg_gen/derivatives/original_620/inactivated-vaccine.jpg.

9.2.3. mRNA Vaccines

The emergence of mRNA vaccines represents a significant advancement in the field of immunisation, particularly highlighted during the COVID-19 pandemic. Rather than using weakened or inactive virus parts, mRNA vaccines tell cells to produce a harmless copy of the SARS-CoV-2 virus's spike protein. It helps the immune system to identify and fight a pathogen if someone is exposed to it in the future. Since these vaccines were quickly distributed and given to many people, it is clear they are both safe and effective, now forming the primary defence against COVID-19 worldwide. With this technology, vaccines are now more effective and could be used against a range of infectious diseases, which is a significant advancement in immunisation. Numerous studies have demonstrated the effectiveness of mRNA vaccines, providing health authorities with reliable guidance. The CDC has said that, according to their interim guidance, children who get a complete primary series of Moderna and Pfizer-BioNTech mRNA vaccines are protected against symptomatic COVID-19. Notably, the effectiveness (VE) of the Moderna vaccine was reported at 60% shortly after the second dose, while the Pfizer-BioNTech vaccine demonstrated a VE of 31% following its third dose. Such data not only underscore the vaccine's role in reducing illness severity but also highlight the importance of timely and appropriate immunisation among vulnerable populations, as a proactive strategy to curb the spread of the virus within communities (Fleming-Dutra et al., 2023). Despite their effectiveness, the rollout of mRNA vaccines has prompted significant challenges related to monitoring adverse drug reactions (ADRs). The agency received a considerable number of ADR reports—103,788—from the COVID-19 vaccine rollout, showing that extra caution is needed in mass vaccination campaigns. For security reasons, decisions were made locally, and robots were used to process the large amount of reports. Also, studies that look for unusual side effects after vaccination point out how challenging it can be to monitor vaccinations, which highlights the importance of strong pharmacovigilance. Such experiences highlight the critical balance between the rapid deployment of innovative vaccines and the necessity of thorough monitoring to ensure public trust, thus enhancing the overall integrity of vaccination programs (Kälkner et al., 2023) (Figure 9.7).

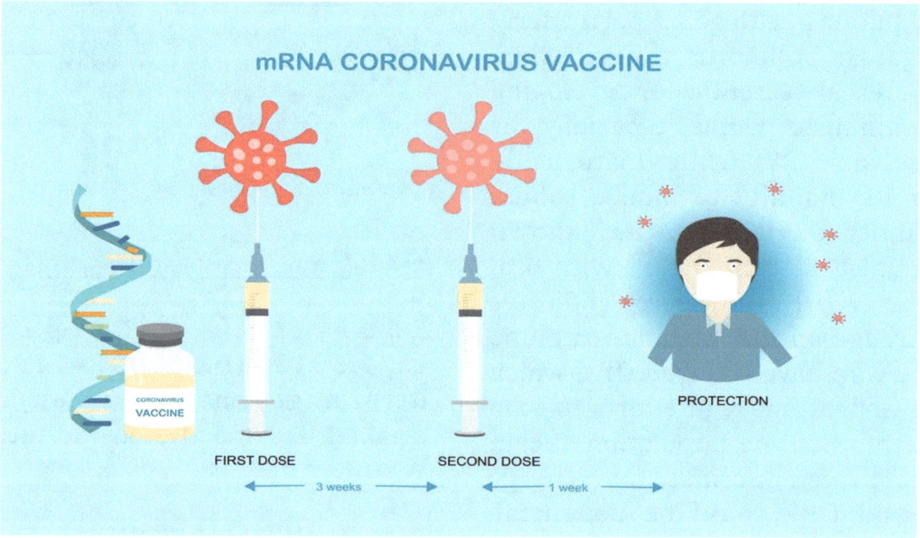

Figure 9.7. mRNA vaccines.

Source: https://media.pri.org/s3fs-public/styles/w2304/public/images/2020/11/mrna-file-20201117-13-k8bxl0.jpg?itok=7FyFPprY.

9.3. Mechanism of Action

The mechanism of action for vaccines is fundamentally grounded in their capacity to mimic pathogen exposure without causing disease. Weakened, inactivated, or broken parts of pathogens in vaccines help the immune system react as it would during a real infection. Antigen-presenting cells are activated and then present the vaccine antigens to T cells. Once T cells detect these antigens, they proliferate and differentiate into various types, which triggers B cells to produce antibodies and memory cells to be formed.

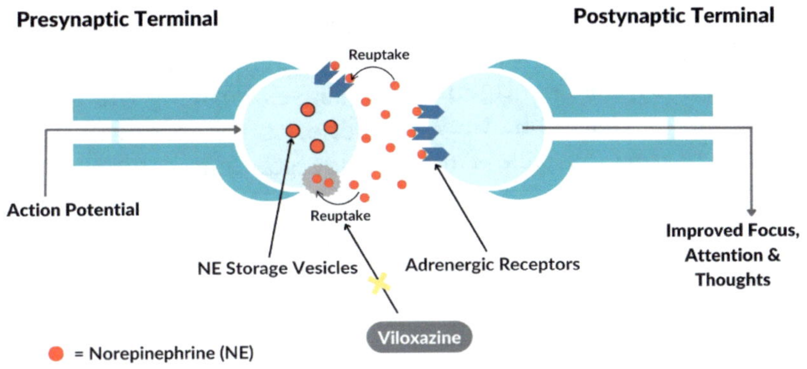

Figure 9.8. Mechanism of action.

Source: https://www.macsenlab.com/wp-content/uploads/2023/06/Mechanism-of-Action-of-Viloxazine.png.

Thus, if a vaccinated person meets the real pathogen in the future, the immune system can quickly respond, stopping the person from getting sick. Taking this step ahead of time demonstrates the importance of vaccines in achieving herd immunity, reducing disease rates, and promoting public health. Factors outside the vaccine itself, such as the environment, can strongly impact how well immunisation programs function. For example, the COVID-19 pandemic made it clear that any disruption in routine vaccination can lower the number of vaccinated people and harm public health. Research on the pandemic's effects on regular immunisation in northern Nigeria found that while some things were improved, shortages of supplies, travel restrictions, and fewer staff at healthcare centres made it harder to provide services. The results indicated that despite efforts to maintain vaccination coverage, the pandemic's influence led to detrimental consequences on the capacity of immunisation programs to operate effectively, underscoring the vulnerability of vaccination initiatives to broader health crises (Aigbogun et al., 2023). In addition, making vaccines available to all populations helps their effectiveness in different settings. The problem of unequal vaccine distribution reveals the weaknesses in the system that can hinder immunization programs. Because pharmaceutical companies are focused on profits, there is now a big difference in vaccine access for people in rich and poor countries. With a limited percentage of fully vaccinated individuals in lower-middle-income and low-income countries, the potential for achieving herd immunity and reducing transmission rates is severely compromised (Borges et al., 2022). Addressing these inequities necessitates a robust international framework that prioritizes human rights and equitable health access, ultimately strengthening global immunization programs and their ability to respond to future pandemics (Figure 9.8).

9.3.1. How Vaccines Stimulate the Immune Response

The process by which vaccines stimulate the immune response is integral to their effectiveness in preventing diseases. Vaccines typically contain antigens derived from pathogens or weakened versions of them. When they are introduced to the body, these antigens trigger the immune system to react, but they do not cause the person to become sick. The first step in fighting infections is the innate immune system, which recognizes the invaders and sends phagocytes to destroy them. The first response triggers adaptive immunity, which makes B cells and T cells more active. B cells produce antibodies for each antigen, while T cells either attack infected cells or assist B cells by releasing cytokines. As a result, the body remembers the pathogen, allowing it to respond faster and more effectively if exposed again, which demonstrates the significant impact of vaccines on public health. Vaccines play a crucial role in strengthening the immune system against specific diseases, as demonstrated by the research on SARS-CoV-2. Knowing the details of how viruses affect the immune system helps improve vaccine development. For example, learning about the SARS-CoV-2 virus has shown that it has certain genomic traits and can evade the immune system, which is used to develop effective vaccines. Vaccines can be made to trigger a strong immune response by using mRNA and viral vectors. Such insights are critical in evolving not only vaccine composition but also in crafting comprehensive immunisation programs that can swiftly adapt to emerging viral threats, thereby highlighting the need for continuous research and innovation in vaccine efficacy (Hu et al., 2020; V'kovski et al., 2020). Also, having immune memory is necessary for vaccines to provide lasting protection. When you get a vaccine, the immune system creates a lasting collection of memory B and T cells. If the body encounters the actual pathogen, memory cells react more quickly and strongly than during the initial infection, significantly reducing the disease's severity or preventing it altogether. Because of this principle, mass vaccination programs are used to safeguard individuals and also to create herd immunity, which prevents infectious diseases from easily spreading among people. When many people are vaccinated, it can eventually eliminate certain diseases, proving the significant immunisation benefits of programs for society. Hence, understanding how vaccines trigger the immune system is crucial for supporting public health and making communities resilient to infectious diseases.

9.3.2. Role of Antigens in Vaccination

The cornerstone of vaccination is the introduction of antigens, which serve as key components in eliciting an immune response. Antigens, which are usually made from weakened or dead pathogens, help the immune system to recognise and handle future infections. Vaccines can be categorised into different groups based on their antigenic composition, including live attenuated, inactivated, and subunit vaccines. Every category uses various features of the antigen to build immunity but not cause the disease. It is crucial for the immune system to remember these antigens; when the actual pathogen is reencountered, the immune system responds quickly to prevent the disease from starting. The success of vaccines depends on antigens triggering the immune system, highlighting the vital role of antigens in vaccination. Also, the development of new vaccines has made it possible to include a wider variety of antigens in immunization programs. Modern techniques, for example, recombinant DNA technology, enable scientists to precisely adjust antigens to increase their effectiveness and lessen the chance of adverse effects. As an example, vaccines that treat HPV infections are being developed by targeting specific proteins from HPV that cause the immune system to attack related cancers. Research has shown that while prophylactic vaccines aim to prevent infections, therapeutic strategies are used to treat diseases that have already developed, which significantly benefits public health. This advances the notion that the role of antigens extends beyond mere prevention; it includes innovative approaches to treat diseases that arise despite prior vaccination efforts, demonstrating their critical function in comprehensive immunization strategies (Zheng et al., 2025). Additionally, the success of vaccination programs often depends on the public understanding how antigens work and the benefits they provide against infectious diseases. Ensuring people are informed about vaccination is crucial, particularly in areas with limited access to vaccines, as evidenced by the impact of COVID-19 on immunization programs worldwide. It illustrates why understanding how vaccines utilise antigens to stimulate the immune system is essential. It is imperative to address the concerns of at-risk groups to reach herd immunity and avoid further outbreaks of VPD. As vaccination campaigns adapt to changing public health landscapes, it is imperative to prioritize education about the science behind antigens and their role in safeguarding community health (Rifqi et al., 2024) (Figure 9.9).

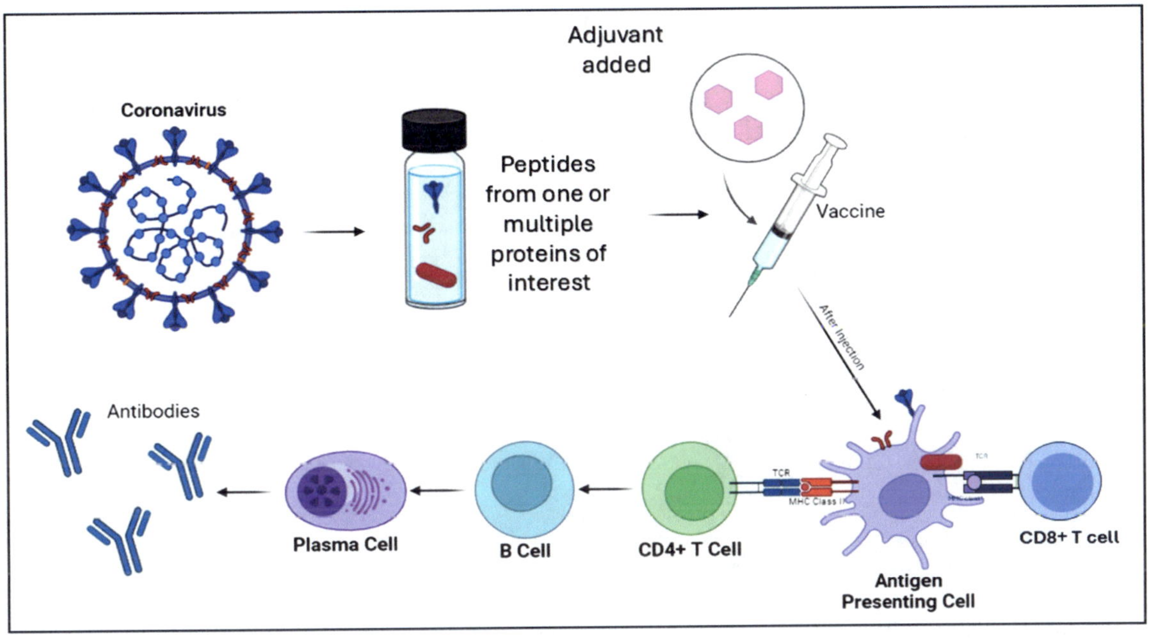

Figure 9.9. Role of antigens in vaccination.

Source: https://www.mdpi.com/vaccines/vaccines-13-00030/article_deploy/html/images/vaccines-13-00030-g001.png.

9.3.3. Memory Cells and Long-Term Immunity

The development and function of memory cells are crucial components of the immune system, particularly in the context of long-term immunity provided by vaccines. Vaccination introduces a harmless part of a pathogen to the immune system, prompting it to respond. At the beginning, B and T cells are activated to recognise and fight the infection. After the primary response, some of the activated lymphocytes become memory cells, which remain in the body even after the infection has resolved. They are educated to identify specific antigens, enabling a quicker and more effective defense when the same pathogen is reencountered. It takes the lasting presence of memory cells for long-term immunity, and these cells can last for years or decades after you are immunised or infected. Several factors can impact the stability of these cells, including the type of pathogen and the immune response it triggers. Memory B cells produce antibodies that stop pathogens, and memory T cells help eliminate infected cells directly. Vaccination programs make use of this process, training the immune system to quickly find and fight off infections, which improves public health. Research into memory cell longevity and functionality is vital, as it informs the design of vaccines that induce lasting immunity, illustrated by the successful deployment of vaccines during the recent pandemic, which emphasized the importance of understanding memory cell responses to emerging strains (Hassan et al., 2024). When memory cells are understood in vaccine development, immunization programs can perform much better. One example is developing vaccines that trigger a strong and varied immune response to deal with problems like changes in antigens and the appearance of new diseases. Improved knowledge of how memory cells are made and maintained can help create better vaccines for different groups or diseases. Adjuvants, which help the immune system respond to vaccines, are also very important for the development of memory cells that last a long time. As highlighted by ongoing research into cancer vaccination, the strategic engagement of immune pathways can not only aid in combating infectious diseases but also in addressing chronic conditions, thereby paving the way for improved healthcare outcomes and disease management (Paul et al., 2024) (Figure 9.10).

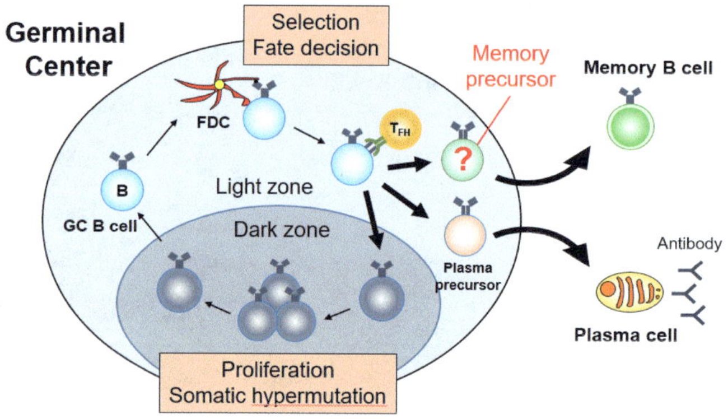

Figure 9.10. Memory cells and long-term immunity.

Source: https://resou.osaka-u.ac.jp/en/research/2020/en/research/files/20201012_1_fig_1.png/@@images/image.

9.4. Benefits of Vaccination

The benefits of vaccination extend far beyond individual immunity, impacting public health on a societal scale. Vaccines have been important in controlling and getting rid of diseases that have caused many cases of sickness and death in the past. As a result of vaccines being widely used, smallpox is almost eradicated, and there are far fewer cases of polio. Public health efforts that support vaccination also help achieve herd immunity, which protects those who are unable to be vaccinated for medical reasons. So, vaccinations are necessary because they help the community stay healthy and save money on treating illnesses that can be prevented. Additionally, vaccination programs help establish systems for monitoring and understanding disease trends. When countries have comprehensive immunization databases, they can regularly check how many people are vaccinated and watch for outbreaks of diseases. For example, Denmark's robust medical databases allow for rigorous epidemiological research and evaluation of vaccination strategies, revealing the long-term benefits of sustained immunization efforts (Schmidt et al., 2019). With this data, it becomes easier to identify outbreaks early and respond to them effectively. Health authorities can use population data to assess the success of vaccination programs and identify ways to reduce barriers to vaccination, thereby improving public health measures. It is essential to consider psychological factors when trying to improve the number of people who get vaccinated. Research has identified various motivations behind vaccine hesitancy, including confidence in vaccines, complacency regarding disease risk, and perceived constraints to vaccination (Betsch et al., 2018). Adjusting how messages are delivered can help more people get vaccinated. Campaigns that highlight the group effort required for vaccination teach people how they can contribute to public health and also foster a sense of community well-being. When public health officials consider these psychological factors, they can effectively address vaccine hesitancy and encourage everyone to get vaccinated, resulting in numerous positive outcomes for society.

9.4.1. Prevention of Infectious Diseases

The prevention of infectious diseases is fundamentally anchored in the development and implementation of effective vaccines and immunization programs. Vaccination is the primary way to protect people from various infections, significantly reducing the risk of serious health issues or death. When many people are vaccinated, herd immunity develops, which helps prevent diseases from spreading widely. This is particularly important for individuals who cannot be vaccinated due to medical reasons. As has been highlighted in different global contexts, adapting immunization strategies to address specific age groups and health profiles ensures a more targeted approach to disease prevention (Anastassopoulou et al., 2024). For example, older people are a group that needs to be considered in the planning of immunization programs. Due to a longer life expectancy, infectious diseases have a bigger effect on older adults, mainly because their immune systems weaken with age and they often have other health problems. Recent studies have found that using vaccines tailored to children can result in better health for them. They usually include new adjuvants and more antigens, which help them work better. Furthermore, differences in vaccine recommendations and implementation strategies, especially between countries in Europe and the United States, underline the necessity of tailored approaches in vaccination programs to optimize protection against diseases such as influenza and pneumococcal disease (Anastassopoulou et al., 2024). China has made significant progress in its vaccination efforts as part of global initiatives to stop the spread of infectious diseases. Since 2007, when the EPI was established, a comprehensive strategy has been implemented to introduce vaccines for various diseases. The fact that about 570 million doses are distributed annually illustrates the program's wide reach and the teamwork of domestic manufacturers to make vaccines available. Better standards for vaccines have made domestic production more like what is used worldwide, making immunisation programs more trustworthy. The robust supervision system covers all stages from research and development to distribution, ensuring that every dose contributes meaningfully to public health and the prevention of infectious diseases (Figure 9.11).

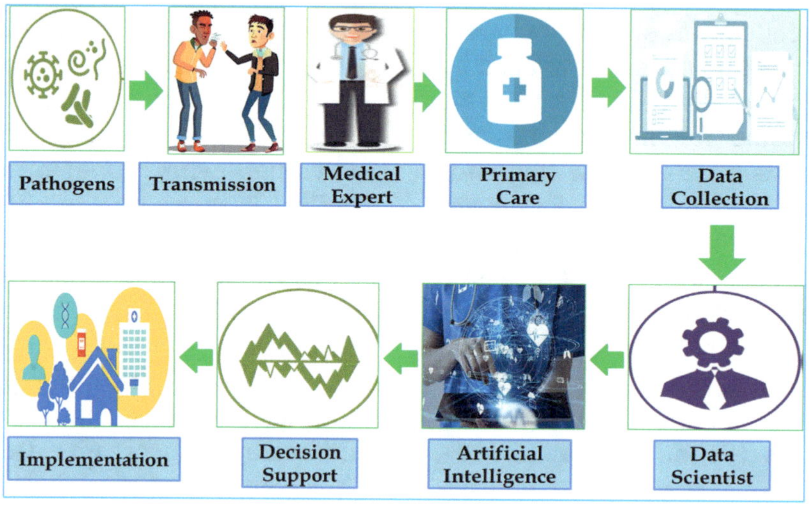

Figure 9.11. Prevention of infectious diseases.

Source: https://www.researchgate.net/publication/359437289/figure/fig1/AS:1147550837018626@1650608848877/nfectious-disease-prevention-principles-must-be-followed-The-series-presents-the-main.png.

9.4.2. Herd Immunity and Community Protection

Achieving herd immunity is a crucial aspect of public health, particularly in the context of vaccines and immunisation programs. Herd immunity occurs when a large number of people are immune to a disease, either through vaccination or prior infection, which helps protect those who are not immune. It helps to control infectious diseases by lowering the amount of virus or bacteria that can spread among people. When many people are vaccinated, herd immunity is established, making it difficult for diseases to spread and helping to safeguard those who cannot be vaccinated, such as infants or individuals with weakened immune systems. Keeping vaccination rates high is crucial for maintaining a strong barrier. In addition to protecting people from disease, herd immunity brings economic benefits, which can be seen in countries that have strongly promoted vaccination. For instance, analyses involving the switch from the quadrivalent human papillomavirus (HPV) vaccination strategy demonstrate substantial public health impacts. Some countries, such as Costa Rica and Panama, have suggested that increasing the use of HPV vaccines could significantly decrease the number of HPV-related diseases. Such analyses often incorporate herd immunity metrics, projecting a marked decrease in the incidence of cancers and related diseases over long time horizons due to increased vaccination rates (Orengo et al., 2025a; Orengo et al., 2025b). The link between more people being vaccinated and achieving herd immunity means that everyone plays a part in maintaining health, which leads to fewer health expenses and a better quality of life for all. Even though the value of herd immunity is obvious, it is still hard to achieve and maintain. Misinformation and a lack of healthcare trust stop many from getting vaccinated which prevents reaching the level of herd immunity needed to protect everyone. Educating the public about the benefits and safety of vaccines through public health campaigns is crucial. Regularly checking and adjusting immunization programs can also help address new health issues and changes in people's opinions about vaccination. By doing this, communities can improve their disease prevention, bring people closer together, and boost public health. The role of vaccines in achieving herd immunity is not just a medical issue; it embodies a shared commitment to safeguarding the health of all individuals within a community (Figure 9.12).

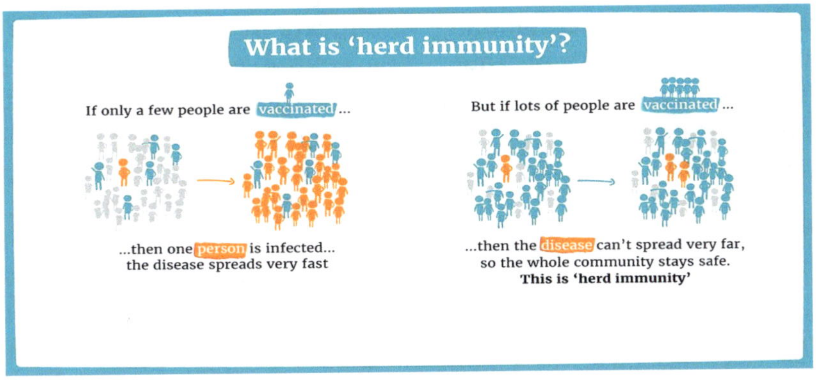

Figure 9.12. Herd immunity and community protection.

Source: https://www.vpslakeshorehospital.com/uploads/blog/whatisherdimmunity-veY49kYc9E88Odn.jpeg.

9.4.3. Economic Impact of Vaccination Programs

The economic impact of vaccination programs extends far beyond the immediate costs of purchasing and administering vaccines. When people become sick with infectious diseases, there are significant financial costs for the healthcare system due to hospitalisation, prolonged care, and lost productivity. When vaccination is effective, the number of cases drops, which also helps reduce health care costs. The transition from using lower-valent pneumococcal conjugate vaccines to PCV20 has been shown to prevent many cases of pneumococcal disease, resulting in substantial savings on direct medical costs. In countries that have delayed adopting PCV20, the cumulative financial losses can reach 100s of millions of euros, highlighting the economic rationale for expediting transitions to more effective vaccination strategies (Perdrizet et al., 2025). It therefore highlights the importance of quickly introducing advanced vaccines into NIPs, ensuring that resources are utilised effectively and public health is improved. Besides saving money, vaccination programs help the economy by improving productivity and quality of life for people, as well as how they work. A healthy community means more people can work, which benefits the economy. Preventing diseases through vaccination is linked to a drop in missed days at school or work and fewer serious illnesses, which helps reduce the costs for families and companies. Moreover, the long-term preventive measures afforded by vaccines such as those targeting Human metapneumovirus can reduce the societal burden posed by respiratory illnesses, particularly for vulnerable populations (Shapovalova, 2025). Assessing how vaccines boost health and labour productivity, policymakers gain a better understanding of the advantages of vaccination. To be successful, vaccination programs rely on public health agencies, healthcare providers, and policymakers working together to implement comprehensive strategies. Overcoming issues such as funding, program rollout, and public persuasion is necessary to achieve the best economic results. When vaccinations are included in health systems, the economy gains from immediate healthcare savings and also from better protection of the community from outbreaks. This holistic approach underscores the connection between immunisation and economic vitality, advocating for robust investments in vaccine development and distribution (Perdrizet et al., 2025). By enhancing public understanding of these benefits, stakeholders can foster greater engagement and support for immunisation initiatives that ultimately promote societal well-being and economic development (Figure 9.13).

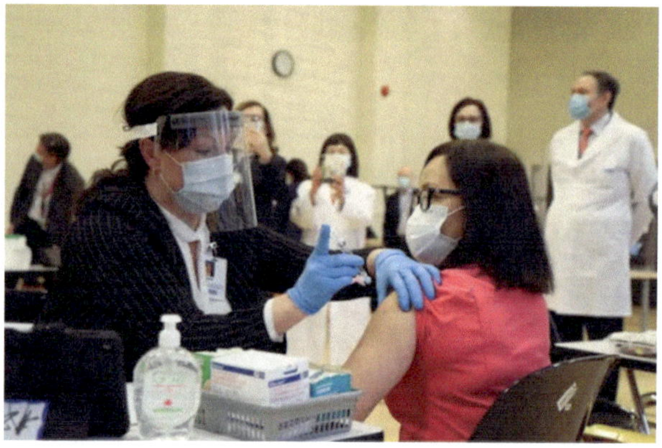

Figure 9.13. Economic impact of vaccination programs.

Source: https://static01.nyt.com/images/2020/12/14/world/14virus-canada-vaccines-1sub/merlin_181249923_582fcf73-56ef-4c6f-87e5-c8a39bd1d79b-articleLarge.jpg?quality=75&auto=webp&disable=upscale.

9.5. Challenges in Immunisation

The challenges associated with immunisation programs are multifaceted and stem from a variety of social, economic, and technological factors. Many people or groups are hesitant about getting vaccinated because they believe false news or doubt the information given by health authorities. Being hesitant about vaccines can significantly diminish the effectiveness of immunisation programs, particularly in areas with limited access to education or reliable information. For example, anti-vaccine opinions frequently grow larger on social media, which leads people to make wrong decisions about vaccines and puts herd immunity at risk. Using targeted methods to communicate and educate people is necessary to increase public acceptance and participation in vaccination programs. Additionally, distributing vaccines is very challenging due to the logistical issues involved. It is difficult for immunization programs in developing countries to overcome problems with transportation, storage, and the lack of healthcare facilities. An example is that vaccines need to be kept at specific temperatures to work correctly, which is a challenge when delivering them in remote places. Shifts in the allocation of funds and resources can also make it difficult to keep vaccines available to all, which makes immunization more challenging. An effective response to these logistical challenges necessitates robust supply chain management and innovative approaches, such as mobile vaccination clinics and community partnerships to ensure that vaccines reach underserved populations and that immunization targets are met (Nur et al., 2024). Creating and using vaccines for diseases such as dengue is also a big challenge in immunization programs. Although vaccines have advanced, there are still challenges in ensuring they are effective and safe for all groups of people. The dengue vaccine situation highlights the challenges, as each serotype has its own issues with the vaccine's effectiveness for individual patients. Additionally, vaccine-induced immunological enhancement poses a risk of complications that can further complicate public acceptance of vaccination initiatives (Mehboob, 2024). We need to continue research, work together globally, and invest significantly in vaccine technology to overcome these obstacles. Working on these aspects can lead to more effective vaccination programs and improved health for everyone worldwide.

9.5.1. Vaccine Hesitancy and Misinformation

Vaccine hesitancy remains a significant barrier to achieving optimal immunisation coverage, deeply intertwined with the proliferation of misinformation. This phenomenon often manifests as a reluctance or refusal to vaccinate despite the availability and accessibility of vaccines. A variety of factors contribute to vaccine hesitancy, including cultural beliefs, a history of mistrust in medical institutions, and a preference for anecdotal evidence over scientific findings. In the context of school-based immunization programs, for instance, parents may exhibit hesitancy primarily due to perceived safety concerns, particularly surrounding vaccines such as the human papillomavirus (HPV) vaccine. This uncertainty can be exacerbated by false stories in the media, which lead people to question whether vaccines are genuinely effective and safe. Understanding these dynamics is crucial for public health strategies aiming to bolster vaccine uptake and reduce misinformation-driven resistance to immunization initiatives (McIndoe et al., 2025). Talking about vaccines in the right way helps to overcome doubts and clear up false information. Having trustworthy healthcare providers involved is very important; studies indicate that people are more willing to get vaccinated when advised by their own general practitioners. Building connections between healthcare workers and the community allows targeted actions to help parents learn about vaccines and dispel any misinformation they may have. Also, making it easier for people to give consent and communicate with health workers can reduce the reasons why some people do not get vaccinated. Public health campaigns that focus on relatable narratives and transparent information about vaccine safety can help navigate the prevailing hesitance, ultimately supporting higher immunisation rates within communities (McIndoe et al., 2025). Where people are reluctant to get vaccinated, cultural beliefs and misinformation can significantly hinder public health programs. As an illustration, the COVID-19 pandemic in Haiti highlighted a significant correlation between public opinion and vaccination rates, with only 5% of the population agreeing to receive a vaccination, despite the availability of numerous vaccine doses provided by donors. In this situation, mistrust in healthcare, religious beliefs, and a lack of clear information all played significant roles. Using mixed-methods research helps understand the unique features and challenges of communities, which allows health interventions to be adjusted appropriately. Engaging religious leaders and healthcare workers in dialogue about vaccination can yield better engagement and trust within communities, ultimately enhancing public health responses to future global health threats (Figure 9.14).

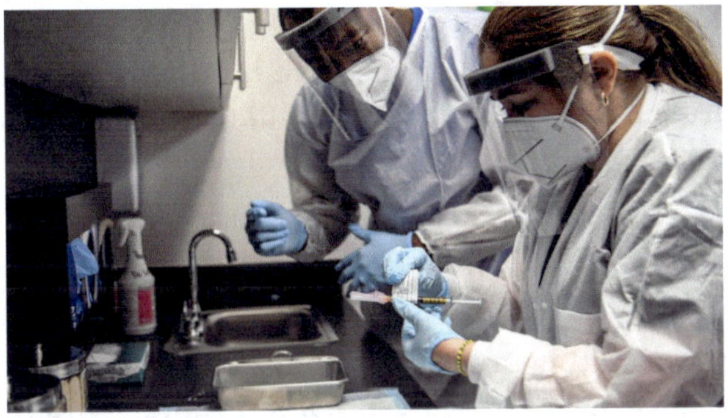

Figure 9.14. Vaccine hesitancy and misinformation.

Source: https://csis-website-prod.s3.amazonaws.com/s3fs-public/publication/GettyImages-1228042254_0.jpg.

9.5.2. Access and Distribution Issues

Access and distribution issues have profoundly impacted the effectiveness of vaccines and immunization programs worldwide. These challenges often stem from socioeconomic disparities, logistical hurdles, and geopolitical factors, leading to significant inequalities in vaccine availability. For instance, during the COVID-19 pandemic, certain regions encountered severe shortages, while wealthier nations secured large quantities of vaccines ahead of low- and middle-income countries (LMICs). Because of this unequal distribution, some people are still at risk of infectious diseases even though modern vaccines are available. In Bhutan, a well-established NIP facilitated the rapid execution of a COVID-19 vaccination strategy, demonstrating how robust infrastructure can mitigate access issues (Phuntsho et al., 2022). Even so, the significant disparities in vaccination rates across countries highlight the barriers that prevent equal access to immunisation. Additionally, administering vaccines to those who need them relies heavily on the existing infrastructure. Those with well-organized healthcare and logistics usually conduct vaccination campaigns more successfully. Bhutan's approach is noteworthy, as it utilized a digital platform for tracking and monitoring vaccinations, which played a crucial role in ensuring high coverage rates (Phuntsho et al., 2022). Effective logistics include delivering vaccines, as well as the necessary equipment and training for healthcare workers. Experience from health emergencies shows that using mobile vaccination teams or joining forces with local groups helps provide healthcare to people who lack access. Having this adaptability is essential for handling the urgent need to protect people against both current and new health problems. Besides logistics and infrastructure, public perceptions of vaccines and their involvement in the process are crucial for vaccine access and distribution. Misinformation often prevents people from getting vaccinated, even when vaccines are available. Due to variants like omicron, people are questioning the effectiveness of vaccines, leading to increased attention on vaccination programs. To address these fears, public health campaigns should be transparent and emphasise that vaccines are essential for preventing the spread of diseases. Ensuring that vaccines are available to all communities is essential, since including them helps achieve immunity for many. Working together with local leaders and health professionals can help communities trust vaccination programs more, which leads to more people participating and fewer gaps in access.

9.5.3. Emerging Infectious Diseases and Vaccine Development

The emergence of infectious diseases represents a significant challenge to global public health, necessitating ongoing vigilance and innovation in vaccine development. It is clear from history that contagious diseases can spread rapidly, often faster than medical efforts can keep pace. Because of vaccination, many infectious diseases have been brought under control, including the complete eradication of smallpox and a significant drop in polio cases. The recent outbreaks of Zika and COVID-19, caused by new pathogens, have highlighted the need for faster vaccine development. They reflect the constant change in pathogens and how we try to protect against them with vaccines. As society navigates these complexities, it becomes essential to strike a balance between responsive measures while fostering public confidence in vaccination programs, ensuring effective herd immunity, and minimizing healthcare costs associated with infectious diseases (Mwende, 2024). Such outbreaks often reveal that existing health systems are not robust enough, underscoring the need for greater effort in vaccine research and development. The Ebola virus disease (EVD) outbreak, particularly the 2014 West African crisis, served as a pivotal moment, accelerating the licensure of vaccines and therapeutics that had previously languished in development phases. Such urgent outbreaks encouraged scientists to develop innovative vaccines, and mRNA vaccines proved to be very fast to produce. It demonstrates that what we learn from earlier epidemics can be applied to future situations, not just with EVD, but with many other diseases as well. As vaccine development progresses, integrating lessons learned from these emergent threats into public health strategies is crucial to mitigate the impacts of future infectious disease outbreaks (Marzi et al., 2024). Also, since vaccine research must respond to EIDs, work together on surveillance, research, and sharing vaccines. During outbreaks, it is common to notice that some people have poorer access to healthcare, highlighting the disparities in global health. Due to limited resources and healthcare systems, developing countries are disproportionately affected by infectious disease outbreaks. Thus, joining forces with private companies and collaborating with other nations on vaccine development can improve how fast we respond to epidemics. Investing in vaccine research and working to dispel myths about vaccines helps public health efforts to handle EIDs. Adopting such strategies not only aims to maintain the success of existing vaccination programs but also prepares society for the unexpected challenges posed by emerging infections in the future (Mwende, 2024) (Figure 9.15).

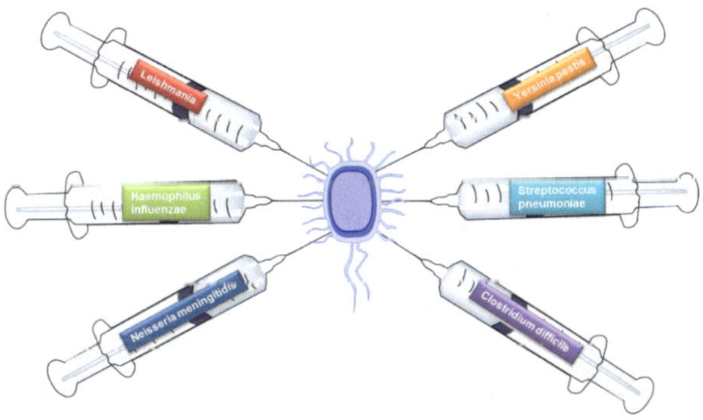

Figure 9.15. Emerging infectious diseases and vaccine development.

Source: https://www.mpikg.mpg.de/192615/teaser-1372934746.jpg.

9.6. Global Vaccination Efforts

Global vaccination efforts serve as a critical component in preventing the spread of infectious diseases, thereby significantly impacting public health. Immunisation programs have been effective in reducing the number of cases of VPD, such as measles, polio, and hepatitis B. Such programs protect people and also help build community immunity, which protects those who cannot get vaccinated for medical reasons. The usefulness of vaccines is evident in their ability to improve health for mothers and children. Vaccines have been found to reduce maternal morbidity and mortality rates by protecting mothers from infectious diseases during pregnancy, ultimately contributing to healthier deliveries and improved neonatal health outcomes (Kumari et al., 2024). Including vaccination in overall healthcare plans highlights that immunisation is connected to the overall health of individuals. In the last few years, both international organisations and governments have worked harder to vaccinate vulnerable people through special campaigns. Gavi, the Vaccine Alliance, and WHO's extended immunisation programs are designed to improve vaccination services for all, especially in places with fewer resources. The goal of these efforts is to help overcome the problems caused by geography and low income, so more people in underserved areas can get and afford vaccines. Also, informing the public and providing healthcare resources help families understand why vaccinations are essential. These campaigns typically emphasise that vaccination can prevent outbreaks and also benefit the overall health and well-being of the entire community. By involving local communities and healthcare workers, these programs help establish a culture in which vaccination is viewed as a key public health measure. Even so, it is not easy to ensure that every country has access to vaccines. Vaccine hesitancy, false information, and logistical obstacles can slow down progress and increase health differences among people. Noticing the barriers related to gender has shown the importance of making immunization more accessible to everyone. Projects like USAID's MOMENTUM aim to overcome these gender barriers by incorporating gender perspectives at every stage of vaccination planning and implementation. By focusing on the unique circumstances faced by women and caregivers in accessing immunization services, the initiative strives to enhance overall service quality and engage both men and women in dialogue about vaccination (Gerber et al., 2024). Addressing these challenges head-on allows for a more robust and equitable vaccination framework, ultimately ensuring that the benefits of immunization are realized by all, regardless of gender or socioeconomic status (Figure 9.16).

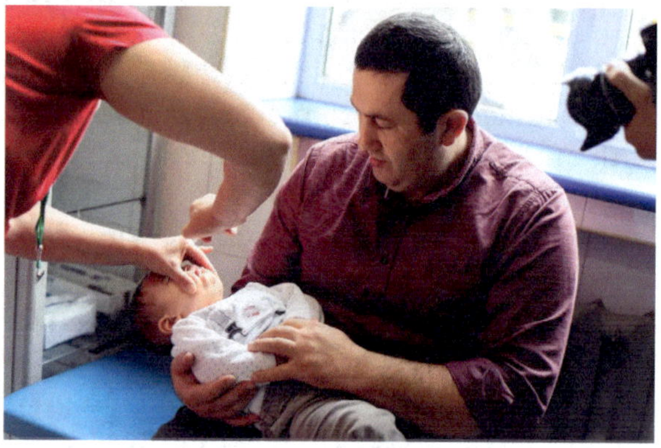

Figure 9.16. Global vaccination efforts.

Source: https://external-content.duckduckgo.com/iu/?u=https%3A%2F%2Fwww.unicef.org%2Farmenia%2Fsites%2Funicef.org.armenia%2Ffiles%2Fstyles%2Fhero_desktop%2Fpublic%2F2018.3.6_UNICEF_Children_089.webp%3Fitok%3DAQjQ-yT7&f=1&nofb=1&ipt=458a8696f4c712f672b78411da0563a9b0215f1810d664e4a959d60911d9e2e2.

9.6.1. World Health Organization Initiatives

The role of the WHO in promoting global vaccine initiatives is critical in the context of safeguarding public health. The WHO has carried out many efforts, and the GPEI is among the most important, as it aims to eliminate polio, which continues to harm communities, mainly in low-income areas affected by conflict. The GPEI employs advanced geospatial technologies through the WHO Regional Office for Africa's Geographic Information System (AFRO GIS) Centre, which was established to enhance vaccine delivery and case tracking. With AFRO GIS, healthcare resources and personnel can be deployed in real-time to combat polio outbreaks, and the system provides essential data to support informed decisions in areas where diseases spread rapidly. This timely response not only aims to eradicate polio but also builds a sustainable framework for managing other health crises encountered in these regions (Kipterer et al., 2024). Apart from working on polio eradication, the WHO also works on boosting immunization efforts by improving NIPs everywhere. A notable example is the collaboration with the Bill & Melinda Gates Foundation to enhance the delivery of vaccines in China. The establishment of the Innovation Laboratory for Vaccine Delivery Research (VaxLab) reflects a strategic move towards addressing systemic issues in immunisation. By conducting thorough research and advocating for policy reforms, VaxLab aims to increase coverage of vital vaccines, including the human papillomavirus vaccine (HPV) and pneumococcal conjugate vaccine (PCV). It is clear from the results that government action and public knowledge are key to helping marginalised communities and those in remote places access vaccines. Such initiatives highlight the WHO's commitment to equitable healthcare across diverse global contexts (Chen et al., 2024). During the COVID-19 pandemic, the quick rollout of vaccines had a significant effect on public health. The WHO has been key in leading the worldwide effort to distribute vaccines, underlining the importance of reliable systems to improve vaccination programs. What was learned from COVID-19 vaccination can be used to enhance future immunisation efforts. Addressing difficulties in vaccine supply, delivery, and public reluctance is best achieved by employing various approaches, and the WHO is well-positioned to take the lead. Working together with government officials, non-governmental organisations, and community leaders can create an environment that supports increasing vaccination rates. Ultimately, the WHO's initiatives serve as a blueprint for effective immunisation programs that not only address current public health challenges but also bolster the resilience of health systems against future crises (Chen et al., 2024).

9.6.2. National Immunisation Programs

NIPs play a crucial role in safeguarding public health by establishing standardised vaccination schedules intended to reduce the incidence of VPD. These programs are often shaped by national health policies that reflect contemporary scientific knowledge and epidemiological data. Universal vaccination programs by NIPs are designed to achieve herd immunity, which helps shield infants and individuals with weakened immune systems from diseases they may not be able to fight with vaccines. Vaccine programs help make vaccines more accessible, which can help reduce health disparities and benefit the entire population. As a result, communities benefit from improved health and reduced costs associated with preventable health issues. Working on and carrying out NIPs generally requires cooperation among government health agencies, healthcare providers, and community organizations. Talking to the public in the right way helps more people participate and voice their concerns about vaccines. For instance, informing the community about vaccines can have a substantial effect on the number of people vaccinated. Educational materials and community outreach can help people feel more comfortable about vaccines and encourage more people to accept them. In Alaska, efforts are underway to make meningitis vaccination mandatory by law, highlighting the importance of collaboration between the government and the community. These efforts underscore the necessity for ongoing education to promote vaccination, catalysing community dialogue surrounding the critical role of immunisation in maintaining public health as recommended by the national Advisory Committee on Immunisation Practices (ACIP) (Hulstine et al., 2017). Additionally, NIPs are evaluated in relation to emerging health issues, which necessitates their ability to incorporate new vaccines and adapt to shifting disease patterns. One can see similarities between vaccinating for bacterial meningitis and vaccinating groups at risk for other infectious diseases, such as those with HIV. By changing national immunization policies based on the newest research, vaccination efforts are kept up to date and work well. Reviewing the experiences of patients and the community after new vaccination strategies are introduced can help improve programs and make preventive care more accessible. As the global landscape of infectious diseases continues to change, so too must the frameworks that guide NIPs to protect public health comprehensively (N/A, 2006).

9.6.3. Case Studies of Successful Vaccination Campaigns

Vaccination campaigns have demonstrated significant successes in controlling and eradicating infectious diseases worldwide. For example, the campaign to eradicate smallpox employed both thorough research and extensive fieldwork. A live vaccine was used, and approaches were adapted to meet the needs of different areas, allowing health workers to reach people who are often missed. It was important that research kept happening during the campaign, which led to better vaccine delivery and immunisation plans. The initiative was shaped by surveillance, which monitored outbreaks and tracked vaccination rates. This comprehensive research and surveillance framework ensured that essential adjustments could be made in real time, exemplifying how evidence-based decision-making is vital in vaccination campaigns, especially as they approach eradication phases (Breman et al., 2011). Polio eradication demonstrates how diverse groups collaborate in vaccination campaigns. The GPEI, which began in 1988, brought together many international efforts to fight polio. It was also a success when it developed methods to find polio in people without symptoms, which helped guide vaccination programs. Also, the campaign recognised the importance of getting communities involved in vaccination. Studies in anthropology and sociology helped explain the local beliefs and customs that made people more willing to get the vaccine. Emphasising community involvement showed that public health strategies should be designed to fit the needs of local people. Through these efforts, polio vaccination campaigns have managed to decrease global incidence significantly, showcasing how essential localized approaches coupled with scientific research are for the success of immunization programs (Breman et al., 2011). The success of vaccination campaigns against measles proves that public health strategies can be very effective. Nations with high immunization rates usually have strong political and institutional systems that help healthcare programs. Research indicates that countries with stable governance and effective bureaucratic systems achieved higher coverage rates for vaccines like the diphtheria-tetanus-pertussis (DTP) and measles vaccines. In fact, epidemics do not usually stop these campaigns from succeeding; instead, strong health policies and involvement with international organizations encourage more people to get vaccinated. It is clear from LMICs that significant changes in global policies can influence immunization rates, which highlights the importance of institutional quality in healthcare programs. This illustrates the impact of socioeconomic factors in determining a nation's vaccination success and highlights avenues for strengthening immunization strategies globally (Figure 9.17).

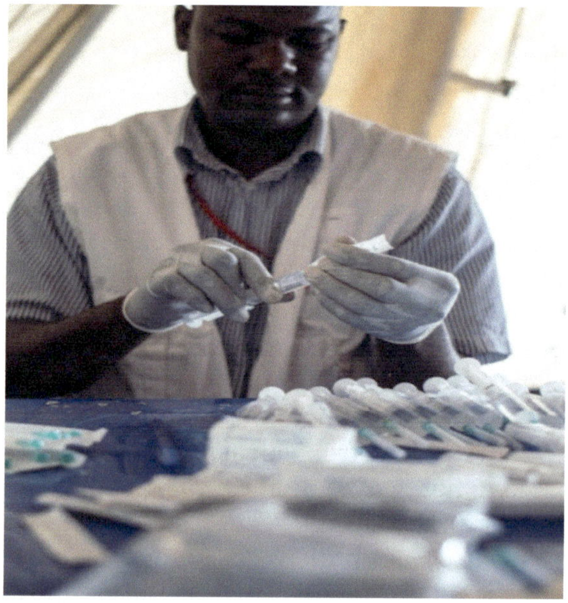

Figure 9.17. Case studies of successful vaccination campaigns.

Source: https://msfaccess.org/sites/default/files/styles/full_default/public/2022-04/Vaccines_Niger_NurseVaccine_Sylavin_Cherkaoui_2015_MSF145893_3800.jpg?itok=jH0Cyv85.

SUMMARY

In concluding the examination of vaccines and immunisation programs, it is clear that the timely implementation of new vaccines, such as the PCV20, is critical to enhancing public health outcomes. Several recent modelling studies point out that if countries do not switch to PCV20 soon, they will miss the chance to prevent many cases of pneumococcal disease and also lose a lot of money in healthcare costs. The results show that the delays lead to thousands of diseases that could have been prevented and significant savings in medical expenses, which is why NIPs should update their vaccination schedules right away.

Thus, the immediate incorporation of advanced vaccines is vital in steering public health toward improved outcomes and reduced disease burden (Perdrizet et al., 2025). Immunization has also shown that it can reduce the number of infectious diseases in many groups, as evidenced by the drop in hepatitis A cases after the EPI was introduced in China. The EPI has effectively reduced hepatitis A cases among target populations by about 80.77% which proves that the program protects vaccinated people and also gives unvaccinated populations some herd immunity. These outcomes underscore the importance of public health efforts to maintain high vaccination rates and effectively monitor diseases. Consequently, the EPIs approach to managing hepatitis A serves as a model for adapting and strengthening immunization efforts globally (Ming et al., 2024). In short, ensuring strong and ongoing vaccination programs is the most effective way to combat infectious diseases. There is strong support for the view that vaccines are essential for public health and for ensuring the security of health worldwide. It is crucial for policymakers, healthcare providers, and stakeholders to focus on vaccination programs, adding new vaccines and widening current efforts to make sure all groups benefit. Achieving lasting success in immunization programs requires people to cooperate in addressing problems, building community trust, and continuing efforts to eliminate diseases and improve public health. We should work actively, use evidence, and focus on the health of future generations.

Vaccination helps to stop diseases and protect the health of people in communities. The recent Adult Immunization Board meeting in April 2024 highlights the need for a well-planned way to introduce vaccines in Europe. Choosing new vaccines primarily depends on the disease burden, their effectiveness, and safety. Also, economic assessments and public support for vaccination are now acknowledged, but they should be included more in decision-making. Thorough planning is necessary for NIPs, which covers setting clear goals, selecting the target population, and improving communication among healthcare workers. Boccalini et al. (2025) highlight that operational NIPs must undergo continual monitoring to assess safety and effectiveness, ensuring that these programs adapt to changing healthcare landscapes and demonstrate measurable health outcomes. The integration of a life course approach (LCA) to vaccination strategies presents another key development in immunization programs. Due to population aging and the impact of COVID-19 on vaccination rates, there is growing interest in improving immunization strategies. As explained by the LCA findings, using this approach helps health systems provide the right vaccines at every stage of life. Balsells et al. (2024) underscore that such an approach not only addresses the immediate need for boosters or catch-up vaccinations but also reinforces lifelong protection against VPD. If health authorities find new ways to administer vaccines, they can better reach a larger number of people and improve the overall health of the population. Vaccination strategies are successful when public health and the community work together. The public, healthcare workers and policymakers must join forces to address reasons why vaccines are not being used. According to the Adult Immunisation Board, more attention should be given to making vaccination benefits and safety clear to everyone. If hesitancy, misinformation, and logistical problems in vaccine delivery are handled, more people may feel comfortable and willing to get vaccinated. Using both evidence-based methods and behavioural understanding will encourage more people to follow vaccination schedules, which helps develop a preventative health culture. Because we still face issues from previous pandemic vaccination programs, it is crucial to work together to support vaccination and help communities resist future health threats.

CLOSER LOOK:

ORAL POLIO VACCINE (OPV):

Oral Polio Vaccine (OPV) is a cornerstone in the global fight against poliomyelitis, a highly infectious viral disease caused by the poliovirus. Developed in the 1950s by Albert Sabin, OPV is a live attenuated vaccine, meaning it contains a weakened form of the virus that is capable of stimulating immunity without causing the disease in healthy individuals. Unlike the Inactivated Polio Vaccine (IPV), which is administered via injection, OPV is given orally, making it easy to administer, especially in mass immunization campaigns. Its ease of use and ability to induce both systemic and intestinal immunity have made it a key tool in the global polio eradication initiative.

The vaccine works by introducing the weakened poliovirus into the gastrointestinal tract. There, it replicates in the gut, prompting the immune system to produce antibodies. This local intestinal immunity is particularly significant because the poliovirus spreads through the fecal-oral route. By preventing viral replication in the intestines, OPV not only protects the vaccinated individual but also reduces viral shedding, thereby contributing to **herd immunity**. This is a critical feature in areas with poor sanitation, where polio can spread rapidly.

OPV comes in three types, corresponding to the three serotypes of poliovirus: type 1, type 2, and type 3. Initially, trivalent OPV (tOPV) containing all three serotypes was widely used. However, after the eradication of wild poliovirus type 2, global vaccination strategies shifted toward bivalent OPV (bOPV), targeting types 1 and 3, to minimize the risk of vaccine-derived poliovirus type 2 (VDPV2) outbreaks. Monovalent OPV (mOPV) is also used in outbreak responses for rapid immunity against a specific serotype.

The advantages of OPV are clear: it is inexpensive, easy to administer, and highly effective at inducing intestinal immunity. Additionally, it can indirectly immunize unvaccinated individuals in a community through secondary spread of the vaccine virus. However, OPV is not without limitations. In very rare cases, the attenuated virus can mutate and regain neurovirulence, leading to **vaccine-associated paralytic poliomyelitis (VAPP).** Moreover, if the vaccine virus circulates extensively in under-immunized populations, it can result in circulating vaccine-derived polioviruses (cVDPVs), which have caused outbreaks in some regions.

Global health organizations, including the World Health Organization (WHO), have relied on OPV as part of large-scale immunization campaigns that have drastically reduced polio incidence worldwide, from hundreds of thousands of cases annually in the 1980s to fewer than 100 reported cases in recent years. The vaccine's role in eradication efforts cannot be overstated, though strategies now increasingly combine OPV and IPV to balance the benefits of intestinal immunity with the safety of inactivated vaccines.

In conclusion, the Oral Polio Vaccine remains a powerful public health tool. Its ease of administration, ability to induce strong gut immunity, and contribution to herd protection have been instrumental in driving the near-eradication of polio. Ongoing vigilance, careful monitoring, and strategic use of OPV alongside IPV are essential to ensure the disease is finally eliminated globally.

REFERENCES

1. Program Directors' Perspectives on global Health Elective Preparation in Canadian Paediatric Residency Programs. (2013). *Paediatrics & Child Health*. https://doi.org/10.1093/pch/18.suppl_a.18aAigbogun, E., Ibrahim, R., Yusufari, Y., Igbokwe, U., Okongwu, C., Abdulkarim, A., Tijanni, H., et al. (2023). Impact of the COVID-19 pandemic on routine immunization programs in Northern Nigeria. *Sustainability*. https://www.semanticscholar.org/paper/6c2e9292684bee9015836fa618bcc67eb3aaf5d3 (accessed on 30th May 2025).
2. Al Kaabi, N. A., Yang, Y., Hussein, S. E., Yang, T., Abdalla, J., Wang, H., Lou, Z., et al. (2023). Efficacy and safety of a booster vaccination with two inactivated SARS-CoV-2 vaccines on symptomatic COVID-19 infection in adults: Results of a double-blind, randomized, placebo-controlled, phase 3 trial in Abu Dhabi. *Vaccines, 11*. https://www.semanticscholar.org/paper/56c6cd6c1df467a1b62959b1a1c4b143d764b83d (accessed on 30th May 2025).
3. Alghamdi, S., Safar, S., Alghamdi, S., Jabbar, S., Alghamdi, H., Shabab, A., & Alghamdi, S. (2024). Advancements in immunization strategies for enhanced infection control: A comprehensive review and future directions. *Power System Technology*. https://www.semanticscholar.org/paper/a75c82ad28a4d88178d62bd09760077afdf48e06 (accessed on 30th May 2025).
4. Anastassopoulou, C., Ferous, S., Medić, S., Siafakas, N., Boufidou, F., Gioula, G., & Tsakris, A. (2024). Vaccines for the elderly and vaccination programs in Europe and the United States. *Vaccines, 12*. https://www.semanticscholar.org/paper/f45aaa31ea4c6f5506b24b2a382c25d76bc7cfb6 (accessed on 30th May 2025).
5. Andrews, N., Stowe, J., Kirsebom, F., Toffa, S., Rickeard, T., Gallagher, E., Gower, C., et al. (2022). COVID-19 vaccine effectiveness against the Omicron (B.1.1.529) variant. *New England Journal of Medicine, 386*, 1532–1546. https://doi.org/10.1056/nejmoa2119451.
6. Anis, E., Davis, D. C., Parker, E. P. K., Ghendon, Y. Z., Glezen, W. P., Herremans, M. M., et al. (2015). Impact of inactivated poliovirus vaccine on mucosal immunity: Implications for the polio eradication endgame. *Expert Review of Vaccines*. https://core.ac.uk/download/77002957.pdf (accessed on 30th May 2025).
7. Balsells, E., Ghiselli, M., Hommes, C., Nascimento, L. De. O., B., Rosado-Valenzuela, A. L., & Vega, E. (2024). Rethinking immunization programs through the life course approach. *Frontiers in Public Health, 12*. https://www.semanticscholar.org/paper/6dbb573bab91356ca8c38f948e98c1c3ac470e4b (accessed on 30th May 2025).
8. Betsch, C., Schmid, P., Heinemeier, D., Korn, L., Holtmann, C., & Böhm, R. (2018). Beyond confidence: Development of a measure assessing the 5C psychological antecedents of vaccination. *PLoS ONE, 13*, e0208601–e0208601. https://doi.org/10.1371/journal.pone.0208601.
9. Bird, J. (2023). *Anti-Vaccination: Addressing Vaccine Hesitancy and its Consequences for Modern Public Health Policy*. https://core.ac.uk/download/568250634.pdf (accessed on 30th May 2025).
10. Boccalini, S., Bechini, A., Del Riccio, M., Weinberger, B., Wysocki, J., Martinelli, D., Wichmann, O., et al. (2025). Strategies for introducing and implementing vaccines for adults into national immunization programs in Europe: Good practices and key insights of the adult immunization board meeting. *Human Vaccines & Immunotherapeutics, 21*(1), 2451487. https://www.semanticscholar.org/paper/0e64741f2321f2741c841ae087599af4ac53c506 (accessed on 30th May 2025).

11. Borges, L. C., De Menezes, H. Z., & Crosbie, E. (2022). More pain, more gain! The delivery of COVID-19 vaccines and the pharmaceutical industry's role in widening the access gap. *International Journal of Health Policy and Management, 11*, 3101–3113. https://www.semanticscholar.org/paper/5f65eee0e400570969999aefa75d171272ff483f (accessed on 30th May 2025).

12. Breman, J. G., De Quadros, C. A., Dowdle, W. R., Foege, W., et al. (2011). The role of research in viral disease eradication and elimination programs: Lessons for malaria eradication. *PLoS Medicine*. https://core.ac.uk/download/12211911.pdf (accessed on 30th May 2025).

13. Bulcha, J., Wang, Y., Ma, H., Tai, P. W. L., & Gao, G. (2021). Viral vector platforms within the gene therapy landscape. *Signal Transduction and Targeted Therapy, 6*. https://doi.org/10.1038/s41392-021-00487-6.

14. Chen, S., Rodewald, L. E., Du, A., & Tang, S. (2024). Advancing the National Immunization Program in an era of achieving universal vaccine coverage in China and beyond. *Infectious Diseases of Poverty, 13*. https://www.semanticscholar.org/paper/740c3be760f0195db88e5dd0506e7d9b285d8748 (accessed on 30th May 2025).

15. Dinleyici, M., Nepesov, M. İ., Sipahi, O., Carman, K., Kilic, O., & Dinleyici, E. (2018). The attitudes, behaviors, and knowledge of healthcare professionals towards the diagnosis, treatment, and prevention of bacterial meningitis in Turkey. *Human Vaccines & Immunotherapeutics, 15*, 134–140. https://www.semanticscholar.org/paper/fa1202636d1c1f48d96f1d217303528c9d0848ae (accessed on 30th May 2025).

16. Etienne-Mesubi, M., Oni, B., Labbe-Coq, N. R., Alcide-Jean-Pierre, M. C., Lamarre, D., Dorestan, D., Bien-Aime, M. A., et al. (2024). Factors that influence COVID-19 vaccine uptake and hesitancy among a population in the West Department of Haiti: Implications for enhancing effectiveness of immunization programs. https://www.semanticscholar.org/paper/59ab2a745ac153f40cdf31705afb9e275432e141 (accessed on 30th May 2025).

17. Fleming-Dutra, K., Ciesla, A., Roper, L., Smith, Z. R., Miller, J. D., Accorsi, E. K., Verani, J., et al. (2023). Preliminary estimates of effectiveness of monovalent mRNA vaccines in preventing symptomatic SARS-CoV-2 infection among children aged 3–5 years — Increasing Community Access to Testing Program, United States, July 2022–February 2023. *Morbidity and Mortality Weekly Report, 72*, 177–182. https://www.semanticscholar.org/paper/4665d939056c86f028defbd52a7ce6faa08dabef (accessed on 30th May 2025).

18. Friedman, A., Walker, D., Bloom, D., Canning, D., O'Brien, J., Privor-Dumm, L., Levine, O., et al. (2025). *The Economic Case for Expanding Vaccination Coverage of Children*. https://core.ac.uk/download/pdf/6617060.pdf (accessed on 30th May 2025).

19. Gauri, V., & Khaleghian, P. (2025). *Immunization in Developing Countries: Its Political and Organizational Determinants*. https://core.ac.uk/download/pdf/6615639.pdf (accessed on 30th May 2025).

20. Gerber, W., Fields, R., Guesela, N., Nuhu, K. A. I., & Manika, E. (2024). Beyond constructs and principles: Addressing gender-related barriers to high, equitable immunization coverage. *Frontiers in Global Women's Health, 5*. https://www.semanticscholar.org/paper/d81ea54939d8128cd670c065ab1f00ea05d27e74 (accessed on 30th May 2025).

21. Goishi-Bessey, L. S. (2016). *The Effectiveness of California Assembly Bill 2109: Personal Belief Exemptions for Kindergarten Immunizations*. https://core.ac.uk/download/70426936.pdf (accessed on 30th May 2025).

22. Hassan, A., El-Adham, K., & Eithar, E. (2024). *The Penetration, Possibility of Protection and Treatment of COVID-19.* https://core.ac.uk/download/636476054.pdf (accessed on 30th May 2025).

23. Hu, B., Guo, H., Zhou, P., & Shi, Z. L. (2020). Characteristics of SARS-CoV-2 and COVID-19. *Nature Reviews Microbiology, 19*, 141–154. https://doi.org/10.1038/s41579-020-00459-7.

24. Hulstine, A. (2017). *Vaccine Implementation: Alaska 2017.* https://core.ac.uk/download/286607590.pdf (accessed on 30th May 2025).

25. Jeon, J., & Kim, E. (2025). Exploring future pandemic preparedness through the development of preventive vaccine platforms and the key roles of international organizations in a global health crisis. *Vaccines, 13.* https://www.semanticscholar.org/paper/b8db63eb8941df18b25b9ff5756fad3ce73c4c86 (accessed on 30th May 2025).

26. Johnston, A. (2020). *Vaccines in Current Culture: The HPV Vaccine Controversy.* https://core.ac.uk/download/322851046.pdf (accessed on 30th May 2025).

27. Kälkner, K., Sundström, A., Nurminen, M. L., Larsson, M., Ljung, R., & Arthurson, V. (2023). Optimizing safety surveillance for COVID-19 vaccines at the Swedish Medical Products Agency. *Drug Safety, 46*, 319–321. https://www.semanticscholar.org/paper/8fa60ae7f6bf8b4188e41d6ef82aeaef5e609898 (accessed on 30th May 2025).

28. Kipterer, J., Touray, K., Godwin, A. U., Cisse, A., Aimee, B. N. M., Busisiwe, N., Demeveng, C. Y., et al. (2024). Geographic information system and information visualization capacity building: Successful polio eradication and current and future challenges in the COVID-19 era for the World Health Organization's African region. *PLOS ONE, 19.* https://www.semanticscholar.org/paper/0b97870c1fc1f4de41c3db3c16ada8c4e8c0a536 (accessed on 30th May 2025).

29. Kumari, P., & Shivom. (2024). Investigating the importance of vaccines and childhood nutrition on improving maternal and child health. *International Journal of Multidisciplinary Research in Science, Engineering and Technology.* https://www.semanticscholar.org/paper/43250fb56deed5041a7f0ee86dd07b1c8f23ffb9 (accessed on 30th May 2025).

30. Larson, H. J., Clarke, R., Jarrett, C., Eckersberger, E., Levine, Z. A., Schulz, W. S., & Paterson, P. (2018). Measuring trust in vaccination: A systematic review. *Human Vaccines & Immunotherapeutics, 14*, 1599–1609. https://doi.org/10.1080/21645515.2018.1459252.

31. Lebdah, M., Abdallah, A., Hamouda, E. E., Elseddawy, N. M., & ElBakrey, R. M. (2024). Protective effectiveness of two vaccination schemes against the prevalent Egyptian strain of Newcastle disease virus genotype VII. *Open Veterinary Journal, 14*, 32–45. https://www.semanticscholar.org/paper/db30e9b90af1fa56e6156bfb07563b1e5ce4989f (accessed on 30th May 2025).

32. Mambetaliyev, M., Kilibayev, S., Kenzhebaeva, M., Sarsenkulova, N., Tabys, S., Valiyeva, A., Muzarap, D., et al. (2024). Field trials of live and inactivated camelpox vaccines in Kazakhstan. *Vaccines, 12.* https://www.semanticscholar.org/paper/fc39ccfee2fe5e5d9df538d1df3a63308c0bed1b (accessed on 30th May 2025).

33. Marzi, A., & Feldmann, H. (2024). Filovirus vaccines as a response paradigm for emerging infectious diseases. *NPJ Vaccines, 9.* https://www.semanticscholar.org/paper/2105ab1d68fe546dd82f60e2d22dd07ad2415d0e (accessed on 30th May 2025).

34. McIndoe, L., Young, A., Davies, C., Vujovich-Dunn, C., Kean, S., Dives, M., & Sheppeard, V. (2025). Provider preference, logistical challenges, or vaccine hesitancy? Analyzing parental decision-making in school vaccination programs: A qualitative study in Sydney, Australia.

Vaccines, 13. https://www.semanticscholar.org/paper/07c7c6af02db2e024b4d29c5374603350b849863 (accessed on 30th May 2025).

35. Mehboob, R. (2024). Advancement of dengue virus vaccine: Progress and challenges. *Pakistan Journal of Health Sciences.* https://www.semanticscholar.org/paper/a8756b0ff8f391f7df96eb55edfba8eec967ac8b (accessed on 30th May 2025).

36. Ming, B. W., Li, L., Huang, H. N., Ma, J. J., Shi, C., Xu, X., Yang, Z., et al. (2024). The effectiveness of national expanded program on immunization with hepatitis A vaccines in the Chinese mainland: Interrupted time-series analysis. *JMIR Public Health and Surveillance, 10.* https://www.semanticscholar.org/paper/108b85926a15f338286dd8e2d59bf90f630c2157 (accessed on 30th May 2025).

37. Mwende, W. G. (2024). The role of vaccination in preventing infectious diseases. *Research Invention Journal of Scientific and Experimental Sciences.* https://www.semanticscholar.org/paper/3f7244a841bf848ad41655f02e5a97f3784a216d (accessed on 30th May 2025).

38. N/A. (2006). *New Approaches to HIV Prevention: Accelerating Research and Ensuring Future Access.* https://core.ac.uk/download/71353396.pdf (accessed on 30th May 2025).

39. N/A. (2012). The update, February 13, 2012. https://core.ac.uk/download/11354793.pdf (accessed on 30th May 2025).

40. Nur, A. F., Rahman, N., & Fadjriah, R. N. (2024). Understanding maternal intentions and behaviors for vaccine preventable diseases (VPD) control: A structural equation modeling analysis. *Jurnal Kesehatan Manarang.* https://www.semanticscholar.org/paper/f9d8b9eed33f4097015d58797260cfbcd873c071 (accessed on 30th May 2025).

41. Orengo, J. C., Rendon, A. M., Lima, B. C., Daniels, V., Saxena, K., Pavelyev, A., & Parellada, C. I. (2025). P-3. Assessing the public health impact of transitioning from a 4-valent to a 9-valent HPV vaccination program in Panama. *Open Forum Infectious Diseases, 12.* https://www.semanticscholar.org/paper/1a384c5783978e596bc39624951dafa31988a023 (accessed on 30th May 2025).

42. Orengo, J. C., Rendon, A. M., Lima, B. C., Pavelyev, A., Daniels, V., Saxena, K., Herrera-Solano, W., et al. (2025a). P-2. Public health and economic impact of implementing gender-neutral vaccination with the 4-valent human papillomavirus vaccine in Costa Rica. *Open Forum Infectious Diseases, 12.* https://www.semanticscholar.org/paper/60ceb04c426ee05ca6c666f2a19fca127f3df60a (accessed on 30th May 2025).

43. Otoguro, T., Wagatsuma, K., Hino, T., The Society of Ambulatory and General Pediatrics, Ichikawa, Y., Purnama, T. B., Sun, Y., et al. (2025b). Antibody responses to mRNA COVID-19 vaccine among healthcare workers in outpatient clinics in Japan. *Vaccines, 13.* https://www.semanticscholar.org/paper/0695cf3a224f8c6067e22b24e5c29730d1bcdd6b (accessed on 30th May 2025).

44. Paul, S. (2024). *Tumor Metastasis: Mechanisms and Prevention.* https://core.ac.uk/download/631531143.pdf (accessed on 30th May 2025).

45. Pavia, G., Branda, F., Ciccozzi, A., Romano, C., Locci, C., Azzena, I., Pascale, N., et al. (2024). Integrating digital health solutions with immunization strategies: Improving immunization coverage and monitoring in the post-COVID-19 era. *Vaccines, 12.* https://www.semanticscholar.org/paper/261415276b6bd0e4a7b88b177a42eaea0bb59b41 (accessed on 30th May 2025).

46. Perdrizet, J. E., Ta, A., Huang, L., Wannaadisai, W., Ilic, A., Hayford, K., & Sabra, A. (2025). Delayed

transition to 20-valent pneumococcal conjugate vaccine in pediatric national immunization programs: Forgone public health and economic benefit. *Infectious Diseases and Therapy, 14*, 501–525. https://www.semanticscholar.org/paper/a3bfcd3914470f8ddf0f441f290b627ed3b82cb1 (accessed on 30th May 2025).

47. Phuntsho, S., Tshokey, T., Gurung, M. S., Wangdi, S., Wangdi, S., & Wangchuk, S. (2022). An exemplary national COVID-19 vaccination: Lessons from Bhutan. *Tropical Medicine and Infectious Disease, 7*, 131–131. https://doi.org/10.3390/tropicalmed7070131.

48. Regan, A. K., & Muñoz, F. M. (2021). Efficacy and safety of influenza vaccination during pregnancy: Realizing the potential of maternal influenza immunization. *Expert Review of Vaccines, 20*, 649–660. https://doi.org/10.1080/14760584.2021.1915138.

49. Rifqi, A. I., Hertiana, Tubuon, Y. N., Hariani, Rahma, S., & Indar. (2024). Ethical dilemma in vaccination in Indonesia: Balance between public health obligations and individual autonomy rights. *Promotif: Jurnal Kesehatan Masyarakat.* https://www.semanticscholar.org/paper/2e8ec41814b6bba3320507e926f4c0eace42eb45 (accessed on 30th May 2025).

50. Sathian, B., Asim, M., Banerjee, I., Roy, B., Pizzaro, A. B., Mancha, M. A., Van Teijlingen, E., et al. (2021). Development and implementation of a potential coronavirus disease 2019 (COVID-19) vaccine: A systematic review and meta-analysis of vaccine clinical trials. *Deleted Journal, 11*, 959–982. https://doi.org/10.3126/nje.v11i1.36163.

51. Schmidt, M., Jóhannesdóttir Schmidt, S. A., Adelborg, K., Sundbøll, J., Laugesen, K., Ehrenstein, V., & Sørensen, H. T. (2019). The Danish health care system and epidemiological research: From health care contacts to database records. *Clinical Epidemiology, 11*, 563–591. https://doi.org/10.2147/clep.s179083.

52. Shapovalova, V. (2025). Human metapneumovirus: Modern challenges for medicine and pharmaceutics. *SSP Modern Pharmacy and Medicine.* https://www.semanticscholar.org/paper/fc6db59542eeb9919d25f073efddf248fa593a5a (accessed on 30th May 2025).

53. Sun, C., Zuo, T., & Wen, Z. (2023). First clinical study of germline-targeting strategy: One step closer to a successful bnAb-based HIV vaccine. *The Innovation, 4*, 100374. https://doi.org/10.1016/j.xinn.2023.100374.

54. Tebruegge, M., Ritz, N., Curtis, N., & Shingadia, D. (2015). Diagnostic tests for childhood tuberculosis. *The Pediatric Infectious Disease Journal, 34*, 1014–1019. https://doi.org/10.1097/inf.0000000000000796.

55. V'kovski, P., Kratzel, A., Steiner, S., Stalder, H., & Thiel, V. (2020). Coronavirus biology and replication: Implications for SARS-CoV-2. *Nature Reviews Microbiology, 19*, 155–170. https://doi.org/10.1038/s41579-020-00468-6.

56. Wang, G. J., & Shao, M. (2022). [Analysis of the development status and trend of vaccines in China's immunization program in the past decade]. *Zhonghua Yu Fang Yi Xue Za Zhi [Chinese Journal of Preventive Medicine], 56*(6), 878–883. https://www.semanticscholar.org/paper/adb3380af0b603932f4b91da7a9f3f66b26ecd5c (accessed on 30th May 2025).

57. Zhang, S., Liu, G., Zhang, Y., Wang, C., Xu, X., Zhao, Y., Xiang, Z., et al. (2024). Investigation of the safety and protective efficacy of an attenuated and marker *M. bovis-BoHV-1* combined vaccine in bovines. *Frontiers in Immunology, 15.* https://www.semanticscholar.org/paper/24fe4fd792674748de614644f0f03496d24ef83c (accessed on 30th May 2025).

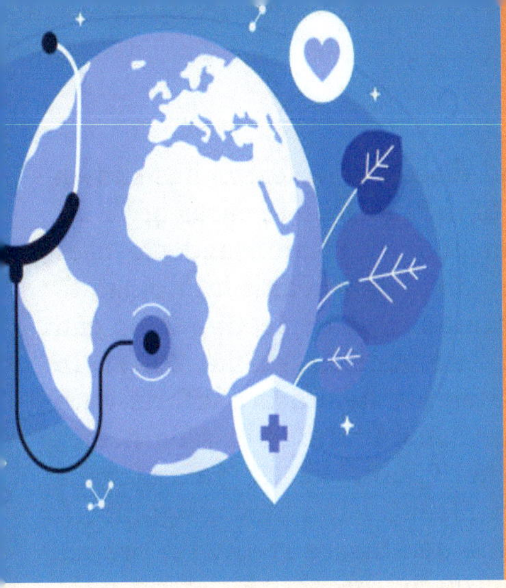

Chapter 10

INFECTIOUS DISEASE AND GLOBAL HEALTH

Contents

Introduction

Infectious diseases have long been a pivotal aspect of global health, exerting a profound impact on populations worldwide. As emerging pathogens continue to threaten public well-being, understanding the complexities of these diseases becomes increasingly critical. The declaration of monkeypox (mpox) as a public health emergency of international concern by the WHO in July 2022 exemplifies the urgent need for global vigilance. By July 2023, there were 88,288 confirmed cases and 149 deaths from mpox, which highlights how these diseases can spread worldwide and put health systems under pressure. The role of frontline healthcare workers, particularly nurses, emerges as a crucial element in addressing such outbreaks, as their resilience and adaptability are tested amid ever-evolving circumstances, thereby highlighting the complexities of managing infectious diseases within the framework of global health (Ahmed et al., 2024). Besides the problems caused by certain infectious diseases, the environment has a significant impact on public health. To develop effective health policies, it is essential to understand how air, water, and soil pollution can cause and spread diseases. Research has shown that environmental damage caused by climate change contributes to the increase in cases of VBDs, such as malaria and dengue fever. Additionally, the link between poor sanitation and diseases such as cholera underscores the importance of incorporating environmental health into plans to combat infectious diseases. Mitigating these ecological risks is paramount, as neglecting them can create a fertile ground for outbreaks and subsequent public health emergencies (Yadika, 2024). To address infectious diseases and environmental issues, we must integrate healthcare efforts with those to protect the environment. Policymakers need to encourage collaboration between health and environmental agencies to develop sustainable measures that help public health. Taking steps to reduce pollution, improve water quality, and upgrade healthcare facilities can play a significant role in stopping infectious diseases. Additionally, providing frontline healthcare staff with proper training and mental health care will better prepare them for future outbreaks. By fostering a holistic understanding of the interconnectedness between infectious diseases and environmental health, a more resilient global health system can be established, better prepared for the challenges of tomorrow (Ahmed et al., 2024; Yadika, 2024) (Figure 10.1).

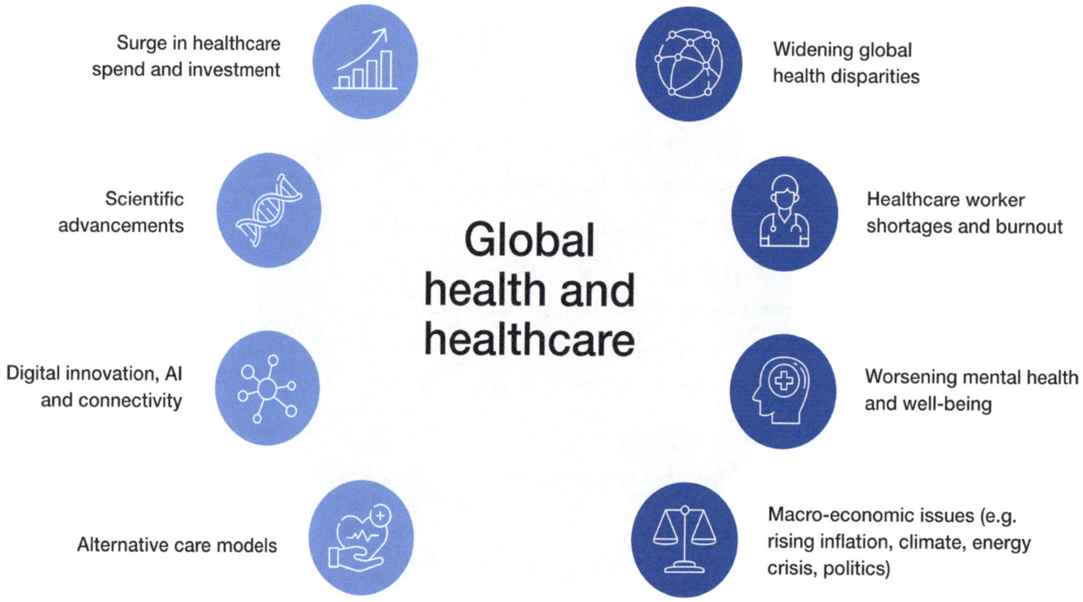

Figure 10.1. Infectious diseases and global health.

Source: https://www.gavi.org/sites/default/files/vaccineswork/2023/Thumbnail/K4WtoM2Z-WyAFpXdzFgrvf3-7kZAKGdBM90ks-w7rDU_h2.jpg.

Definition of Infectious Diseases

Infectious diseases are ailments caused by pathogenic microorganisms, including bacteria, viruses, fungi, and parasites. These diseases can be transmitted between individuals or environmental sources, leading to substantial morbidity and mortality on a global scale. How diseases are transmitted can be very different, including direct contact, airborne spread, or through insects, which makes it harder for public health to stop outbreaks. Respiratory viruses such as those responsible for influenza and COVID-19 can quickly infect large numbers of people and result in worldwide health emergencies. Additionally, to understand how infectious diseases function, we must examine both the pathogens and the environmental and social conditions that influence their spread and impact. Besides medical outcomes, infectious diseases are tied to major public health concerns. AMR is now a significant problem, making infections more common and severe around the world. In fact, a landmark study estimated that in 2019, there were approximately 4.95 million deaths associated with bacterial AMR, illustrating the profound health risks that resistant pathogens pose to populations (Murray et al., 2022). Additionally, the pressure is heaviest in regions with limited resources, as their healthcare systems may not be adequately prepared to handle both the infections and their drug-resistant forms. Dealing with AMR is essential to reduce the number of infectious diseases and deaths, and it involves improving infection prevention. A multifaceted understanding of infectious diseases must also consider the commercial determinants of health (CDoH) that influence their prevalence and management. Recent scholarly work highlights the significance of market forces in shaping health outcomes, revealing that economic conditions, access to healthcare, and policy decisions play crucial roles in addressing infectious disease outbreaks (Freudenberg et al., 2021). If public health experts consider commercial factors when thinking about contagious diseases, they can develop more effective strategies to manage both infectious and noninfectious diseases. It highlights the interconnectedness of health problems and advocates for collaboration among different sectors to enhance global health. So, to define infectious diseases means considering the ways pathogens, healthcare and social and economic factors interact.

Importance of Global Health

The significance of global health is underscored by its direct impact on the prevention and control of infectious diseases, which transcend borders and affect populations worldwide. Due to highly contagious pathogens, nations must unite and establish effective surveillance and response systems. By acknowledging the interconnectedness of global health, policymakers can work towards enhancing frameworks such as the International Health Regulations (IHR 2005), which serve to mitigate the spread of diseases. They improve health services in the area and help protect the world from future outbreaks, benefiting everyone. The governance mechanisms surrounding these regulations can often dictate the level of preparedness nations have against infectious threats, highlighting the essential role of international cooperation in safeguarding global health (Anaemene et al., 2016). Furthermore, disease surveillance networks (DSNs) have emerged as pivotal components in the global health landscape, especially in light of the challenges presented by EIDs. Programs like the DSN have been necessary because they encourage cooperation between many sectors and fields, which is required to understand how diseases change over time. Such networks are reported to improve the speed at which diseases are identified and managed. Strong cooperation between countries within these frameworks can make disease surveillance more effective and accurate, which helps control outbreaks rapidly and lowers the rates of sickness and death. As noted in assessments of the DSN Initiative, the strategic deployment of philanthropic resources can further optimise these networks, paving the way for a more resilient global health infrastructure (Kimball et al., 2011). Last but not least, including global health initiatives in national plans is extremely important. Health governance in countries should be based on global guidelines and also fit the needs of local communities. Ebola Virus Disease in Nigeria demonstrated that having strong health systems and flexible laws is crucial. Improving these systems is necessary for countries to handle future public health emergencies well. Continued support for laws, teamwork among institutions, and new policies is needed to enable countries to both deal with current diseases and be ready for unexpected ones. Thus, addressing the importance of global health is not merely an academic exercise; it is a practical necessity that hinges on collective actions and shared responsibilities in the interconnected world (Anaemene et al., 2016) (Figure 10.2).

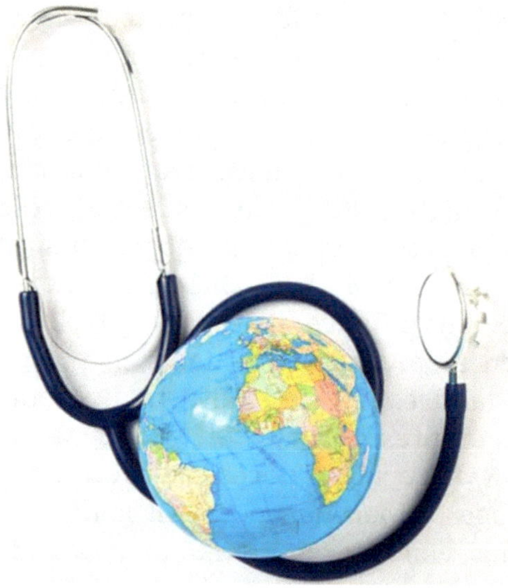

Figure 10.2. Global health.

Source: https://thumbor.forbes.com/thumbor/fit-in/900x510/https://www.forbes.com/advisor/wp-content/uploads/2023/05/global-health.jpeg.jpg.

10.1. Historical Context of Infectious Diseases

Throughout history, infectious diseases have played a significant role in shaping human societies, affecting populations, economies, and public health policies. Major pandemics like the Black Death in the 14th century resulted in many deaths and had a significant impact on society. Because the plague killed approximately one-third of Europeans, there were fewer workers, which led to the decline of feudalism and the emergence of a new economic system. This pandemic also highlighted the interconnection between global health and public health systems, as well as areas for improvement. Such historical events emphasize the crucial need for equitable healthcare access and disease preparedness, as the impact of infectious diseases is often disproportionately felt by marginalized communities, reflecting systemic inequalities that persist today (Domingo, 2020). In recent years, the emergence of new infectious diseases has made it clear how pandemics have occurred and repeated themselves throughout history. In the early 2000s, several outbreaks of infectious diseases occurred, including the SARS epidemic in 2003 and the H1N1 influenza pandemic in 2009. Both events demonstrated that different nations were not equally prepared, which had an impact on global health governance. This also showed that globalization and increased travel increase the speed of disease spread, so nations must cooperate to handle the problem effectively. The COVID-19 pandemic has brought these historical lessons to the forefront, illustrating that despite advanced medical technologies and knowledge, societies remain vulnerable to infectious disease threats due to inequities in healthcare systems (Bashshur et al., 2020). Understanding the history of infectious diseases highlights the importance of addressing social issues in addition to treating the illness directly. Examining past pandemics, it is evident that socio-economic factors, including healthcare, education, and living conditions, have a significant impact on the unequal outcomes of infectious diseases. Furthermore, examining past epidemiological data can support current public health measures, informing risk messages, vaccination plans, and community engagement strategies. As we navigate the complexities of global health in the wake of the COVID-19 pandemic, learning from past epidemics is essential for formulating policies that not only mitigate the impact of infectious diseases but also promote health equity on a global scale (Domingo, 2020) (Figure 10.3).

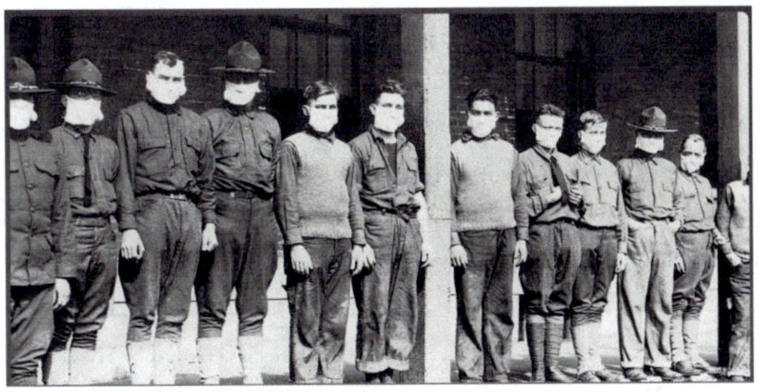

Figure 10.3. History infectious diseases.

Source: https://www.google.com/search?q=Historical+Context+of+Infectious+Diseases&sca_esv=d204c5fe6303d08c.

10.1.1. Major Pandemics in History

Throughout history, pandemics have had a profound impact on societies, economies, and public health systems. The Black Death, which spread through Europe in the 14th century, is remembered as one of the worst pandemics, taking away an estimated 25 million lives and leaving many communities destroyed. As a result, the population underwent changes, social and economic systems were altered, and significant changes occurred in healthcare. During the 1918 influenza pandemic, which affected approximately one-third of the world's population and resulted in over 50 million deaths, similar trends emerged. Both pandemics highlighted the crucial role that public health measures and interventions play during outbreaks. Policymakers learned that understanding disease transmission and implementing rapid responses are vital components in combating infectious diseases and safeguarding global health, as emphasized in several analyses of prior pandemics (Sirleaf et al., 2021). In more contemporary times, the Ebola and Zika viruses (ZIKV) exemplify the ongoing challenges of EIDs. During the Ebola outbreak in West Africa from 2014 to 2016, over 11,000 people died, and the event made it clear that health systems should be ready for epidemics. It revealed that the healthcare infrastructure was insufficient and that countries must cooperate more effectively in managing outbreaks. At the same time, the ZIKV epidemic caused many people to fear it because it was linked to severe birth defects. They demonstrated that understanding disease vectors, the mechanisms by which diseases are spread, and engaging with the community are essential for effective prevention. The lessons drawn from these experiences align with the recommendations from the Independent Panel for Pandemic Preparedness and Response, which stress the need for integrated health strategies essential for both current and future infectious disease threats (Rogerson et al., 2020). The COVID-19 pandemic, for instance, demonstrated that global health crises have widespread and complex effects. Because SARS-CoV-2 spread so quickly, many countries have seen that their healthcare systems are not fully ready for pandemics and are now reconsidering their preparedness. Late responses and the fact that some people cannot get vaccines have added to the health disparities seen during earlier pandemics. The crisis also highlighted that when resources are stretched, gains in controlling other diseases, such as malaria, can be easily lost. COVID-19 responses are causing disruptions to health initiatives that fought malaria, which could result in serious public health issues. Ultimately, understanding these historical and current health emergencies is paramount in shaping effective global health strategies aimed at preventing future pandemics from inflicting similar devastation (Rogerson et al., 2020; Sirleaf et al., 2021).

10.1.2. Evolution of Public Health Responses

The evolution of public health responses to infectious diseases reflects a dynamic interplay between societal needs, scientific advancements, and global interconnectivity. Typically, efforts to combat contagious diseases are initiated only after a major outbreak has occurred. The appearance of cholera in the 19th century spurred the development of public health systems, which contributed to the establishment of modern epidemiology. In the past few decades, the appearance of SARS and Ebola has shown that traditional public health approaches are not enough. These outbreaks demonstrated that existing protocols needed to evolve to address complexities arising from global travel, urbanization, and ecological distress, which are now recognized as key factors in disease transmission (Borda et al., 2022). Due to these transformations, it is evident that enhanced teamwork is necessary to ensure prompt responses and effective resource utilisation. Given the world's current challenges with numerous infectious diseases, including COVID-19, it is evident that public health policies must be flexible. The pandemic made it clear that rapid analysis of data and teamwork among countries are key to successful public health actions. Experiences from previous epidemics, such as Ebola, have shown that trust and involvement of communities are crucial for effective public health measures. In such circumstances, mathematical models are crucial for predicting the spread of diseases and for informing policy decisions. By analyzing past failures and successes, researchers advocate for an integrated approach that combines technological advancements with community-based strategies (Ali et al., 2023). Given that infectious diseases can change unexpectedly, policies need to be flexible and use data. Emerging technologies, such as artificial intelligence (AI), are poised to profoundly reshape the landscape of public health responses. Using AI in disease surveillance systems can significantly enhance the way data is collected, analysed, and utilised for immediate public health action. It can help predict outbreaks and build early warning systems that respond better to new infectious diseases. At the same time, the use of AI in public health raises concerns about who makes decisions and how much control individuals have. The examples of COVID-19 and other recent outbreaks show that technology and public health policy must be considered together. Addressing these challenges requires a responsible AI framework that considers the ethical implications while ensuring agile and data-informed responses to health emergencies (Borda et al., 2022; Ali et al., 2023). Balancing innovative technological applications with community needs is paramount for effective and equitable public health outcomes in the context of our interconnected world (Figure 10.4).

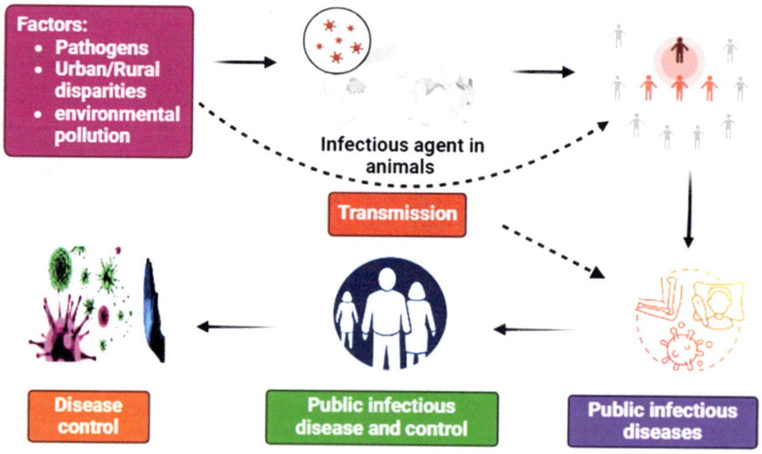

Figure 10.4. The evolution of public health responses.

Source: https://www.frontiersin.org/files/Articles/1423191/fpubh-12-1423191-HTML/image_m/fpubh-12-1423191-g001.jpg.

10.1.3. Impact of Historical Outbreaks on Society

The impact of historical outbreaks on society is profound and multifaceted, often reshaping demographic, social, and economic landscapes. Notably, the Black Death of the 14th century created a demographic void in Europe, leading to significant shifts in labour dynamics and social structures. Due to the sudden population decline, a shortage of workers emerged, prompting surviving workers to demand better pay and job conditions. The major shift in society and the economy led to the decline of feudalism and the rise of a market-based system. Furthermore, the mental impact of these epidemics led to significant changes in how society viewed health, which in turn encouraged progress in medicine and public health. Due to these lessons, current societies must adopt flexible health policies and effective strategies for managing future infectious disease outbreaks. Epidemics can influence both culture and politics in addition to affecting people's health. As another example, the 1918 influenza pandemic resulted in millions of deaths and prompted people to reassess public health systems and policies, emphasising the need for prevention and monitoring. Because nations recognised the need for prepared healthcare, they established health commissions and collaborated with other countries, which remains essential today. In the past, outbreaks have led to shifts in political beliefs, which have often granted authorities greater power to enforce public health regulations. Many people continue to discuss the balance between civil liberties and the use of technology to track public health during modern epidemics. These examples prove that the way societies are organized plays a big part in how infectious diseases develop, and past outbreaks still have a lasting impact on how public health is managed today. Additionally, the social and cultural aspects of responding to epidemics underscore the critical role that science and community involvement play in tandem. Often, historical outbreaks make it clear that marginalized people are more affected than the rest of the population. The outbreaks of Ebola in West Africa made it clear that communities were dealing with health problems and also with doubts and false information, which slowed down the efforts to control the disease. Handling such emergency calls requires detailed scientific modeling and also a respect for local customs and beliefs to motivate the community to take part in health activities. Integrating traditional ways and local customs into public health plans makes them more culturally appropriate and effective. The historical context of infectious disease responses emphasizes that overcoming health crises necessitates a collaborative approach, where science and society work hand in hand to build resilience against future outbreaks, as highlighted by the imperative of comprehensive infectious disease modelling, which integrates both technical and sociocultural narratives (Huang et al., 2024; Macauley, 2024).

10.2. Current Global Infectious Diseases

The prevalence and spread of infectious diseases on a global scale have become increasingly complex due to various interrelated factors, particularly climate change. Climate change has caused malaria and dengue to be found in more areas of Asia, sub-Saharan Africa, and South America. Due to climate change, there is growing concern that certain diseases may spread into temperate regions if greenhouse gas emissions remain high. The 2018 West Nile virus outbreak in Europe was exacerbated by early spring temperatures, highlighting the need for public health systems to respond to such changes. As climate change continues to drive alterations in disease distribution, understanding and addressing these influences is crucial to implementing effective global health responses to infectious diseases (Semenza et al., 2022). Because of the COVID-19 pandemic, it is now more evident that knowing how the virus spreads is important for public health. Airborne transmission seems to be a significant factor in spreading SARS-CoV-2, which means that only considering droplet and surface transmission is no longer sufficient. It is now clear that infectious aerosols may remain in the air for a long time, making some safe-looking places still risky. It means that earlier public health practices, which mainly focused on direct contact and disinfection, now need to be reconsidered. So, governments and health organisations should prioritise better ventilation, encourage wearing masks, and make sure there are fewer people indoors at the same time. Such a shift is crucial to mitigate transmission risks and reinforce public health initiatives aimed at mitigating the pandemic's global impact (Greenhalgh et al., 2021).

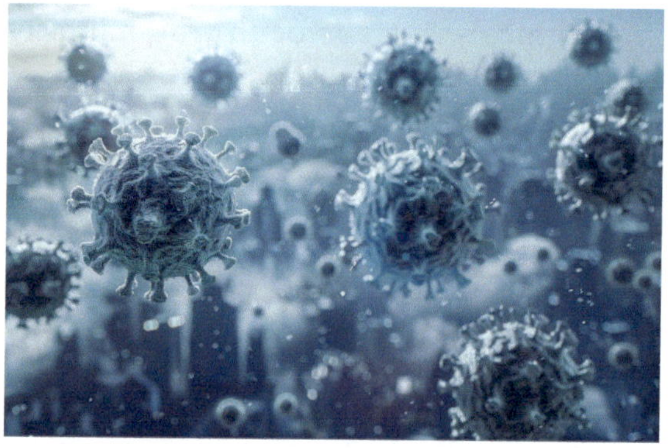

Figure 10.5. Current global infectious diseases.

Source: https://scitechdaily.com/images/Global-Virus-Pandemic-Concept-1536x1024.jpg.

Because climate change and infectious diseases are connected, global health requires a joint and active strategy. Changes in weather patterns can help diseases like schistosomiasis and those spread by ticks to spread, and they can also cause a rise in waterborne diseases that have been in decline. A combination of climate change, population migration, urban expansion, and international trade leads to a situation where health impacts can include many outbreaks. Global health systems need to encourage interdisciplinary teams of experts to understand how environmental changes impact the spread of infectious diseases. By fostering resilience in public health infrastructure, countries can improve their preparedness for future challenges posed by infectious diseases exacerbated by climate variability (Semenza et al., 2022) (Figure 10.5).

10.2.1. Overview of Prevalent Infectious Diseases

Infectious diseases represent a significant challenge to global health, with a range of pathogens causing widespread morbidity and mortality across diverse populations. Pneumonia and influenza are still important causes of death, mainly in countries where access to healthcare is limited. When new diseases emerge and older ones evolve, it is crucial to focus on their spread and develop effective responses. The COVID-19 pandemic made it clear that global health systems are not robust enough, as the disease can quickly impact daily life, the economy, and healthcare services. Municipal waste, particularly plastic and infectious waste generated during such outbreaks, has placed additional pressure on environmental management systems, highlighting the intersection between public health and ecological sustainability (Septiariva et al., 2022). AMR is becoming a bigger problem that makes infectious diseases more challenging to manage. In 2019, it was believed that nearly 4.95 million people died due to bacterial AMR, and lower respiratory infections played a significant role. AMR-related deaths are often caused by various antibiotic-resistant bacteria, which points to the urgent need for solutions to address them. Areas with a lack of clean water, sanitation, and proper medical care suffer the most from AMR, which increases health inequalities worldwide. This situation necessitates rigorous public health policies that prioritise infection prevention, antibiotic stewardship, and the development of new therapeutics (Murray et al., 2022). Dealing with AMR requires using local approaches and collaborating globally to ensure equal access to healthcare. Socio-economic issues, like poverty, crowding, and not having enough access to healthcare, help infections spread. Tuberculosis, malaria, and HIV/AIDS mainly affect people from marginalised groups, which helps maintain poverty and poor health. The presence of communicable diseases highlights the importance of healthcare strategies that address social and economic factors. Moreover, when vaccination programs improve and countries cooperate for disease monitoring, infectious diseases have less of an effect in places with limited resources. By fostering comprehensive public health initiatives and addressing structural inequalities, the global community can work towards reducing the burden of infectious diseases, ultimately improving the overall health status of populations across the globe (Figure 10.6).

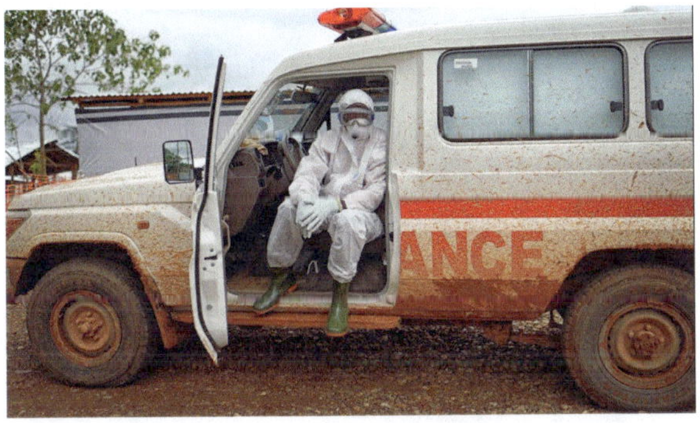

Figure 10.6. Infectious diseases represent a significant challenge to global health.

Source: https://cdn.who.int/media/images/default-source/big-stories/ten-threats-to-global-health/emergencies.tmb-1200v.jpg?sfvrsn=881196a4_4.

10.2.2. Geographic Distribution and Demographics

The geographic distribution of infectious diseases illustrates significant disparities influenced by environmental, climatic, and socio-economic factors. Regions that support high densities of human or animal populations are particularly vulnerable to outbreaks, as seen with the recent emergence of Highly Pathogenic Avian Influenza (HPAI) in the United States. This outbreak, which involved 232 cases and resulted in $950 million in economic damage, underscores that certain regions, such as the Midwest and coastal areas, are more susceptible to these diseases. Making detailed suitability maps with species distribution modelling can help detect risks linked to infectious agents. Consequently, understanding these demographic patterns becomes critical for effective interventions and enhancing preparedness, as data not only reflect current distributions but also guide future preventive strategies against similar outbreaks (Alkhamis et al., 2016). The way infectious diseases spread is strongly linked to One Health, which highlights the importance of human, animal, and environmental health together. As we learn more about how these areas relate, it is essential to understand geographic differences in order to effectively address global health problems. It is clear from the One Health approach that where a population resides, such as in rural or urban areas, can shape the ways diseases are transmitted and the associated risks. Due to urbanisation and climate change, the distribution of infectious diseases will also shift. Consequently, integrating demographic data from human populations, animal health indicators, and environmental assessments becomes vital for developing effective surveillance and intervention strategies (COHERE Expert Review Group et al., 2017). Seeing the big picture is crucial for addressing the challenges posed by infectious diseases worldwide. Using both geographic and demographic information, public health professionals can design strategies that address the issues of each region. For example, places with a high chance of zoonotic diseases should receive special attention with focused surveillance and early action programs that involve the community. Health authorities use demographic data and changes in the environment, such as climate and landscapes, to predict when diseases might spread. Also, combining knowledge from different fields and including the views of experts in human and veterinary medicine greatly improves the study of disease patterns. These approaches establish a foundation for robust evidence-based public health recommendations aimed at protecting both human and animal populations while maintaining environmental integrity (Alkhamis et al., 2016; COHERE Expert Review Group et al., 2017).

10.2.3. Emerging Infectious Diseases and Their Threats

Emerging infectious diseases (EIDs) pose a significant threat to global health, characterised by the rapid evolution of pathogens and their ability to exploit ecological changes. Urbanisation, changes in climate, and globalisation help these diseases to appear and spread, sometimes making it possible for them to jump between different species as humans move into areas where wildlife lives. The chances of zoonotic diseases such as Ebola and COVID-19 rise. Healthcare and illness management now pay particular attention to how modern biomedical technologies interact with newly found pathogenic microbes.

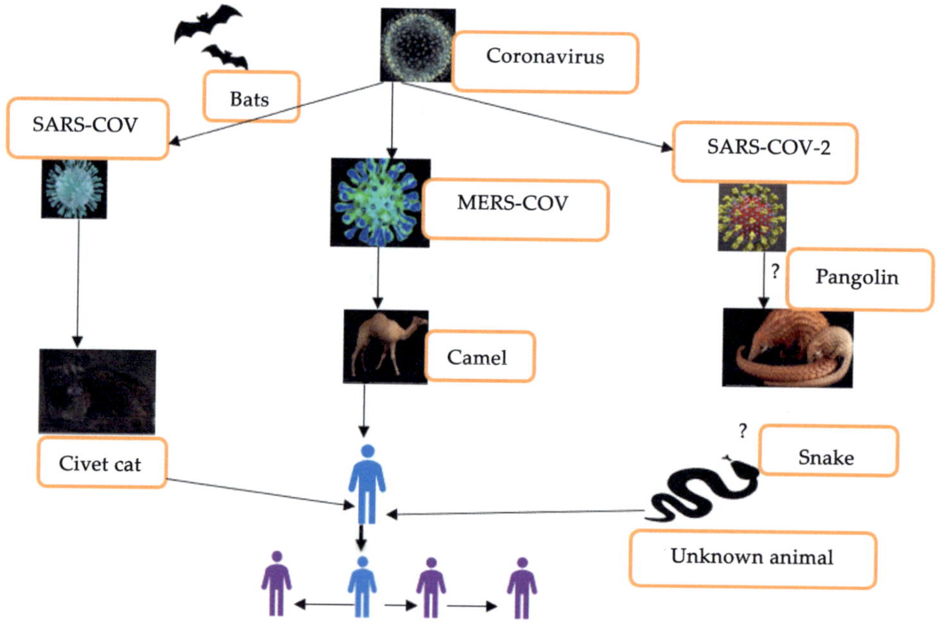

Figure 10.7. Emerging infectious diseases pose a significant threat to global health.

Source: https://www.clinmedjournals.org/articles/ijva/ijva-7-067-004.jpg.

While advances in medical science offer promising diagnostic tools and treatments, they also reveal vulnerabilities in the ability to predict and respond to emerging infectious threats, emphasising the need for an adaptive and comprehensive public health strategy (Umesh et al., 2024). Epidemiological tools are essential for controlling EIDs, especially where resources are limited. Ecological and socio-economic factors in Zambia make the infectious disease landscape there quite distinct. Scientists use detailed methods, such as analysing space and studying genes, to determine how common and easily transmitted these diseases are. Using this approach, investigators assess whether these tools are effective and apply them, providing valuable information for informed public health decisions. Even so, having enough resources and reliable data remains a problem that complicates the response to infectious disease outbreaks. Consequently, there is a need for the ongoing refinement and adaptation of these epidemiological tools to effectively address emerging health threats, particularly in regions most affected by these diseases (Arthur et al., 2023). Working together, technology and public health policies are crucial in mitigating the risks of EIDs. New techniques in genomic sequencing and data analysis can help us spot new pathogens more quickly and correctly. However, this should be supported by a robust infrastructure that enables countries and regions to respond quickly and collaborate effectively. In addition, telling the public about the risks of new diseases is crucial for preventing them. If global health experts use teamwork, technology, epidemiology, and community support, they can better face and reduce the impacts of EIDs. Overall, a multidisciplinary approach is necessary to successfully tackle these public health challenges and protect vulnerable populations globally (Figure 10.7).

10.3. Transmission and Prevention

The dynamics of transmission are critical when understanding the spread of infectious diseases, particularly in the context of global health. There are many ways pathogens can spread, including through droplets from the mouth and nose, contaminated water, and insects such as mosquitoes. Such transmission routes are affected by the environment, the density of population in an area, and people's habits. A detailed study reveals that traditional tracing methods often overlook the complex aspects of these interactions in mixed populations. Pertinently, developments like the Heterogeneous Hypergraph Attention Network (HHAN) model have emerged to address these complexities better. The model can account for different ways diseases can spread, which helps public health officials to predict outbreaks more accurately. By identifying and analysing these transmission routes, researchers can formulate more effective and targeted interventions, ultimately transforming our approach to epidemic management (He et al., 2025). It is necessary to employ various methods to prevent infectious diseases, considering the ways they are spread and the different local conditions worldwide. Among all preventative steps, vaccination is beneficial for respiratory diseases, since airborne infections can quickly cause outbreaks. Still, the effectiveness of these interventions can vary significantly, typically depending on the accessibility of healthcare in different regions and the level of public compliance. For instance, in many low- and middle-income countries (LMICs), the challenge lies not only in vaccine availability but also in public education and healthcare infrastructure. Besides vaccines, actions such as controlling insects and improving cleanliness are also crucial for controlling malaria and cholera, which are spread through the environment. This necessitates a tailored approach in prevention strategies that reflect local contexts while also considering global disparities in healthcare access (Almatrood et al., 2024). Along with making vaccines and sanitation available, it is essential to involve the community to sustain prevention efforts. Influencing people about disease prevention and transmission is best done through behavioural change initiatives. Educating the community about the ways infections spread and the value of good hygiene can give them more control. Also, local influencers can help communities become more open to health messages. Incorporating local traditions and experiences into health promotion plans can make these efforts more effective and more welcomed by the community. As the landscape of infectious diseases evolves with globalisation and climate change, these community-centred approaches offer a promising avenue for sustaining public engagement and advancing global health outcomes (Almatrood et al., 2024; He et al., 2025).

10.3.1. Modes of Transmission

Understanding the modes of transmission is vital for comprehending how infectious diseases spread globally. Infectious agents can be transmitted through multiple pathways, including direct contact, vector-borne transmission, airborne routes, and more. When pathogens are spread from one person to another through direct contact, such as touching, hugging, or sexual contact, this is known as direct contact transmission. Close personal contact is significant for transmitting HIV/AIDS and other sexually transmitted infections. Additionally, public health measures such as informing the public and vaccinating individuals can significantly reduce the spread of infections through contact during outbreaks. In addition to being transmitted directly, some diseases can also be spread by insects and ticks, posing a significant problem in tropical and subtropical regions. Vectors, such as mosquitoes, ticks, and fleas, transmit pathogens from one host to another, making diseases like malaria, dengue, and Crimean-Congo Hemorrhagic Fever (CCHF) notorious for their global impact. The interaction between vectors, human behavior, and environmental conditions adds to the complexity of disease transmission. For example, CCHF is primarily transmitted through tick bites and contact with infected animal blood. Individuals who work with animals, such as livestock workers and those in slaughterhouses, are at a higher risk of contracting it. This underscores the need for a multi-faceted approach to public health, emphasising vector control and awareness of the risks associated with certain occupations (Srivastava et al., 2024). Vaccinating people is an effective way to prevent diseases from being transmitted through various means. The dynamics of vaccination can drastically alter the landscape of infectious disease spread, as evidenced in models assessing the impact of vaccination against diseases like hand, foot, and mouth disease (HFMD). They demonstrate that strategic immunisation can reduce the number of infections and the rate at which the disease spreads, thereby helping healthcare systems cope. Vaccination benefits individuals and helps prevent the spread of diseases among community members. By prioritizing vaccination in public health agendas, countries can bolster their defenses against endemic and epidemic scenarios, particularly in regions where diseases exhibit complex transmission patterns (Alqahtani et al., 2025) (Figure 10.8).

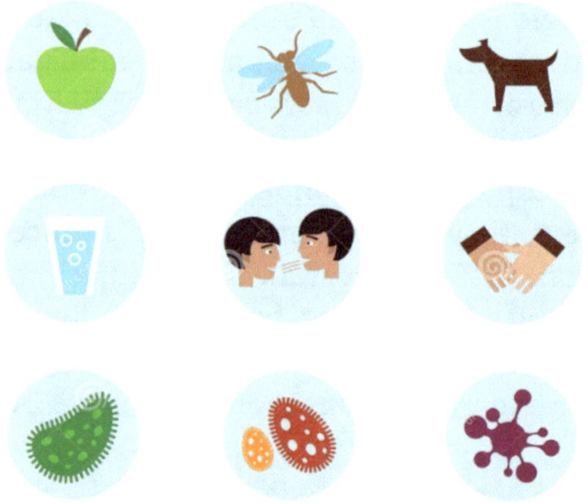

Figure 10.8. Mode of transmission.

Source: https://thumbs.dreamstime.com/z/viral-diseases-modes-transmission-icons-their-vector-illustration-96854324.jpg.

10.3.2. Vaccination and Immunisation Strategies

Vaccination and immunisation strategies are vital components in addressing infectious diseases globally, particularly as the world grapples with emerging pathogens. These methods have shown strong results in stopping diseases such as measles, polio, and COVID-19. Vaccination campaigns need to support strong healthcare systems and fair policies for everyone. For example, when countries allocate more resources to healthcare, they tend to have a higher vaccination rate, which in turn reduces the number of cases of contagious diseases. Furthermore, these infrastructures not only facilitate the administration of vaccines but also support education efforts that help mitigate misinformation surrounding immunisation, ultimately leading to better public health outcomes (Gadelha et al., 2021). New ways to produce and distribute vaccines are essential for developing good immunisation plans. The rapid development of mRNA vaccines for COVID-19 demonstrates the power of biotechnology in responding to health emergencies. It illustrates why investing in research and development for vaccines is essential to be ready for future infectious disease outbreaks. Suppose public health and pharmaceutical companies work together. In that case, collaborate, it can help make vaccines more affordable and accessible in areas with limited resources. Addressing the technological and economic disparities in vaccine production is crucial for achieving universal immunisation coverage, as this can avert potential crises similar to the widespread impacts of COVID-19 (Evanega et al., 2020). Tackling the misinformation about vaccines is very important for successful immunisation plans. The pandemic has made it clear that misinformation about vaccines can prevent many from getting vaccinated, which can severely affect public health. Health authorities should utilise precise and reliable information to explain vaccination programs, thereby helping people regain trust in them. The difficulty lies in addressing misinformation and disinformation, as these can significantly influence how people perceive vaccines and decide whether to get them. If public health officials use clear messages and involve community leaders, they can help people accept vaccines more easily. Ultimately, a collective effort that integrates education, research, and transparent communication will fortify global immunization strategies, ensuring healthier populations worldwide (Evanega et al., 2020) (Figure 10.9).

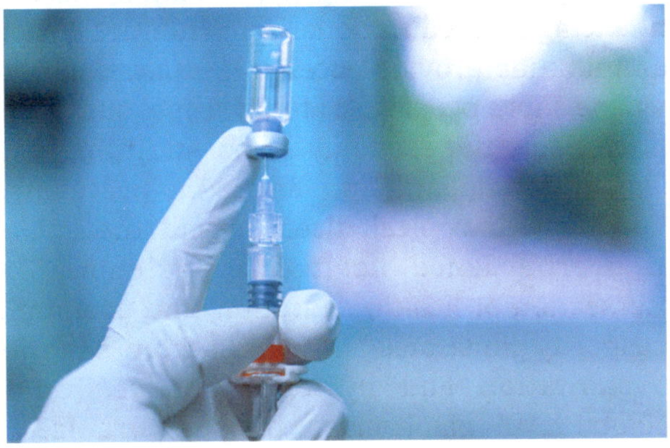

Figure 10.9. Vaccination and immunization strategies.

Source: https://research.unimelb.edu.au/_data/assets/image/0008/4497605/Vaccine Rabies NeedleMedical DoctorHospitalShutterstock.jpg.

10.3.3. Role of Sanitation and Hygiene in Prevention

Sanitation and hygiene play a crucial role in preventing infectious diseases, serving as fundamental public health measures. If people have clean water, proper toilets, and good hygiene habits, it becomes much less likely for diarrhoea, cholera, and dysentery to spread. These diseases are most common in areas where people live in poverty, and they strongly affect children and women. Global health organisations emphasise that poor sanitation and hygiene facilitate the spread of diseases, hindering progress in health and development. The integration of sanitation measures into communal living advancements and the education of individuals regarding hygiene practices can shift the trajectory of public health in regions plagued by infectious diseases, underlining the necessity of investment in WASH (Water, Sanitation, and Hygiene) initiatives that focus on sustainable and equitable access to these essential services (Mills et al.,

2016). Besides fighting immediate diseases, sanitation and hygiene help improve the social and economic conditions of people. For example, improved sanitation helps children, especially girls, stay in school during menstruation, thereby enhancing their educational opportunities. When communities provide accessible sanitation and hygiene, more people can attend school and learn, which helps the economy grow. Additionally, a clean environment helps reduce the prevalence of neglected tropical diseases and the strain on overburdened healthcare systems. The intersection of health, education, and economic prosperity illustrates the multifaceted benefits of sanitation and hygiene practices on a societal level, emphasising their importance in global health strategies (Harris et al., 2013). Besides allocating resources, it is important to encourage people in communities to change their behaviours. The promotion of good hygiene in public health campaigns, such as teaching how to wash hands and handle food safely, is vital for the community. Any such initiative should be tailored to the culture and needs of each community to be effective. Collaborative efforts between governments, non-governmental organisations (NGOs), and local stakeholders are necessary to create a culture of hygiene that prioritises education and sustainable practices. If communities prioritise sanitation, they can better combat infectious diseases. Thus, the role of sanitation and hygiene extends beyond mere prevention; it is integral to building healthier, more resilient societies committed to overcoming public health challenges (Mills et al., 2016).

10.4. Global Health Organisations and Initiatives

Global health organisations play a critical role in addressing infectious diseases that transcend national borders. Organisations like the WHO are key to leading international actions against health crises. They develop guidelines for stopping diseases, organise vaccination programs, and campaign to get more resources. Working together is essential for handling outbreaks, as was the case with the Ebola and Zika epidemics. In addition, NGOs and philanthropic organisations play a significant role in these achievements. Programs funded by sources such as those outlined in Mutima (2004) demonstrate how financial support for health-related activities can bolster local healthcare systems in regions most affected by infectious diseases. So, these organisations and initiatives are essential for the worldwide response to health emergencies. Along with well-known organisations, new initiatives have appeared to boost disease surveillance and response. One notable example is the Disease Surveillance Networks (DSN) Initiative, which was evaluated by the Rockefeller Foundation, as described in Kimball et al. (2011). Its purpose is to develop international networks that allow countries to work together when dealing with infectious diseases. The DSN Initiative explains that working together across different sectors can enhance the reporting of diseases and the implementation of responses. Such reviews assess the effectiveness of the initiatives and explain the key factors that support successful cross-border cooperation. Such projects help different sectors work together, which improves the preparedness and resilience of health systems globally. Additionally, the coordination of funding, research, and implementation strategies is crucial for the success of global health initiatives. Through targeted investments, such as those highlighted in Mutima (2004), health organisations can focus on combating infectious diseases that disproportionately affect low-income countries. The money can be used to create health clinics and laboratories necessary for detecting and addressing outbreaks. Meanwhile, research projects, which are often backed by government and private groups, help develop new methods for diagnosis, treatment, and vaccines. This demonstrates that having sufficient funds and a well-planned strategy is essential for handling global health challenges. By ensuring that resources are effectively allocated and partnerships are nurtured, stakeholders can enhance their capacity to control infectious diseases and ultimately improve global health outcomes (Figure 10.10).

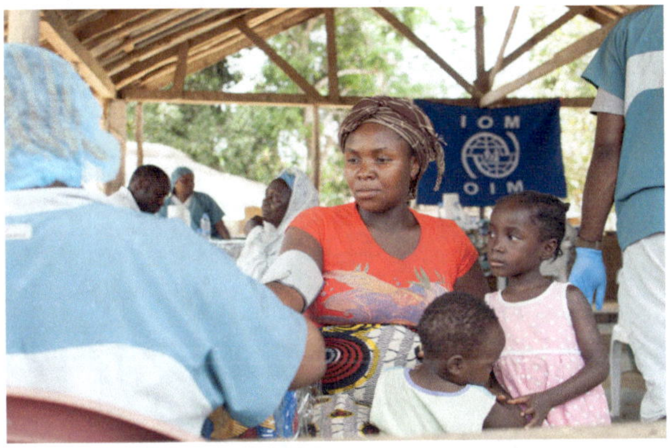

Figure 10.10. Global health organizations.

Source: https://borgenproject.org/wp-content/uploads/16369812974_83ba830af2_k.jpg.

10.4.1. Role of the World Health Organization (WHO)

The WHO plays a crucial role in the global health field, primarily by combating infectious diseases. Established in 1948, the WHO is responsible for coordinating global public health initiatives and advising countries on how to manage epidemics and pandemics. This role is especially vital in the context of diseases that can cross borders rapidly, such as tuberculosis (TB) and COVID-19. For example, the WHO has not only established guidelines for the management of TB, adjudicating new therapies like pretomanid in conjunction with other anti-TB agents, but has also emphasised the necessity for multi-drug regimens to tackle multi-drug resistant strains of tuberculosis effectively (Stancil et al., 2021). The WHO works to encourage research, provide funding, and share up-to-date treatment guidelines, which help member states cooperate and are key in tackling persistent infectious diseases. After the COVID-19 pandemic began, people are paying more attention to the WHO's work. When the organisation declared COVID-19 a global pandemic, it assumed the role of coordinating worldwide research and response, underscoring the importance of combating the disease globally. The WHO has helped disseminate information about the virus and its spread, enabling countries to take immediate action.

They have also campaigned for equal access to vaccines and treatments, which is crucial as health disparities widen across different countries. Correspondingly, ongoing studies have highlighted potential therapeutic targets against SARS-CoV-2, such as specific seleno compounds, bolstered by the WHO's encouragement of scientific research to combat the pandemic effectively (Rakib et al., 2021). The various approaches employed by the WHO demonstrate its commitment to safeguarding the world against health threats. The WHO is also responsible for creating international health standards and developing plans for addressing new health problems caused by infectious diseases. It means developing strategies that cover prevention, fast assessment, and emergency action plans. The WHO achieves this by utilising its extensive network to share and compare experiences with infectious disease outbreaks from various countries. These initiatives help improve health systems worldwide and also make them more prepared for future health emergencies. It emphasises the use of surveillance and reporting tools to quickly identify outbreaks, enabling prompt action. Thanks to its efforts in supporting global health infrastructure, the WHO helps countries prepare for infectious diseases and makes a big difference in improving global health and well-being as health threats keep changing.

10.4.2. International Health Regulations and Agreements

The International Health Regulations (IHR), established by the WHO, represent a crucial framework for global health governance, particularly in the realm of infectious disease control. These legally binding regulations obligate 196 signatory countries to monitor and report potential public health emergencies effectively. As more contagious diseases emerge, the IHR's role in fostering global cooperation and responsibility has become increasingly important. This role is crucial in preventing outbreaks from escalating into pandemics. The importance of the IHR is underscored by its practical implications for public health practice, which include the establishment of surveillance systems, response strategies, and the integration of health resources across borders, all of which are essential for comprehensive outbreak management and response (Anne MacFarlane et al., 2024). The IHR highlights the One Health approach, which emphasises the interconnectedness of human, animal, and environmental health. This way of thinking is significant for zoonotic diseases, as many new pathogens originate from animals. The IHR requires nations to develop key skills for managing and monitoring animal diseases, underscoring the need for veterinary care for animals with infectious diseases. By ensuring that countries adhere to these regulations, the IHR aims to mitigate health risks associated with globalisation and increased trade, which can lead to the introduction and spread of new pathogens (Martinho et al., 2024). The continuous talks among nations about the IHR are essential for making it more effective and handling the problems that existed in disease prevention and response before. The IHR's role in travel medicine has been recognised more, mainly due to the COVID-19 pandemic, as international travel can significantly impact the spread of diseases. Ensuring that vaccines are distributed well and health rules are followed helps keep people safe and supports travel worldwide. However, there are still difficulties, such as the lack of a standard way to evaluate and insufficient research on how travel medicine fits into the IHR framework. Health professionals, legal authorities, and policymakers must cooperate in addressing these issues. By fostering a multidisciplinary approach to health regulations, the IHR can adapt to current and future infectious disease threats while promoting global health preparedness and resilience (AnneMacFarlane et al., 2024; Martinho et al., 2024) (Figure 10.11).

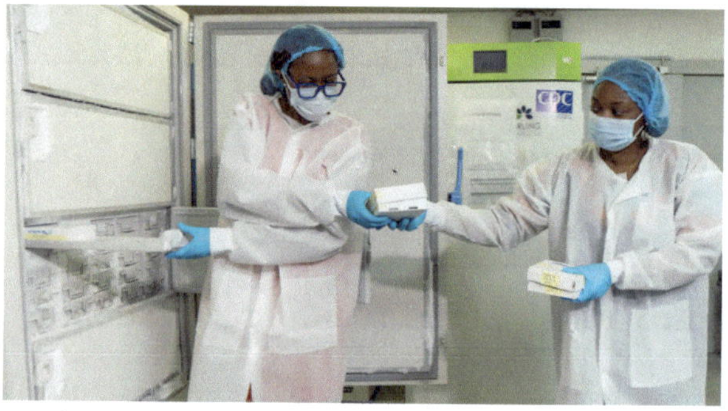

Figure 10.11. The international health regulation.

Source: https://www.cdc.gov/global-health/media/images/nigeria_partner_to_increase_covid19_vaccination_photo_006.jpg.

10.4.3. Non-Governmental Organizations (NGOs) and Their Contributions

NGOs play a critical role in addressing infectious diseases and promoting global health initiatives. Their contributions often bridge the gaps left by governments and international bodies, particularly in resource-limited settings where health systems may be fragile or underfunded. NGOs employ methods such as community outreach, policy advocacy, and direct service provision, all of which are crucial for addressing diseases among vulnerable populations. As an illustration, through programs that teach about hygiene and prevention, NGOs support communities in learning about infectious diseases and lowering their spread. Engaging local people in health activities encourages them to take responsibility, which can help health programs remain effective over time. In addition to providing preventive education, NGOs are often key in supplying healthcare to people living in remote or underserved areas. Many organizations have mobilized healthcare workers to implement community case management (CCM) strategies effectively, enabling local populations to access timely medical care for diseases like malaria.

A systematic review found that community health workers (CHWs) can deliver high-quality malaria care, provided they receive appropriate training and are supported through guidelines and supervision. Such efforts demonstrate that NGOs can significantly enhance community health and address the pressing issues posed by infectious diseases. This model not only enhances immediate health outcomes but also strengthens the overall healthcare system by integrating services and fostering collaborations among various healthcare stakeholders (Buj et al., 2014). NGOs play a major role in funding, especially for research and efforts to control infectious diseases around the world. Between 2000 and 2002, U.S.-based foundations played a significant role in funding health-related projects in Africa, marking a concerted effort to address pressing health challenges on the continent (Mutima, 2004). The financial support enables NGOs to implement and sustain programs for disease prevention, treatment, and health education. They also utilize their funds to support policy reforms and bring together community assets, thereby increasing their impact. When NGOs align their work with international health goals, they contribute to controlling infectious diseases and play a vital role in enhancing public health worldwide.

10.5. Socioeconomic Factors Affecting Infectious Diseases

The interplay between socioeconomic factors and infectious diseases is a critical aspect influencing global health outcomes. Individuals in LMICs often face a range of challenges that exacerbate their vulnerability to infectious diseases. A lack of healthcare, poor sanitation, and insufficient access to foodsignificantly increase the health problems in these groups. The health of a community is influenced by its economic stability, which in turn affects its ability to implement effective health policies and provide quality public health services. A lack of resources makes it harder for the healthcare system to respond to disease outbreaks and prevent illnesses, resulting in more cases of sickness and death. For example, diseases in working equids in LMICs highlight how social and economic factors can endanger both animals and humans. Such vulnerabilities can destabilise livelihoods and food security, reinforcing a cycle of poverty and illness that is difficult to escape (Anderson et al., 2023). The presence of AMR introduces a new dimension to how social and economic factors influence infectious diseases, particularly in regions with high agricultural activity. The increased use of antimicrobials in livestock is primarily driven by the high demand for animal products, which can lead to serious public health issues due to the rise of resistant bacteria. In LMICs, the healthcare system often does not have the means to fight against the growing problem of AMR. As more resistance mechanisms emerge, the effectiveness of treatments for infectious diseases decreases, resulting in increased healthcare expenses and reduced productivity. Antimicrobial use should be rationalized by bringing together actions from agriculture, human health, and wildlife conservation. These interdisciplinary strategies are essential to mitigate the widespread impacts of AMR and to foster a holistic understanding of the interconnectedness of health issues (Ducrot et al., 2017). Socioeconomic health factors make it clear that a comprehensive approach is necessary to address infectious diseases. To address these issues, we should develop policies and interventions that ensure everyone has equal access to healthcare and enhance the community's capacity to withstand disease outbreaks. When policymakers recognise the impact of socioeconomic conditions, they can develop targeted policies to support the most vulnerable. In addition, using the One Health framework will bring together human, animal, and environmental health, making it clear how these areas are connected. This way of thinking can result in better disease prevention and control, mainly in places where diseases are common and resources are scarce. Ultimately, a concerted effort to address these socioeconomic factors is imperative to improve global health outcomes and reduce the impact of infectious diseases across diverse populations (Anderson et al., 2023; Ducrot et al., 2017) (Figure 10.12).

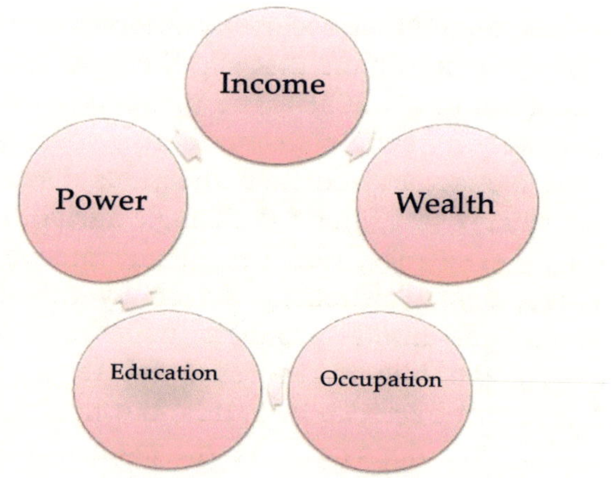

Figure 10.12. Socioeconomic factors and infectious diseases.

Source: https://slideplayer.com/slide/4509483/15/images/6/Five+Determinants+of+Socioeconomic+Status.jpg.

10.5.1. Impact of Poverty on Disease Prevalence

The intricate relationship between poverty and the prevalence of infectious diseases can be observed through various lenses, including access to healthcare, nutritional status, and preventive measures. Many living in low-income areas struggle to get good healthcare, which means they are less able to prevent or treat diseases. The problem is exacerbated by the lack of money, which prevents many from accessing the medical care and drugs they need. Because of this, there is an increase in untreated infectious diseases, which leads to a cycle where poor health makes poverty worse. It is clear from studies that some diseases, such as tuberculosis and hepatitis, which could be prevented by vaccines or early action, primarily impact people living in poverty, so there is a pressing need for public health strategies that focus on these issues in global health. The nutritional value of a person's diet can significantly impact how poverty contributes to disease. Weakened immune systems in children and pregnant women caused by malnutrition make them more likely to get infected with diseases. The COVID-19 pandemic has exacerbated these conditions by severely disrupting food systems, resulting in increased levels of malnutrition among vulnerable populations in low- and middle-income countries (LMICs). It is estimated that because of the pandemic, 6.7 million children under five years may suffer from severe wasting, which makes them more likely to die from infectious diseases because their immunity is weakened. Such alarming trends underscore the interconnectedness of nutrition and health, necessitating comprehensive approaches to enhance both dietary quality and access to healthcare services in resource-constrained settings (Headey et al., 2020). The conditions that come with poverty help spread infectious diseases. In poor communities, too many people living together, inadequate sanitation, and little access to clean water help diseases such as cholera, malaria, and HIV/AIDS to spread. As shown in different studies, marginalised groups such as women and ethnic minorities are more heavily affected by infectious diseases. A lack of health information and support for disease prevention among these groups can lead to numerous infections, which may spread throughout the community and exacerbate public health issues. Thus, eradicating poverty is not solely a matter of economic development; it is also a foundational element for enhancing global health outcomes by reducing disease prevalence and improving population resilience (Burton et al., 2021) (Figure 10.13).

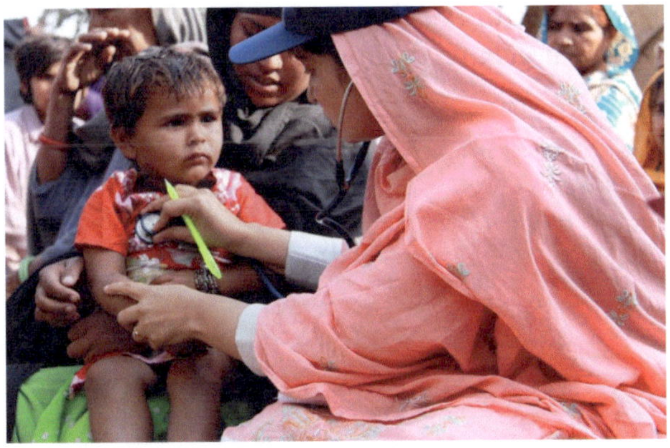

Figure 10.13. The intricate relationship between poverty and the prevalence.

Source: https://www.borgenmagazine.com/wp-content/uploads/2019/11/The-Top-4-Diseases-of-Poverty-Worldwide-e1581553810215.jpg.

10.5.2. Access to Healthcare and Its Implications

Access to healthcare is a fundamental determinant of public health, particularly in the context of infectious diseases that transcend geographic and socioeconomic boundaries. Where healthcare is not readily available, people are more likely to catch and spread illnesses, which may cause more cases of sickness and death. Inadequate access becomes very clear during disease outbreaks, as was seen during the recent COVID-19 pandemic. Those in low-resource areas faced greater difficulties accessing vaccination and medical care, which further exacerbated the public health situation. Additionally, the pressure on healthcare systems in these areas often leads to problems for people needing help with other health issues, exacerbating the situation and is referred to as the "collateral damage" of the pandemic. Because there are many barriers to healthcare access, special policies are needed to ensure that all groups have equal chances for good health. Restricted access to healthcare leads to issues that extend beyond infectious diseases, affecting society and the economy. If there are not enough healthcare services, people may postpone seeking care until their illness worsens, which could have been prevented by earlier treatment. Lack of access to care can make it harder for vulnerable groups to avoid the infection and its complications.

A model used during COVID-19 found that cutting down on essential health services could result in much higher rates of maternal and child deaths, mainly in LMICs that do not have many resources. The rise in poverty and social disturbances exacerbates these problems, underscoring the need for equal access to healthcare for all. It is essential to understand the many effects of healthcare access when making global health policies and practices. AMR indicates that a lack of equitable access to healthcare can exacerbate public health issues. Regions with inadequate healthcare infrastructure often lack essential resources, such as antibiotics, which contributes to the emergence of drug-resistant infections that spread unchecked (Murray et al., 2022). So, to address public health issues, actions should focus on increasing access to healthcare, tackling AMR and making health systems stronger. Also, during the COVID-19 crisis, it was clear that ensuring people have stable finances and access to quality education is crucial for improving access to healthcare services. Ultimately, a holistic approach to healthcare access can foster resilience in global health systems, ensuring preparedness for future infectious disease outbreaks and challenges (Yoshikawa et al., 2020).

10.5.3. Education and Awareness in Disease Prevention

Education and awareness play a crucial role in disease prevention, particularly in the context of infectious diseases at a global level. Informing people about the risks of infectious diseases and how to prevent them significantly reduces the spread of these diseases. Public health organizations are now focusing on informing the public about vaccines, especially after the COVID-19 pandemic started. Pharmacists in Nigeria have become crucial in addressing the doubts and misleading information that deter people from getting vaccinated. Because they are nearby and trusted by the community, they can give important advice and education on vaccines, which encourages people to have confidence in them. Effective health education can lead to improved health outcomes, making it an essential component of any comprehensive response to infectious disease threats (Rasaq et al., 2021). It is also crucial for global disease prevention to address the new dangers brought by globalisation. When people move and travel more, there is a greater chance of infectious diseases emerging in areas where they are not typically found.

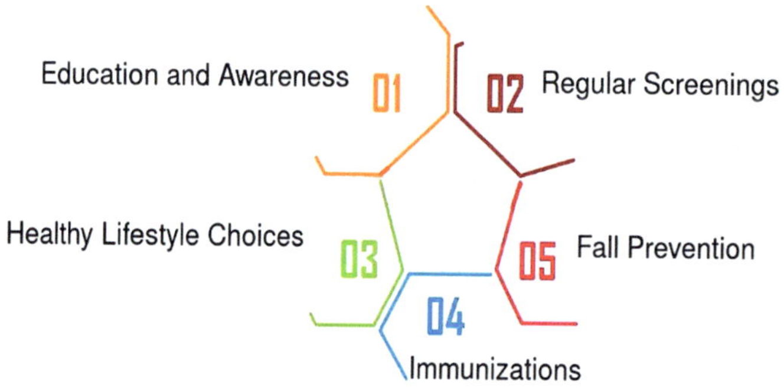

Figure 10.14. Education and awareness play a crucial role in disease prevention.

Source: https://fastercapital.co/i/Geriatric-care-service-Innovative-Strategies-for-Marketing-Geriatric-Care-Services-to-Seniors--Promoting-Preventive-Health-Measures.webp.

For example, due to increased international travel and trade, diseases that were once confined to tropical regions can now emerge in China. It shows that health education is essential for travellers and migrant workers to know about the health risks linked to common diseases in their new places. Increasing awareness about the importance of vaccination and health screenings before travel can help prevent the spread of diseases. Furthermore, to ensure timely diagnosis and treatment, a system of continued education for medical professionals in non-endemic countries is imperative, enabling them to recognise and respond to imported diseases effectively (Zhou et al., 2018). For educational strategies to be effective, the government health agencies, schools, and community groups must cooperate. If education programs are culturally sensitive and liked by the local community, it will be easier for them to accept and use health information. Also, programs that focus on particular community worries, such as doubts about vaccine safety, can help reduce vaccine hesitancy. When trust and openness are present, these educational steps help people manage their own health decisions. Ultimately, comprehensive education and awareness campaigns should be a central focus of global health initiatives aimed at preventing infectious diseases, ensuring the establishment of a healthier future for communities worldwide (Rasaq et al., 2021) (Figure 10.14).

10.6. Technological Advances in Disease Management

Technological advances have significantly transformed the landscape of disease management, particularly in the realm of infectious diseases. Digital health technologies, including telemedicine and mobile health apps, are now crucial for improving the way healthcare is delivered. They enable patients and healthcare providers to communicate in real time, thereby increasing access to care for individuals living far from medical centers. In the COVID-19 pandemic, telehealth played a crucial role in enabling healthcare systems to treat patients while minimizing face-to-face contact. Besides, new technologies in data analytics and AI allow healthcare workers to analyze extensive epidemiological data, which helps them respond to public health issues and control diseases. As highlighted by ongoing research, these technological innovations play a pivotal role in preparing for future pandemics and global health challenges (Miranda et al., 2022). Besides improving healthcare, new technologies are also transforming the detection of infectious diseases. The integration of polymerase chain reaction (PCR) testing has significantly improved the speed and accuracy of disease diagnosis, enabling quicker interventions and treatment options. Also, point-of-care devices that use microfluidics and lab-on-a-chip technology can produce results quickly, which is very important during outbreaks. They enable healthcare providers to access information quickly, facilitating fast actions such as contact tracing and vaccination. The SARS-CoV-2 pandemic demonstrated the effectiveness of rapid testing, with widespread testing being crucial in controlling the outbreak. Such progress highlights the importance of ongoing investment in diagnostic technologies to enhance disease surveillance and management efforts worldwide (Burton et al., 2021). Innovative approaches to treating infections made possible by technology are now changing the way infectious diseases are handled. AMR is increasing in concern, but ML and genomics are assisting in finding new ways to treat infections and improve existing drugs. With genetic testing of pathogens, doctors can design treatments that are more likely to work for each patient. New technologies in vaccine development, such as those used for COVID-19 vaccines, have helped make vaccines available more quickly, which has been important in preventing infectious disease outbreaks. It is also thanks to new manufacturing and distribution systems that vaccines can be quickly distributed to those who need them. As we look to the future, leveraging these technological breakthroughs will be essential in addressing the challenges presented by infectious diseases in a globalized world (Miranda et al., 2022).

10.6.1. Innovations in Diagnostics and Treatment

The transformation in diagnostics and treatment methods has become essential to combat infectious diseases and improve global health outcomes effectively. The COVID-19 pandemic highlighted the importance of robust diagnostic systems everywhere, but many areas, particularly in low- and middle-income countries, still face significant challenges with access and capabilities. Advances in health technology, such as rapid testing and diagnostics conducted on-site, have become crucial for quickly identifying infectious agents. Due to these advances, it is now easier to respond rapidly to disease outbreaks and also make diagnostics available to those who need them most. According to Fleming et al. (2021), nearly half of the global population struggles to access reliable diagnostics, emphasising that innovations must be coupled with efforts to improve health infrastructure and resource allocation to bridge this gap effectively. Besides diagnostics, new treatments have made it easier to control infectious diseases. The rise of antimicrobial resistance (AMR) poses a significant threat to public health, necessitating innovative treatment approaches that integrate new therapies with traditional antimicrobial agents. Personalised medicine and targeted therapies may help treatments work better and reduce the chance of resistance. With genetic and molecular profiling, doctors can design treatments tailored to each patient, resulting in improved outcomes and fewer side effects. Emerging treatment modalities, such as monoclonal antibodies and novel vaccine platforms, especially in response to outbreaks like COVID-19, point to a growing understanding of infection dynamics and the importance of rapid research and development in crises, as emphasized in studies by Kruk et al. (2018). Innovation in diagnostics and treatment can be made sustainable by bringing together different stakeholders. All these groups should join forces to establish a system that supports research, development, and distribution of health technologies. Ensuring that healthcare workers are trained is as important as introducing the new technologies. Also, when health care policies focus on fairness, it can lead to changes that help diagnostics and treatments reach more people in different communities. The necessity of a coordinated effort to address health disparities reinforces (Fleming et al., 2021) findings that effective diagnostics and treatment are fundamental to achieving universal health coverage, ultimately offering a blueprint for comprehensive public health strategies in mitigating the impact of infectious diseases globally (Figure 10.15).

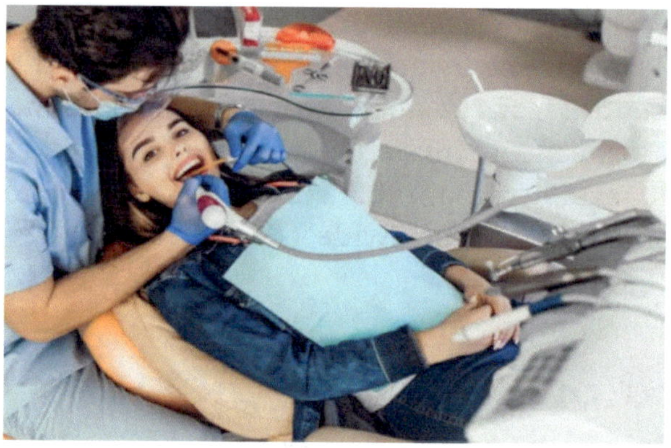

Figure 10.15. The transformation in diagnostics and treatment infectious diseases.

Source: https://klinikabymagicstyle.ae/wp-content/uploads/2023/11/Latest-Innovations-in-Dental-Treatment-494x344.png.

10.6.2. Role of Telemedicine in Global Health

Telemedicine is now an essential part of global health, mainly because infectious diseases can spread across the world. With the help of video conferencing, mobile apps, and remote monitoring, healthcare providers can deliver essential services to many people in regions where healthcare infrastructure is underdeveloped. This is particularly important during outbreaks of infectious diseases, as seen during the COVID-19 pandemic, as telemedicine enabled patients to consult quickly and safely. Remote care enables quick interventions, benefiting health in areas with insufficient medical staff or those that are difficult to reach. Telemedicine is a creative and effective way to address logistical challenges as global health efforts strive to expand access to basic healthcare services. The role of telemedicine is further highlighted when addressing the long-term effects of infectious diseases, such as post-acute sequelae of SARS-CoV-2 infection (PASC). Many people with long COVID deal with lasting symptoms such as tiredness and trouble with thinking, and these can be managed with ongoing medical support. Telemedicine facilitates regular follow-up meetings, allowing doctors to observe symptoms, adjust the treatment plan, and instruct patients on how to manage their condition effectively. Moreover, using remote care services reduces the need for patients to travel, which can be very difficult for those with health problems. To keep patients with chronic illnesses from infectious diseases, global health organisations rely on telemedicine, which strengthens the link between health technology and patient health. Telemedicine is very helpful, but it does not solve the problem of health equity on a global scale.

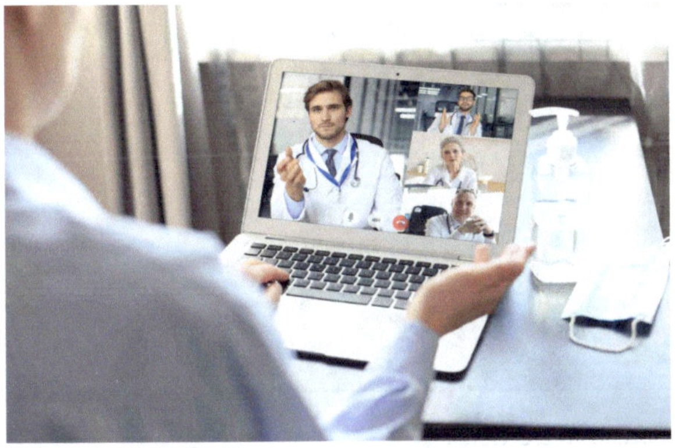

Figure 10.16. Role of telemedicine in global health.

Source: https://xpresshealth.ie/wp-content/uploads/2025/02/215_12_11zon.jpg.

When some people lack access to technology or a reliable internet connection, telemedicine may not be an effective option for them and could exacerbate existing inequalities. To ensure that telemedicine benefits everyone in global health, we need to implement policies that provide equal access and facilitate the integration of these technologies into the current healthcare system. It involves teaching healthcare workers how to use telemedicine and ensuring that individuals requiring additional support can participate in virtual healthcare. Creating an inclusive and accessible system enables global health initiatives to maximize the benefits of telemedicine for infectious disease care, benefiting diverse patients. The future of healthcare greatly depends on our ability to implement equitable telemedicine solutions across varied contexts, fostering resilience in the face of global health challenges (Figure 10.16).

10.6.3. Data Analytics and Disease Tracking

The integration of data analytics in disease tracking has become increasingly vital in the context of global health. Governments and health groups are using advanced technology and large data to find and watch for infectious diseases. Using predictive analytics, stakeholders can anticipate when an outbreak may occur and take prompt action. By using this approach, we can both closely monitor pathogens and make informed choices in public health, which helps improve responses. The use of social media, health information, and environmental data provides more information, which strengthens the analytical models to identify trends and unusual cases. As a result, data analytics enables the real-time monitoring of diseases, allowing health authorities to more effectively implement preventive measures, ultimately benefiting the global health system. Mobile computing and portable DNA sequencing are changing how diseases are tracked. Field conditions can now be used for DNA sequencing, thanks to the Oxford Nanopore MinION which helps identify and track infectious agents quickly. They enable the instant diagnosis of infection cases at the outbreak site. There are still issues with using mobile systems, including the need for high data transmission and intense processing, which can be hard to maintain in changing connectivity settings. Tackling these issues is crucial for making the most of portable technology in disease tracking, which means that technology and algorithms should be carefully co-designed to support fast health interventions. Because of this, combining portable sequencing with data analytics has the potential to transform the way we address infectious diseases worldwide, making us more proactive rather than reactive. Data analytics facilitates the study of disease epidemiology by collecting and analyzing large amounts of data. The Journal of Global Health has included research that stresses the importance of accurate epidemiological estimates for public health. Numerous research outputs have contributed to the analytics field, encouraging different sectors to collaborate for effective infectious disease tracking. Sharing research findings widely people to discuss health issues and participate in policy-making, leading to more effective health strategies. Because of the focus on data, understanding and interpreting complex data will be essential for fighting EIDs worldwide. Enhanced collaboration coupled with advanced analytical methodologies aims to establish an integrated response network, paving the way for improved health outcomes worldwide (Bornmann et al., 2014; Ko et al., 2017) (Figure 10.17).

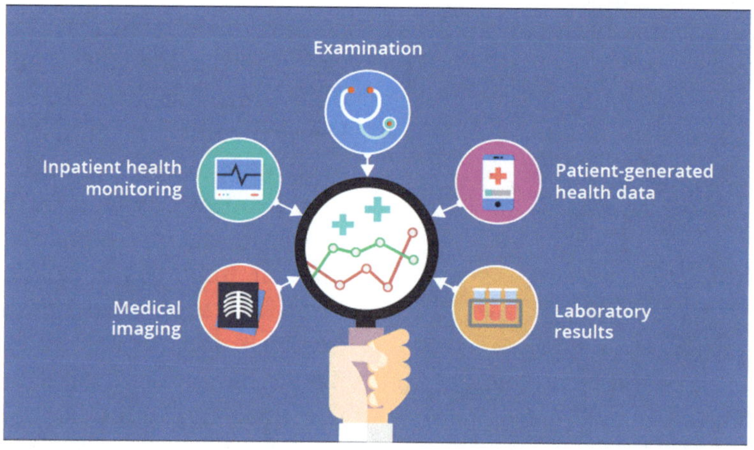

Figure 10.17. The integration of data analytics in disease tracking.

Source: https://www.scribbledata.io/wp-content/uploads/2023/01/Data-cycle-analytics-01-2.jpg.

SUMMARY

Examining infectious diseases in global health reveals the need for improved surveillance and response. The pandemic has made it clear that several nations are not well-prepared to detect and control infectious outbreaks. Countries with strong public health systems handled the crisis better, whereas countries with weak health systems, especially those in the Infectious Disease Vulnerability Index, struggled a lot. It is clear from comparing response efforts that countries must cooperate in public health planning, since new infections can spread quickly around the world. As highlighted in recent studies, the lack of timely intervention can lead to exponentially rising cases and fatalities, emphasizing the importance of prompt and coordinated public health initiatives (Tuite et al., 2020).

Global health experts should focus on increasing capacity in poorer countries, as they are often the most severely affected by infectious diseases. During the pandemic, the gap in healthcare resources has been glaring, resulting in numerous deaths and illnesses in areas unprepared to handle them. Partnerships and financial support from other nations can help improve local health systems, enabling these countries to detect and manage outbreaks more effectively. In addition, implementing effective vaccination campaigns and improving healthcare services will significantly reduce the risk of infectious diseases among those who are at risk. This proactive approach not only enhances local health outcomes but also serves to safeguard global health security, as the interconnectedness of our world means that infectious threats easily transcend borders (Roth et al., 2018). The experiences from COVID-19 and previous outbreaks should be turned into practical policies that help global health. The need for improved data sharing, enhanced teamwork in research, and equitable access to vaccines and treatments is more evident than ever. Stronger communication between countries and public health bodies may result in a unified plan that helps everyone resist future threats. Stressing both prevention and treatment will play a key role in combating infectious diseases. Moving forward, a commitment to global health equity and the integration of infectious disease management into broader health initiatives will significantly bolster our collective defences against emerging pathogens, ultimately leading to a healthier, more prepared global population (Tuite et al., 2020).

The intricate relationship between infectious diseases and global health has become increasingly urgent in light of recent pandemics, particularly the simultaneous challenges posed by tuberculosis (TB) and COVID-19. Studies show that having more than one infection at the same time can lead to worse health results, higher rates of respiratory failure and more deaths among patients. A study at an Italian infectious disease hospital found that about 9.4% of TB patients were also infected with COVID-19. Those who are coinfected often suffer from chronic conditions like diabetes and severe lung issues, which highlights the need for integrated care that manages many infections together. These findings compel healthcare systems worldwide to strengthen their preparedness and response strategies to address not only individual diseases but also the complexities of coinfection in a global health context (Bari et al., 2025). Being involved with the community is crucial for improving health responses in public health emergencies. The pandemic has highlighted the importance of community-based initiatives. An evaluation in Laos found that participation in community health activities encouraged villagers to seek health services more frequently and to receive vaccinations against COVID-19. Additionally, these programs help create a supportive environment that enables vulnerable individuals to manage their health issues more effectively. Thus, integrating community engagement into national health agendas is crucial for addressing both current infectious diseases and emerging threats such as AMR (Haenssgen et al., 2025). Moreover, the COVID-19 pandemic has shown that quick diagnosis and management of infectious diseases is essential. The TB-COVID-19 study revealed that patients with multiple pathogens often have worse outcomes, which stresses the need for quick action. As COVID-19 becomes a more persistent presence, it remains crucial to investigate how it affects and is influenced by other diseases. Since infectious diseases are constantly changing, it will be crucial to focus on community engagement and integrated care models in the global health response. Further studies and effective policies guided by these findings are necessary to strengthen healthcare systems to better handle future infectious diseases.

CLOSER LOOK:

BESIDES VACCINES:

Vaccines are widely recognized as one of the most effective tools in preventing infectious diseases. Yet, while they play a critical role in public health, they are only one part of a broader strategy for disease prevention and health promotion. Understanding the complementary measures that support immunity and reduce the spread of illness is crucial, especially in the context of emerging diseases and global health challenges.

One major area beyond vaccines is **hygiene and sanitation.** Simple practices such as regular handwashing, safe food handling, and proper disposal of waste have historically reduced the incidence of infectious diseases, sometimes even before vaccines were widely available. Clean water and sanitation infrastructure, for example, have dramatically decreased the prevalence of waterborne diseases such as cholera and typhoid in many regions. These preventive measures act at the community level and reduce the overall exposure to pathogens, complementing the protection offered by vaccines.

Another critical component is **healthy lifestyle and nutrition.** A well-balanced diet rich in vitamins and minerals strengthens the immune system, making it better equipped to respond to infections. Adequate sleep, regular physical activity, and stress management also contribute to immune resilience. While vaccines provide targeted immunity against specific pathogens, a robust immune system supports the body in fighting off a wide range of infections and can improve the effectiveness of vaccines themselves.

Public health measures such as quarantine, social distancing, and mask-wearing have also proven effective, particularly during outbreaks. These interventions limit the spread of contagious diseases and protect vulnerable populations while vaccines are being developed or distributed. Additionally, **antiviral and antibiotic treatments** serve as critical tools to manage infections once they occur, reducing morbidity and mortality even when prevention is not possible.

Finally, **education and awareness** empower individuals and communities to adopt preventive behaviors and make informed health decisions. Public campaigns on hygiene, nutrition, and disease prevention can create lasting societal changes that reduce disease burden across populations.

In conclusion, while vaccines remain a cornerstone of disease prevention, a holistic approach that includes hygiene, nutrition, lifestyle, public health measures, treatment, and education is essential for comprehensive health protection. Combining these strategies not only prevents illness but also builds stronger, more resilient communities capable of facing both current and emerging health challenges.

REFERENCES

1. Ahmed, S. K., Dabou, E. A., Ibrahim, F. M., Mohammed, M. G., Chandran, D., Basit, J., Chakraborty, S., Emran, T. B., Islam, M. R., & Dhama, K. (2024). Challenges and counteracting strategies including optimum health service practices for frontline nurses during the MPOX outbreak and Futuristic Vision. *SAGE Open Nursing, 10.* https://doi.org/10.1177/23779608241256209Ali, G. S., Garud, S. K., Nashte, A., Patil, et al. (2023). *Public Health Policy and Infectious Disease Control: Lessons from Recent Outbreaks.* https://core.ac.uk/download/599214703.pdf (accessed on 30th May 2025).
2. Alkhamis, M. A., Belkhiria, J., & Martínez-López, B. (2016). Application of species distribution modeling for avian influenza surveillance in the United States considering the North America migratory flyways. https://core.ac.uk/download/323068666.pdf (accessed on 30th May 2025).
3. Almatrood, M. A., Alharbi, A. K. S., Al Harbi, A. R., Almousa, A. N., & Moqbel, A. M. (2024). The global burden of infectious diseases: A comparative analysis of transmission modes and prevention strategies. *European Chemical Bulletin.* https://www.semanticscholar.org/paper/d4644d1dc6c830858c62c871481375f6c4471fa8 (accessed on 30th May 2025).
4. Alqahtani, Z., DarAssi, M. H., AbuHour, Y., & Almuneef, A. (2025). Assessing the role of vaccination in the control of hand, foot, and mouth disease transmission. *Mathematics.* https://www.semanticscholar.org/paper/0d012bc6c61931949c1d426ea068b7c26d2f6ed9 (accessed on 30th May 2025).
5. Anaemene, B. U. (2016). Localizing the global: The WHO International Health Regulations and domestic health governance mechanisms of infectious diseases in Nigeria. https://core.ac.uk/download/157771930.pdf (accessed on 30th May 2025).
6. Anderson, N., Bonsi, M., & Carder, G. (2023). The socioeconomic impact of diseases on working equids in low and middle-income countries: A critical review. https://core.ac.uk/download/595732107.docx (accessed on 30th May 2025).
7. Arthur, C., Banda, H., Chazya, R., Chijoka, et al. (2023). Epidemiological tools in focus: A comprehensive assessment of their role in addressing infectious disease challenges in Zambia. https://core.ac.uk/download/597862448.pdf (accessed on 30th May 2025).
8. Bashshur, R. L., Doarn, C. R., Frenk, J., Kvedar, J. C., & Woolliscroft, J. O. (2020). Telemedicine and the COVID-19 pandemic, lessons for the future. *Telemedicine Journal and e-Health, 26,* 571–573. https://doi.org/10.1089/tmj.2020.29040.rb.
9. Bibbins-Domingo, K. (2020). This time must be different: Disparities during the COVID-19 pandemic. *Annals of Internal Medicine, 173,* 233, 234. https://doi.org/10.7326/m20-2247.
10. Borda, A., Kostkova, P., Molnar, A., Neesham, et al. (2022). *Ethical Issues in AI-Enabled Disease Surveillance: Perspectives from Global Health.* https://core.ac.uk/download/519722062.pdf (accessed on 30th May 2025).
11. Bornmann, L., Casadevall, A., Falagas, M., Golubic, R., Hirsch, J., & van Leeuwen, T. (2014). The first three years of the *Journal of Global Health*: Assessing the impact. https://core.ac.uk/download/28977936.pdf (accessed on 30th May 2025).
12. Buj, V., Kedenge, S., Kim, J., Ngongo, et al. (2014). Community health workers and stand-alone or integrated case management of malaria: A systematic literature review. https://core.ac.uk/download/19452714.pdf (accessed on 30th May 2025).

13. Burton, M. J., Ramke, J., Marques, A. P., Bourne, R., Congdon, N., Jones, I., Ah Tong, B. A. M., et al. (2021). The Lancet Global Health Commission on global eye health: Vision beyond 2020. *The Lancet Global Health, 9*, e489–e551. https://doi.org/10.1016/s2214-109x(20)30488-5.

14. COHERE Expert Review Group, Cole, S., Conti, L., Davis, M. F., et al. (2017). *Checklist for One Health Epidemiological Reporting of Evidence (COHERE).* https://core.ac.uk/download/323070004.pdf (accessed on 30th May 2025).

15. Di Bari, V., Cerva, C., Libertone, R., Carli, S. M., Musso, M., Goletti, D., Aiello, A., et al. (2025). Impact of severity of COVID-19 in TB disease patients: Experience from an Italian infectious disease referral hospital. *Infectious Disease Reports, 17.* https://www.semanticscholar.org/paper/1cc4dffb7a945d645a008e5b9320e5ec4c2cca8f (accessed on 30th May 2025).

16. Ducrot, C., & Roger, F. (2017). *Antimicrobials in Agriculture: Reducing Their Use While Limiting Health and Socioeconomic Risks in the Countries of the South.* https://core.ac.uk/download/154377163.pdf (accessed on 30th May 2025).

17. Evanega, S., Lynas, M., Adams, J., & Smolenyak, K. (2020). Coronavirus misinformation: Quantifying sources and themes in the COVID-19 'infodemic' (Preprint). https://doi.org/10.2196/preprints.25143.

18. Fleming, K. A., Horton, S., Wilson, M. L., Atun, R., DeStigter, K., Flanigan, J., Sayed, S., et al. (2021). The Lancet Commission on diagnostics: Transforming access to diagnostics. *The Lancet, 398*, 1997–2050. https://doi.org/10.1016/s0140-6736(21)00673-5.

19. Freudenberg, N., Lee, K., Buse, K., Collin, J., Crosbie, E., Friel, S., Eisenkraft, K. D., et al. (2021). Defining priorities for action and research on the commercial determinants of health: A conceptual review. *American Journal of Public Health, 111*, 2202–2211. https://doi.org/10.2105/ajph.2021.306491.

20. Gadelha, C. A. G., Braga, P. S. C., Montenegro, K. B. M., & Cesário, B. B. (2021). Access to vaccines in Brazil and the global dynamics of the Health Economic-Industrial Complex. *Figshare.* https://doi.org/10.6084/m9.figshare.14280906.

21. Greenhalgh, T., Jiménez, J. L., Prather, K. A., Tüfekçi, Z., Fisman, D. N., & Schooley, R. T. (2021). Ten scientific reasons in support of airborne transmission of SARS-CoV-2. *The Lancet, 397*, 1603–1605. https://doi.org/10.1016/s0140-6736(21)00869-2.

22. Haenssgen, M., Elliott, E. M., Bode, S., Souksavanh, O., Xayyahong, T., Okabayashi, H., & Kubota, S. (2025). Community engagement to support public health: Mixed-method evaluation evidence on COVID-19 attitudes and practices in Lao PDR. *Global Health Action, 18*(1), 2485523. https://www.semanticscholar.org/paper/26daab05542a920000229156ef45ff5d7e6d9cb6 (accessed on 30th May 2025).

23. Harris, M., Martin, A., & Rhodes, T. (2013). Taming systems to create enabling environments for HCV treatment: Negotiating trust in the drug and alcohol setting. Social Science & Medicine.

24. He, Q., Bao, Y., Fang, H., Lin, Y., & Sun, H. (2025). HHAN: Comprehensive infectious disease source tracing via heterogeneous hypergraph neural network. Proceedings of the AAAI Conference on Artificial Intelligence. https://www.semanticscholar.org/paper/2d522b94a1cc22ce47b76d85b4942e6cb7b65409 (accessed on 30th May 2025).

25. Headey, D., Heidkamp, R., Osendarp, S., Ruel, M. T., Scott, N., Black, R. E., Shekar, M., et al. (2020). Impacts of COVID-19 on childhood malnutrition and nutrition-related mortality. *The Lancet, 396*, 519–521. https://doi.org/10.1016/s0140-6736(20)31647-0.

26. Herrera, J. E., Niehaus, W., Whiteson, J., Azola, A., Baratta, J. M., Fleming, T. K., Kim, S. Y., et al. (2021). Multidisciplinary collaborative consensus guidance statement on the assessment and treatment of fatigue in postacute sequelae of SARS-CoV-2 infection (PASC) patients. *PM&R, 13*, 1027–1043. https://doi.org/10.1002/pmrj.12684.

27. Huang, J., & Morris, J. S. (2024). Infectious disease modeling. *Annual Review of Statistics and Its Application*. https://www.semanticscholar.org/paper/496f4eb667233035d01beb193251887f743ef348 (accessed on 30th May 2025).

28. Jeon, J., & Kim, E. (2025). Exploring future pandemic preparedness through the development of preventive vaccine platforms and the key roles of international organizations in a global health crisis. *Vaccines, 13*. https://www.semanticscholar.org/paper/b8db63eb8941df18b25b9ff5756fad3ce73c4c86 (accessed on 30th May 2025).

29. Johnson, S. E., & Clark, H. (2021). Report of the independent panel for pandemic preparedness and response: Making COVID-19 the last pandemic. *The Lancet, 398*, 101–103. https://doi.org/10.1016/s0140-6736(21)01095-3.

30. Kimball, A. M., Gugerty, M. K., Abernethy, N., & Curran, S. (2011). *Disease Surveillance Networks Initiative Global: Final Evaluation*. https://core.ac.uk/download/86445037.pdf (accessed on 30th May 2025).

31. Ko, S. Y., Sassoubre, L., & Zola, J. (2017). *Applications and Challenges of Real-Time Mobile DNA Analysis*. http://arxiv.org/abs/1711.07370.

32. Kruk, M. E., Gage, A., Arsenault, C., Jordan, K., Leslie, H. H., Roder-DeWan, S., Adeyi, O., et al. (2018). High-quality health systems in the Sustainable Development Goals era: Time for a revolution. *The Lancet Global Health, 6*, e1196–e1252. https://doi.org/10.1016/s2214-109x(18)30386-3.

33. Macauley, M. (2024). Infectious disease modeling. *Annual Review of Statistics and Its Application*. https://www.semanticscholar.org/paper/b012e36220dec79707a3a5dd6bc59347cf769088 (accessed on 30th May 2025).

34. MacFarlane, A., Sá, R., & Silva, C. (2024). 2.Y.2. International Health Regulations – Role on disease control and global challenges. *The European Journal of Public Health, 34*. https://www.semanticscholar.org/paper/e467673f0d25f1029463a3807c9ac7c2635d76fa (accessed on 30th May 2025).

35. Martinho, J., Diogo, E., Mateus, R., Fernandes, S., Carvalho, T., Díonisio, J., Santos, M. A., et al. (2024). International Health Regulations' role in zoonosis prevention, and intersection with travel medicine. *The European Journal of Public Health, 34*. https://www.semanticscholar.org/paper/5ca30a926c1576fb9bc67bed6f5c120e32174acb (accessed on 30th May 2025).

36. Mills, J. E., & Cumming, O. (2016). *The Impact of Water, Sanitation, and Hygiene on Key Health and Social Outcomes: Review of evidence*. https://core.ac.uk/download/75761114.pdf (accessed on 30th May 2025).

37. Miranda, M., Pingarilho, M., Pimentel, V., Torneri, A., Seabra, S. G., Libin, P., & Abecasis, A. (2022). A tale of three recent pandemics: Influenza, HIV and SARS-CoV-2. *Frontiers in Microbiology, 13*. https://doi.org/10.3389/fmicb.2022.889643.

38. Murray, C. J. L., Ikuta, K. S., Sharara, F., Swetschinski, L. R., Robles, A. G., Gray, A. P., Han, C., et al. (2022). Global burden of bacterial antimicrobial resistance in 2019: A systematic analysis. *The Lancet, 399*, 629–655. https://doi.org/10.1016/s0140-6736(21)02724-0.

39. Mutima, N. (2004). *Funding for Health in Africa: Mapping the U.S. Foundation Landscape, 2000–2002.* https://core.ac.uk/download/75779536.pdf (accessed on 30th May 2025).

40. Pandey, B. D., Shah, Y., Tun, M. M. N., & Morita, K. (2025). Current landscape and future directions for dengue vaccines: Addressing a global health challenge. *Europasian Journal of Medical Sciences.* https://www.semanticscholar.org/paper/ab6d56199431cc16134e11664d10a1de0b1f6601 (accessed on 30th May 2025).

41. Rakib, A., Nain, Z., Sami, S. A., Mahmud, S., Islam, M. A., Ahmed, S., Siddiqui, A. B. F., et al. (2021). A molecular modelling approach for identifying antiviral selenium-containing heterocyclic compounds that inhibit the main protease of SARS-CoV-2: An *in silico* investigation. *Briefings in Bioinformatics, 22*, 1476–1498. https://doi.org/10.1093/bib/bbab045.

42. Rasaq, K. O., Afeez, B. O., Olajide, A., Monisola, I., & Kudirat, A. A. (2021). COVID-19 vaccine hesitancy: Maximizing the extending roles of community pharmacists in Nigeria in driving behavioral changes in public health interventions. *Journal of Infectious Diseases and Epidemiology*. https://www.semanticscholar.org/paper/30dda95f835f1e7870fa6810e645bc3a79e46e64 (accessed on 30th May 2025).

43. Rogerson, S. J., Beeson, J. G., Laman, M., Poespoprodjo, J. R., William, T., Simpson, J. A., Price, R. N., et al. (2020). Identifying and combating the impacts of COVID-19 on malaria. *BMC Medicine, 18*. https://doi.org/10.1186/s12916-020-01710-x.

44. Roth, G. A., Abate, D., Abate, K. H., Abay, S. M., Abbafati, C., Abbasi, N., Abbastabar, H., et al. (2018). Global, regional, and national age-sex-specific mortality for 282 causes of death in 195 countries and territories, 1980–2017: A systematic analysis for the Global Burden of Disease Study 2017. *The Lancet, 392*, 1736–1788. https://doi.org/10.1016/s0140-6736(18)32203-7.

45. Roth, G. A., Mensah, G. A., Johnson, C. O., Addolorato, G., Ammirati, E., Baddour, L. M., Barengo, N. C., et al. (2020). Global burden of cardiovascular diseases and risk factors, 1990–2019. *Journal of the American College of Cardiology, 76*, 2982–3021. https://doi.org/10.1016/j.jacc.2020.11.010.

46. Semenza, J. C., Rocklöv, J., & Ebi, K. L. (2022). Climate change and cascading risks from infectious disease. *Infectious Diseases and Therapy, 11*, 1371–1390. https://doi.org/10.1007/s40121-022-00647-3.

47. Septiariva, I. Y., Suryawan, I. W. K., Sarwono, A., & Ramadan, B. S. (2022). Municipal infectious waste during COVID-19 pandemic: Trends, impacts, and management. *International Journal of Public Health Science (IJPHS), 11*, 552. https://doi.org/10.11591/ijphs.v11i2.21292.

48. Srivastava, S., Kumar, S., Sharma, P. K., Rustagi, S., Mohanty, A., Donovan, S., Henao-Martínez, A., et al. (2024). Control strategies for emerging infectious diseases: Crimean-Congo hemorrhagic fever management. *Health Science Reports, 7*. https://www.semanticscholar.org/paper/0070505be9f28cb5bfef53d331b24da065a5ce2c (accessed on 30th May 2025).

49. Stancil, S. L., Mirzayev, F., & Abdel-Rahman, S. M. (2021). Profiling Pretomanid as a therapeutic option for TB infection: Evidence to date. *Drug Design Development and Therapy, 15*, 2815–2830. https://doi.org/10.2147/dddt.s281639.

50. Tuite, A. R., Bogoch, I. I., Sherbo, R., Watts, A., Fisman, D. N., & Khan, K. (2020). Estimation of coronavirus disease 2019 (COVID-19) burden and potential for international dissemination of infection from Iran. *Annals of Internal Medicine, 172*, 699–701. https://doi.org/10.7326/m20-0696.

51. Umesh, L., & Verma, S. (2024). *Modern Biomedical Technologies Versus Emerging Pathogenic Microbes: Insights into the Confronting Situation*. https://core.ac.uk/download/618266512.pdf (accessed on 30th May 2025).

52. Yadika, A. D. N. (2024). Environment that causes diseases: Article review. *Jurnal Ilmiah Kesehatan Sandi Husada*. https://www.semanticscholar.org/paper/f316ef32520ad8722b4d36c10f5b6e6cb68be85f (accessed on 30th May 2025).

53. Yoshikawa, H., Wuermli, A. J., Rebello, B. P., Dreyer, B. P., Leckman, J. F., Lye, S. J., Ponguta, L. A., et al. (2020). Effects of the global coronavirus disease-2019 pandemic on early childhood development: Short- and long-term risks and mitigating program and policy actions. *The Journal of Pediatrics, 223*, 188–193. https://doi.org/10.1016/j.jpeds.2020.05.020.

54. Zhou, X., Qian, M., Priotto, G., Franco, J., & Guo, J. (2018). Tackling imported tropical diseases in China. *Emerging Microbes & Infections, 7*. https://www.semanticscholar.org/paper/b87a3b8ae6a38ef5a6600ded803b03dfdb7327f1 (accessed on 30th May 2025).

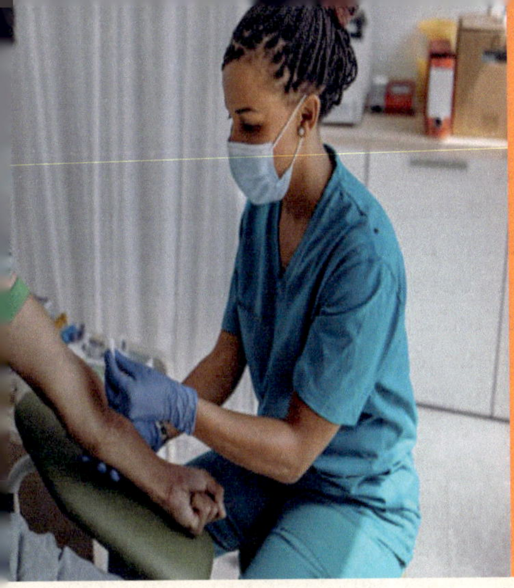

Chapter 11

RISK ASSESSMENT AND MODELLING IN INFECTIOUS DISEASE

Contents

Introduction

Infectious disease risk assessment serves as a critical foundation in public health, guiding strategies for prevention, control, and response to outbreaks. This process involves the systematic identification and evaluation of potential hazards associated with infectious diseases, assessing the probability of occurrence and the severity of their health impacts. By applying statistical modelling and epidemiological methods, researchers can determine the number of cases, the level of infection, and deaths related to a disease. Such quantitative assessments play a pivotal role in allocating healthcare resources effectively and implementing timely public health interventions, especially in regions disproportionately affected by specific pathogens (Rudd et al., 2020). By understanding the risk factors of infectious diseases, health organisations can determine the most effective actions and advise on policies that help mitigate global health issues. Epidemiological modelling helps assess the risk of contagious diseases by showing how the disease might spread and what effects interventions could have. Researchers can use compartmental models, agent-based models, and network models to study how diseases spread and how different control methods, such as vaccination and quarantine, can affect these spreads. For instance, by using data derived from the Global Burden of Diseases, Injuries, and Risk Factors Study (GBD, 2017), researchers can analyze patterns in disease incidence and mortality across different demographics and geographical regions. Such detailed analyses not only enhance the understanding of how factors like age and sex influence disease burden but also reflect broader public health trends over time (James et al., 2018). As a result, being able to model infectious disease risk is crucial for addressing new threats, especially in today's global world. Using data from many sources in infectious disease risk assessment makes the results more reliable and valuable for practical purposes. Researchers can build detailed risk profiles by incorporating clinical data, surveillance reports, and hospital records, which consider both social and economic factors, as well as access to healthcare. Because of this approach, it becomes easier to see which groups are most affected by infectious diseases. Additionally, the ongoing efforts to improve data quality and detail within risk assessment frameworks contribute to more accurate predictors of disease trends and their associated impacts on health systems (Rudd et al., 2020). As public health initiatives evolve, the continuous refinement of infectious disease risk assessment methodologies will be vital for addressing emerging challenges and ensuring preparedness against future outbreaks (Figure 11.1).

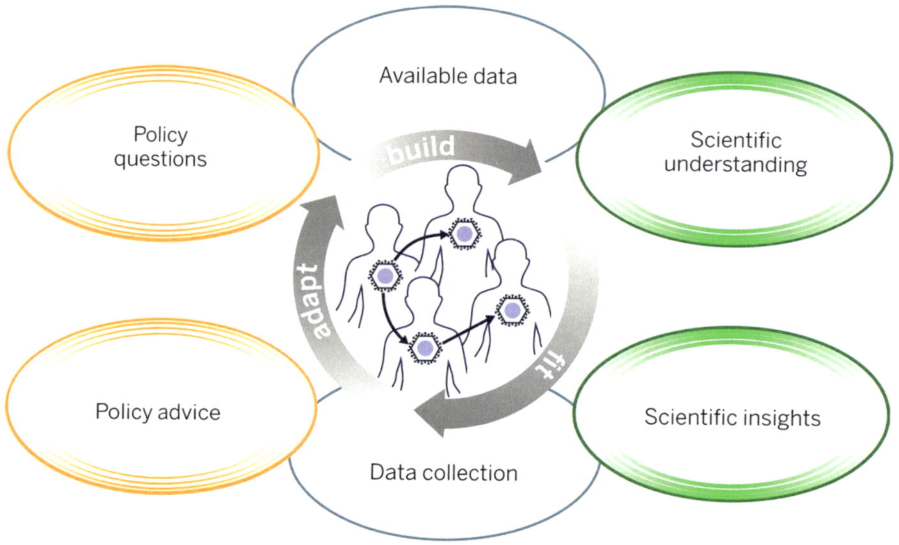

Figure 11.1. Risk assessment and modelling in infectious disease foundation in public health.

Source: https://www.science.org/cms/10.1126/science.aaa4339/asset/07500115-cbd2-4198-8bf1-a86c41ee7601/assets/graphic/347_aaa4339_fa.jpeg.

Definition of Risk Assessment in Public Health

The concept of risk assessment in public health is foundational to understanding and controlling infectious diseases. This systematic process involves identifying potential hazards, evaluating the likelihood and severity of adverse effects, and determining the overall risk to populations. Public health officials use knowledge about pathogen transmission, the prevalence of the disease, and who is most likely to contract it to determine the appropriate actions. Because the threats from infectious diseases are constantly evolving, it is essential to continually update risk models to reflect new pathogens and altered disease patterns. By being proactive, public health can ensure policies and resources are used to address risks, which strengthens communities during outbreaks. Risk assessment greatly depends on strong data analysis and predictive modeling. Public health practitioners can use numbers to predict possible outbreaks and measure the impact of different actions. For example, using information about population density, the number of people who have been vaccinated, and past data on disease spread, models can judge the impact of vaccination programs and if quarantines are needed. This helps shape both quick public health actions and plans for stopping the disease in the future. Moreover, effective communication of these risks to the public is essential, as it cultivates awareness and fosters public cooperation in adhering to recommended health measures (Cesario, 2016). Including risk assessment in public health affects how resources are managed and how strategies are planned, mainly for infectious diseases. Understanding the risk level of different public health threats helps plan which interventions have the most significant effect on reducing disease and death. It matters most in areas with limited resources, where health services must serve a large number of people. In such cases, proper risk assessment helps decision-makers improve healthcare for everyone and make sure vulnerable groups are not left behind. Furthermore, as the burden of infectious diseases intersects with non-communicable diseases, understanding these multifaceted risks leads to a more holistic approach to community health (Turillazzi et al., 2016). For this reason, it is essential to conduct thorough risk assessments to maintain public health programs and enhance the health of the population.

Importance of Infectious Disease Modelling

The modelling of infectious diseases plays a critical role in understanding and mitigating the spread of pathogens within populations. Researchers can use simulations to learn about the causes of outbreaks and evaluate how different ways to stop the disease might work. Being able to predict cases is essential for public health authorities who want to respond quickly with control measures. For example, eco-epidemiology studies the environmental and ecosystem factors that contribute to increased disease cases, and it relies on geographic risk maps to predict where future outbreaks may occur. This approach highlights the importance of integrating ecological data with public health strategies, as exemplified by diseases such as cutaneous leishmaniasis, where anthropogenic factors have significant implications for disease risk assessment and management (Chavy et al., 2019). Also, since infectious diseases are constantly changing, it is necessary to use advanced modeling approaches that consider many different factors. The Global Burden of Diseases, Injuries, and Risk Factors Study (Brown et al., 2017) showcases how detailed statistical models correlate prevalence, incidence, and disability metrics across various populations. They are necessary for tracking shifts in disease rates, identifying individuals at the greatest risk, and managing resources effectively. The use of new data and advanced methods, such as Bayesian meta-regression, enables disease modelling to provide detailed insights into both infectious and non-infectious diseases. Consequently, insights gained from such modelling not only inform local public health policies but also shape global health initiatives aimed at reducing morbidity and mortality across diverse populations (James et al., 2018). With advanced modelling of infectious diseases, there are significant effects on policy and practice. The use of various types of data, including environmental, demographic, and clinical, facilitates a comprehensive risk assessment that informs the development of strategies to prevent and control diseases. Identifying groups that may be affected and the outcomes of different interventions helps decision-makers. It is essential in the event of

EIDs, because fast and informed actions can prevent outbreaks from getting worse. Ultimately, the importance of infectious disease modelling cannot be overstated; it serves as a cornerstone for effective public health surveillance, resource allocation, and ultimately, the protection of global health (Spencer James et al., 2018; Chavy et al., 2019) (Figure 11.2).

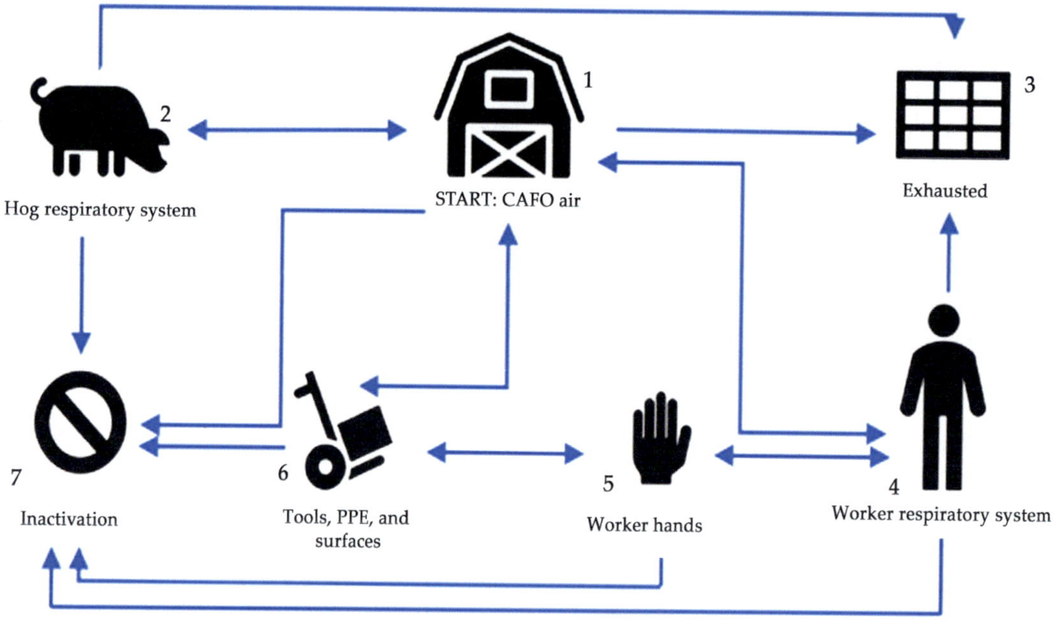

Figure 11.2. Modeling of infectious diseases.

Source: https://duckduckgo.com/?q=Importance+of+infectious+disease+modeling+The+modeling+of+infectious+diseases+plays+a+critical+role+in+understanding+and+mitigating+the+.

Overview of Key Concepts and Methodologies

Understanding risk assessment and modelling in infectious diseases requires a comprehensive grasp of the fundamental concepts and methodologies that underpin these processes. The central part of risk assessment is to evaluate the risks posed by pathogens, which can be caused by their own activities and by other factors that influence their spread. It is essential to find out how microbes enter food to prevent people from getting sick. The framework of Hazard Analysis Critical Control Points (HACCP) and Good Manufacturing Practices (GMP) provides a structured approach to identifying critical points in the production chain where interventions can be most effective. Moreover, the dynamic nature of pathogens, alongside their ability to adapt and proliferate, necessitates an ongoing reassessment of risks, highlighting the importance of predictive models that can forecast where and when infections may occur, as articulated in Brul et al. (2025). It is essential to employ multiple methods to model infectious diseases and understand changes in epidemiology. To simulate the spread of diseases, assess the influence of interventions, and inform public health decisions, mathematical and statistical models are highly useful. They consist of various types, for example, compartmental models group people as susceptible, infected, and recovered, and network models focus on how people interact in their social networks. The use of these methods has enabled the prediction and management of outbreaks more effectively, allowing for a more precise response during major outbreaks. Furthermore, the integration of real-time data collection, epidemiological studies, and molecular typing of pathogens enhances the precision of these models, enabling researchers to tailor interventions with greater accuracy and effectiveness, as noted in Cameron et al. (2017). Therefore, the progress in risk assessment and modelling for infectious diseases depends on knowledge from microbiology, epidemiology, and statistics. A holistic approach encourages scientists, public health workers, and policymakers to communicate and cooperate, which is essential for implementing effective disease control strategies. Additionally, the growing complexity of food systems and the ways diseases spread underscore the need for innovative methods to assess risks that address the numerous challenges posed by modern infectious diseases. Methods such as using molecular markers to detect outbreaks and find the source help experts better understand the pathogens and choose the best response options. Hence, the ongoing refinement of methodologies must align with emerging global health demands, ensuring that risk assessment remains robust and responsive in the face of evolving infectious threats, as emphasized in the discussions captured by Brul et al. (2025).

11.1. Historical Context of Infectious Disease Modelling

The historical context of infectious disease modeling is vital in understanding the evolution of public health responses to epidemics. Early models, such as the SIR (susceptible, infectious, recovered) and SEIR (susceptible, exposed, infectious, recovered) frameworks, emerged from the need to represent the mathematical spread of diseases. They demonstrated how infection rates can lead to outbreaks, which in turn helped drive more innovations. Due to the cholera and influenza epidemics of the 19th and early 20th centuries, public health officials began to utilise these models to predict and control the spread of diseases. With these models, experts could measure the spread of diseases and use that information to manage resources and plan how to stop the outbreaks, which led to the first use of numbers in epidemiology due to real-world events. With the progress of infectious disease modelling, advanced statistical methods were used more often. New approaches, such as stochastic modelling and network analysis, became popular, enabling researchers to study more detailed and changing ways in which diseases spread. We can see this evolution most clearly in how public health responded to the COVID-19 pandemic, which required strong models to give up-to-date information for health interventions. Thanks to new technology, scientists can now handle extensive amounts of data, which has led to new models that show the details of human behaviour and how diseases spread. Such progress made it possible for scientists to use more detailed models that helped them deal with the uncertainties in infectious disease outbreaks. They have greatly helped improve the handling of EIDs. People are paying more attention to the ethical issues related to infectious disease modelling today. Because of ML and big data analytics in modelling, concerns about privacy, consent, and representation have become more noticeable. Such matters gain importance when models are used to guide public health policies that can have a significant effect on communities. During outbreaks, predictive models must ensure accuracy and consider the ethical implications related to data collection and use. In addition, delivering risk information from these models is not easy, since public health messages must be both understandable and useful. As the field grows, it is essential to make the modeling process clear and ensure that all people are included, to keep the public trust and ensure infectious disease management remains effective.

11.1.1. Early Models and Their Impact on Public Health

The early models of infectious disease risk assessment laid crucial groundwork for modern public health initiatives. These pioneering frameworks emerged as the necessity to comprehend disease patterns and their transmission dynamics became more apparent, particularly following the outbreaks of various epidemics. With mathematical and statistical tools, early models enabled public health officials to forecast how diseases would spread and how interventions might be effective. Having the ability to predict helped in handling outbreaks and taking steps to prevent further problems in public health. Improvements in modelling methods greatly benefited public health systems react better, proving that it is essential to understand epidemiological trends early on to limit the effect of infectious diseases on people.

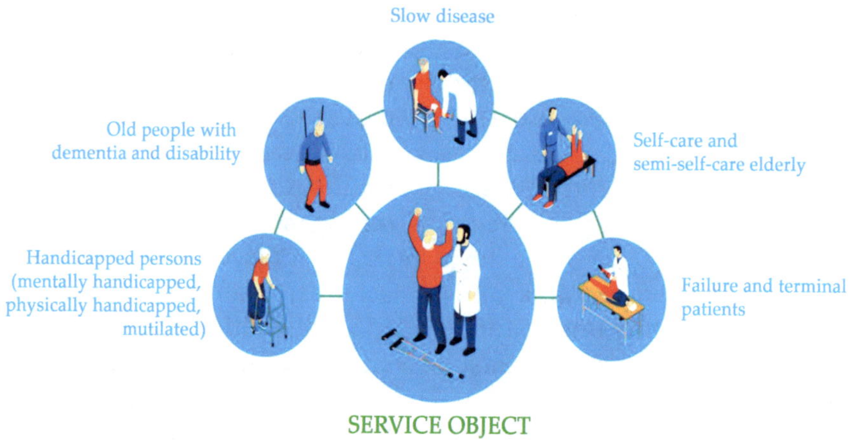

Figure 11.3. Early models of infectious disease risk assessment.

Source: https://www.mdpi.com/sustainability/sustainability-14-16505/article_deploy/html/images/sustainability-14-16505-g001.png.

These early models played a significant role in shaping policies and improving practices within public health departments. Having a structure for studying outbreaks made it easier to identify the social, economic, and environmental factors contributing to disease transmission, which emphasised the need for integrated health intervention strategies. As public health officials used models to assess and change their responses to new threats, it was noticed that modelling also helped engage stakeholders in discussions about how to use health resources and decide on the most critical actions. Such models helped to apply the theory of infectious diseases to practice, which was an essential step for protecting people who were at risk of infection. Additionally, as early models evolved, it became increasingly clear to professionals that public health challenges are more complex, particularly when addressing infodemic situations. These models helped us understand how diseases spread, and they also highlighted the importance of addressing misinformation and public attitudes during health emergencies. It was recognised that data modelling and effective communication strategies go together, so health departments should improve their skills in crisis management and risk communication. This development is necessary for public health to leverage its past experiences and develop improved strategies for handling future pandemics. By advancing statistical modeling techniques and integrating them into comprehensive public health strategies, officials can foster enduring resilience against infectious disease outbreaks, as emphasized in recent assessments of health department capabilities in crisis emergency risk communication and infodemic management (Izah et al., 2024; Tahir et al., 2025) (Figure 11.3).

11.1.2. Evolution of Modelling Techniques Over Time

The evolution of modelling techniques in the field of infectious disease has been marked by significant advances in both theory and application. Initially, models relied on straightforward statistics to forecast disease spread, primarily using data from previous outbreaks. With a better understanding of infectious diseases, researchers began to use more sophisticated models, such as compartmental models that represent how populations move between susceptible, infected, and recovered compartments. Using these models has enhanced our understanding of epidemics and informed public health actions to control them. The rise in complexity in modelling is part of a larger move to handle complexity in biology to improve how we assess and manage risks in infectious diseases. The use of advanced computing has dramatically boosted the progress of modelling approaches. For the last two decades, the rise of high-throughput data and ML algorithms has changed how models are built and adjusted. New methods, such as computational toxicology and in silico models, enable scientists to study various environmental and pharmacological scenarios without the need for animal testing. Due to these new techniques, models can utilise large amounts of data to make more accurate predictions and assess risks. They also enable the real-time monitoring and addressing of infectious disease outbreaks, which is crucial in our interconnected world. Because of this, the field of modelling now includes new ways of thinking that fit our updated knowledge about how diseases are transmitted and how risk is calculated. Pandemics like COVID-19 have prompted researchers to refine and enhance the modelling techniques used for infectious diseases. During the pandemic, various modelling tools, including agent-based and network models, were utilised to understand the spread and inform public health recommendations. The studies in Guatemala highlighted the value of local epidemiological models, demonstrating how diseases varied across different regions and which human activities increased the risk of spreading them. It was clear that effective risk mapping was necessary, and models played a crucial role in facilitating resource distribution and prevention in the event of an outbreak. As the field grows, it becomes clear that modeling will be essential for risk management, continually evolving to provide valuable insights for future epidemic planning and response.

11.1.3. Case Studies of Significant Outbreaks and Responses

The response to significant outbreaks such as the COVID-19 pandemic has underscored the critical importance of practical risk assessment and modelling in infectious disease management. Through careful examination of case studies, public health authorities have developed a deeper understanding of how urban environments can exacerbate transmission rates. For instance, the implementation of disaster risk management (DRM) frameworks has been highlighted as a vital strategy in fostering resilient urban settings. It means looking at all aspects, including city structures and economic and social risks. All parts of the response phase emphasize the importance of implementing changes, including the use of smart city features and new technologies, to control disease spread. They demonstrate how urban planning can be adapted to address future epidemics, thereby improving the community's health preparedness. In studying the SARS-CoV-2 outbreak, experts have gathered basic information about the virus and its significant impact on global health. Examining the virus, the symptoms it causes, and the patterns of its spread explains how it is transmitted and the health problems that arise in epidemics. Case studies have shown that past experiences with coronaviruses inform our approach to new viruses, emphasising the importance of being prepared and acting quickly. For example, new public health policies based on modelling help officials devise ways to prevent the disease from spreading further. This comparison approach supports current actions and helps prepare for future work, which can assist with a unified response to other pandemics. It is just as important in urban resilience to continually review the causes of disease outbreaks and plan effective ways to address them. It is now clear that cities must focus on environmentally friendly city planning and have plans in place for responding to disasters, utilising lessons learned from previous health emergencies. There is now a focus on creating environments that proactively address health risks through community planning and involvement. Urban resilience can be improved by using new tools and encouraging people to be ready for emergencies. Integrating health and urban planning aims to improve crisis management now and ensure the city can adapt and survive over the long run due to EIDs. Understanding and implementing these insights will be crucial in shaping future frameworks for managing public health risks in urban environments, ultimately leading to more effective responses to future outbreaks (Figure 11.4).

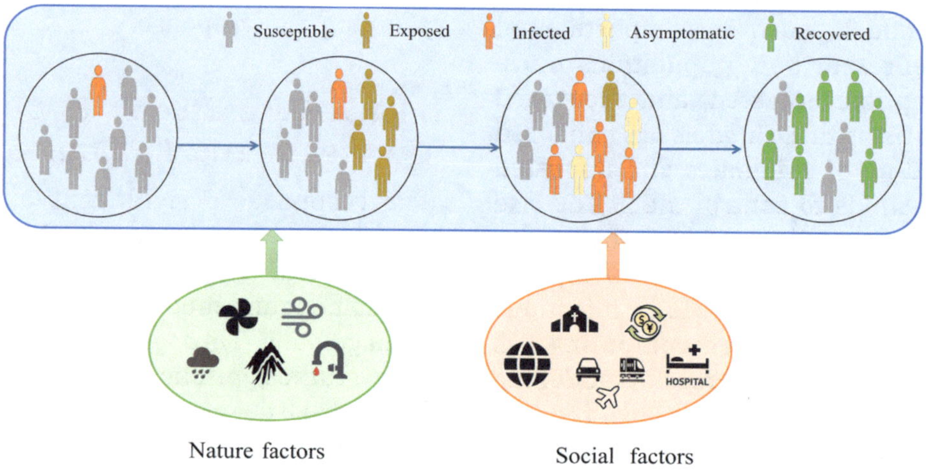

Figure 11.4. Modeling in infectious disease management.

Source: https://media.springernature.com/lw1200/springer-static/image/art%3A10.1186%2Fs40249-024-01195-3/MediaObjects/40249_2024_1195_Fig2_HTML.png.

11.2. Types of Infectious Disease Models

In the realm of infectious disease modelling, various frameworks serve to quantify and analyse the dynamics of disease spread, each tailored to address specific epidemiological questions. Among these, the SEIR (Susceptible, Exposed, Infectious, Removed) model stands out for its ability to incorporate the incubation period of diseases, thereby providing a more nuanced representation than simpler models like SIR. Using compartments, the SEIR framework helps track how individuals move through the different stages of infection, which makes it easier to understand the spread of disease. Being able to adapt demonstrates how complex real-life outbreaks require attention to many groups and different actions. However, using these models can be challenging because it is difficult to accurately select parameters that accurately represent the disease's traits and how the population behaves, as these factors significantly influence predictions about control and public health actions. To improve on compartmental models, it is possible to include details like demographics and different transmission rates, which allows for a more detailed analysis of outbreaks. The SEIR model illustrates how susceptibility can change due to age, frequency of exposure, and other key factors in modern epidemiology. Besides, it enables the use of interventions like vaccination or isolation, helping experts better understand how to control disease spread. Even so, it isn't easy to fit these complex models to the available data because the numerous parameters can easily lead to the model overfitting. This highlights the ongoing requirement for robust data collection methods that can enhance model reliability, ultimately aiding in the formulation of practical risk assessments in infectious disease scenarios (Getz et al., 2019). Additionally, since disease models are constantly evolving, it is essential to regularly review the assumptions that guide them. A central issue with these models is that they assume all people in a population mix evenly, which is not how fundamental social interactions actually happen. During outbreaks, this problem becomes more noticeable because social networks and the movement of people play a big part. Researchers suggest including unpredictable factors and possible obstacles in models to improve how they handle disease management. When these details are included in the models, researchers are better able to imitate the unpredictable nature of outbreaks and measure how different methods compare in terms of their effectiveness and ability to withstand change. Such refinements not only improve predictions but also highlight the critical need for adaptive management approaches to emerge from the enhanced understanding of epidemiological processes (Brown et al., 2017) (Figure 11.5).

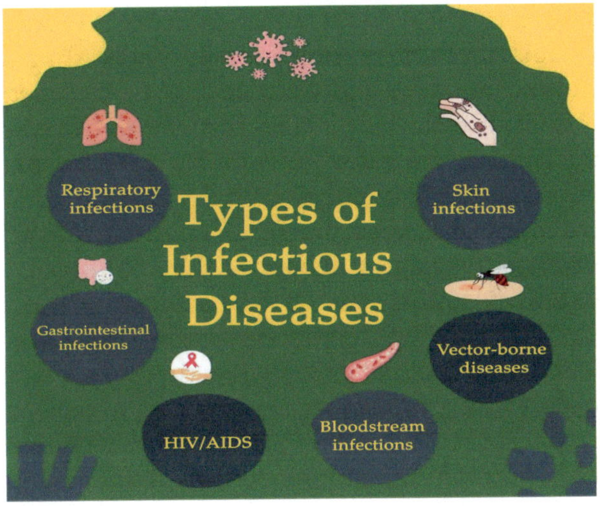

Figure 11.5. Types of infectious disease modeling.

Source: https://ihms.edu.pk/wp-content/uploads/2023/07/Beige-Types-of-coffee-Instagram-Post.jpg.

11.2.1. Deterministic Versus Stochastic Models

In the field of infectious disease modelling, distinguishing between deterministic and stochastic models is crucial. Deterministic models believe that outcomes can be predicted and repeated if you know the initial conditions. These models are typically configured with fixed parameters that enable them to make precise predictions about how infections will spread over a specified period. For instance, compartmental models, such as the SIR (Susceptible, Infectious, Recovered) model and its derivatives, present a structured approach to understanding epidemic behaviour. However, the idealistic nature of these models often overlooks the complexities inherent in real-world scenarios, as outlined in recent findings that emphasise the need for extended models incorporating external frictions and robustness measures in the management of epidemics (Brown et al., 2017). Thus, even though deterministic frameworks help predict results, their straightforwardness can cause people to miss the fact that infectious diseases are often unpredictable. Alternatively, stochastic models include randomness to show that biological systems are rarely predictable. Because they account for the randomness of interactions among individuals, these models can simulate how outbreaks may occur and estimate risks more accurately. These approaches help to assess changes in the rates of contact, the risk of getting sick, and environmental conditions, which are common influences on how infections spread. This becomes important when diseases are evolving rapidly, as the factors influencing transmission can also change. The ability to account for these variables enhances the robustness of model predictions, making stochastic modelling a critical component of risk assessment in infectious disease management, as represented in studies examining extensive outbreak scenarios, such as Ebola (Getz et al., 2019). The fact that both deterministic and stochastic models are used in risk assessment and epidemic forecasting leads to further exploration of their uses. Deterministic models are easy to understand; however, because they do not effectively handle real-world issues, stochastic elements are necessary to make predictions more accurate. With the progress in infectious disease modeling, researchers are increasingly encouraged to combine the benefits of both types of approaches. Recognising the complexity of infectious diseases and acknowledging the limitations of some frameworks enables researchers to address disease transmission and management more effectively. This integration not only augments the computational complexity of model analysis, as highlighted in recent studies, but also enhances the understanding of epidemic dynamics, leading to more informed decision-making and effective public health interventions (Brown et al., 2017).

11.2.2. Compartmental Models (SIR, SEIR)

Compartmental models, such as the SIR (Susceptible, Infectious, Recovered) and SEIR (Susceptible, Exposed, Infectious, Recovered) frameworks, serve as pivotal tools in understanding the dynamics of infectious disease spread. Models that separate the population into compartments allow for an easier study of how diseases are spread and how interventions work. For example, the SIR model groups people according to whether they have the disease, which helps study how the disease spreads over time. Alternatively, the SEIR model includes an extra group for people who have been infected but are not yet capable of spreading the disease, which helps understand diseases with a long incubation period. Because of this approach, predictions about infection rates are more accurate and can guide public health responses, mainly when the disease is spreading rapidly. When emergencies like the Russian invasion of Ukraine occur, compartmental models are beneficial for understanding the risks from infectious diseases. Emergencies can force large groups of people to move, which can lead to the spread of more contagious diseases. Using the SIR and SEIR models, researchers can study how these interruptions change the spread of the disease and its numbers when a crisis occurs. They enable the combination of data on demographics, the environment, and healthcare, facilitating close monitoring of disease spread. The adaptability of compartmental models to various contexts is crucial for understanding the epidemic threats posed by emergencies and guiding public health decisions aimed at mitigating risks (Chumachenko et al., 2024a). Additionally, employing ML algorithms and other advanced computational methods can enhance the effectiveness of traditional compartmental models. For example, using hybrid models that connect compartments with data on time and space helps more accurately simulate how infectious diseases are affected by climate. According to studies, diseases transmitted by insects, such as malaria, are susceptible to environmental changes; therefore, models must be able to adapt to them. The VECTRI model, which employs a grid-distributed approach alongside a simple SEIR framework, exemplifies this integration, demonstrating its effectiveness in simulating malaria transmission in response to fluctuating climatic factors (Fall et al., 2022). Improved compartmental models with advanced approaches make them more dependable for modeling infectious diseases which helps with risk assessment and encourages early public health actions.

11.2.3. Agent-Based Models and Their Applications

In the context of infectious disease risk assessment, agent-based models (ABMs) serve as a powerful tool for simulating interactions among individuals within a population, thereby facilitating a nuanced understanding of disease transmission dynamics. They portray each individual as a self-governing agent who makes decisions based on set rules and inputs from their surroundings. Because ABMs represent a wide range of behaviours, they can explain the possible outcomes of actions such as social distancing or vaccination on infectious diseases. Furthermore, their adaptability allows for the integration of complex variables, including travel behaviours and environmental influences, making ABMs particularly suitable for scenarios where traditional models may fall short, such as during outbreaks in densely populated areas or alongside other risk factors present (Kone et al., 2024). Besides exploring ideas, ABMs can be used to guide public health strategies and decisions. For instance, they have proven effective in modelling the impact of interventions during epidemics, such as the transmission dynamics of respiratory diseases exacerbated by interactive behaviours in confined spaces, like airports (Kone et al., 2024). They help health authorities forecast possible outbreaks based on the actions taken and assess the effectiveness of those actions. Through running tests in various conditions, those in charge can learn about how elements impact the risk of infection and the outcomes of disease control methods, which helps them manage resources and plan their response to infectious diseases. In addition, agent-based models help explain how contagious agents spread during foodborne illness incidents. Utilising techniques like quantitative microbial risk assessment (QMRA), researchers can simulate the behaviour of pathogens, thereby estimating risk levels associated with food consumption and handling practices, as demonstrated in scenarios involving Salmonella and Listeria contamination. ABMs help by creating detailed models that include how food is distributed, what people eat, and the environment, which leads to valuable insights on how to decrease foodborne diseases. Ultimately, these efforts contribute to a more proactive approach toward managing public health risks associated with infectious diseases, indicating that agent-based models are invaluable in both elucidating disease mechanisms and aiding in effective risk management strategies (Figure 11.6).

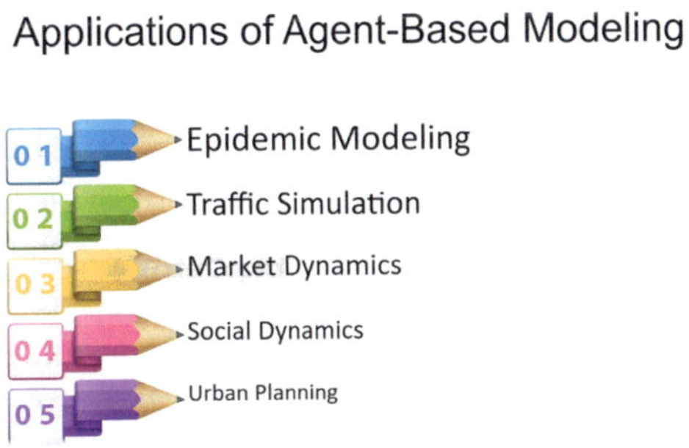

Figure 11.6. Agent-based models and their applications.

Source: https://fastercapital.co/i/Agent-Based-Modeling--Exploring-Complex-Systems-with-Agent-Based-Model-Simulation--Applications-of-Agent-Based-Modeling.webp.

11.3. Data Collection and Analysis in Risk Assessment

Risk assessment for infectious diseases depends on proper data collection and analysis. Through these processes, researchers and public health authorities can determine how diseases are spreading, assess the effectiveness of interventions, and predict when new outbreaks may occur. To illustrate, the Oxford COVID-19 Government Response Tracker, which records government responses, gives essential insights into the effects of various policies on disease spread. This helps understand how well containment policies worked and when they were most effective, which supports real-time decision-making. By integrating behavioural and epidemiological indicators with policy data, researchers can construct a more nuanced understanding of the interplay between human actions and disease dynamics, thus enhancing overall risk assessment methodologies (Hale et al., 2021). In addition, the growth of ML and data analytics has dramatically improved how data is gathered and analysed for the risk of infectious diseases. Using data with many dimensions, scientists can discover important information about diseases and the behaviour of pathogens. They are significant for studying plant and animal stress from diseases that might affect food supply, as they allow scientists to detect and sort out stress factors at all levels, from individual organisms to the entire ecosystem. ML algorithms that work well can identify relationships between different variables, which helps improve the reliability of disease prediction and care strategies. The integration of automated data collection methods, such as unmanned aerial systems (UAS), alongside ML-driven analysis, creates a robust framework for ongoing surveillance and rapid response to emergent infectious disease threats (Singh et al., 2020). Substantial data collection and analysis support not only short-term risk management but also guide long-term public health planning. Thanks to the use of complete data and robust analysis, public health officials can predict the spread of infectious diseases, assess the risks from new pathogens, and develop more effective ways to address them. When a global pandemic occurs, fast and accurate data can determine if the virus spreads or is controlled. Also, standardising how data is collected helps various groups, such as government agencies and research institutions, to work together and share information about diseases. Ultimately, robust data practices in risk assessment not only inform effective responses but also contribute to the resilience of public health systems in an increasingly interconnected world (Hale et al., 2021) (Figure 11.7).

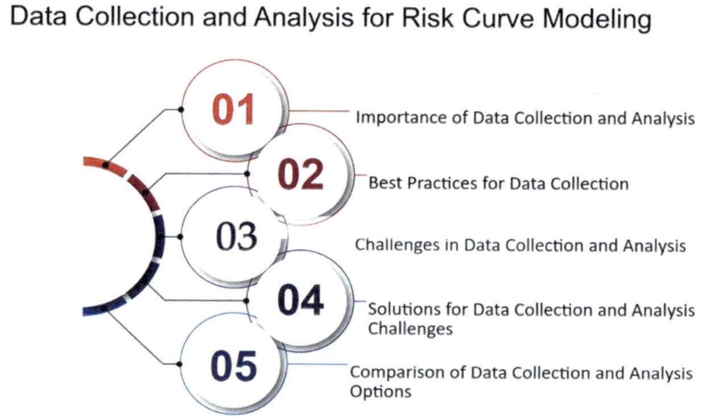

Figure 11.7. Effective data collection and analysis are fundamental components of risk.

Source: https://fastercapital.co/i/Risk-curve-modeling--Navigating-uncertainties-for-better-decision-making--Data-Collection-and-Analysis-for-Risk-Curve-Modeling.webp.

11.3.1. Sources of Data for Infectious Disease Modelling

In infectious disease modelling, the integration of diverse data sources is critical for producing accurate risk assessments. Long-standing disease surveillance systems at public health agencies, such as the Centres for Disease Control and Prevention, help gather data. These systems heavily rely on routine data regarding diseases, potential exposures, and the population. The establishment of an environmental public healthtracking (EPHT) network is a recent initiative aimed at enhancing these connections. Connecting collected disease data with ecological information enables the EPHT to better understand chronic diseases and improve the accuracy of infectious disease forecasts.

Additionally, the incorporation of real-time data allows for timely responses to emerging infectious threats, ensuring that public health strategies are informed by current evidence and environmental contexts (Balmes et al., 2004). Molecular and digital information is another primary source of data used in infectious disease modelling. With better genomic sequencing technologies and bioinformatics, researchers can now study the genes of pathogens in greater detail. With information from social media and mobile health apps, this system allows real-time tracking of infectious disease outbreaks. Using these data with standard models helps make forecasts more accurate and also identifies those who might be most vulnerable to epidemics. As the field evolves, innovators in infectious disease epidemiology are called upon to refine analytical techniques that can incorporate such novel data, ultimately advancing both research and public health strategies (Lewnard et al., 2019).

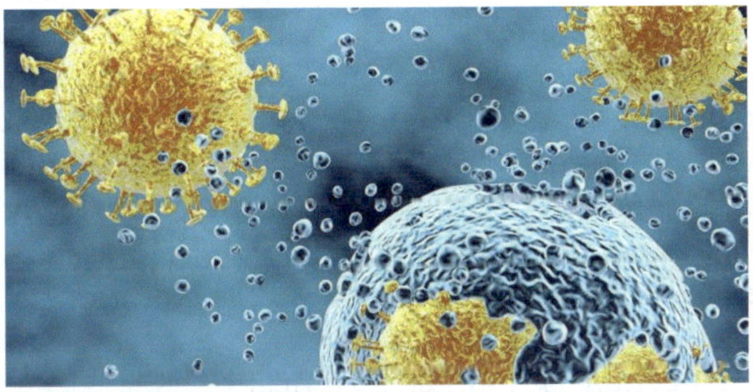

Figure 11.8. The data of infectious disease modeling.

Source: https://www.corning.com/media/worldwide/cls/images/cls%20Applications/cls-disease-modeling-infectious-disease-resources-engineering-viral-infections-ls.jpg.transform/retina-704/img.jpg.

By combining different types of data, infectious disease modelling highlights how the field is always progressing. As new pathogens emerge and existing ones evolve, the field must continually adapt and generate new ideas. Researchers must create frameworks that utilise all these types of data to enhance the accuracy of risk assessment and modelling. Examining existing statistical methods closely and incorporating a broader range of data sources enables us to gain a deeper understanding of how infectious diseases behave. This comprehensive approach not only enhances the predictive power of models but also ensures that public health interventions are data-driven and responsive to the multifaceted nature of infectious disease threats (Lewnard et al., 2019; Balmes et al., 2004) (Figure 11.8).

11.3.2. Statistical Methods Used in Data Analysis

In the realm of risk assessment and modelling in infectious disease, statistical methods play a crucial role in deriving actionable insights from complex datasets. Among the most used techniques is logistic regression, which helps find links between risk factors and the outcomes of infectious diseases. For example, logistic regression can analyse the chances of infection considering sex, age, and immunological factors. In a study on systemic lupus erythematosus, the odds ratio calculated through logistic regression revealed significant disparities in infection risk between male and female patients, underscoring how statistical analysis can illuminate critical health disparities (Borrelli et al., 2025). In addition, using goodness-of-fit tests, such as the Hosmer-Lemeshow test, confirms that the models are a good fit for the observed data, which helps researchers draw reliable conclusions. Descriptive statistics and correlation analyses are also crucial in statistical methods because they provide fundamental insights into data and its variables. Descriptive statistics are used in these studies to summarise the population and assess the perceived risk of infectious diseases. For instance, an empirical study in Russia utilised descriptive statistics alongside odds ratio calculations to explain behaviours associated with infectious disease management

(Lebedeva-Nesevria et al., 2024). They show not only what the typical perception is, but also the differences in risk assessments among various groups. Statistical analysis provides a clearer picture of the data, which helps in designing effective and responsive public health strategies and interventions for communities. Additionally, employing advanced statistical techniques, such as factor analysis, enhances the detail of data analysis in infectious disease research. It helps to identify the main patterns in large datasets and categorise variables based on their connections. It can be beneficial for learning about behavioral methods to control infectious diseases. The research cited previously illustrated how factor analysis identified key action groups—information seeking, creating protective spaces, and external interactions—representing shared behaviors among urban populations (Lebedeva-Nesevria et al., 2024). By painting a clearer picture of how individuals respond to perceived risks, factor analysis equips public health officials and researchers with the knowledge needed to design targeted interventions that resonate with specific populations, ultimately improving health outcomes in the face of infectious threats (Figure 11.9).

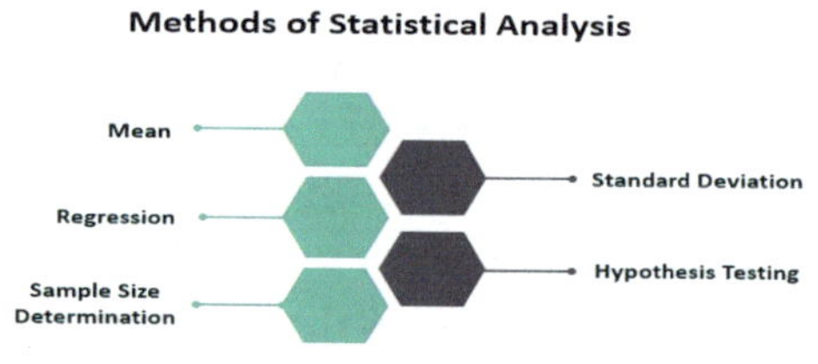

Figure 11.9. The statistical data analysis.

Source: https://wallstreetmojo-files.s3.ap-south-1.amazonaws.com/2022/05/Methods-of-Statistical-Analysis.jpg.

11.3.3. Challenges in Data Collection and Accuracy

The success of risk assessment and modelling in infectious diseases depends a lot on the quality and accuracy of the collected data. There is a significant challenge here because data can come from many different sources, including clinical and genetic records. Because of this inconsistency, the data used for modelling can be various. For instance, when applying deep learning in medical diagnostics, errors in medical imaging data can lead to incorrect predictions. Furthermore, many datasets lack the diversity necessary to generalize findings across different demographics, further complicating the task of generating reliable models that can be extended to broader populations, as evidenced in the ongoing research in Argentina (Elena, 2025). Another critical issue is integrating data, particularly when using ML for public health tasks like contact tracing. Their success is based on handling various types of data, such as personal health information and data on human movement. Not collecting data properly can result in missing some contacts or not having complete risk profiles, which reduces the trust in the model. Additionally, questions about data privacy complicate matters; it is necessary to establish robust privacy measures that safeguard sensitive data while enabling effective public health actions. The importance of data quality and integration cannot be overstated, as it forms the foundational basis for building accurate and effective ML models (Siddiq, 2023). Additionally, ensuring a reliable method for ongoing data verification is another significant challenge. As diseases change, the models that explain their effects should also change. It is essential to keep collecting data and giving feedback, but many public health institutions find it difficult to manage this process. The situation worsens due to insufficient resources, technological issues, and the urgent need to respond quickly upon the onset of an outbreak. Because of this, when data accuracy is not maintained, the predictions from the model may become less reliable. Addressing these challenges is crucial for ensuring that risk assessment frameworks remain effective and can adapt to the evolving landscape of infectious diseases (Siddiq, 2023; Elena, 2025) (Figure 11.10).

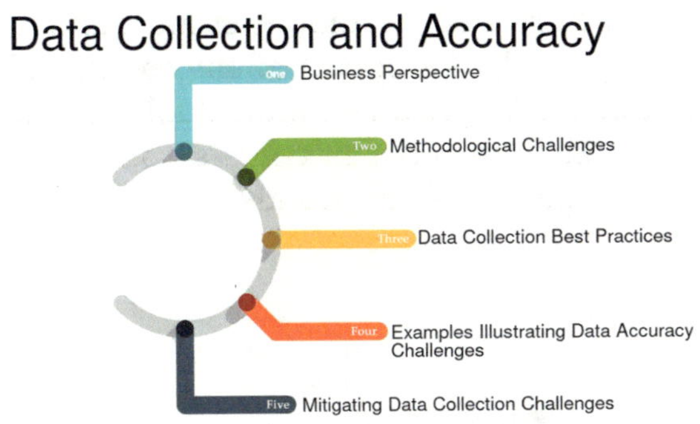

Figure 11.10. Challenges in data collection and accuracy.

Source: https://fastercapital.co/i/Market-Share-Analysis-Challenges--How-to-Overcome-the-Common-Challenges-of-Market-Share-Analysis--Data-Collection-and-Accuracy.webp.

11.4. Risk Factors in Infectious Disease Spread

It is essential to understand the risk factors that help infectious diseases spread to assess and model risks properly. Climate change, urbanisation, and societal shifts are key factors in how hosts, pathogens, and the environment interact. For instance, if the weather changes, mosquitoes may be able to live in more places, which can result in more cases of malaria and ZIKV. In addition, cities growing too quickly can lead to overcrowding, which increases contact and reduces cleanliness, thereby facilitating the spread of infectious diseases. Because of these factors, it is essential to use models that consider the whole situation in which these diseases appear and spread, which helps guide prevention and public health policies. Many infectious diseases are transmitted from animals to humans, making zoonotic transmission a vital means of their spread. Many significant pandemics, such as HIV/AIDS and SARS, are caused by viruses that move from animals to humans because of changes in the environment and human actions. To deal with this challenge, one must understand the relationships among human, animal, and environmental health. Deforestation and the trade of wild animals can increase the risk of zoonotic diseases being transmitted to humans and causing outbreaks. Using surveillance at these interfaces is essential for identifying and assessing risks, which helps protect global health. New mathematical modelling techniques have emerged that can locate and report previously unknown pathogens, thereby providing opportunities to mitigate the risks of future pandemics (Carroll et al., 2012). Additionally, the methods we use to manage epidemics must evolve to keep pace with the complexities of current diseases. Ebola and H1N1 are recent examples that demonstrate the need for more detailed theories to reflect how outbreaks are handled accurately. Extending epidemic models to cover management processes and include unpredictable challenges in the response is necessary for better procedures and organisational actions. Including robustness and risk measures in their assessments allows stakeholders to handle the complexities of infectious disease spread. As models become more complicated, they become increasingly difficult to analyze and utilize with computers. Developing streamlined approaches to simplify this analysis will be crucial for effective epidemic management and risk assessment (Brown et al., 2017).

11.4.1. Environmental Factors Influencing Disease Transmission

The interplay between environmental factors and disease transmission is multifaceted, significantly impacting the epidemiology of infectious diseases. Vectors like mosquitoes and other pathogens thrive in habitats made possible by temperature, humidity, and precipitation. An increase in temperature can cause parasites in the vectors to develop more rapidly, leading to a higher number of humans being infected. Additionally, the amount and timing of rainfall can determine whether there is standing water, which malaria vectors, such as Anopheles mosquitoes, need for their breeding grounds. Satellite data are now used to study the impact of environmental factors on malaria, providing detailed insights into how weather changes affect individuals at risk. Satellites provide rich data sources that can assess the relationships between climate conditions and malaria occurrence, revealing critical insights into seasonal and long-term trends that influence infection rates (Wimberly et al., 2021).

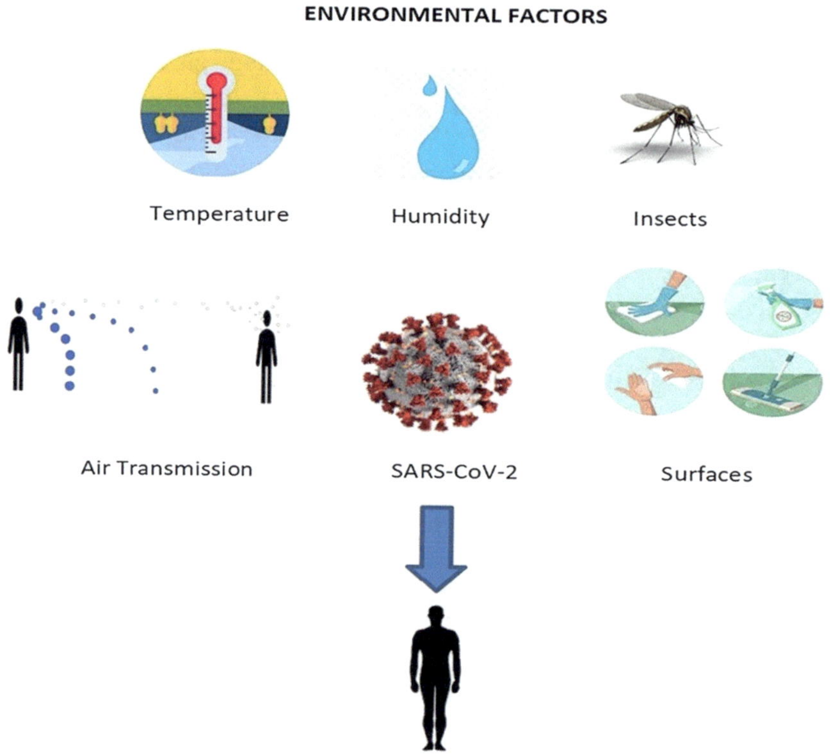

Figure 11.11. Environmental factors and disease transmission.

Source: https://media.springernature.com/lw1200/springer-static/image/art%3A10.1007%2Fs10311-022-01418-9/MediaObjects/10311_2022_1418_Fig1_HTML.png.

Changes in land use are essential factors in influencing how diseases are spread. Deforestation, city growth and more farming change the environment in ways that encourage diseases to appear. For example, irrigation in farming can provide suitable habitats for vectors, thereby increasing the likelihood of malaria transmission. In some places, urbanisation can cut down on malaria by destroying the usual breeding sites, but it can also cause more cases in areas where urban-adapted mosquitoes live. These challenges can be managed well with the help of spatial decision support systems, which allow environmental data to be included in strategies against malaria. By analysing land use patterns and integrating them with epidemiological data, interventions can be better targeted to high-risk areas (Chen et al., 2020). Additionally, the latest developments in remote sensing and big data analysis are enabling us to better understand the environmental effects on infectious diseases. With high-quality satellite images and land temperature data, it is possible to watch for changes in the environment over different periods. Because of these improvements, researchers can better link climate change to disease spread, which helps build a stronger model for risk assessment. For example, research shows that both precipitation and temperature are essential factors in how mosquitoes behave, which affects the spread of malaria. Also, because satellite data and cloud computing are now available for free, anyone can use geospatial information for malaria research and control activities. Therefore, ongoing collaboration between environmental scientists and public health professionals is critical to develop effective, evidence-based strategies for infectious disease mitigation (Wimberly et al., 2021) (Figure 11.11).

11.4.2. Socioeconomic Determinants of Health

Understanding the socioeconomic determinants of health is essential for conducting accurate risk assessments and developing effective models in infectious disease epidemiology. These determinants encompass a range of factors, including income, education, living conditions, and access to healthcare, all of which significantly influence health outcomes and vulnerability to diseases. If epidemiological models do not account for these factors, their predictions may be inaccurate and lead to ineffective policies, particularly during infectious disease outbreaks, where social disparities can impact the effectiveness of response plans. Some social groups may suffer more from diseases because they are denied access to the medical care and resources they need. Consequently, integrating socioeconomic factors into modelling efforts enhances the predictive capability of these models and ensures that they address the needs of diverse populations (Ali et al., 2024). Additionally, research has shown that social factors play a significant role in explaining why certain groups are at higher risk and experience worse outcomes from diseases. For example, a study examining cancer patients revealed that race and socioeconomic status (SES) significantly influenced the stages at which diagnoses were made and the time to metastasis or death. Those from poorer communities were more likely to experience dangers and worse results than people from richer areas. The results demonstrate that socioeconomic factors are crucial for health and should be taken into account in models that assess risks from infectious diseases. By accurately reflecting these disparities, modellers can tailor public health interventions that holistically address the underlying causes of health inequities (Osterland et al., 2024). Socioeconomic factors must be considered in infectious disease modelling because it is necessary for fair healthcare access. Decisions made from models that do not consider this can perpetuate health disparities, which is detrimental to public health.

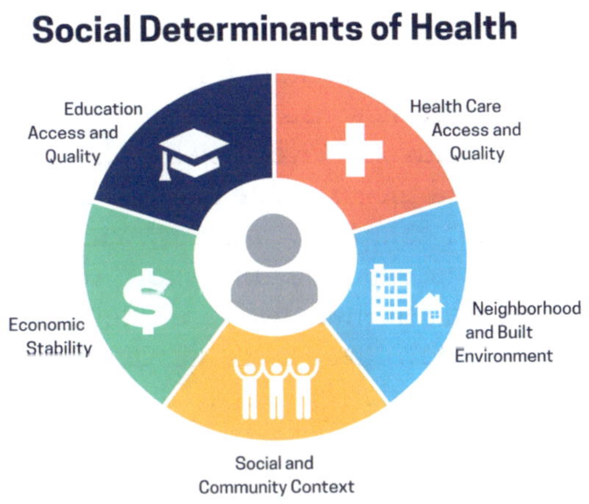

Figure 11.12. Socioeconomic determinants of health.

Source: https://www.cancer.gov/rare-brain-spine-tumor/sites/g/files/xnrzdm226/files/styles/cgov_article/public/cgov_image/media_image/2024-06/Healthy%20People%202030%20SDOH%20Graphic%20Domain%20Labels_0.png?h=b8ebcc01&itok=jegVom05.

If public health strategies acknowledge that health risks vary across socioeconomic groups, they can be more effective in supporting those at risk. By using this approach, the models for economic forecasting during outbreaks are more accurate, and resources are distributed to support health equity. Therefore, as policymakers navigate the complexities of infectious disease management, it is imperative that socioeconomic determinants of health are front and center in model formulations to drive effective and just health interventions (Ali et al., 2024) (Figure 11.12).

11.4.3. Behavioural Factors and Public Compliance

The intersection of behavioural factors and public compliance plays a critical role in managing infectious disease outbreaks, influencing the effectiveness of public health interventions. The extent to which people follow vaccination, hygiene, and social distancing largely depends on their perception of risk and their social environment. People who think they might get sick are much more likely to follow health advice. Nevertheless, when people misunderstand the risks due to misinformation, they may not comply with rules, which could lead to the disease spreading more widely. To make sure health messages are effective, it is essential to know these dynamics and use them to create strategies that suit the needs and habits of different groups. They can guide the evaluation of risks and play a role in designing effective public health actions. Additionally, social factors can significantly impact how effectively people follow guidelines in managing infectious diseases. SES, education, and access to healthcare significantly influence whether someone follows public health advice. Those who are vulnerable often have difficulties getting the necessary information and resources, which may cause health inequalities. Due to both trust issues and practical hurdles, individuals from lower socioeconomic backgrounds were less likely to comply with masking and vaccination during the COVID-19 pandemic. Taking care of these social factors improves compliance among everyone, especially those who are marginalised. When these factors are incorporated into risk assessment models, public health officials can more easily identify ways to encourage people to follow health advice and mitigate the impact of infectious diseases. Using behavioural insights when designing public health interventions is crucial for encouraging people to follow the rules during infectious disease outbreaks. It suggests that understanding the factors that influence choices can help identify more effective ways to encourage compliance. For example, making small changes in the environment, such as placing hand sanitizer in public places, can encourage people to get vaccinated or wash their hands. Sharing information promptly and openly by health authorities can improve how the public views risks and encourages them to cooperate.

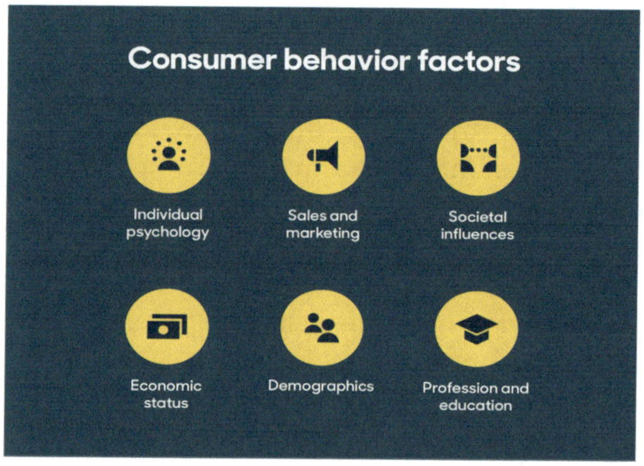

Figure 11.13. Behavioral factors and public compliance.

Source: https://d1eipm3vz40hy0.cloudfront.net/images/AMER/consumerbehavior44.png.

As illustrated in the context of the Russian invasion in Ukraine, where health systems face significant challenges, the application of a framework like the Capacity, Vulnerability, and Risk Assessment (CVRA) can help identify both behavioral and systemic barriers to compliance in conflict zones. This multidimensional approach highlights the need for a nuanced understanding of public behavior to maximize the efficacy of infectious disease modeling and risk assessment initiatives, thereby promoting better health outcomes in diverse contexts (Chumachenko et al., 2024b; Izah et al., 2024) (Figure 11.13).

11.5. Applications of Risk Assessment in Public Health

Risk assessment plays a crucial role in public health, particularly when managing infectious diseases. Various models and approaches enable public health officials to assess the risks associated with spreading pathogens, which helps them plan for managing and preventing outbreaks. One of the best-known strategies in this area is QMRA, which uses different disciplines to determine and predict infection risks. According to recent workshops, the field identifies important research areas that include improving dose-response studies and exposure measurements. Furthermore, it emphasises the necessity of a collaborative research community that can harmonise environmental monitoring efforts with QMRA, ultimately strengthening public health responses worldwide (Hamilton et al., 2024). Working together is crucial for the progress of risk assessment and better informing both policymakers and the public about risks. Seasonal infectious diseases require risk assessment to be adjusted to the particular ways in which pathogens are transmitted. Since outbreak potential changes with the seasons, it is essential to understand when and how pathogens might infect people. Traditionally, the Case Epidemic Risk (CER) has been utilised to gauge these probabilities; however, limitations exist, particularly regarding pathogens that may become extinct due to temporal constraints on transmission opportunities. For example, if a pathogen is only present during certain seasons, the CER can give wrong information about its ability to cause an outbreak. To address this, researchers have introduced the Threshold Epidemic Risk (TER), which estimates the likelihood that an outbreak will exceed a certain infection threshold before becoming extinct, providing more contextually relevant assessments for public health planning (Kaye et al., 2024). Besides using technology, risk assessment in public health also requires the application of scientific knowledge to inform new policies. Using new approaches such as molecular tools in QMRA, demonstrates that the industry is dedicated to making data more accurate and reliable. With information on co-exposure risks and by using consistent modelling, health authorities are better prepared for new infectious disease outbreaks. Additionally, creating strong communication plans and securing the necessary funds for research are crucial for advancing public health initiatives. As the body of knowledge surrounding infectious disease risks evolves, public health frameworks must remain flexible and responsive to incorporate these advancements for improved health outcomes (Hamilton et al., 2024).

11.5.1. Informing Policy Decisions and Resource Allocation

The role of risk assessment and modelling in informing policy decisions and resource allocation cannot be overstated, especially in the context of infectious diseases. Oxford COVID-19 Government Response Tracker data indicate that swift and effective government actions were crucial during the pandemic. Monitoring policies in over 180 nations allows users to compare approaches and discover which methods have been most helpful for infection control. Such analytical frameworks enable the evaluation of the impacts of different interventions on the spread of COVID-19, ultimately contributing to more informed decision-making that can save lives and allocate resources effectively within healthcare systems (Hale et al., 2021).

In addition, it is essential to assess the risk among specific groups, such as frontline healthcare workers, to guide the appropriate interventions and protect them adequately. Research examining the risk of COVID-19 among healthcare professionals compared to the general community highlights the need to integrate personal protective equipment (PPE) guidelines into policy frameworks. Data on PPE and infection risk help determine where to allocate resources, ensuring that health workers handling outbreaks are protected. By utilising this evidence base, policymakers can craft tailored strategies that not only preserve front-line workers but also maintain healthcare system functionality during crises (Nguyen et al., 2020). Policymakers must take into account epidemiological indicators, healthcare resources, and socio-economic factors. It is essential to understand the economic effects of different actions during infectious disease outbreaks to decide how to use resources best. For example, tough lockdowns may help stop the spread of disease, but they can seriously harm local businesses and add pressure to social services. Using models that measure both health and economic factors, policymakers can find a good balance between controlling the virus and maintaining the economy. Informed policies based on solid risk assessments can show how health, economy, and society are connected, which helps prepare for future infectious disease threats.

11.5.2. Outbreak Prediction and Management Strategies

The effective prediction and management of infectious disease outbreaks hinge on the incorporation of advanced statistical models and comprehensive data analytics. Because there is a lack of data on EIDs, traditional epidemiological models struggle to assess the risks involved. One way to address this challenge is by utilising SpatMCDA, which incorporates spatial multi-criteria decision analysis to enhance risk prediction. By using standardized risks and weighting them according to their importance, SpatMCDA helps identify areas at high risk, even with limited data. Furthermore, its application in mapping areas at risk for diseases such as West Nile virus in China highlights the model's potential utility in understanding transmission patterns and guiding targeted public health interventions, thereby fostering a proactive approach to outbreak management (Wang et al., 2024). Besides modelling, the use of specialised infrastructure is crucial for dealing with infectious disease outbreaks. The ISTARI 1B isolation tent case in Uganda during the 2022 Sudan ebolavirus outbreak clearly demonstrates that utilising specific resources can significantly enhance how cases are managed and infection is prevented. The ISTARI 1B, which promotes safe and standardised care, is a practical method for helping in high-risk areas. Through a collaborative effort involving local health authorities and institutions, comprehensive site assessments were conducted across various health facilities, ensuring that the infrastructure met the necessary standards for effective isolation and treatment (Broadhurst et al., 2024). Utilising such strategies enhances healthcare systems and makes the country better equipped to respond to outbreaks. In the end, combining predictive modelling with strategic infrastructure provides a comprehensive approach to handling and predicting outbreaks. By employing advanced approaches and situating interventions within the healthcare context, public health officials can gain valuable insights that enable them to respond promptly to potential outbreaks. For example, using SpatMCDA data together with current health services can help people better understand how diseases spread, which allows communities to improve their response to them. This multifaceted strategy ensures that resources are allocated effectively and that health systems are prepared for emergent threats, affirming the importance of foresight and adaptability in managing infectious diseases in an increasingly interconnected world (Figure 11.14).

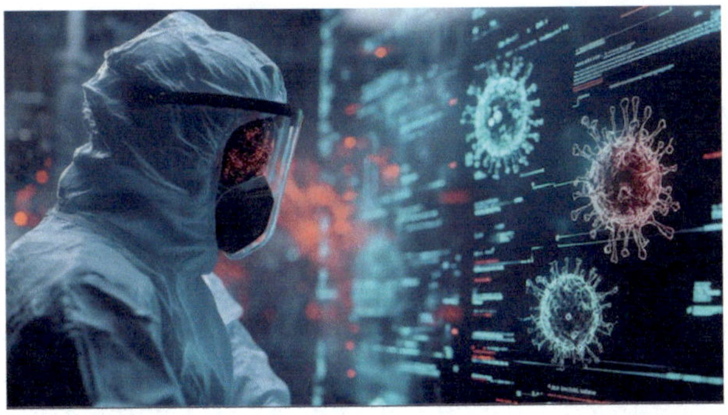

Figure 11.14. The effective prediction and management of infectious disease outbreaks.

Source: https://img.freepik.com/premium-photo/aipowered-epidemic-outbreak-prediction-digital-interface-showing-realtime-predictions-epidemic-outbreaks_1230253-18826.jpg.

11.5.3. Vaccination Strategies and Their Modelling

Vaccination strategies play a crucial role in controlling and preventing infectious diseases, especially in the context of fluctuating immunity. Traditional models, such as the SIR (susceptible-infected-recovered) framework, have long been utilised to examine the dynamics of disease transmission. However, as vaccination efforts evolve, the introduction of models like the SIRSV (susceptible-infected-recovered susceptible-vaccinated) allows for a more nuanced understanding of how vaccinated populations influence transmission dynamics. When immunity weakens over time, the risk of infection can increase for some individuals, potentially leading to new outbreaks. By integrating individual and society-based risk assessments (SB-RA) within these models, researchers can derive effective reproduction numbers that inform public health interventions and vaccination strategies to mitigate the impact of infectious diseases (Meng et al., 2025). Modelling vaccination strategies also helps look at how people choose to be vaccinated, which can change the results of public health efforts. When vaccination rates differ among groups, the level of immunity in the population can be uneven, which may influence the spread of diseases. Researchers can simulate models that examine the effects of individuals' vaccination decisions on the spread of disease within the community using probabilistic methods. Such a detailed study is essential to understand the results of strategies aimed at achieving herd immunity.

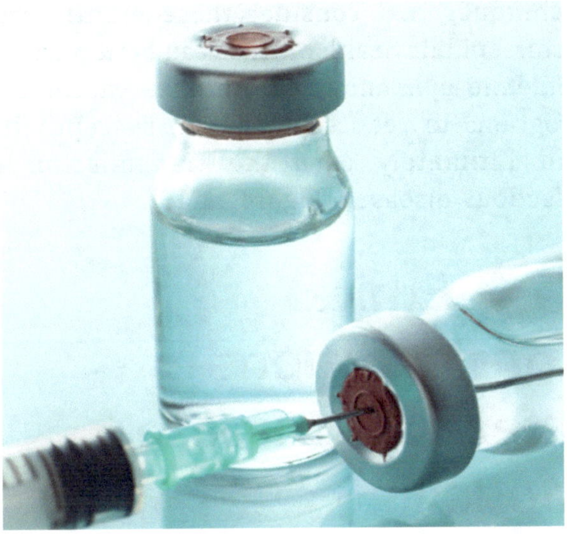

Figure 11.15. Vaccination strategies and their modeling.

*Source:*https://explore.research.ufl.edu/wp-content/uploads/2021/05/Morris-influenza-vaccine-770x770.jpg.

The incorporation of risk assessment methods, such as the individual-based risk assessment (IB-RA) and SB-RA, enables a comprehensive evaluation of both localised and global perspectives on vaccination, promoting the formulation of effective public health strategies tailored to population needs (Meng et al., 2025). Additionally, recent research on airborne transmission highlights the importance of considering environmental factors in vaccine modelling. Recent research indicates that airborne pathogens, which persist in the air, can lead to increased infections, particularly on the International Space Station. Because of these insights, we should consider using an approach that covers both biology and environmental and social factors when modelling vaccinations. For this reason, it is essential to use vaccination strategies that consider how well the immune system works and how much risk of exposure there is to manage the spread of infectious diseases. By leveraging advanced modeling techniques that consider these multifaceted factors, public health officials can better predict epidemic dynamics and optimize vaccination programs to reduce population susceptibility and ultimately curb the transmission of infectious diseases (Figure 11.15).

11.6. Ethical Considerations in Infectious Disease Modelling

The ethical considerations surrounding infectious disease modelling are critical to ensuring that public health initiatives are effective and just. Transparency is an essential ethical principle, meaning people should be aware of the modelling methods and the underlying assumptions. If data is misrepresented or oversimplified, it can lead to incorrect decisions in health policy, potentially exacerbating health inequalities. For example, models that focus solely on certain groups may lead to unfairness in the distribution of resources and healthcare. As discussed in ethical frameworks, sharing model results in a way that is easy for everyone to understand helps build trust and encourages people to participate. Hence, ethical modelling practices necessitate a commitment to open dialogue and the equitable distribution of information (Adefemi et al., 2023). Another significant ethical consideration involves privacy and data security. Many infectious disease models rely on extensive health data about individuals, which raises concerns about how this information is collected, stored, and utilised. Trouble arises when models utilise sensitive data without obtaining proper consent, which can infringe upon people's rights and erode trust in the system. The integration of ML and artificial intelligence (AI) in disease surveillance exemplifies this challenge;. At the same time, these technologies offer enhanced predictive capabilities, they also risk compromising patient confidentiality if not managed appropriately. Therefore, establishing robust protocols for data protection and ensuring that ethical guidelines govern the use of personal information in modeling practices are paramount to responsible research in public health (Siddiq, 2023). Also, the impact of infectious disease modeling must be examined with a focus on social justice. Issues of ethics arise in both the technical aspects of these models and in their impact on policy and the community. For instance, biased models may lead healthcare responses to overlook the needs of those who are most vulnerable. Because of this concern, community representatives should be involved in the modeling to make sure their voices and experiences are included in the research and policies. Bringing diverse perspectives into the modeling discourse facilitates equitable public health strategies that reflect the realities of all community members, thereby enhancing the effectiveness and ethical grounding of infectious disease interventions (Adefemi et al., 2023).

11.6.1. Ethical Implications of Predictive Modelling

The ethical implications of predictive modelling in the context of infectious disease are multifaceted and deeply significant. The primary concern is ensuring the accuracy and reliability of model predictions, as this directly affects public health decisions. If predictive models fail to accurately predict outcomes or overlook new factors, they may lead to misguided actions, increased panic, and the wasteful use of resources. It becomes especially noticeable in cases of infectious diseases, for example, the COVID-19 pandemic, where the risks are very high and quick decisions are necessary. If predictions are not accurate, it can worsen health inequities since marginalised communities are often affected by policies that result from wrong data interpretation. Thus, rigorous adherence to transparency and standardised reporting practices, such as those outlined in the ARRIVE guidelines, becomes essential in upholding ethical standards in research and application of predictive modelling (du Sert et al., 2020). Also, some people worry that predictive modelling techniques may introduce bias. Often, these models utilise information from the past, which may include biases prevalent in healthcare and society. Using biased historical details usually leads to keeping inequalities in place, mainly with regard to race, SES, and health care access. When managing infectious diseases, biased models may cause essential groups of people to be overlooked by the interventions. As articulated in the findings of recent research, models that fail to account for variance in demographic data can lead to catastrophic public health failures, manifesting in higher rates of morbidity and mortality in underrepresented groups (Guzik et al., 2020). So, taking steps to include all groups in data and testing models ensures fairness in health outcomes. Lastly, predictive modelling must be responsible for privacy and obtaining informed consent from people. The use of sensitive health data for predictions raises doubts about the freedom of individuals and populations whose data is used. To be ethical, predictive modeling must take strong steps to guard privacy and be clear about the use of data. Besides, individuals need to be aware of and agree to take part in data gathering that could guide public health policies. During an infectious disease crisis, the need for quick action can lead to giving more weight to public health than to people's privacy. To navigate this conundrum, researchers and policymakers must strive for a balance that respects individual rights without compromising the broader goal of public health safety, ensuring ethical integrity under the pressures of urgent decision-making (du Sert et al., 2020) (Figure 11.16).

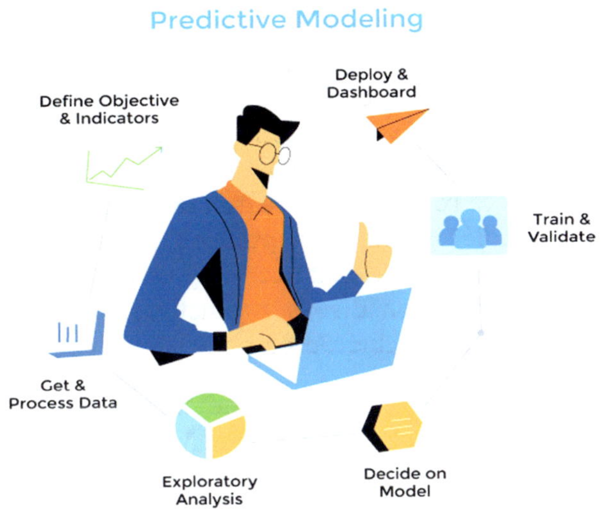

Figure 11.16. Ethical implications of predictive modeling.

Source: https://cdn.prod.website-files.com/620d42e86cb8ec4d0839e59d/6230f046627012226ca691ed_61c9f5e9334bd82512b86cda_predictive-modelling-diagram.png.

11.6.2. Balancing Public Health and Individual Rights

The tension between public health imperatives and individual rights has emerged as a significant concern, particularly during infectious disease outbreaks. Mandatory vaccinations and quarantine are usually supported because they can help stop the spread of disease and protect those who are most at risk. Still, such actions can limit personal freedoms, leading to debates about autonomy and rights. The issue became particularly clear during the COVID-19 pandemic, when countries worldwide implemented restrictions to curb the spread of the virus. Understanding this balance requires a nuanced discussion of risk assessment methodologies, such as those detailed in the Public Health Agency of Canada's framework, which integrates qualitative risk assessments to guide public health responses while considering individual impacts and the broader societal context (Anand et al., 2024). Also, personal beliefs and social trends often influence how people respond to public health requirements. When people in specific communities doubt the effectiveness of vaccinations, fewer individuals get vaccinated, which may allow preventable diseases to return and threaten the community as a whole. Vaccination policies present this issue, as they must balance the goal of keeping everyone safe from disease against each person's choice to be vaccinated or not.

During the COVID-19 pandemic, Indonesia saw that problems with vaccination programs made it more likely for diseases like measles to spread because fewer people were getting vaccinated. Here, the tension between governmental public health obligations and individual autonomy illustrates the complexities involved in policymaking (Rifqi et al., 2024). Achieving a good balance between public health and individual rights requires using strategies that focus on teaching and engaging the community. Talking openly about the role of public health measures allows stakeholders to clear up any doubts or misunderstandings people may have. As a result, individuals may trust public health more and follow its advice, such as getting vaccinated. Improving how vaccines are delivered and communicating with people in remote areas can address some of the ethical issues created by these competing interests. As societies grapple with these issues, employing robust risk assessment models will be essential in guiding equitable policy decisions that respect individual rights while safeguarding public health (Anand et al., 2024; Rifqi et al., 2024) (Figure 11.17).

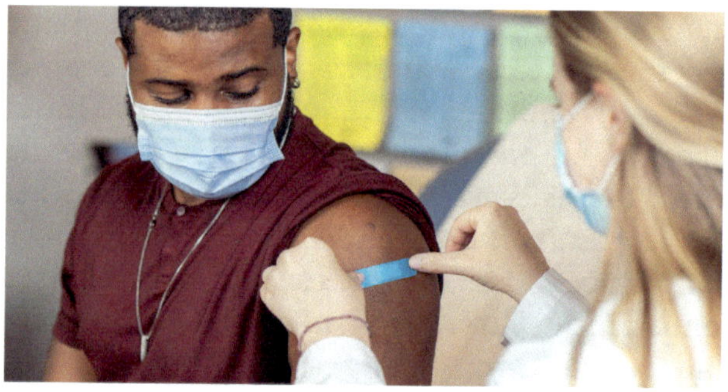

Figure 11.17. Balancing public health and individual right.

Source: https://assets.openstax.org/oscms-prodcms/media/original_images/PH_Figure_15_00_001_Splash.jpg.

11.6.3. Transparency and Communication of Risk

Effectively communicating risks associated with infectious diseases is pivotal in guiding public perception and behaviour. Health authorities need to be transparent to gain trust, mainly during outbreaks. If health organisations share reliable, easy-to-understand and timely information, people and other stakeholders are more likely to trust them. It matters most during epidemics because uncertainty can lead to panic or misguided decisions. Investing in data analysis, teamwork, and prevention is crucial for establishing a robust health communication system. As evidenced by recent reforms in food safety initiatives across several countries, better data handling can significantly improve risk management practices; these insights can be applied to infectious disease models to optimize communication efforts and ultimately enhance public health outcomes (N/A, 2010). Also, to manage risk, it is necessary to communicate information and recognise the complex aspects of infectious diseases. Ebola and H1N1 outbreaks have highlighted that traditional approaches to managing epidemics overlook the possibility of random outcomes. It is essential to add non-deterministic aspects and frictions to how risks are communicated. Awareness of the uncertainties and difficulties in disease transmission enables health officials to be better prepared and to communicate effectively. This approach requires extending existing models to encapsulate the nuances of epidemic management, reinforcing the notion that clear communication must adapt to encompass evolving evidence and dynamic variables within disease outbreaks (Brown et al., 2017). In addition, being open about risks is not only necessary but also the right thing to do, especially during public health emergencies. Policymakers, healthcare workers, and the public should be aware of the fundamental concepts and limitations underlying risk assessments derived from mathematical modelling. If stakeholders can view detailed risk assessments that explain potential issues in an outbreak, they can participate more effectively in group decision-making. As risk models become more advanced, their explanations to stakeholders must also improve to remain clear and informative. Ultimately, fostering an environment of transparency will empower communities to respond to health threats with increased resilience and informed agency (Brown et al., 2017; N/A, 2010).

SUMMARY

The examination of risk assessment and modelling in infectious diseases reveals the critical need for comprehensive methodologies that can adapt to various emergencies, particularly in conflict-affected regions like Ukraine. Recent research demonstrates that emergencies have a significant impact on the transmission dynamics of infectious diseases, due to disruptions in healthcare systems and societal structures (Chumachenko et al., 2024b). It shows that continuous assessments should use current data and advanced analysis. When using ML models together with conventional epidemiology, public health officials can more accurately predict when diseases will outbreak and how to handle them during emergencies. Therefore, such approaches underscore the importance of having robust systems in place to address sudden public health issues. Moreover, the integration of information and communication technology (ICT) into healthcare systems presents both opportunities and risks, particularly in the realm of telemedicine (D-won et al., 2020). Even though telemedicine makes healthcare available in emergencies, its introduction creates new risks that should be carefully examined. Because cybersecurity threats can seriously impact patient safety and data, risk assessment frameworks should include them. Using attack trees and similar models helps healthcare providers organise risks and respond to them before they become serious. Working on both types of problems allows researchers and public health officials to develop comprehensive approaches that help healthcare and protect against new threats. In brief, handling complex health emergencies today relies heavily on practical risk assessment and modelling of infectious diseases. Emphasising both infectious disease management and the protection of telemedicine systems gives a complete solution to public health. Healthcare systems can be better prepared for emergencies by using advanced methods like combining ML with strong cybersecurity. The results highlight a strong connection between health security and technology, indicating the need for further research and collaboration to enhance these models. We can see that understanding these areas better helps us to respond more effectively to infectious disease outbreaks in a world where things are less predictable.

In the study of risk assessment and modelling in infectious diseases, key findings reveal the critical role of environmental and anthropogenic factors in the emergence of EIDs. From 1975 to 2020, it is clear that proximity to forests increases the likelihood of zoonotic transmission, where diseases move from animals to humans. It means that when cities expand into natural habitats, the likelihood of outbreaks increases, highlighting the importance of using models that address both biodiversity loss and population density. The research highlights the complexity of EID emergence, demonstrating that traditional models may overlook significant variables, which necessitates a nuanced approach to public health policy and proactive measures to mitigate risks associated with habitat encroachment (Massaro et al., 2024). Moreover, advancements in diagnostic technologies such as metagenomic next-generation sequencing (mNGS) significantly enhance the identification of pathogens responsible for lower respiratory tract infections (LRTIs). The comparative analysis illustrates the superiority of mNGS over conventional microbiological testing (CMT), revealing higher sensitivity and specificity in detecting pathogens such as Epstein-Barr virus and *Klebsiella pneumoniae*. The discovery is important and significant because it allows for early medical care, which in turn may help save the lives of infected individuals. The study indicates that timely mNGS implementation can improve diagnostic outcomes, especially for patients with complex LRTIs, underscoring the importance of integrating cutting-edge diagnostic tools into risk assessment frameworks in infectious disease modeling (Gao et al., 2024). In the end, risk assessment and predictive modeling play a key role in handling the prognosis of patients with infectious diseases. Building a mortality prediction model using variables identified through careful analysis demonstrates the role of statistics in helping doctors make informed treatment decisions. Nomograms facilitate the assessment of patient risk by healthcare workers, taking into account both their medical history and the timing of diagnostic tests. These models are designed to facilitate understanding of epidemiology and inform the development of specific strategies for managing patients with infectious diseases. Ultimately, the findings advocate for the continued evolution of risk assessment methodologies to incorporate advanced diagnostic and predictive modeling techniques, essential for navigating the complexities of infectious disease management (Gao et al., 2024; Massaro et al., 2024).

CLOSER LOOK:

ENVIRONMENTAL MONITORING

Environmental monitoring is the systematic collection of data to assess the state of the natural environment and detect changes over time. It plays a critical role in understanding the impact of human activities, climate change, and natural processes on ecosystems. By providing accurate and timely information, environmental monitoring helps policymakers, scientists, and the public make informed decisions about conservation, resource management, and pollution control. One of the primary objectives of environmental monitoring is to track air and water quality. Air monitoring involves measuring pollutants such as carbon monoxide, nitrogen oxides, particulate matter, and volatile organic compounds. These measurements are essential to understanding urban air pollution, identifying industrial emissions, and protecting public health. Water monitoring, on the other hand, focuses on parameters such as pH, dissolved oxygen, heavy metals, and microbial contaminants. Monitoring rivers, lakes, and groundwater sources helps ensure safe drinking water, preserves aquatic life, and prevents ecosystem degradation.

Soil monitoring is another crucial aspect. By analyzing soil composition, nutrient content, and contamination levels, scientists can detect agricultural runoff, heavy metal accumulation, and other forms of land degradation. This information is vital for sustainable farming, preventing desertification, and maintaining soil health. Similarly, biodiversity monitoring tracks the abundance and diversity of species within an ecosystem. Changes in species populations can serve as early warning signs of environmental stress or habitat loss, guiding conservation strategies. Technological advancements have greatly enhanced environmental monitoring capabilities. Remote sensing through satellites and drones allows large-scale observation of forests, oceans, and glaciers. Sensors and Internet of Things (IoT) devices provide real-time data on air quality, water levels, and soil conditions. Geographic Information Systems (GIS) help visualize and analyze spatial patterns, making it easier to detect trends and respond to environmental threats promptly.

Environmental monitoring also supports regulatory frameworks and sustainable development initiatives. Governments and organizations rely on monitoring data to enforce environmental standards, evaluate the effectiveness of policies, and plan urban development with minimal ecological impact. Public access to monitoring data fosters environmental awareness and encourages community involvement in conservation efforts.

In conclusion, environmental monitoring is a vital tool for understanding, protecting, and managing our natural world. By combining scientific research, technological innovation, and public engagement, it helps safeguard ecosystems, ensure human health, and promote sustainable development for future generations.

REFERENCES

1. Adefemi, N. A., Ukpoju, N. E. A., Adekoya, N. O., Abatan, N. A., & Adegbite, N. a. O. (2023b). Artificial intelligence in environmental health and public safety: A comprehensive review of USA strategies. *World Journal of Advanced Research and Reviews, 20*(3), 1420–1434. https://doi.org/10.30574/wjarr.2023.20.3.2591Afrin, S., Chowdhury, F. J., & Rahman, M. M. (2021). COVID-19 pandemic: Rethinking strategies for resilient urban design, perceptions, and planning. *Frontiers in Sustainable Cities, 3*. https://doi.org/10.3389/frsc.2021.668263.
2. Ali, S., Li, Z., Moqueet, N., Moghadas, S., Galvani, A. P., Cooper, L. A., Stranges, S., et al. (2024). Incorporating social determinants of health in infectious disease models: A systematic review of guidelines. *Medical Decision Making, 44*, 742–755. https://www.semanticscholar.org/paper/af2b60e1528a713ec848b81ade2a9cc0bcbe26fb (accessed on 30th May 2025).
3. Anand, S. P., Tam, C. C., Calvin, S., Ayache, D., Slywchuk, L., Lambraki, I., Ahmad, R., et al. (2024). Estimating public health risks of infectious disease events: A Canadian approach to rapid risk assessment. *Canada Communicable Disease Report, 50*, 282–293. https://www.semanticscholar.org/paper/9ce687568cb65b79221efc207988ca75d48a0962 (accessed on 30th May 2025).
4. Balmes, J., Ritz, B., & Tager, I. (2004). Can lessons from public health disease surveillance be applied to environmental public health tracking? *Environ. Health Perspect.* https://core.ac.uk/download/pdf/3775836.pdf (accessed on 30th May 2025).
5. Belau, M. H., Boenecke, J., Ströbele, J., Himmel, M., Dretvić, D., Mustafa, U. K., Kreppel, K., et al. (2025). Integrated rapid risk assessment for dengue fever in settings with limited diagnostic capacity and uncertain exposure: Development of a methodological framework for Tanzania. *PLOS Neglected Tropical Diseases, 19*. https://www.semanticscholar.org/paper/542fa28b032daa1f5228f48dc211b956e2bb4060 (accessed on 30th May 2025).
6. Borrelli, R., Nicola, S., Corradi, F., Badiu, I., Lo Sardo, L., Rashidy, N., Quinternetto, A., et al. (2025). Impact of sex on infection risk in patients with systemic lupus erythematosus. *Bioengineering, 12*. https://www.semanticscholar.org/paper/391780c6f62964e300e6343afd2ac16a541cd108 (accessed on 30th May 2025).
7. Broadhurst, M. J., Ayebare, R., Brett-Major, D. M., Carroll, S. M., Lacore, J., Laskey, A. D., Lawler, J. V., et al. (2024). Feasibility assessment of a novel isolation care tent in Uganda during the 2022 Sudan ebolavirus outbreak. *Health Security*. https://www.semanticscholar.org/paper/73f707ac9d8d64e0cd68a78b3d244b7f04cc8e8f (accessed on 30th May 2025).
8. Brown, A. E. X., Ch'ng, Q. L., Currie, M., & Grundy, et al. (2017). *Some Remarks About the Complexity Of Epidemics Management.* http://arxiv.org/abs/1705.02612 (accessed on 30th May 2025).
9. Brul, S., Havelaar, A. H., De Jong, A. E. I., et al. (2025). *Future Challenges to Microbial Food Safety*. https://core.ac.uk/download/pdf/29244275.pdf (accessed on 30th May 2025).
10. Cameron, A., Drakeley, C., & Stresman, G. (2017). *Freedom from Infection: Confirming Interruption of Malaria Transmission.* https://core.ac.uk/download/74229811.pdf (accessed on 30th May 2025).
11. Carroll, D., Daszak, P., Karesh, W. B., Lipkin, et al. (2012). *Prediction and Prevention of the Next Pandemic Zoonosis.* https://core.ac.uk/download/323071111.pdf (accessed on 30th May 2025).

12. Cesario, A. (2016). *Current Pharmaceutical Design*. https://www.semanticscholar.org/paper/3b04cd9382c4c7b95715a565425e205bcec850fa (accessed on 30th May 2025).

13. Chavy, A., Dales, N. A. F., Bessa, L. S. L., Ramírez, J. D., Herrera, G., Dos, S. T. V., Ginouvès, M., et al. (2019). Ecological niche modelling for predicting the risk of cutaneous *Leishmaniasis* in the Neotropical moist forest biome. *PLoS Neglected Tropical Diseases, 13*, e0007629–e0007629. https://doi.org/10.1371/journal.pntd.0007629.

14. Chen, C., Gao, G., Xu, Y., Pu, L., Wang, Q., Wang, L., Wang, W., et al. (2020). SARS-CoV-2–positive sputum and feces after conversion of pharyngeal samples in patients with COVID-19. *Annals of Internal Medicine, 172*, 832–834. https://doi.org/10.7326/m20-0991.

15. Chumachenko, D., Bazilevych, K., Butkevych, M., Meniailov, I., Parfeniuk, Y., Sidenko, I., & Chumachenko, T. (2024a). Methodology for assessing the impact of emergencies on the spread of infectious diseases. *Radioelectronic and Computer Systems*. https://www.semanticscholar.org/paper/8c34f2e252daa4ba003aceb5c1a2e6c9113b5ccd (accessed on 30th May 2025).

16. Chumachenko, T. O., & Chumachenko, D. (2024b). Assessing infectious disease simulation in combat zones through capacity, vulnerability, and risk framework. *Ukrainian Journal of Military Medicine*. https://www.semanticscholar.org/paper/9cba36e3e6bf5b57f5593cb2ace4db61cdd5ffb2 (accessed on 30th May 2025).

17. Colella, J. P., Bates, J., Burneo, S. F., Camacho, M. A., Carrion Bonilla, C., Constable, I., D'Elía, G., et al. (2021). Leveraging natural history biorepositories as a global, decentralized, pathogen surveillance network. *PLoS Pathogens, 17*. https://www.semanticscholar.org/paper/36776dc39f457ce3d1f2a52144b47e4f10be33cd (accessed on 30th May 2025).

18. Elena, P. (2025). Role of deep learning in enhancing medical diagnosis accuracy in Argentina. *International Journal of Technology and Systems*. https://www.semanticscholar.org/paper/8f36e589f5baf8547525107896a4378bf1081c32 (accessed on 30th May 2025).

19. Fall, P., Diouf, I., Deme, A., & Sène, D. (2022). Assessment of climate-driven variations in malaria transmission in Senegal using the VECTRI model. *Atmosphere*. https://www.semanticscholar.org/paper/29d3aeb98d62d2501a48d0aa386a7c1d86466192 (accessed on 30th May 2025).

20. Gao, Q., Li, L., Su, T., Liu, J., Chen, L., Yi, Y., Huan, Y., et al. (2024). A single-center, retrospective study of hospitalized patients with lower respiratory tract infections: Clinical assessment of metagenomic next-generation sequencing and identification of risk factors in patients. *Respiratory Research, 25*. https://www.semanticscholar.org/paper/a7e83ce3501ba0c71a2fe8505270695eb8dc8a4d (accessed on 30th May 2025).

21. Getz, W. M., Mgbara, W., & Salter, R. (2019). Adequacy of SEIR models when epidemics have spatial structure: Ebola in Sierra Leone. *Philos. Trans. R Soc. Lond. B Biol. Sci.* https://core.ac.uk/download/287623859.pdf (accessed on 30th May 2025).

22. Guzik, T. J., Mohiddin, S., Dimarco, A., Patel, V., Savvatis, K., Marelli-Berg, F. M., Madhur, M. S., et al. (2020). COVID-19 and the cardiovascular system: Implications for risk assessment, diagnosis, and treatment options. *Cardiovascular Research, 116*, 1666–1687. https://doi.org/10.1093/cvr/cvaa106.

23. Hale, T., Angrist, N., Goldszmidt, R., Kira, B., Petherick, A., Phillips, T., Webster, S., et al. (2021). A global panel database of pandemic policies (Oxford COVID-19 Government Response Tracker). *Nature Human Behavior, 5*, 529–538. https://doi.org/10.1038/s41562-021-01079-8.

24. Hamilton, K. A., Harrison, J. C., Mitchell, J., Weir, M. H., Verhougstraete, M., Haas, C. N., Nejadhashemi, A., et al. (2024). Research gaps and priorities for quantitative microbial risk assessment (QMRA). *Risk Analysis: An Official Publication of the Society for Risk Analysis.* https://www.semanticscholar.org/paper/ad97577b841027b44ebf97b0dddce459df96cf42 (accessed on 30th May 2025).

25. Hu, B., Guo, H., Zhou, P., & Shi, Z. L. (2020). Characteristics of SARS-CoV-2 and COVID-19. *Nature Reviews Microbiology, 19*, 141–154. https://doi.org/10.1038/s41579-020-00459-7.

26. Izah, S. C., Udofia, A. S., Johnson, I. U., & Etim, N. G. (2024). Risk assessment and behavioral health statistics: Modeling lifestyle factors and exposure impacts on public health outcomes. *Greener Journal of Epidemiology and Public Health.* https://www.semanticscholar.org/paper/b16c412f2538811f26c94057b4fc369c0e1bfb13 (accessed on 30th May 2025).

27. James, S. L., Abate, D., Abate, K. H., Abay, S. M., Abbafati, C., Abbasi, N., Abbastabar, H., et al. (2018). Global, regional, and national incidence, prevalence, and years lived with disability for 354 diseases and injuries for 195 countries and territories, 1990–2017: A systematic analysis for the Global Burden of Disease Study 2017. *The Lancet, 392*, 1789–1858. https://doi.org/10.1016/s0140-6736(18)32279-7.

28. Kaye, A. R., Guzzetta, G., Tildesley, M. J., & Thompson, R. N. (2024). Quantifying infectious disease epidemic risks: A practical approach for seasonal pathogens. *PLOS Computational Biology, 21.* https://www.semanticscholar.org/paper/8c643fd3378fa2757106f6db5759a6e587061347 (accessed on 30th May 2025).

29. Kim, D. W., Choi, J. Y., & Han, K. H. (2020). Risk management-based security evaluation model for telemedicine systems. *BMC Medical Informatics and Decision Making, 20.* https://www.semanticscholar.org/paper/7cec507bbf131c157cb778aa9f5e62ab3881cd90 (accessed on 30th May 2025).

30. Kone, T. C., Ghinet, S., Dana, S. A., & Grewal, A. (2024). Speech detection models for effective communicable disease risk assessment in air travel environments. *The Journal of the Acoustical Society of America.* https://www.semanticscholar.org/paper/f00742bcb7f6ed5d8e0fb18e599a998a9215ac90 (accessed on 30th May 2025).

31. Lebedeva Nesevria, N., Sharypova, S., & Kornilitsyna, M. D. (2024). Risks of infectious diseases in the subjective perception of metropolitan residents: From assessment to management strategy. *Kuban Scientific Medical Bulletin.* https://www.semanticscholar.org/paper/be8a3495a591ab84004971ada09dd97d96978d7a (accessed on 30th May 2025).

32. Lewnard, J. A., & Reingold, A. L. (2019). *Emerging Challenges and Opportunities in Infectious Disease Epidemiology.* https://core.ac.uk/download/323082106.pdf (accessed on 30th May 2025).

33. Macauley, M. (2024). Infectious disease modeling. *Annual Review of Statistics and Its Application.* https://www.semanticscholar.org/paper/b012e36220dec79707a3a5dd6bc59347cf769088 (accessed on 30th May 2025).

34. Massaro, E., Fanelli, A., Cescatti, A., Riccetti, N., Debois, G., Robuchon, M., Szewczy, W., et al. (2024). Human-forest proximity and the risk of infectious diseases in a changing world. *The European Journal of Public Health, 34.* https://www.semanticscholar.org/paper/fe5ded56f2c7e80213771840d41b227d99aaadb7 (accessed on 30th May 2025).

35. Meng, X., Fan, Y., Qiao, Y., Lin, J., Cai, Z., & Si, S. (2025). Evolutionary analysis of a coupled epidemic-voluntary vaccination behavior model with immunity waning on complex networks. *Risk Analysis: An Official Publication of the Society for Risk Analysis*. https://www.semanticscholar.org/paper/3fc7227a68b3b4380f609f224386465125050e13 (accessed on 30th May 2025).

36. N/A. (2010). Building the science foundation of a modern food safety system: Lessons from Denmark, the Netherlands, and the United Kingdom on creating a more coordinated and integrated approach to food safety information. https://core.ac.uk/download/71349712.pdf (accessed on 30th May 2025).

37. Nguyen, L. H., Drew, D. A., Graham, M. S., Joshi, A. D., Guo, C. G., Ma, W., Mehta, R. S., et al. (2020). Risk of COVID-19 among front-line health-care workers and the general community: A prospective cohort study. *The Lancet Public Health, 5*, e475–e483. https://doi.org/10.1016/s2468-2667(20)30164-x.

38. Osterland, A., Wang, Y., Wilson, T. W., Paulus, J. K., Patton, G., Firozvi, K., & Desai, K. (2024). Assessment of social determinants of health (SDOH) in patients with non-metastatic cancer: Real-world evidence from a large geographically representative community oncology network. *JCO Oncology Practice*. https://www.semanticscholar.org/paper/0a89fda26ec8ea3dac8a86e8cd41c51e2e65dd13 (accessed on 30th May 2025).

39. Park, J. S., Park, S. Y., Moon, J. W., Kim, K., & Suh, D. (2025). Artificial intelligence models for pediatric lung sound analysis: Systematic review and meta-analysis. *Journal of Medical Internet Research, 27*, e66491. https://www.semanticscholar.org/paper/3d124d272c80f7dbc9c731751c696fc0f7f8255c (accessed on 30th May 2025).

40. Percie Du, S. N., Ahluwalia, A., Alam, S., Avey, M. T., Baker, M., Browne, W. J., Clark, A., et al. (2020). Reporting animal research: Explanation and elaboration for the ARRIVE guidelines 2.0. *PLoS Biology, 18*, e3000411–e3000411. https://doi.org/10.1371/journal.pbio.3000411.

41. Ponciano, J., Chang, J., Abdalah, M., Facey, K., & Ponciano, J. (2022). COVID-19 regional waves and spread risk assessment through the analysis of the initial outbreak in Guatemala (preprint). https://www.semanticscholar.org/paper/94754da64c62bf1b144317e2a94672cf37970173 (accessed on 30th May 2025).

42. Rana, S. V. S. (2024). Metamorphosis of human health risk assessment with artificial intelligence (AI) – A new paradigm in pharmaco-toxicological sciences. *Journal of Environmental Biology*. https://www.semanticscholar.org/paper/1586089455cc5bc593cf9ecf82470cfc072740a5 (accessed on 30th May 2025).

43. Rifqi, A. I., Hertiana, Y. N. T., Hariani, S. R., & Indar, S. (2024). Ethical dilemma in vaccination in Indonesia: Balance between public health obligations and individual autonomy rights. *Promotif: Jurnal Kesehatan Masyarakat*. https://www.semanticscholar.org/paper/2e8ec41814b6bba3320507e926f4c0eace42eb45 (accessed on 30th May 2025).

44. Rudd, K. E., Johnson, S. C., Agesa, K. M., Shackelford, K. A., Tsoi, D., Kievlan, D., Colombara, D. V., et al. (2020). Global, regional, and national sepsis incidence and mortality, 1990–2017: Analysis for the Global Burden of Disease Study. *The Lancet, 395*, 200–211. https://doi.org/10.1016/s0140-6736(19)32989-7.

45. Salazar, L. E. J., Cobos, M. F. J., Caicedo, H. L., & Vera, S. M. (2024). Microbiological risk assessment of high-demand food from three major cities in Ecuador. *Bionatura Journal, 2.*

https://www.semanticscholar.org/paper/96b2f814ad0e07bdbab85000a2555aa266cedc2d (accessed on 30th May 2025).

46. Sararat, C., Jiravejchakul, N., Nawattanapaiboon, K., & Modchang, C. (2024). *Modeling the Risk of Airborne Transmission of Respiratory Viruses in Microgravity*. https://www.semanticscholar.org/paper/838b8e91644fe174b2c3e04f49be5b9f068e2f20 (accessed on 30th May 2025).

47. Siddiq, M. (2023). Exploring the role of machine learning in contact tracing for public health: Benefits, challenges, and ethical considerations. *American Journal of Economic and Management Business (AJEMB), 2*, 99–110. https://www.semanticscholar.org/paper/c55a051fcd1e7c1616bba97b9ca7f436cef792fb (accessed on 30th May 2025).

48. Singh, A., Jones, S. E., Ganapathysubramanian, B., Sarkar, S., Mueller, D. S., Sandhu, K. S., & Nagasubramanian, K. (2020). Challenges and opportunities in machine-augmented plant stress phenotyping. *Trends in Plant Science, 26*, 53–69. https://doi.org/10.1016/j.tplants.2020.07.010.

49. Tahir, M., Haq, I., Zakki, S. A., & Akbar, F. (2025). Infodemic management and public health emergency preparedness capacities — Khyber Pakhtunkhwa, Pakistan, 2024. *China CDC Weekly, 7*, 368–373. https://www.semanticscholar.org/paper/3c6e3be0c9f813212fa4e3e6a204d0c99f5aac56 (accessed on 30th May 2025).

50. Turillazzi, E., Fineschi, V., Palmiere, C., & Sergi, C. (2016). Cardiovascular involvement in sepsis. *Mediators of Inflammation, 2016*. https://www.semanticscholar.org/paper/756a3f9ae9900e29796b3c15ae2a3856176c9b27 (accessed on 30th May 2025).

51. Wang, H., Zeng, J., Gao, X., Wang, H., & Xiao, J. (2024). SpatMCDA: An R package for assessing areas at risk of infectious diseases based on spatial multi-criteria decision analysis. *Methods in Ecology and Evolution*. https://www.semanticscholar.org/paper/99bf66dc6c32af1c36b73479b348902b756c6756 (accessed on 30th May 2025).

52. Wimberly, M. C., de Beurs, K. M., Loboda, T., & Pan, W. (2021). Satellite observations and malaria: New opportunities for research and applications. *Trends in Parasitology, 37*, 525–537. https://doi.org/10.1016/j.pt.2021.03.003.

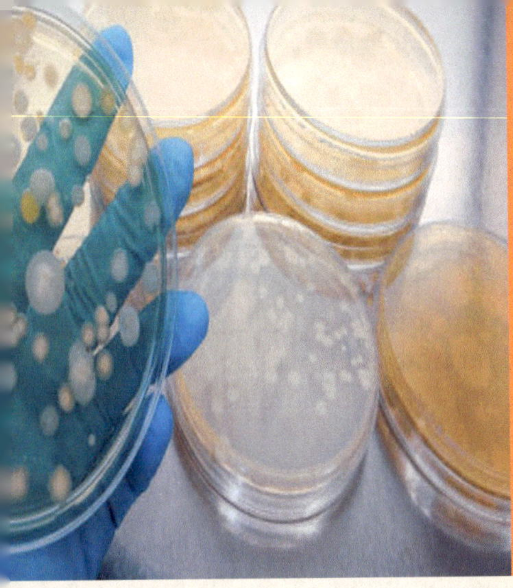

Chapter 12

ANTIMICROBIAL RESISTANCE AND PUBLIC HEALTH

Contents

Introduction

The issue of antimicrobial resistance (AMR) poses a significant threat to public health globally, transcending geographic and economic boundaries. When bacteria become resistant to antibiotics, infections that could once be treated may now become very serious, causing complications during surgery and the management of chronic diseases. In Vietnam and similar areas, the situation is clear because antibiotic resistance is caused by people taking them incorrectly or using them too often. Because AMR is now a primary concern for health security in Vietnam, the government is investigating local practices around antibiotic use, especially in communities. When public health officials understand the specific factors that influence antibiotic use, they can design targeted interventions that are effective and appropriate for the community, thereby reducing AMR and improving health outcomes. People's opinions about antibiotics influence their health decisions and their understanding of AMR. In many places, people view antibiotics as necessary, largely due to their past experiences. Based on qualitative research, Vietnamese people are careful about choosing antibiotics, yet they often prefer quick relief from symptoms over knowing the correct medical way to use them. Such perspectives usually depend on the advice from the community and the economic and social environment in which people live. If people misunderstand the capabilities of antibiotics, it may weaken public health efforts to address AMR, indicating a need for more education about the risks of unsupervised antibiotic use. Interventions must address these deeply held beliefs and explain how resistance forms, as well as its implications for both personal and public health. AMR encompasses not only personal habits but also various aspects of public health, including monitoring, rule creation, and public education. When dealing with AMR, we must consider several factors, including access to healthcare and knowledge about antibiotic use. There is a clear need to watch AMR more closely, as the high number of sepsis cases which resistant infections can cause, leading to significant death and illness. In fact, it was estimated that in 2017, about 11 million people died from sepsis, showing how AMR affects important health problems. As efforts to confront AMR intensify, fostering collaborative initiatives that bring together health professionals, policymakers, and the public will be essential in mitigating this growing threat, protecting both individual patients and broader public health systems (Figure 12.1).

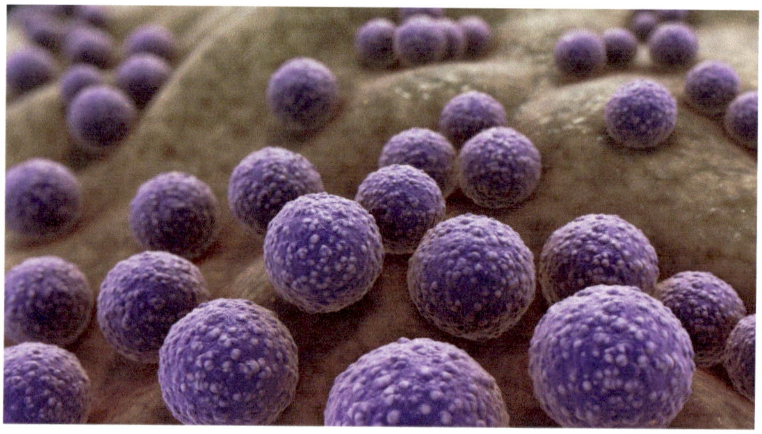

Figure 12.1. Antimicrobial resistance and public health.

Source: https://biology.mit.edu/wp-content/uploads/2020/08/SciPol.png.

Definition of Antimicrobial Resistance (AMR)

AMR refers to when microorganisms, for example, bacteria, viruses, fungi, and parasites, become resistant to drugs that are used to kill or control them. These pathogens develop resistance when they undergo mutations or acquire new resistance genes from other microbes. As a consequence, standard treatments are less successful, which causes people to be sick for a longer period, spend more on healthcare, and have a higher risk of dying. The WHO believes that AMR is a significant problem for global health and requires everyone to work together to address it. AMR is defined as encompassing the biological aspects of resistance, as well as highlighting the associated health risks, which underscores the need for monitoring, research, and the development of new methods to address resistance in various environments. Rising AMR seriously affects public health and how infectious diseases are managed worldwide. Because more infections are now resistant to drugs, there is a growing number of illnesses and deaths, mainly in areas where getting effective antimicrobials is already tricky. For example, the use of bedaquiline to combat drug-resistant tuberculosis shows the difficulties public health authorities have in controlling AMR. It is essential to monitor the spread of multidrug-resistant strains, particularly in areas where a large number of people are affected by diseases. As highlighted in studies involving genomic surveillance, the meticulous tracking of resistance patterns can inform public health interventions and alert authorities to potential outbreaks of resistant infections, thus facilitating timely responses to safeguard community health (Marcon et al., 2025). New approaches are needed to address AMR, which means reconsidering how antimicrobials are managed and applied in healthcare. Many traditional models reward companies for selling more antimicrobials, which can encourage doctors to prescribe them too often. Evaluating how antimicrobials affect public health, as ceftazidime-avibactam is being assessed in the NHS, can promote better use and investment in new treatments. Focusing on how antimicrobials benefit the population encourages better resource utilisation, improved patient outcomes, and a reduced likelihood of resistance. Therefore, addressing the definition of AMR is not solely a matter of understanding resistance dynamics; it requires a comprehensive approach that encompasses public health strategy, economic evaluation, and collaborative efforts to ensure the sustainability of antimicrobials for future generations (Harnan et al., 2024).

Importance of AMR in Public Health

The issue of AMR in public health cannot be overstated, as it presents significant challenges for healthcare systems worldwide. Because of AMR, people may get sick for longer, medical bills may become higher, and their chances of getting sick, ill, or dying increase. The World Health Organisation (WHO) has recognised AMR as one of the top 10 global public health threats, emphasising the urgent need for effective strategies to combat this issue. As multidrug-resistant organisms become more common, it is increasingly complex to treat infections that were once easily manageable, resulting in higher failure rates and challenges during surgeries. The impact of AMR extends beyond individual patient care, as it poses a threat to public health by compromising the efficacy of antimicrobial treatments, which are fundamental for managing both infectious diseases and cancer therapies (Oliveira et al., 2024). Addressing AMR requires intense surveillance and stewardship programs, which are central to public health. Implementing robust antimicrobial stewardship programs (ASPs) encourages the responsible use of antibiotics, promoting optimal prescribing practices that can minimize the development of resistance. For this reason, education should be provided to healthcare workers as well as patients. When stewardship is effective, both patient results and the use of antibiotics improve, which helps to slow down the rise of drug-resistant germs. Furthermore, public health authorities must integrate data from surveillance systems to monitor resistance patterns, allowing tailored interventions based on local epidemiological trends (Graham et al., 2021). They are necessary to keep current antibiotics working and to enable healthcare providers to fight infections in the future. Because AMR affects both the economy and society, it is even more critical in public health discussions. In addition to endangering health, AMR poses significant economic challenges for healthcare systems and the economies of many countries. More money is spent on healthcare because patients require costly alternative treatments, more extended hospital stays, and assistance managing the side effects of unsuccessful therapies. In addition, AMR mainly affects those who are already vulnerable, which widens health gaps and makes it harder for low-resource areas to develop. In this context, different fields need to cooperate through One Health to address AMR at the same time. Addressing AMR through comprehensive interventions will not only improve health outcomes but also enhance the overall resilience of healthcare systems globally (Oliveira et al., 2024) (Figure 12.2).

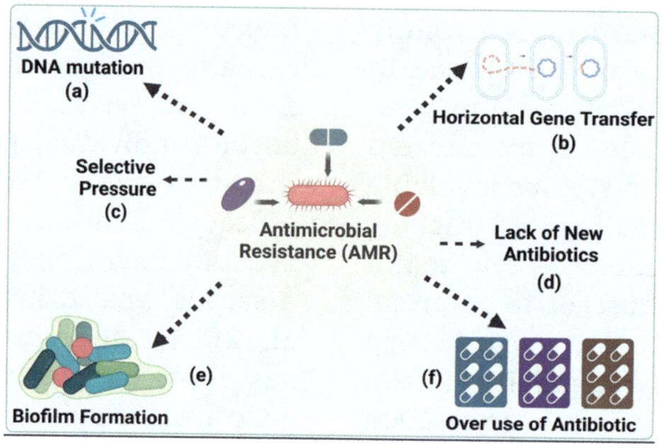

Figure 12.2. Antimicrobial resistance (AMR).

Source: https://www.teagasc.ie/media/website/animals/amr/how-does-antimicrobial-resistance-occur.png.

Historical Context of Antimicrobial Resistance

The historical context of AMR is crucial for understanding its present ramifications on public health. As soon as antibiotics were discovered in the early 20th century, AMR started to spread because these drugs were not always used correctly. Antibiotics were once seen as wonders, and people used them for both bacterial and viral diseases, even though they don't help with viruses. This indiscriminate use has accelerated the evolution of resistant strains, leading to the emergence of multidrug-resistant (MDR) bacteria such as *E. coli* and *Staphylococcus aureus*. Consequently, each breakthrough in antibiotic therapy was met with the onset of new resistance mechanisms, highlighting an unfortunate cycle that has jeopardised both treatment success and public health outcomes (Sharma et al., 2024). As more people began using antibiotics worldwide, especially in the latter part of the 20th century, it became more evident that AMR was a serious problem. More resistant strains emerged as infection rates increased, creating severe difficulties for healthcare providers. Hospitals saw more cases of tough-to-treat infections, which caused patients to stay longer and increased the number of deaths. In addition, AMR puts a strain on the economy by reducing the amount of work people can do and by increasing healthcare spending. The broader implications of AMR prompted health organisations to establish surveillance systems aimed at monitoring its prevalence and facilitating collaboration between human health and veterinary domains, as the misuse of antibiotics in agriculture also contributes to this public health crisis (Sharma et al., 2024). Recently, public health efforts have focused on reducing AMR by encouraging people to get vaccinated. The approval of the 20-valent pneumococcal conjugate vaccine (PCV20) exemplifies these efforts, particularly in addressing diseases that often lead to antibiotic prescriptions. Analysis shows that a catch-up vaccination program can reduce both the use of antibiotics and the number of antibiotic-resistant infections. Implementation of these programs could prevent thousands of cases of invasive pneumococcal disease, save lives, and reduce the costs associated with AMR. As public health strategies advance, it is more crucial than ever to integrate vaccination programs with educational efforts that teach people about the responsible use of antibiotics and the enduring significance of AMR for public health.

Discovery of Antibiotics and Their Initial Impact

The discovery of antibiotics marked a transformative era in medical history, fundamentally altering the treatment landscape for bacterial infections. Alexander Fleming's accidental finding of penicillin in 1928 led to the rise of antibiotics. Following its initial use in World War II, penicillin significantly reduced the number of deaths from bacterial infections, prompting doctors to use it more frequently in hospitals. Afterwards, the creation of tetracyclines and macrolides as antibiotic classes increased the range of treatments that healthcare providers could use. With these improvements, it became possible to perform more complex surgeries and organ transplants, which were once considered too risky because of infection. Because antibiotics were so successful at first, public health recognized how important they are for modern medicine. As more antibiotics were administered to patients, it became increasingly clear what this meant for public health. Because bacterial infections could be treated, the number of diseases decreased, and people started living longer, as serious conditions could now be effectively managed. Still, depending too much on antibiotics led to the worrying rise of AMR. Bacteria that came into contact with low antibiotic doses and incorrect prescriptions developed resistance, which put the progress made with antibiotics at risk. Because resistant infections remain a significant threat to public health, efforts are now underway to promote the responsible use of antibiotics and prevent their misuse. Admitting this is necessary to strike a balance between the use of antibiotics and the growing threat of resistance. Tackling AMR brings a focus to the need for responsible use and innovative ideas in creating new antibiotics. There is now a stronger push for public health to reduce inappropriate prescriptions, as ASPs are expanding in many healthcare settings. They work to ensure antibiotics are used wisely, which reduces resistance and improves patient outcomes by using methods suited to the way healthcare is delivered. The PASTEUR Act, among other legislative efforts, is designed to encourage more economic support for the creation of new antibiotics, since AMR requires new approaches. As the landscape of infectious disease management continues to evolve, a multifaceted approach that incorporates stewardship, novel therapeutics, and public education remains critical for sustaining the effectiveness of antibiotics and protecting global public health against the threat of resistance (Burton et al., 2023; Gyasi-Darko et al., 2024) (Figure 12.3).

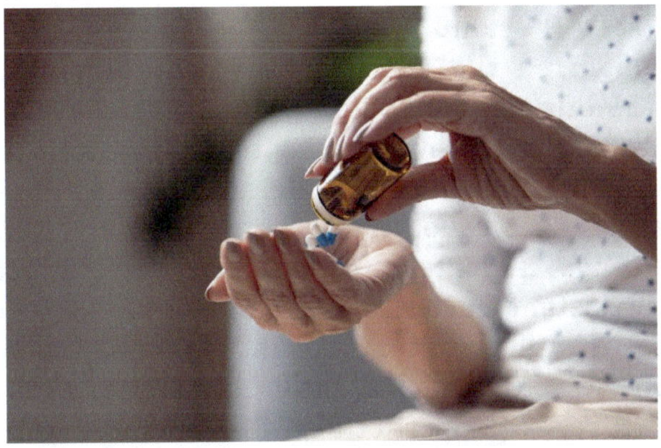

Figure 12.3. The discovery of antibiotics and their initial impact.

Source: https://d2jx2rerrg6sh3.cloudfront.net/images/Article_Images/ImageForArticle_22702_16558138940082493.jpg.

Early Cases of Resistance and Their Implications

The emergence of AMR has its roots in early cases where bacterial adaptations outpaced the effectiveness of available antibiotics. Antibiotics were widely used starting in the 1940s, but not long afterwards, cases of resistance were already being documented, showing how fast bacteria can adapt. For example, the use of penicillin to treat bacterial infections significantly reduced deaths; however, this soon led to *Staphylococcus aureus* becoming resistant to penicillin. This alarming trend suggested that bacteria could acquire resistance through mechanisms such as gene mutations and horizontal gene transfer (HGT), underscoring the need for vigilant monitoring and effective treatment strategies. They revealed that antibiotics are not always reliable and that public health is threatened, which is why it is crucial to continue funding AMR research and policies that help maintain current antibiotics and develop new treatments. Besides affecting clinical results, early resistance cases also shape global public health policies and efforts to use antibiotics wisely. As more and more *Escherichia coli* and *Staphylococcus aureus* became resistant, health officials recognised the need for new guidelines on antibiotic use immediately. Initial studies, for example, those investigating the level of AMR in pregnant women in East Africa, found shocking results that called for targeted action. These findings indicated a concerning prevalence of resistant bacterial isolates, reinforcing the idea that antibiotic misuse and poor healthcare infrastructure significantly contribute to the AMR crisis (Mehari et al., 2025). So, including AMR surveillance in regular clinical care is now crucial to guide prescribing and design public health actions that address the different resistance patterns found in various regions. The ongoing challenge of AMR necessitates a multi-faceted approach that includes not only robust surveillance and stewardship but also innovative solutions such as artificial intelligence (AI). Because AIs can review large amounts of data, they may help detect resistance markers early, which supports quick action and better treatment choices. For example, AI can facilitate the identification of effective antibiotics based on local resistance patterns, thereby enhancing patient outcomes (Branda et al., 2024). Also, using AI in drug development can result in the creation of new antimicrobial agents that can overcome existing resistance. They are important for treating today's infections and also for preserving antibiotics as resistance grows. As the public health landscape evolves, fostering collaborations among healthcare providers, researchers, and technologists will be essential in addressing the complex challenges posed by AMR (Figure 12.4).

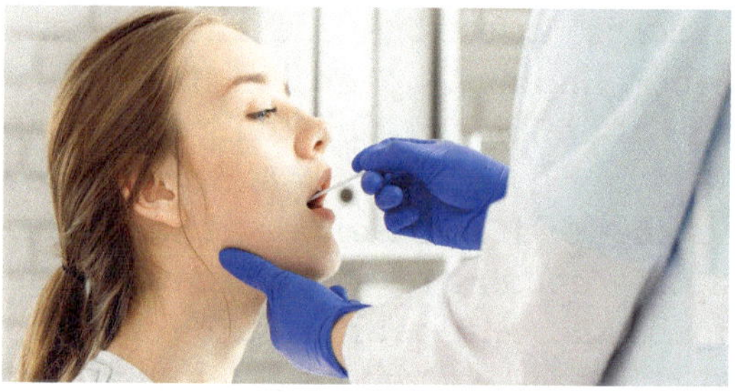

Figure 12.4. Early cases of resistance and their implications antimicrobial resistance (AMR).

Source: https://www.pgeu.eu/wp-content/uploads/2019/03/COVER-1300x607.jpeg.

Evolution of AMR Over the Decades

The evolution of AMR over the decades has marked a distressing trajectory, with resistance rates significantly escalating since the early 2000s. According to recent global studies, there has been a 65% increase in resistant infections from 2000 to 2023, which has caused about 4.95 million deaths each year due to AMR. These trends are particularly alarming in low- and middle-income countries (LMICs), where resistance rates are observed to be three to four times higher than in high-income nations. This indicates that there are significant issues within the system, including a lack of proper healthcare facilities and the improper use of antibiotics for both humans and animals. The consequences of these challenges have been profound, affecting not only individual health outcomes but also burdening public health systems with increased morbidity and economic strain, emphasising the pressing need for comprehensive interventions to combat global AMR (Alomari et al., 2024). Due to the presence of multidrug-resistant organisms, such as the

ESKAPE pathogens, the challenge of dealing with AMR has become even greater. These pathogens are adept at avoiding the effects of conventional antibiotics, leading to treatment failures and higher mortality rates in healthcare-associated infections (HAIs). The emergence of drug-resistant strains has complicated patient treatment and increased healthcare costs, further straining limited resources. Since AMR is a systemic problem, multiple approaches are necessary to address its various causes. Actions range from strict infection control to encouraging ASPs to use antibiotics wisely. These initiatives seek to reduce the selective pressure that has historically driven the evolution of resistance, thereby safeguarding current and future treatment options (Ravi et al., 2024). As AMR becomes a more significant issue, the global health community must unite and cooperate more effectively in surveillance, research, and policy development. Investment in technological innovations, such as machine learning (ML) for predicting resistance patterns, has shown promise in enhancing AMR management. Additionally, international cooperation will play a crucial role in disseminating knowledge about the proper use of antimicrobials and infection control, particularly in regions where resistant infections are prevalent. Responding well to ABR means keeping healthcare workers and the public informed about the importance of using antibiotics correctly. Ultimately, addressing the evolution of AMR is imperative for protecting public health and ensuring that effective therapeutic options remain available for the future (Alomari et al., 2024; Ravi et al., 2024).

12.1. Mechanisms of Antimicrobial Resistance

The emergence of AMR is a complex phenomenon influenced by various mechanisms that allow pathogens to evade the effects of antibiotics. Among the most significant are antibiotic-inactivating enzymes, which alter or inactivate antimicrobial drugs, rendering them ineffective. Bacteria such as *Campylobacter* display enzymatic resistance, which developed as a response to antibiotics used in farming. Certain bacteria modify their drug targets, which helps them continue to multiply when antibiotics are present. Because bacteria can adapt, it is urgent to review the way antibiotics are used in livestock farming, as this greatly leads to resistance. Understanding these mechanisms will aid in developing targeted strategies to combat AMR, ultimately safeguarding public health in an era where antibiotic efficacy is increasingly jeopardized (Almeida et al., 2023). Another aspect of AMR is HGT, which enables bacteria to share resistance traits. HGT facilitates the rapid transfer of antibiotic resistance genes from one bacterium to another through transformation, transduction, and conjugation. This is especially important for *Campylobacter* species, particularly when they are linked to human infections in livestock. Tetracycline-resistant *Campylobacter jejuni* is often associated with the use of antibiotics in agriculture for both growth and disease prevention. Thus, the ongoing connection between farming and AMR poses a significant problem for both animal and human health, as bacteria can transfer from animals to humans. Addressing these mechanisms through improved biosecurity and judicious antibiotic use in agriculture will be vital for curbing the spread of AMR (Algamody et al., 2023). Besides enzymatic resistance and HGT, the ability to tolerate antibiotics also facilitates the spread of AMR. Bacteria may adapt physically to survive antibiotics without becoming resistant. For example, some microbes form protective biofilms, making it difficult for antibiotics to reach them. Biofilms are a significant issue in hospitals, as they can develop on medical devices and cause infections that are difficult to eradicate. Also, the connection between tolerance and resistance makes it clear that research and policy-making should involve multiple viewpoints. Understanding these intricate mechanisms will contribute to the formulation of effective therapeutic strategies and public health initiatives aimed at mitigating the impact of AMR in healthcare settings and the broader community (Almeida et al., 2023) (Figure 12.5).

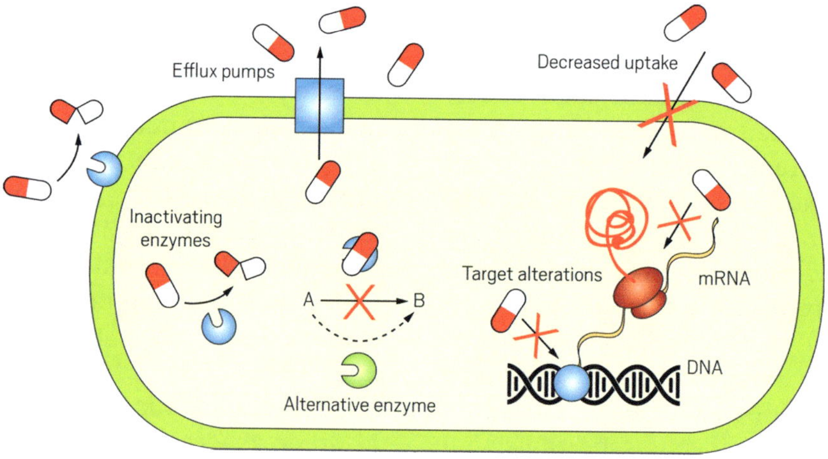

Figure 12.5. Mechanism of antimicrobial resistance.

Source: https://www.reactgroup.org/wp-content/uploads/2016/09/Resistance-mechanisms_Erik-Gullberg.png.

12.1.1. Genetic Mutations in Microorganisms

Changes in the genes of microorganisms are key to the rise and spread of AMR which is causing a growing public health issue. They may occur randomly while the DNA is being copied or in response to environmental factors, including the presence of antibiotics. As microbes multiply, certain changes can strengthen some strains, helping them survive, while also making weaker strains less common. In areas where antibiotics are frequently used, such as hospitals, natural selection can rapidly lead to the development of resistant strains. Because microorganisms can adapt and evolve, they are now able to resist the drugs used to treat infections, which makes it harder to treat these diseases and increases the number of deaths and cases. The dynamics of microbial evolution necessitate a comprehensive understanding of genetic mutations to effectively address the challenges posed by AMR and safeguard public health (Khan et al., 2025). HGT is also a significant way for AMR genes to be shared among different microorganisms. Resistant genes can be transferred to other species through transformation, transduction, and conjugation, exacerbating the problem of resistance development. For example, bacteria can acquire resistance genes from plasmids, which are small, circular pieces of DNA that can replicate independently. Such exchanges are most common in environments where multiple microbes coexist, such as in the human body or on farms. As a result of HGT, resistance traits can spread rapidly, making it more challenging to treat diseases conventionally. Case studies, particularly in foodborne pathogens like Salmonella, highlight how genetic mutations and gene transfer contribute to the emergence of multidrug-resistant strains of bacteria, necessitating a One Health approach to monitoring and managing AMR across various ecosystems (Amal et al., 2025). Understanding genetic mutations in microorganisms is crucial for controlling AMR. Thanks to new developments in molecular microbiology, we now understand the genetic basis of resistance and how these mutations are transmitted among microbes. Public health measures need to try to prevent the spread of infections. Realizing that antibiotics are used in farming and in hospitals can inform changes in policies and support the responsible use of antibiotics. Further research is needed to investigate the relationship between genetic changes, environmental exposure, and the evolution of resistance. Enhanced understanding will inform the development of novel therapies and interventions, ultimately serving to mitigate the threat posed by antimicrobial-resistant microorganisms to public health (Khan et al., 2025)

12.1.2. Horizontal Gene Transfer Among Bacteria

The study of HGT among bacteria is critical to understanding how AMR proliferates and poses risks to public health. HGT helps bacteria exchange genes, which allows them to get resistance genes that help them survive when exposed to antibiotics. It occurs through transformation, transduction, and conjugation, which enable bacteria to quickly adapt to new conditions, especially when antibiotics are used frequently. Because HGT is so common, it often results in bacteria becoming resistant to many antibiotics, which makes it difficult to treat infections effectively. Biofilms significantly increase the chances of bacteria sharing genes, which can lead to more AMR. Biofilms are groups of microorganisms that adhere to surfaces, creating an environment that facilitates genetic exchange. Antibiotics applied to biofilms can cause some bacteria to survive, potentially increasing the transfer of genes among bacteria. This is particularly important in healthcare facilities and refugee camps, where poor sanitation can lead to biofilm formation in the water. As bacteria interact within biofilms, they form hidden reservoirs of resistance genes that can be passed on during outbreaks, which shows why biofilms should be considered in public health strategies for controlling AMR. The environment also affects how HGT occurs and what consequences it has for public health in water systems.

In agriculture and aquaculture, antibiotics can introduce bacteria that are resistant to drugs, and these can transfer their genes to the native microbes in the water. For instance, bacterial extracellular vesicles (BEVs) have emerged as vehicles that can carry resistance genes, amplifying the spread of AMR in these environments. It has been found that BEVs contain genes like blaCTX-M and tetA, which highlight their part in spreading antibiotic resistance. To effectively combat this crisis, it is critical to adopt a multidisciplinary approach that encompasses comprehensive monitoring of aquatic ecosystems and robust wastewater treatment protocols, as well as innovative interventions targeting the sources of resistance (Barathan et al., 2024; Nahum et al., 2025) (Figure 12.6).

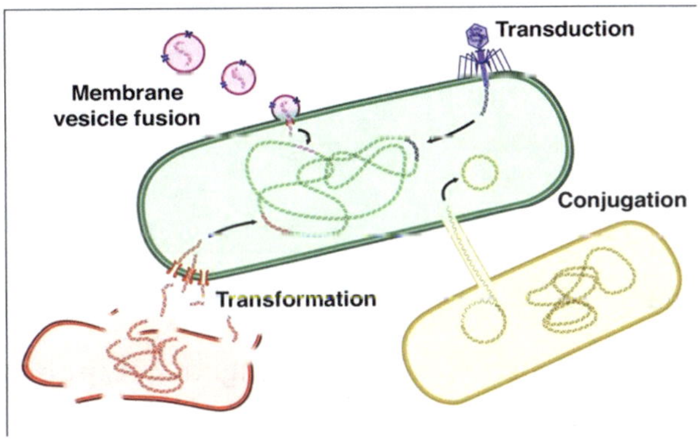

Figure 12.6. The study of horizontal gene transfer among bacteria.

Source: https://acinetobacterbaumannii.no/____impro/1/onewebmedia/HGT.jpg?etag=W%2F%2262cf5-62d03cc2%22&sourceContentType=image%2Fjpeg&ignoreAspectRatio&resize=623%2B411&extract=0%2B0%2B621%2B401&quality=85.

12.1.3. Biofilm Formation and Its Role in Resistance

Biofilm formation is a critical aspect of microbial life that significantly impacts the dynamics of AMR. Biofilms are complex communities of microorganisms, encased in a protective matrix composed of extracellular polymeric substances (EPS). This matrix provides the bacteria with support and blocks antimicrobial agents, thereby reducing the effectiveness of treatment. In hospitals, biofilms commonly grow on medical equipment, wounds, and tissues, which helps infections to last longer. The underlying process of biofilm formation reveals that bacteria employ a unique method to survive both the host's immune system and antibiotic treatment.

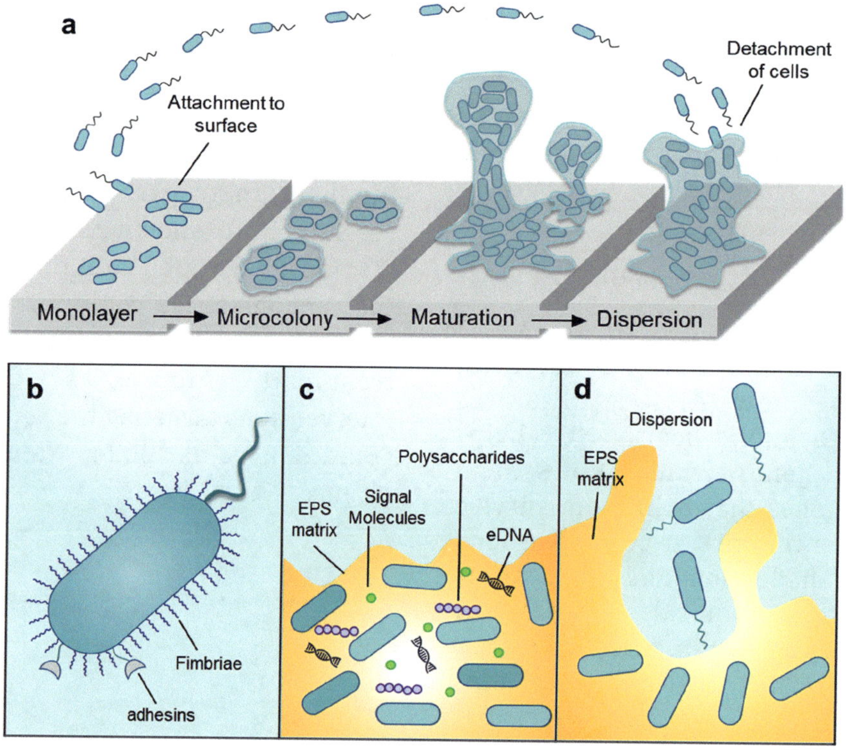

Figure 12.7. Biofilm formation and its role in resistance.

Source: https://www.researchgate.net/publication/371377482/figure/fig2/AS:11431281170568807@1687840167316/Biofilm-formation-stages-and-mechanism-a-Biofilm-formation-stages-b-Adhesins-and.png.

Because biofilms are complex to treat, there is an urgent need for new techniques that can break up these structures and enhance the effectiveness of existing antibiotics. It is crucial to tackle biofilm-related resistance because it helps control the serious public health threat of AMR, which affects both healthcare and health systems. Besides shielding pathogens, biofilms can also serve as a platform where pathogens exchange genetic material. Because of their flexible genomes, biofilm-forming bacteria can acquire resistance genes, making it harder to treat them. *P. aeruginosa* is a good example of a pathogen that uses biofilm formation to avoid being killed by antimicrobial drugs. The organism can form multidrug-tolerant cells within biofilms, which makes it able to resist antibiotics. This makes it more difficult to treat infections, often leading to recurring infections, which require patients to undergo long-term treatment. Because biofilm formation and AMR are closely linked, better monitoring and focused actions are needed in healthcare to address this issue. It is necessary to use different methods to handle biofilm formation and its effects on AMR. Biofilms can be disrupted with biocides or enzymes, which may enhance the effectiveness of traditional antibiotics. Examining various therapeutic approaches, including bacteriophage therapy and antimicrobial peptides, has also yielded promising results in preliminary studies. Taking these innovative steps, along with tight infection control and better antibiotic stewardship, is crucial for addressing AMR caused by biofilm formation. Public health efforts should focus on educating people about the dangers of biofilms and their link to the rise in AMR. By fostering a deeper understanding of the mechanisms at play, stakeholders can better equip healthcare professionals and the public to implement effective responses against biofilm-related infections, ultimately reducing the burden of AMR on society at large (Figure 12.7).

12.2. Factors Contributing to Antimicrobial Resistance

The emergence of AMR has become a pressing global public health concern, primarily driven by the overuse and misuse of antibiotics. This misuse is prevalent in both human medicine and agriculture; the latter often employs antibiotics for growth promotion in livestock, inadvertently fostering the development of resistant strains. In East Africa, there is clear evidence that pregnant women and those who are vulnerable are affected by many bacterial infections. Research has shown that people who have taken antibiotics before are twice as likely to develop infections. Other factors that increase the risk, such as poor sanitation and diabetes, are also important, highlighting the relationship between human actions and the evolution of bacteria. Addressing these risks through improved antibiotic stewardship and hygiene practices is crucial to mitigating the impact of AMR on public health (Mehari et al., 2025). Besides healthcare, environmental factors are also very important in the development of AMR. If sanitation is poor, sewage is handled poorly, and water sources are polluted, people are more likely to encounter resistant pathogens. In many cases, the relationship between environmental factors and AMR bacteria is crucial, particularly when sanitation is not well established. It is clear from the connection between socioeconomics and public health that people who lack access to clean water or proper hygiene are more likely to contract resistant infections. Steps to improve sanitation and encourage adequate hygiene are essential to stop the spread of AMR. Furthermore, incorporating education on the consequences of antibiotic misuse can empower communities to become active participants in combating this crisis (Mehari et al., 2025). The emergence of previously uncommon pathogens makes AMR more challenging to manage. *Streptococcus suis*, which was previously connected to zoonotic transmission and mostly affected adults, is now being found more often in infants with severe conditions like meningitis and sepsis. There is now evidence of strains that hold genes that make them resistant to necessary antibiotics. It has been found that an increasing number of bacteria are becoming resistant to important antimicrobials, such as tetracyclines and macrolides. This highlights the importance of understanding the resistance patterns of these pathogens. Public health needs to respond rapidly to these new threats by strengthening surveillance, designing targeted treatments, and urging the responsible use of antibiotics everywhere.

12.2.1. Overuse and Misuse of Antibiotics in Healthcare

The overuse and misuse of antibiotics in healthcare are significant reasons for the global AMR crisis. This problem is made worse by people who get antibiotics without a doctor's prescription, which causes them to use the drugs incorrectly and not finish the treatment. A study in District Rawalpindi found that around half of the respondents used medicine without a prescription, and about 35% did not complete their prescribed antibiotic course. Although 90% of people understood that using antibiotics too often leads to antibiotic resistance, only 70% had participated in AMR-related public health activities, highlighting an essential lack of education. When people do not engage with antibiotics, it often reflects cultural misunderstandings and expectations put on healthcare providers, which increases the problem of misusing these drugs. Antibiotic overuse in healthcare systems can cause significant harm to patients and also significantly threaten the health of entire communities. Using antibiotics too often encourages the development of antibiotic-resistant pathogens which causes infections that are more difficult to treat and can result in greater sickness and death. The problem is further increased by weak rules that let antibiotics be sold and distributed without regulation, which often causes doctors to come across drug-resistant strains that reduce treatment choices. According to (Ifedinezi et al., 2024), controlling AMR requires concerted efforts across various sectors, emphasizing the need for developing robust antimicrobial stewardship (AMS) programs and implementing strict regulatory systems. They are designed to ensure that antibiotics are used wisely, so that the existing supply is not wasted and people are aware of the link between personal and public health. It is essential to employ a range of measures to address the problem of overusing or misusing antibiotics. Informing the public is essential to teach healthcare providers and patients how to use antibiotics wisely and the risks of AMR. Also, providing thorough training for healthcare professionals on antimicrobial stewardship can significantly affect their prescribing practices and the effectiveness of treatment. Recent studies suggest that when health workers have information about AMR, they are less likely to give in to patient requests for medications they do not really need. To strengthen these efforts, initiatives such as the Global Antimicrobial Resistance and Use Surveillance System (GLASS) and the Access, Watch, and Reserve (AWaRe) classification are vital tools for monitoring antibiotic use and resistance patterns (Ifedinezi et al., 2024). Ultimately, a coordinated, multidisciplinary approach that encompasses education, regulation, and surveillance is paramount to mitigate the impact of AMR and ensure the efficacy of antibiotics in combating infectious diseases (Figure 12.8).

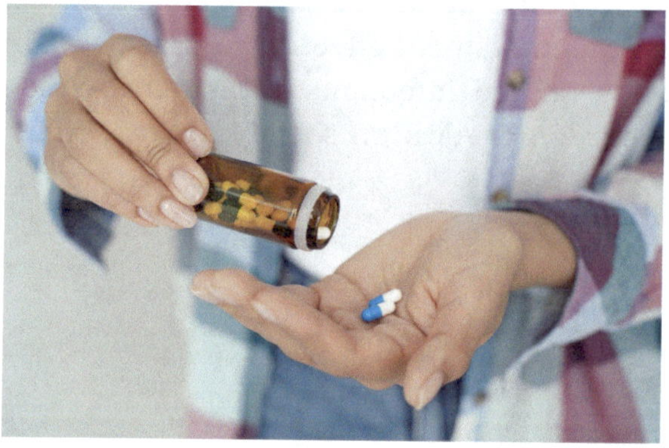

Figure 12.8. The overuse and misuse of antibiotics in healthcare.

Source: https://www.bu.edu/sph/files/2022/10/antibiotics-scaled.jpg.

12.2.2. Agricultural Practices and Antibiotic Use in Livestock

The intersection of agricultural practices and antibiotic use in livestock is a crucial area for understanding the broader implications of AMR on public health. Often, small-scale livestock producers depend on antimicrobials to help their animals grow and live. Dependence on technology is necessary to boost productivity, which in turn helps ensure a stable food supply and a stable economy. Still, if these drugs are used excessively, it can lead to the emergence of resistant pathogens, which are harmful to both animals and humans. In small-scale food animal production systems, where animals are raised in proximity to human communities, the risk of human exposure to antimicrobial-resistant organisms is significantly increased, underscoring the need for vigilant oversight of antibiotic use practices in agriculture (Eisenberg et al., 2017). Besides health issues, the use of antimicrobials in livestock also has economic and societal effects. It is often considered essential to use these drugs in farming to guarantee both safe food and good animal care. With more cases of AMR, the effectiveness of antibiotics and other medicines decreases, which can lead to public health crises. It demonstrates the link between farming success and the unintended consequences of excessive antibiotic use. We need robust policies to manage antimicrobials, particularly as we strive to maintain food security and public health. Understanding this multifaceted relationship is essential in guiding future practices that mitigate the risks associated with AMR (Ferreira et al., 2025). To address AMR, it is essential to rethink agriculture, especially in how antibiotics are used in livestock. By adopting sustainable practices such as improved healthcare and animal management, farmers can reduce the need for drugs to promote animal growth. It is also important to provide farmers with education and training on the safe use of antibiotics. Policymakers should focus on finding additional ways to manage diseases, such as by studying vaccines and probiotics. As a result, public health is improved because there are fewer resistant pathogens, and farming methods are brought in line with new global health standards. Ultimately, a concerted effort across multiple sectors is essential to combat AMR while continuing to support food production systems effectively (Eisenberg et al., 2017; Ferreira et al., 2025) (Figure 12.9).

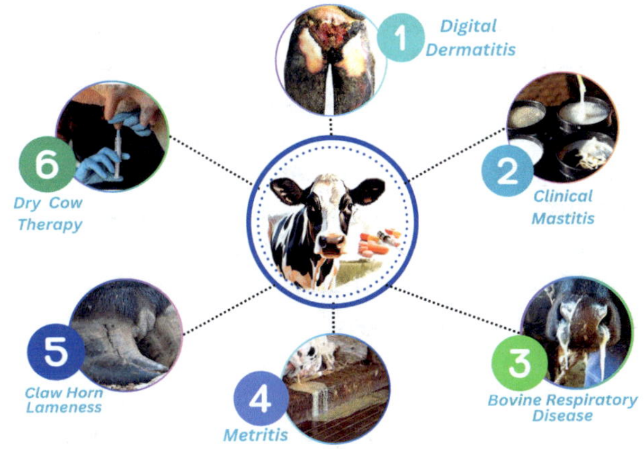

Figure 12.9. The intersection of agricultural practices and antibiotic use in livestock.

Source: https://www.mdpi.com/antibiotics/antibiotics-13-00634/article_deploy/html/images/antibiotics-13-00634-g001.png.

12.2.3. Lack of New Antibiotic Development

The challenge of AMR is intricately linked to the alarming stagnation in new antibiotic development. Over recent years, there has been a significant decline in the pharmaceutical industry's interest in developing new antibiotics. The primary reasons for this decline are the high costs of research and development, as well as the complex nature of regulations. In addition, the profit from antibiotics is usually seen as less attractive than that from chronic disease drugs, which can provide ongoing returns. As a result, the scarcity of new antibiotics makes it more challenging for healthcare providers to treat infections that were once responsive to treatment. As a result of this stagnation, more bacteria are becoming resistant to antibiotics, which necessitates new ideas and increased focus on antibiotic research by both the public and private sectors. Addressing the shortage of new antibiotics requires the combined use of science and effective policies. It is clear from the literature that countries should focus on efforts to boost antibiotic development. One promising strategy is the implementation of financial incentives for pharmaceutical companies, such as grants, tax breaks, or rewards upon successful development of new innovative therapies (Sultana et al., 2024). They can help reduce the financial risks that now discourage investment in research on antibiotics. Additionally, public health agencies should strengthen their partnerships with industry to enhance the efficiency of clinical testing and the approval process for new treatments. By joining forces and sharing risks, different groups can enhance the process of developing antibiotics and help overcome the obstacles that hinder new innovations, ultimately leading to more tools for combating AMR. Besides encouraging new antibiotic research, it is essential to teach people about the proper use of existing antibiotics. People do not fully understand AMR and its results, which has caused a lack of urgency about the issues.

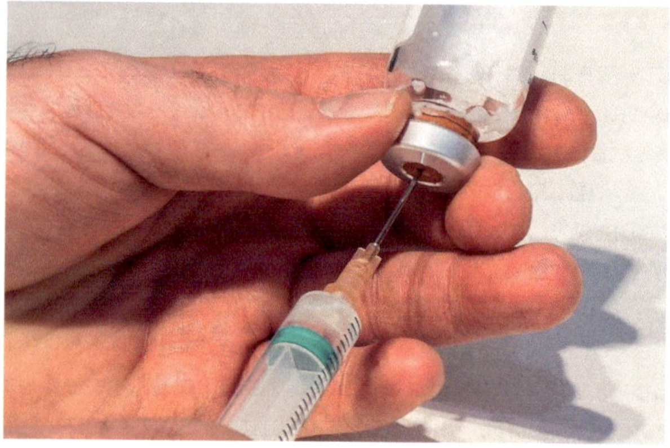

Figure 12.10. Lack of new antibiotic development.

Source: https://cdnph.upi.com/svc/sv/i/2731505923335/2017/1/15059249343290/WHO-warns-of-lack-of-new-antibiotics-under-development.jpg.

As evidenced in recent studies, many individuals hold misconceptions about the efficacy of antibiotics against viral infections, which contributes to the inappropriate prescription and overuse of these medications (Neculai-Valeanu et al., 2024). For this reason, bringing educational campaigns into healthcare can support informed decisions by both healthcare workers and their patients. These strategies can help promote careful use of antibiotics, which is essential for slowing the growth of resistant bacteria. In addition, efforts to create alternative therapies and additional treatments, such as vaccines and phage therapy, should be supported along with antibiotic research. This comprehensive strategy not only addresses the immediate crisis but also lays the groundwork for a reimagined approach to infectious disease management in a landscape increasingly marred by AMR (Figure 12.10).

12.3. Global Impact of Antimicrobial Resistance

The global impact of AMR represents a profound challenge to public health systems around the world. When bacteria develop resistance, the effectiveness of current antimicrobials decreases, resulting in more severe cases of illness and increased mortality from infections that were once treatable. The situation gets worse because antibiotics are used too often in healthcare and farming. In several LMICs, because regulations are not as strict, using antibiotics without care is common, which speeds up the development of drug-resistant bacteria. The CDC notes that urgent, serious, and concerning threats necessitate the use of robust public health measures to prevent and control them. If countries do not respond together, AMR might result in more infections after surgeries and cancer treatments, which could cause medical progress to regress. Besides, the COVID-19 pandemic has introduced more complications in the fight against AMR. The CDC's Special Report highlights that the pandemic has made it more challenging to combat AMR, primarily because hospitals have increased their use of antibiotics to treat secondary infections associated with COVID-19. Due to this setback, there is now a need to reassess the public health measures being used to address AMR. A combination of strategies is necessary, including improving disease detection, developing new medicines, and enhancing disease monitoring. They address the current threats posed by resistant pathogens and ensure public health is prepared to face future challenges. While dealing with the effects of the pandemic, healthcare experts must continue to employ strategies that have proven effective in managing AMR. To tackle the global impact of AMR, different sectors, especially agriculture, must work together because the use of antimicrobials in farming makes a significant contribution to the problem. Because of the rising demand for meat, antibiotics are often given to livestock, which can harm both animals and humans.

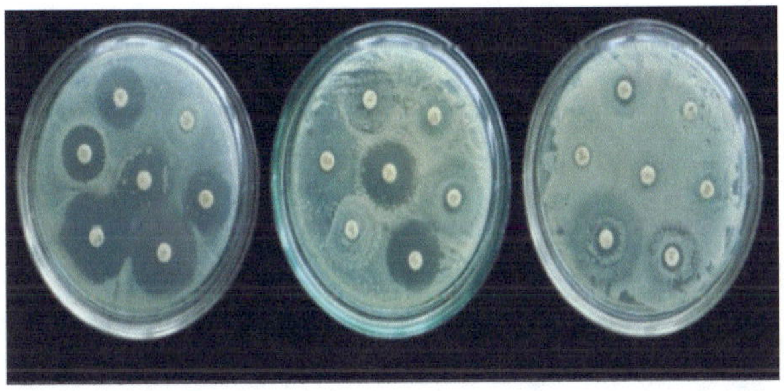

Figure 12.11. The global impact of antimicrobial resistance.

Source: https://media.springernature.com/lw725/springer-cms/rest/v1/content/26527070/data/v1.

As we have seen, bacteria that resist antimicrobials can transfer from animals to humans, making it more challenging to treat infections. It becomes evident that people from different fields must work together to reduce antibiotic overuse in farming, mainly in developing countries. As nations strive to balance agricultural productivity with public health considerations, addressing AMR should become a central tenet of any comprehensive health policy—both to safeguard current public health achievements and to prevent future crises stemming from resistant infections (Figure 12.11).

12.3.1. Statistics on AMR-Related Morbidity and Mortality

AMR poses a significant threat to global public health, leading to increased morbidity and mortality rates associated with bacterial infections. It is estimated that AMR leads to 1.27 million deaths annually, and another 4.95 million deaths happen because of infections where AMR was involved. Such statistics indicate that we must act swiftly to combat AMR, as the effectiveness of current antibiotics is declining. More resistant pathogens lead to increased health issues and place a greater burden on healthcare systems, resulting in longer hospital stays and higher healthcare costs. Examining AMR morbidity and mortality statistics is crucial for informing public health actions that halt the spread of resistant infections and safeguard population health. The ongoing evolution of AMR is making it increasingly difficult to control and prevent diseases using traditional methods. Bovine respiratory disease, which is common in livestock, becomes much more challenging to treat because of AMR. A study demonstrated that while whole-genome sequencing has enabled researchers to identify and catalog AMR genes within bacterial pathogens, there remains a substantial discordance between predicted resistance (genotype) and observed resistance (phenotype). Because of this, it is vital to use comprehensive antimicrobial susceptibility tests to assess the full impact of resistance on health and mortality rates in both animals and humans. Having such insights may help develop treatments that are more tailored to the current situation and lead to better treatment outcomes. Additionally, utilizing advanced data analytics to analyze AMR trends has become increasingly important. New approaches in infectious disease epidemiology demonstrate that we need innovative ways to address the challenges of resistance. Adapting current statistical methods is helping to explore the relationship between AMR and clinical results, which supports better decisions in public health. With various study methods and digital health information, researchers can make accurate models that predict the spread and resistance of pathogens. This evolution in research methodology enhances the landscape of public health surveillance. It provides critical data to policymakers aimed at combating AMR comprehensively, thereby reducing its associated morbidity and mortality rates and protecting population health more effectively (Figure 12.12).

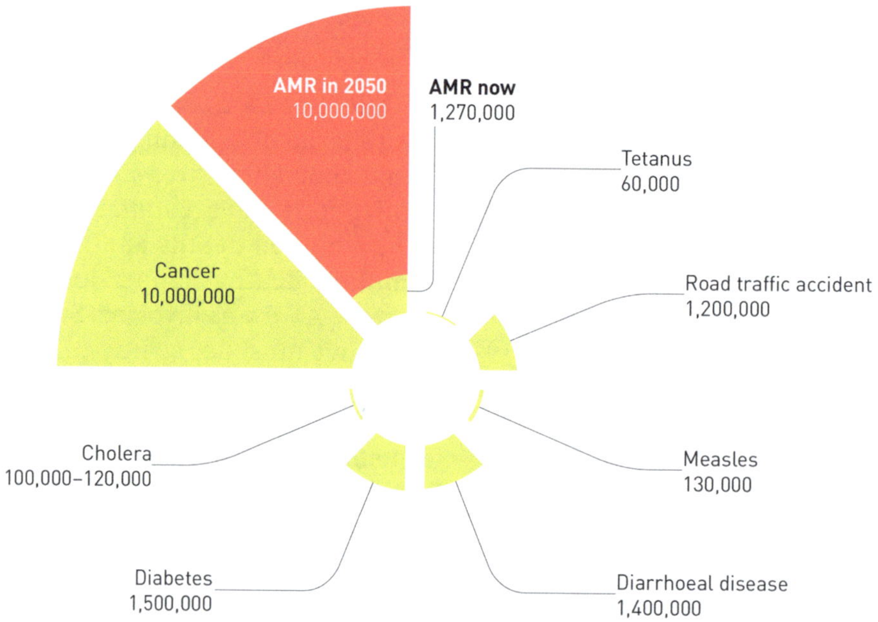

Figure 12.12. Statistics on antimicrobial resistance morbidity and mortality.

Source: https://healthpolicy-watch.news/wp-content/uploads/2023/02/Screenshot-2023-02-06-at-14.35.42.png.

12.3.2. Economic Burden on Healthcare Systems

The cost of AMR to healthcare systems is severe and involves many aspects. Because of AMR, healthcare costs rise, as treating resistant infections usually requires more extended stays in hospitals, more complex care, and stronger medicines. Recent estimates indicate that the worldwide costs of AMR each year are approximately $100-150 billion, and these costs could reach $300 billion by 2030. LMICs face greater difficulties from these costs because resistant infections are much more common in these countries than in richer nations. The growing economic implications challenge healthcare systems that are already operating under constrained budgets, creating a cycle where insufficient resources further exacerbate the problem of AMR, undermining public health initiatives and response strategies (Alomari et al., 2024). AMR has effects that extend beyond financial considerations, as it can impact the health of individuals within a community. Resistant pathogens are often responsible for higher rates of sickness and death, particularly in elderly individuals or children. Age-stratified data indicate that the risk of infection is 2.5 times higher in older adults and 1.8 times higher in pediatric cases, compounding the social and economic impact (Alomari et al., 2024). The additional pressure on healthcare systems may lead to reduced productivity and could result in more people becoming disabled and leaving the workforce. Additionally, healthcare systems face challenges in allocating sufficient effort and resources to ASPs and surveillance systems, which may be overlooked due to rising healthcare costs, thereby exacerbating the problem. Addressing the economic consequences of AMR requires global cooperation and long-term solutions. Healthcare policy needs to use economic analyses to demonstrate that preventive actions such as vaccination and biosecurity, are cost-effective in stopping infections.

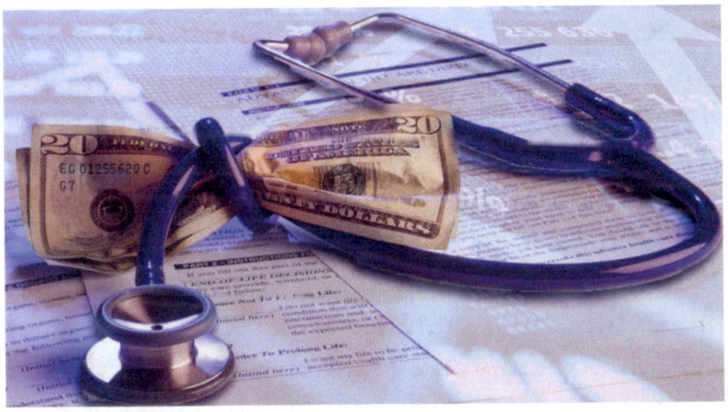

Figure 12.13. Economic burden on healthcare systems.

Source: https://xe.gold/wp-content/uploads/2024/01/Economic-Burden-of-Chronic-Diseases-A-Global-Perspective2_11zon.webp.

It is often challenging to implement effective strategies in low-income countries due to limited resources and underdeveloped healthcare systems. In addition, because diseases such as salmonellosis and campylobacteriosis are still a problem, it is clear that cooperation between the agricultural and healthcare sectors is necessary to find solutions for AMR. By prioritizing investments in research, hospital management, and community education, healthcare systems can begin to alleviate the economic burden posed by AMR, ultimately improving public health and fostering equitable health outcomes for all populations (Figure 12.13).

12.3.3. Effects on Global Health Security

The impact of AMR on global health security is profound and multifaceted. As more resistant pathogens emerge, regular medical treatments are becoming less effective, posing a significant challenge to controlling infectious diseases. This makes it harder to carry out regular procedures, from minor to extensive surgeries, resulting in higher rates of illness and death. Because of AMR, treating diseases becomes more difficult and puts a heavy strain on healthcare systems everywhere. Extended hospital stays and heightened demand for healthcare resources result in escalating medical costs, diverting attention and funding away from other critical health initiatives as health systems struggle to cope with this secondary crisis (Sultana et al., 2024). Besides affecting healthcare, AMR also has economic consequences for each country. Extended stays in the hospital and higher healthcare costs place a significant financial burden on people and healthcare systems, which leads to fewer people being able to work due to their illness. The link between AMR and stable societies is exacerbated by the lack of clean water, proper sanitation, and essential medicines, all of which are crucial in combating infections and preventing resistance. Consequently, weak health infrastructures in LMICs leave populations vulnerable, hampering progress towards achieving sustainable development goals (SDGs) centred around health and well-being (Sharma et al., 2024). Ignoring AMR could ultimately lead to harm for public health, as well as for the economy and society as a whole. To address AMR and maintain global health security, many countries must develop strong and united strategies. Using One Health approaches, which focus on people, animals, and the environment, is a good way to manage this complicated issue. For such efforts to succeed, epidemiological surveillance is needed to watch for resistance and guide effective treatment plans. Furthermore, if public health education tells both healthcare providers and consumers about AMR, it can encourage them to use antimicrobials wisely. Supporting new ways to develop drugs and strengthening rules for using antibiotics helps countries create healthcare systems that can handle AMR. Ultimately, a united global response is necessary to mitigate the effects of this public health crisis and safeguard future generations (Sultana et al., 2024) (Figure 12.14).

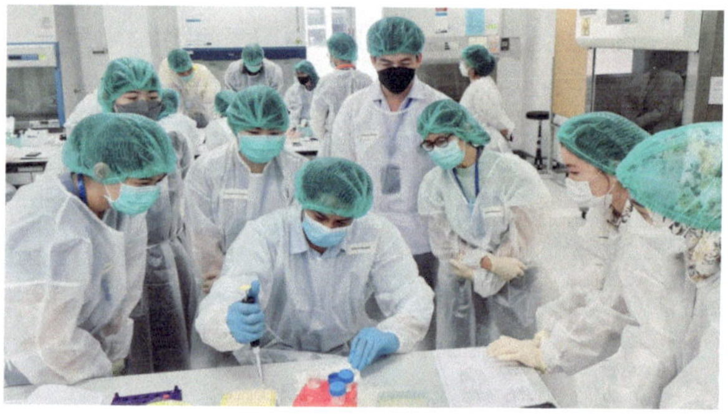

Figure 12.14. Effect on global health security.

Source: https://www.cdc.gov/global-health/media/images/Laboratory_workers.jpg.

12.4. Strategies to Combat Antimicrobial Resistance

The multifaceted challenge of AMR necessitates a comprehensive approach encompassing various strategies. One critical approach is to use ASPs, which encourage doctors and nurses to use antibiotics wisely. The main goals of such programs are to ensure correct prescribing, encourage reducing therapy when appropriate, and emphasise the importance of adhering to treatment guidelines. As a result of these steps, the number of unnecessary antibiotic prescriptions decreases, which helps control the development of resistant strains. Furthermore, integrating education and training on infection prevention measures, such as rightful drug use and healthcare waste management, is vital for increasing health professionals' engagement in AMR containment strategies, as evidenced by findings that identify institutional culture as a critical factor in effective intervention (Sorato, 2025). Informing the public is also crucial in the fight against AMR, as it provides communities with knowledge about the dangers of misusing antibiotics. Such campaigns can explain how antibiotics are used, correct misinformation about their ability to fight viruses, and emphasise the importance of using them as directed. If patients are encouraged to ask questions and participate in their treatment discussions, public health efforts can help prevent inappropriate prescribing and foster a responsible attitude towards antibiotics. Additionally, collaboration between healthcare providers, patients, and policymakers is vital, as evidenced by studies demonstrating that informed public involvement can significantly enhance adherence to national treatment guidelines (Ahmed et al., 2025). The use of One Health is key to handling AMR in human, animal, and environmental health fields. Due to this approach, healthcare providers, veterinarians, and environmental scientists are encouraged to collaborate to prevent infections. For instance, efforts to reduce the use of antibiotics in farming benefit public health and also prevent environmental pollution by pharmaceuticals. Additionally, research on alternative methods, the development of new antibiotic types, and the establishment of reliable monitoring systems are crucial for understanding how resistance develops and responding accordingly. As the body of evidence grows regarding the effectiveness of collaborative strategies, the integration of these efforts will be paramount in the battle against AMR (Ahmed et al., 2025; Sorato, 2025).

12.4.1. Promoting Responsible Antibiotic Use

The promotion of responsible antibiotic use is vital in fighting the looming crisis of AMR, which poses significant challenges to public health. As pathogens evolve mechanisms to counteract the effects of antibiotics, the need for effective Antibiotic Stewardship Programs (ASPs) becomes increasingly apparent. These programs aim to limit the use of antibiotics, so they are only administered when necessary and the correct medication is used for each infection. Thus, healthcare systems worldwide are acknowledging that clinical pharmacists play a crucial role in guiding antibiotic use according to the latest resistance patterns and clinical guidelines. By adhering to evidence-based practices, ASPs can enhance patient outcomes while also mitigating the development of resistant strains, thereby underscoring the crucial connection between responsible antibiotic use and public health initiatives (Ramanisankar et al., 2025). Informing the public is crucial for promoting the responsible use of antibiotics by patients and healthcare providers. Some individuals think that antibiotics can treat viral illnesses like the common cold or flu, which is not true. Making the public and medical staff aware of the proper use of antibiotics can help prevent the unnecessary use of these drugs, which contributes to the rise of AMR. Moreover, including antibiotic education in medical education can help future healthcare workers understand the implications of their prescribing decisions. By fostering a culture of judicious antibiotic use, such initiatives can instill a sense of responsibility among prescribers and patients, recognizing that every unnecessary prescription contributes to the broader public health crisis posed by AMR (Oliveira et al., 2024). Working together in different fields and areas is essential for managing AMR by using antibiotics wisely. The One Health approach, which integrates human, animal, and environmental health, employs the necessary strategies to address this issue. It calls for healthcare professionals, veterinarians, and environmental specialists to collaborate in establishing comprehensive AMR surveillance and effective antibiotic use strategies. Additionally, public health policies should support these collaborations by making responsible use mandatory and promoting research into alternative treatment options. By emphasizing a unified response to AMR, stakeholders can better ensure the sustainability of antibiotics, ultimately safeguarding public health for current and future generations (Ramanisankar et al., 2025).

12.4.2. Enhancing Infection Prevention and Control Measures

The enhancement of infection prevention and control (IPC) measures is critical in the global fight against AMR and its associated public health implications. IPC measures that work help prevent HAIs, which are a key reason for AMR, as they allow resistant bacteria to multiply. It is essential to utilise comprehensive IPC protocols to address these concerns, particularly in healthcare settings that face resource shortages. Such protocols involve routine training for healthcare workers, emphasising knowledge, attitudes, and practices (KAP) regarding IPC measures. In Faranah, Guinea, for example, targeted IPC training and visual reminders significantly improved hand hygiene compliance and triaging practices among healthcare workers, illustrating the potential for IPC programs to enhance both theoretical knowledge and practical application in combating infectious diseases, thereby lessening the burden of AMR (Landsmann et al., 2024). Also, dealing with AMR calls for IPC protocols that are standardised and based on guidelines from respected health organisations.

The WHO outlines the key actions that IPC programs should take to prevent and control HAIs effectively. They help establish robust IPC measures, focusing on good hygiene, the proper use of personal protective equipment, and maintaining a clean environment. Areas with insufficient IPC measures are more at risk of HAIs, which cause higher rates of sickness and death, along with a rise in AMR. The integration of these minimum standards across healthcare facilities can lead to significant improvements in patient outcomes, while concurrently mitigating the risk of developing resistant strains of pathogens (Gilham et al., 2024). Lastly, local efforts that improve IPC measures are crucial in addressing AMR. Due to COVID-19, there is now a greater emphasis on infection control, which has highlighted both the advantages and disadvantages of the current healthcare system. Doing IPC well helps control outbreaks and also prepares healthcare systems to tackle AMR in the future. If hand sanitisers and other essential supplies are made locally, healthcare facilities will still be able to use them when supplies are low worldwide. By fostering a culture of safety, training healthcare workers, and reinforcing awareness of IPC standards, health systems can create resilient responses to infection prevention that are critical in the ongoing battle against AMR (Gilham et al., 2024; Landsmann et al., 2024) (Figure 12.15).

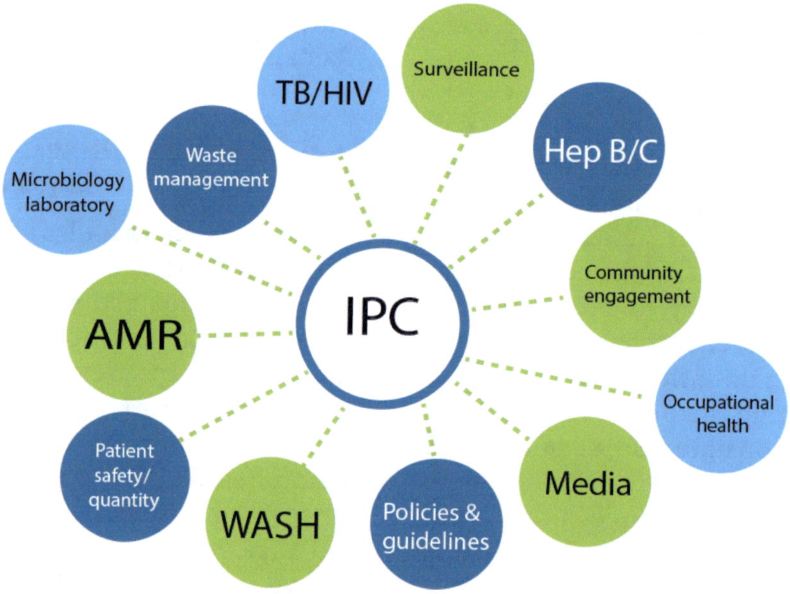

Figure 12.15. The enhancement of infection prevention and control measures.

Source: https://depts.washington.edu/edgh/app-ipc/web/project-images/otherProgrammes.jpg.

12.4.3. Investing in Research and Development of New Treatments

The urgency of investing in research and development (R&D) for new antimicrobial treatments cannot be overstated, especially in the context of rising AMR. AMR poses a significant threat to the health of individuals as well as the functioning of public health systems worldwide. If we do not develop new treatments as microbial pathogens evolve, infections that we can currently control could come back. Given the constant need for new antimicrobial agents, it is clear that R&D funding should be used to discover and utilize new reagents. Because microbial evolution is complex and AMR is varied, it is essential to carry out research that helps outpace resistant strains and restores the usefulness of older treatments. Investing in R&D can ultimately alleviate the burdens of AMR on healthcare systems and improve patient outcomes (Sahgal et al., 2024). In addition, working together, the public and private sectors are vital for the advancement of new antimicrobial treatments. Working together makes it easier for companies to combine their resources, knowledge, and finances for research and development (R&D) purposes.

For example, the launch of zoliflodacin as the first oral antibiotic from a public-private partnership underscores the potential benefits of such partnerships. The drug, which has shown promise in the treatment of uncomplicated urogenital gonorrhea, underscores the importance of strategic R&D investment in creating effective solutions in the face of growing resistance to existing therapies (Pascual et al., 2024). If stakeholders focus on developing new treatment approaches, they can all work together to handle AMR and give healthcare providers what they need to fight resistant infections. Additionally, it is crucial to have a robust system for introducing and monitoring new medical treatments. Strategic use of new antimicrobials in healthcare is necessary to benefit from their effects and avoid the growth of resistance. Using ASPs, it is possible to make sure that new drugs like zoliflodacin are appropriately used so they stay effective for a long time.

Also, closely monitoring how bacteria respond to treatment and the outcomes of those treatments will help guide future drug development. By creating a comprehensive ecosystem that integrates R&D investments with practical implementation strategies, the public health community can establish a sustainable approach to minimizing the threats posed by AMR and protecting global health (Pascual et al., 2024).

12.5. Role of Public Health Organisations

Public health organisations serve as crucial entities in the global struggle against AMR, facilitating coordinated efforts to curb this growing crisis. These organisations, such as the WHO and the Centres for Disease Control and Prevention (CDC), play a pivotal role in monitoring and analysing AMR trends. By highlighting the patterns of resistance, these organisations inform public health actions and shape health policies. They also organise educational activities for healthcare staff and the general public, highlighting the correct use of antibiotics. By working with governments, non-governmental organisations, and research institutions, public health organisations encourage people to cooperate. By working together, we can improve surveillance and management, which helps address AMR and protect the effectiveness of current antibiotics. Besides keeping an eye on health and educating people, public health organisations help develop and research new antibiotics and alternative treatments. As many antibiotics are losing their effectiveness due to widespread resistance, there is a strong need for the development of new drugs. The Global Fund and many public-private partnerships play a crucial role in financing and supporting research on these challenges. By supporting clinical trials and fostering collaboration among companies, universities, and government, they increase the chances of finding new answers to fight infections. Additionally, they help disseminate knowledge about research and best practices, ensuring that healthcare providers are informed about the latest guidance on prescribing and new treatments. Using a variety of methods makes it more likely that AMR can be dealt with effectively and that new solutions fit with public health goals. crucial for public health organisations to cooperate effectively to address the numerous challenges posed by AMR. Since this issue is global, these organisations must team up internationally and talk with each other to use shared resources at both national and international levels. For example, the GLASS project helps countries adopt common ways to gather and exchange data, which allows them to follow resistance patterns accurately. They help people understand what is happening around the world and also support practical actions for each region. Public health organisations emphasise the importance of unity in addressing AMR to bolster healthcare systems, particularly in LMICs, where the issue is particularly concerning. Ultimately, the role of public health organizations is indispensable in nurturing a collaborative framework that mobilizes resources, knowledge, and action to effectively combat AMR and safeguard public health for future generations (Figure 12.16).

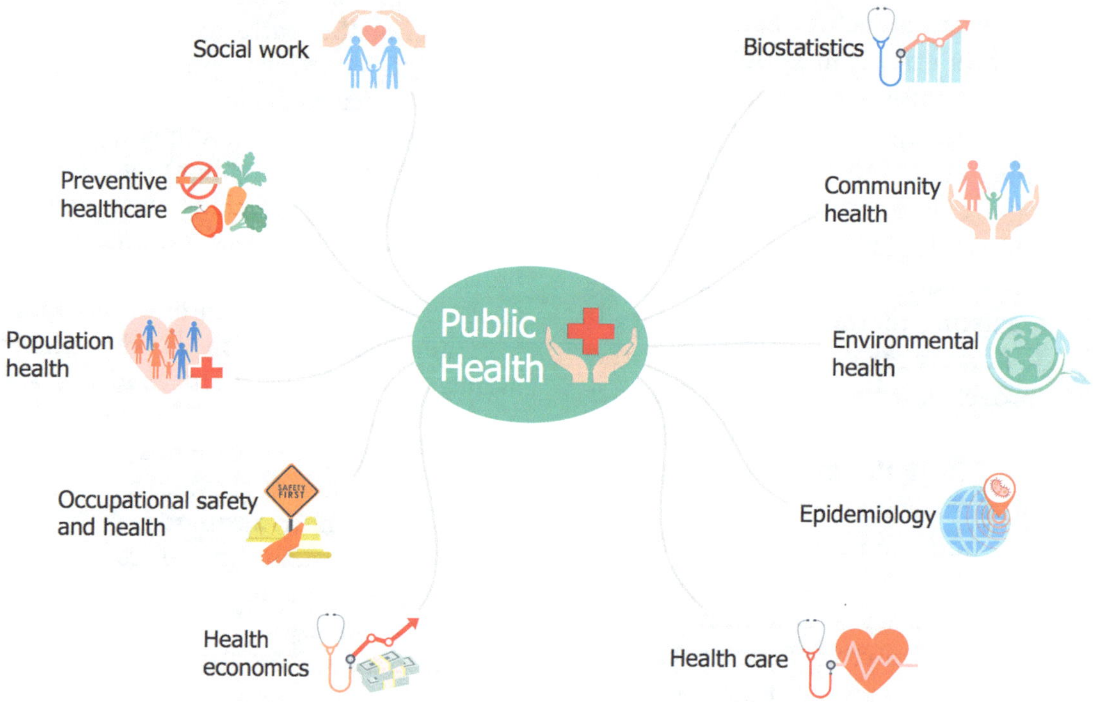

Figure 12.16. Role of public health organizations.

Source: https://www.conceptdraw.com/How-To-Guide/picture/Health-Sciences-Public-Health.png.

12.5.1. Surveillance and Monitoring of AMR Trends

Effective surveillance and monitoring of AMR trends play a crucial role in addressing public health challenges posed by antibiotic-resistant pathogens. The use of clinical samples, laboratory results, and environmental studies allows health authorities to understand how different bacteria are resistant. The integration of traditional epidemiological methods with innovative approaches, such as wastewater surveillance (WWS), can enhance the detection of AMR across communities. Wastewater can be used to track biological threats, and when handled properly, it can complement current AMR monitoring systems. As highlighted by current advancements in WBE, the collection and analysis of sewage can provide valuable insights into the circulation of resistant strains and inform public health decision-making during outbreaks and beyond (Chavarria et al., 2023). Surveillance systems specifically targeting AMR, such as the National Antimicrobial Resistance Monitoring System (NARMS), are integral in tracking resistance trends among foodborne pathogens. They help gather information on the number of cases, who is affected, and the patterns of resistance over the years. The fact that Campylobacter infections are a concern in the United States underscores the importance of surveillance. Data reveal that while the incidence of Campylobacter infections has remained stable, resistance to critical antibiotics, such as ciprofloxacin and erythromycin, has steadily increased (Ahart et al., 2019). This development poses a significant concern for public health, as standard treatments are less effective, prompting healthcare providers to explore alternative methods for treating infections. It is essential to employ a range of methods, including reviewing patient records and monitoring the environment, to continue studying AMR trends. Both laboratory monitoring and environmental studies can provide a clearer understanding of what contributes to the spread of AMR. By using this method, public health officials can identify areas with high risk, understand how infections are transmitted, and implement the appropriate measures. Working together closely is essential for environmental scientists, microbiologists, and epidemiologists to maintain and improve surveillance. As antibiotic resistance continues to evolve, persistently revising and strengthening these surveillance systems will be imperative for protecting public health and ensuring the sustainability of effective antimicrobial therapies (Ahart et al., 2019; Chavarria et al., 2023).

12.5.2. Public Awareness Campaigns and Education

Informing the public through campaigns is very important for tackling AMR. They are designed to educate people on how to use antibiotics properly and what can happen if they are misused. As indicated by recent literature, outreach initiatives such as the WHO's AMR Awareness Week and the CDC's U.S. Antibiotic Awareness Week have been pivotal in enhancing public awareness of AMR (Whitman et al., 2025). Even with these actions, public awareness about cancer is much lower than in other health areas, which means more effort is needed to improve messaging and reach out to people. Addressing this issue can help individuals make informed decisions and support public health, potentially decreasing both antibiotic misuse and the development of resistant pathogens. Evaluating the success of public awareness campaigns is necessary to determine their impact on people's actions regarding antibiotics. Several studies have highlighted how campaigns targeting various demographics, particularly adult populations, have been successful in improving knowledge and altering attitudes toward AMR (Gilham et al., 2024). Nevertheless, many of these campaigns struggle to bring about significant changes in behaviour because AMR's messaging is very complex. It is essential to use criteria for evaluating campaigns, as this helps ensure more accurate results about how much the public is involved and what they recall. Targeted messages, mass media, and improved communication between healthcare professionals and patients are all beneficial for achieving campaign goals; therefore, employing multiple strategies may enhance the effectiveness of these initiatives. Public awareness efforts should also be adjusted to match the new trends in healthcare communication. Many campaigns are less effective because their design and execution are not always consistent, and many interventions have been evaluated using observational studies rather than randomised controlled experiments. Strengthening evaluation frameworks for these campaigns will enable developers to refine their strategies and enhance their reach (Gilham et al., 2024). It is essential to establish methods for quickly adjusting messaging in response to public perceptions and the evolving nature of AMR. A commitment to continuous improvement in public education and outreach will be essential to combat AMR comprehensively, ensuring that these campaigns resonate with diverse audiences and lead to actionable change within communities (Figure 12.17).

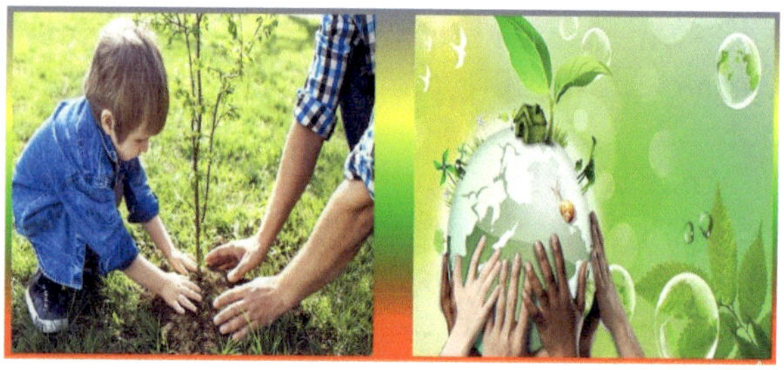

Figure 12.17. Public awareness campaigns and education.

Source: https://i.ytimg.com/vi/t1rNRyKOM_Q/maxresdefault.jpg.

12.5.3. Collaboration Between Countries and Organisations

The complexity of antimicrobial resistance (AMR) necessitates a robust collaborative framework between countries and organisations to address public health challenges effectively. Cooperate. Different nations need to cooperate in sharing important essential resources, data, and best ways of doing things. Working together enables countries to track changes in AMR, apply successful approaches, and develop new technologies to combat resistant pathogens. As an example, the WHO and similar health organizations help spread information and offer advice on how countries should respond to AMR. When countries collaborate on their policies, they can respond more effectively to infectious diseases and address the various aspects of AMR as a global health issue. This international coalition fosters an environment where member states can respond more swiftly and cohesively to the evolving patterns of drug resistance, thereby mitigating risks to public health on a broader scale (Putri, 2024). Additionally, partnerships between countries and organisations extend to sector-specific collaborations, particularly in areas such as Water, Sanitation, and Hygiene (WASH). It is most noticeable in areas where inadequate sanitation facilities contribute to the spread of AMR. For example, a study examining WASH practices in Nigeria and the United Kingdom reveals that collaboration helps reduce the spread of AMR through improved sanitation and hygiene. Although Nigeria faces numerous challenges in WASH, primarily aimed at preventing disease, the UK has benefited from strategies that focus on AMR. When nations collaborate in research and training, they benefit from each other's achievements and lessons learned, which enables them to develop effective solutions for various situations. Such international collaboration not only addresses immediate public health concerns but also establishes a foundation for long-term sustainability in combating AMR (Ezugwu et al., 2024).

Collaborative projects will be more effective if governmental bodies, NGOs, and private sector entities work together. When experts and resources come together, it becomes easier to develop complete plans for handling AMR and to introduce new ways of treating and preventing it. In addition, teaming up for training can enhance the skills of healthcare workers worldwide, ensuring that the best practices for using antimicrobials are shared globally. They can also help people in the community become aware of AMR, which plays a key role in changing attitudes and actions toward using antibiotics. Ultimately, the success of these collaborations hinges on a shared commitment to sustain and enhance global health, demonstrating that collective action is paramount in reversing the tide of AMR and safeguarding public health for future generations (Putri, 2024).

SUMMARY

In conclusion, the crisis of antimicrobial resistance (AMR) poses a significant threat to public health globally, necessitating urgent and coordinated responses across various sectors. Besides harming individuals, AMR also influences healthcare services, finances, and social stability. Recent studies, such as those conducted in China during the COVID-19 pandemic, suggest that while emergency actions can alter AMR trends, it remains crucial to manage antimicrobial use effectively. This underscores the need for consistent monitoring and effective stewardship programs to mitigate the rise of multidrug-resistant infections, as observed in the increasing instances of specific resistant strains, even amid crisis management efforts (Li et al., 2024).

Furthermore, tackling AMR requires a multifaceted approach that addresses environmental drivers, particularly in low and middle-income countries (LMICs). It has been found that the use of specific farming methods and pollution helps resistant pathogens to appear and spread. We should use a One Health approach, which emphasises how human, animal, and environmental health are all linked. Promoting careful use of antimicrobials and better control of pollution can decrease the causes of AMR. Raising public awareness and strengthening public health infrastructures will also play a pivotal role in combating this escalating threat (Nashwan et al., 2024). Afterwards, governments, health organisations, and communities should join forces to address AMR. This can be achieved by adopting policies that help manage antimicrobial use, funding new research, and promoting global efforts to monitor and record AMR cases. Emphasising responsible use of antimicrobials in both healthcare and farming will help stop misuse. For effective treatments to be available in the future and for public health to be safe, everyone must be committed to tackling AMR.

A critical examination of antimicrobial resistance (AMR) reveals significant insights into its escalating public health threat, particularly as identified in recent studies. According to the findings, bacterial AMR was responsible for about 4.95 million deaths worldwide in 2019, and about 1.27 million of those were due to resistance. It emphasises how important it is to tackle AMR, which is a major contributor to deaths worldwide. Additionally, western sub-Saharan Africa bears the most significant burden, underscoring the connection between the state of health services and the spread of diseases. More than 1.5 million deaths were caused by lower respiratory infections, which were the main AMR-related syndrome. Understanding these dynamics is crucial for developing effective public health strategies that mitigate the impact of AMR on diverse populations (Murray et al., 2022). Besides causing more deaths, AMR also affects healthcare spending and the way resources are managed.

It is becoming harder for hospitals and healthcare systems because drug-resistant infections often need stronger treatment, and patients stay in the hospital longer. It is more challenging for healthcare systems in low-resource areas to manage infections and prevent resistance, which exacerbates the financial burden. It is crucial to utilise resources effectively to address AMR, particularly in regions with underdeveloped healthcare systems. Emphasising the need for infection prevention, monitoring, and control programs is vital for bolstering health systems and enhancing patient outcomes amidst the rising tide of AMR (Murray et al., 2022). A combination of steps is necessary to tackle AMR, including monitoring, informing the public, and conducting research and development. Data collection should be improved, especially in resource-limited areas, because a lack of data on antibiotic resistance makes it challenging to create effective policies. Local contexts must be considered, and policies should reflect the different ways people resist in each area. Working together with healthcare providers, policymakers, and research institutions can encourage the development of new vaccines and antibiotics. As we strive to counteract AMR, integrating insights from ongoing research into actionable policies will be pivotal in safeguarding public health and ensuring equitable access to essential medical interventions (Murray et al., 2022).

CLOSER LOOK:

WASTEWATER SURVEILLANCE (WWS):

Wastewater surveillance (WWS) is an innovative public health tool that monitors the presence of pathogens, chemicals, and other biological markers in community sewage systems. By analyzing wastewater, scientists can detect the circulation of infectious diseases, monitor drug use, and even track the spread of antimicrobial resistance. WWS provides a non-invasive, cost-effective, and near real-time method to assess population-level health, complementing traditional clinical surveillance.

One of the most prominent applications of WWS is in tracking viral infections. During the COVID-19 pandemic, wastewater analysis became a vital method for detecting the presence of SARS-CoV-2 in communities, often identifying outbreaks days before clinical testing indicated a rise in cases. This early-warning capability allows health authorities to respond quickly with targeted interventions, such as testing campaigns, vaccination drives, or public advisories. Beyond COVID-19, WWS has been used to monitor other viruses, including influenza, norovirus, and poliovirus, helping to prevent large-scale outbreaks.

Wastewater surveillance is not limited to infectious diseases. It can detect chemical contaminants, including pharmaceuticals, personal care products, and industrial pollutants, providing insight into community exposure and environmental risks. Monitoring illicit drug metabolites in wastewater also allows public health officials to track trends in drug use, guiding prevention programs and resource allocation. Furthermore, WWS can identify antimicrobial resistance genes circulating within populations, offering a crucial tool in the fight against resistant pathogens.

The effectiveness of WWS relies on advanced sampling and analytical techniques. Wastewater samples are collected from treatment plants or sewer networks and analyzed using molecular methods such as polymerase chain reaction (PCR) and genomic sequencing. These methods enable the detection of low concentrations of pathogens and the identification of specific variants or strains. Data collected through WWS can be integrated with geographic information systems (GIS) and statistical models to provide spatial and temporal insights, helping authorities focus interventions where they are most needed.

Despite its advantages, WWS faces challenges, including variability in sewage composition, dilution factors, and the need for standardized protocols. However, ongoing research and technological advancements are improving its accuracy, reliability, and scalability.

In conclusion, wastewater surveillance is a powerful tool for modern public health. By offering a population-level view of infectious diseases, chemical exposure, and antimicrobial resistance, WWS enables proactive health management, supports early warning systems, and strengthens community resilience. Its integration into public health strategies promises to transform how societies detect and respond to emerging health threats.

REFERENCES

1. Owen, J. R., Noyes, N., Young, A. E., Prince, D. J., Blanchard, P. C., Lehenbauer, T. W., Aly, S. S., Davis, J. H., O'Rourke, S. M., Abdo, Z., Belk, K., Miller, M. R., Morley, P., & Van Eenennaam, A. L. (2017). Whole-Genome Sequencing and Concordance Between Antimicrobial Susceptibility Genotypes and Phenotypes of Bacterial Isolates Associated with Bovine Respiratory Disease. *G3 Genes Genomes Genetics*, *7*(9), 3059–3071. https://doi.org/10.1534/g3.117.1137Adams, J., Aidara-Kane, A., Alvarez, J., Amidon, G., Andersson, D. I., Andremont, A., Andremont, et al. (2016). *Veterinary Medicine Needs New Green Antimicrobial Drugs.* https://core.ac.uk/download/76980785.pdf (accessed on 30th May 2025).
2. Ahart, L. (2019). *Trends in Antimicrobial Resistance of Campylobacter Infections—United States, 2005–2017.* https://core.ac.uk/download/215176884.pdf (accessed on 30th May 2025).
3. Ahmad, R., Holmes, A., McLeod, M., Micallef, et al. (2019). A whole-health-economy approach to antimicrobial stewardship: Analysis of current models and future direction. *PLoS Med.* https://core.ac.uk/download/323306206.pdf (accessed on 30th May 2025).
4. Ahmed, S. K., Hussein, S., Qurbani, K., Ibrahim, R. H., Fareeq, A., Mahmood, K. A., & Mohamed, M. G. (2024). Antimicrobial resistance: Impacts, challenges, and future prospects. *Journal of Medicine Surgery and Public Health, 2*, 100081. https://doi.org/10.1016/j.glmedi.2024.100081.
5. Ahmed, S., Ahmed, R., & Adam, R. (2025). A comprehensive outline of antimicrobial resistance, antibiotic prescribing, and antimicrobial stewardship in South Africa: A scoping review protocol. *PLOS ONE, 20*. https://www.semanticscholar.org/paper/86357160d248be445428 2cb66a008710c9704f86 (accessed on 30th May 2025).
6. Algamody, S., Elzen, A., & Shamsi, S. S. (2023). Antibiotic resistance in *Campylobacter*: Mechanisms, resistance emergence, therapy, and future perspective. *Future Microbiol.* https://core.ac.uk/download/595555054.pdf (accessed on 30th May 2025).
7. Almeida, A., Antunes, P., Novais, C., Peixe, et al. (2023). Unraveling the role of metals and organic acids towards bacterial antimicrobial resistance in the food chain. *Antibiotics.* https://core.ac.uk/download/580105523.pdf (accessed on 30th May 2025).
8. Alomari, R., Abdel-Razeq, A., & Shamiah, H. (2024). Comprehensive assessment of the global burden of antimicrobial resistance: Trends and insights from 2000 to 2023. *American Journal of BioMedicine.* https://www.semanticscholar.org/paper/905a9887ee87347ae5a7ec6f6a409 de492b45396 (accessed on 30th May 2025).
9. Amal, U. K., Somanath, S., & Athul, U. K. (2025). Emerging antibiotic resistance in *Salmonella*: Implications for public health and veterinary medicine. *Annual Research & Review in Biology.* https://www.semanticscholar.org/paper/6baadfc2a097fb95ecca05ffc510442f2d3a3ba8 (accessed on 30th May 2025).
10. Barathan, M., Ng, S. L., Lokanathan, Y., Ng, M. H., & Law, J. (2024). Unseen weapons: Bacterial extracellular vesicles and the spread of antibiotic resistance in aquatic environments. *International Journal of Molecular Sciences, 25.* https://www.semanticscholar.org/paper/d2256f88f5ab23b4a3a614f11e9a0e9d9ea88900 (accessed on 30th May 2025).
11. Bhagwandin, N., Jenner, A., & Kowalski, S. P. (2017). Antimicrobial resistance (AMR) and multidrug resistance (MDR): Overview of current approaches, consortia and intellectual property issues. https://core.ac.uk/download/215505935.pdf (accessed on 30th May 2025).

12. Branda, F., & Scarpa, F. (2024). Implications of artificial intelligence in addressing antimicrobial resistance: Innovations, global challenges, and healthcare's future. *Antibiotics, 13*. https://www.semanticscholar.org/paper/d50dea4c6e67029f063c91b89638a6c0e43ea62a (accessed on 30th May 2025).

13. Burton, F., Grazia, L., Sisti, C., Rizzo, S., & Surgery, et al. (2023). Association between influenza vaccination and antibiotic prescription in pediatric population. *The European Journal of Public Health, 33*. https://www.semanticscholar.org/paper/bc0cedb344b8b6c5683a39295d34bf7626787b0a (accessed on 30th May 2025).

14. Chavarria, C. A., Gitter, A., Godbole, A. R., Hanson, et al. (2023). *Not a Waste: Wastewater Surveillance to Enhance Public Health*. https://core.ac.uk/download/561051174.pdf (accessed on 30th May 2025).

15. Desai, V., Kumar, S., Patel, B., Patel, S. N., Patadiya, H., Asawa, D., Pathan, M. S. H., et al. (2025). Navigating antimicrobials and combating antimicrobial resistance: Challenges, impacts, and strategies for global action. *Cureus, 17*. https://www.semanticscholar.org/paper/25eaeacf2c74ab469ebd5d09b70f5ab5c75ebb96 (accessed on 30th May 2025).

16. Ducrot, C., & Roger, F. (2017). Antimicrobials in agriculture: Reducing their use while limiting health and socioeconomic risks in the countries of the South. Perspective. https://core.ac.uk/download/154377163.pdf (accessed on 30th May 2025).

17. Eisenberg, J. N. S., Graham, J. P., Johnson, T. J., Trueba, et al. (2017). Small-scale food animal production and antimicrobial resistance: Mountain, molehill, or something in-between? *Environ. Health Perspect.* https://core.ac.uk/download/323081556.pdf (accessed on 30th May 2025).

18. Ezugwu, N. V., Gayle, A., & Anyamene, C. (2024). Epidemiology of antimicrobial resistance and the WASH project: Averting a potential public health crisis in Nigeria using the United Kingdom as a case study. *International Journal of Tropical Disease & Health*. https://www.semanticscholar.org/paper/a06ef1e72d73da5309d8f33117f7004d2cc3c034 (accessed on 30th May 2025).

19. Ferreira, J. P., Rushton, J., SAFOSO, Switzerland, Staerk, et al. (2025). *Antimicrobial Resistance: The Use of Antimicrobials in the Livestock Sector.* https://core.ac.uk/download/36777949.pdf (accessed on 30th May 2025).

20. Fusco, G., Paradiso, R., Cardillo, L., Salvia, M. A., Dodaro, S., Del Monaco, V., Scarpelli, G., et al. (2025). *Streptococcus suis*-associated neonatal meningitis and sepsis: Characterization, antimicrobial resistance, and public health implications. *Frontiers in Microbiology, 16*. https://www.semanticscholar.org/paper/8e0dcd7a23d3a858483bf9adbdc08236cff65557 (accessed on 30th May 2025).

21. Gilham, E., Pearce-Smith, N., Carter, V., & Ashiru-Oredope, D. (2024). Assessment of global antimicrobial resistance campaigns conducted to improve public awareness and antimicrobial use behaviors: A rapid systematic review. *BMC Public Health, 24*. https://www.semanticscholar.org/paper/de0f0269d63833e4194a363dfb80f596792f0bc0 (accessed on 30th May 2025).

22. Grace, D., Knight-Jones, T. J. D., Melaku, A., Alders, R., & Jemberu, W. (2024). The public health importance and management of infectious poultry diseases in smallholder systems in Africa. *Foods, 13*. https://www.semanticscholar.org/paper/c3deddc7ba59ad563d6ff215ea783ddf143b921e (accessed on 30th May 2025).

23. Graham, D. Y., & Liou, J. M. (2021). Primer for development of guidelines for *Helicobacter pylori* therapy using antimicrobial stewardship. *Clinical Gastroenterology and Hepatology, 20*, 973–983.e1. https://doi.org/10.1016/j.cgh.2021.03.026.

24. Gyasi-Darko, K., Amofah, A. D., Ugwu, D., Apaflo, J. N., & Oware, E. (2024). Initiatives to promote the responsible use of antibiotics and the development of new antimicrobial agents. *World Journal of Advanced Research and Reviews*. https://www.semanticscholar.org/paper/d32c7e67b4a76536348b8805a888d493f310ad77 (accessed on 30th May 2025).

25. Hanif, M. S., Sultan, M. A., Raza, A., Asad, M. J., Hussain, M. I., & Wajid, U. (2025). Antibiotics overuse and its consequences: Raising awareness and promoting responsible use. *History of Medicine*. https://www.semanticscholar.org/paper/ba784812a06982ebd2d5ff981aa762ec50590e0b (accessed on 30th May 2025).

26. Harnan, S., Kearns, B., Scope, A., Schmitt, L., Janković, D., Hamilton, J., Srivastava, T., et al. (2024). Ceftazidime with avibactam for treating severe aerobic Gram-negative bacterial infections: Technology evaluation to inform a novel subscription-style payment model. *Health Technology Assessment, 28*(73), 1–230. https://www.semanticscholar.org/paper/8a004c1400aa538d454fd701110319e57416aa3f (accessed on 30th May 2025).

27. Ifedinezi, O. V., Nnaji, N., Anumudu, C. K., Ekwueme, C., Uhegwu, C. C., Ihenetu, F. C., Obioha, P., et al. (2024). Environmental antimicrobial resistance: Implications for food safety and public health. *Antibiotics, 13*. https://www.semanticscholar.org/paper/523c18254227266da93b9f9bb35ca8c382580978 (accessed on 30th May 2025).

28. Khan, J., Ali, S., Usman, M., Asif, H., Ahmad, M., Waheed, S. F., Rauf, U., et al. (2025). Role of microbiology in tackling antimicrobial resistance: Implications for food safety and public health. *Indus Journal of Bioscience Research*. https://www.semanticscholar.org/paper/effe47d361e4f76a0f8b7fad549ea62753143270 (accessed on 30th May 2025).

29. Kothari, A., Kherdekar, R. S., Mago, V., Uniyal, M., Mamgain, G., Kalia, R. B., Kumar, S., et al. (2023). Age of antibiotic resistance in MDR/XDR clinical pathogen of *Pseudomonas aeruginosa*. *Pharmaceuticals, 16*, 1230. https://doi.org/10.3390/ph16091230.

30. Landsmann, L., Borodova, A., Rocha, C., Diallo, A. A., Diallo, K. M., Borchert, M., Arvand, M., et al. (2024). Healthcare workers' knowledge, attitude and practices on infection prevention and control in the context of the COVID-19 pandemic at the Faranah regional hospital and associated healthcare centers, Guinea. *Antimicrobial Resistance and Infection Control, 13*. https://www.semanticscholar.org/paper/f57cfd8a34feaf66c3551a9860ad03317c74361b (accessed on 30th May 2025).

31. Lewnard, J. A., & Reingold, A. L. (2019). *Emerging Challenges and Opportunities in Infectious Disease Epidemiology*. https://core.ac.uk/download/323082106.pdf (accessed on 30th May 2025).

32. Li, W., Yang, X., Liu, C. N., Liu, X., Shi, L., Zeng, Y., Xia, H., et al. (2024). Multiple impacts of the COVID-19 pandemic and antimicrobial stewardship on antimicrobial resistance in nosocomial infections: An interrupted time series analysis. *Frontiers in Public Health, 12*. https://www.semanticscholar.org/paper/fb3013909bfc3fa41c8cd7a627a50b666bc79049 (accessed on 30th May 2025).

33. Marcon, D., Sharma, A., Souza, A. B., Barros, R. B. B., Andrade, V. G. D. G. D., Guimarães, R. J. D. P. S., Lima, L. N. G. C., et al. (2025). Comprehensive genomic surveillance reveals

transmission profiles of extensively drug-resistant tuberculosis cases in Pará, Brazil. *Frontiers in Microbiology, 15*. https://www.semanticscholar.org/paper/53711359e0d2f0fa7e6624015c8db0d842c2776d (accessed on 30th May 2025).

34. McKinn, S., Trinh, D. H., Drabarek, D., Trieu, T. T., Nguyen, P., Cao, T. H., Dang, A. D., et al. (2021). Drivers of antibiotic use in Vietnam: Implications for designing community interventions. *BMJ Global Health, 6*, e005875–e005875. https://doi.org/10.1136/bmjgh-2021-005875.

35. Mehari, M. G., Yeshiwas, A. G., Esubalew, D., Azmeraw, Y., Delie, A., Limenh, L. W., Worku, N., et al. (2025). Dominance of antimicrobial resistance bacteria and risk factors of bacteriuria infection among pregnant women in East Africa: Implications for public health. *Journal of Health, Population, and Nutrition, 44*. https://www.semanticscholar.org/paper/b77ce0e860fb7354efdca469d2a4f3190bbea4b8 (accessed on 30th May 2025).

36. Murray, C. J. L., Ikuta, K. S., Sharara, F., Swetschinski, L. R., Robles, A. G., Gray, A. P., Han, C., et al. (2022). Global burden of bacterial antimicrobial resistance in 2019: A systematic analysis. *The Lancet, 399*, 629–655. https://doi.org/10.1016/s0140-6736(21)02724-0.

37. N/A. (2025). *COVID-19: U.S. Impact on Antimicrobial Resistance, Special Report 2022*. https://core.ac.uk/download/556240361.pdf (accessed on 30th May 2025).

38. Nahum, Y., Muhvich, J., Morones-Ramírez, J. R., Casillas-Vega, N. G., & Zaman, M. H. (2025). Biofilms as potential reservoirs of antimicrobial resistance in vulnerable settings. *Frontiers in Public Health, 13*. https://www.semanticscholar.org/paper/17a87ecd6429219160f2024cf69b9658dc4f1c93 (accessed on 30th May 2025).

39. Nashwan, A., Shah, H. H., Hussain, T., Rauf, S. A., & Ahmed, S. K. (2024). Environmental drivers of antimicrobial resistance in low- and middle-income countries: The impacts of a changing world. *Environmental Health Insights, 18*. https://www.semanticscholar.org/paper/bfdb4a9c16c4f7612d372e17e46022d1a8d71305 (accessed on 30th May 2025).

40. Neculai-Valeanu, A., Ariton, A., Radu, C., Porosnicu, I., Sanduleanu, C., & Amariții, G. (2024). From herd health to public health: Digital tools for combating antibiotic resistance in dairy farms. *Antibiotics, 13*. https://www.semanticscholar.org/paper/2ff6f9e098bd02da70c40e17f55a40f7b8d1c64a (accessed on 30th May 2025).

41. Oliveira, M., Antunes, W., Mota, S., Madureira-Carvalho, Á., Dinis-Oliveira, R. J., & Dias Da, S. D. (2024). An overview of the recent advances in antimicrobial resistance. *Microorganisms, 12*, 1920. https://www.semanticscholar.org/paper/2f4d8ae10c939874c82c48902e474e482064bf37 (accessed on 30th May 2025).

42. Panwar, D. (2024). *Role of Biotechnology in Combating Antibiotic Resistance*. https://core.ac.uk/download/636456668.pdf (accessed on 30th May 2025).

43. Pascual, F., Au, C., Chikwari, C. D., Daram, P., Deal, C. D., Miranda, A. E., Grad, Y., et al. (2024). Recommendations for the optimal introduction of novel antibiotics to treat uncomplicated gonorrhoea in the face of increasing antimicrobial resistance: A case study with zoliflodacin. *BMC Global and Public Health, 2*. https://www.semanticscholar.org/paper/cc3da2cc86795d1c4d5dfb111c63c1760f5e5cd2 (accessed on 30th May 2025).

44. Putri, T. (2024). Tantangan dan solusi terkini dalam penanganan penyakit menular. *Surabaya Biomedical Journal*. https://www.semanticscholar.org/paper/a02fd13f8f354ce47271c6716a304bdde29df5fc (accessed on 30th May 2025).

45. Ramanisankar, A., Nirenjen, S., Maheswari, P., Neena, P. E. M., Prathap, A. S., Raj, D. S., & Dharshne, P. T. (2025). Antimicrobial resistance patterns and the role of antibiotic stewardship in a secondary care hospital. *Recent Advances in Anti-Infective Drug Discovery*. https://www.semanticscholar.org/paper/bda86305fa76e018db18a4ed7a727fd32cac0dce (accessed on 30th May 2025).

46. Ravi, K., & Singh, B. (2024). ESKAPE: Navigating the global battlefield for antimicrobial resistance and defense in hospitals. *Bacteria*. https://www.semanticscholar.org/paper/0c3cc1849e979547a688606272b77aaa5e171677 (accessed on 30th May 2025).

47. Rozenbaum, M. H., Huang, L., Cane, A., Arguedas, A., Chapman, R., Dillon-Murphy, D., Tort, M. J., et al. (2024). Cost-effectiveness and impact on infections and associated antimicrobial resistance of 20-valent pneumococcal conjugate vaccine in US children previously immunized with PCV13. *Journal of Medical Economics*. https://www.semanticscholar.org/paper/a34b6c105070e61ee8668b5bc9a96a02645107a4 (accessed on 30th May 2025).

48. Rudd, K. E., Johnson, S. C., Agesa, K. M., Shackelford, K. A., Tsoi, D., Kievlan, D., Colombara, D. V., et al. (2020). Global, regional, and national sepsis incidence and mortality, 1990–2017: Analysis for the Global Burden of Disease Study. *The Lancet, 395*, 200–211. https://doi.org/10.1016/s0140-6736(19)32989-7.

49. Sahgal, S., & Srivastava, D. (2024). Antimicrobial resistance and innovation in the development of antimicrobial reagents. *Pharmaceutical Science and Technology*. https://www.semanticscholar.org/paper/17d28f47ab918cb904223a352a4a6673fbc26d72 (accessed on 30th May 2025).

50. Sharma, S., Chauhan, A., Ranjan, A., Mathkor, D., Haque, S., Ramniwas, S., Tuli, H., et al. (2024). Emerging challenges in antimicrobial resistance: Implications for pathogenic microorganisms, novel antibiotics, and their impact on sustainability. *Frontiers in Microbiology, 15*. https://www.semanticscholar.org/paper/6268b8b41c82428b85806dc7031cdf573e2699b7 (accessed on 30th May 2025).

51. Sorato, M. M. (2025). Health professional and facility engagement in antimicrobial resistance prevention and containment strategic initiatives at public hospitals in Southern Ethiopia: Facility-based cross-sectional study. *BMJ Public Health, 3*. https://www.semanticscholar.org/paper/e8df5acc25ba40eb053f00d5c0c57fa8509fcf0d (accessed on 30th May 2025).

52. Sultana, M., Perves, N., Uddin, N., Chowdhury, M. E. E., & Amin, N. (2024). The vicious impact of antimicrobial resistance on global public health security and the role of healthcare systems and policy in combating AMR. *World Journal of Public Health*. https://www.semanticscholar.org/paper/67a094fc5755c7be7d117f710d5c385bf9f890d4 (accessed on 30th May 2025).

53. Swanson, K. S., Gibson, G. R., Hutkins, R., Reimer, R. A., Reid, G., Verbeke, K., Scott, K. P., et al. (2020). The International Scientific Association for Probiotics and Prebiotics (ISAPP) consensus statement on the definition and scope of synbiotics. *Nature Reviews Gastroenterology & Hepatology, 17*, 687–701. https://doi.org/10.1038/s41575-020-0344-2.

54. Ünüvar, G. K. (2024). Infection prevention and control program in healthcare facilities: Minimum requirements. *Lokman Hekim Health Sciences*. https://www.semanticscholar.org/paper/0d23599d16f8c7066d61ff1d5eb94a72ea3dbbb6 (accessed on 30th May 2025).

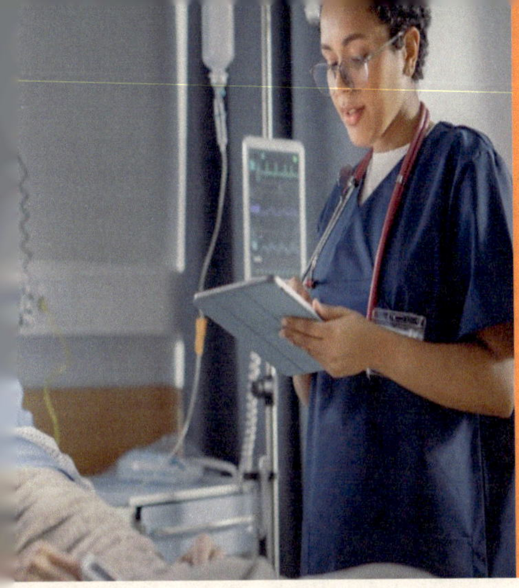

Chapter 13

ETHICAL CONSIDERATIONS IN INFECTIOUS DISEASE EPIDEMIOLOGY

Contents

Introduction

In the realm of public health, ethical considerations play a foundational role in addressing infectious disease epidemiology. The quick and widespread arrival of contagious diseases such as COVID-19, highlights the need for a strong set of ethical principles for epidemiology. They ensure transparency, respect for each person's rights, and social justice as they address challenges posed by disease outbreaks. While studying infectious diseases, researchers must ensure that they consider both the health of the public and the dignity of every individual. Ethical frameworks ensure that the data collected and used serve not only scientific and public health interests but also the overarching goal of fostering trust and compliance among affected populations, which is crucial for effective mitigation strategies during health crises (Soroye et al., 2024). Talking about this topic, we must also consider the role of ethical governance in research and data management during infectious disease outbreaks. In such cases, public health officials should develop policies that balance privacy protection with effective surveillance and response efforts. It becomes an ethical dilemma when health interventions for many people clash with people's personal rights, forcing health practitioners to handle these situations skillfully. For example, using contact tracing and quarantines to stop the spread of disease may limit people's rights, so their ethical impact should be carefully examined. The principles of autonomy and justice come into play, demanding that populations affected by these measures are engaged and informed, ensuring that interventions are both fair and effective (Freeman, 2018). Additionally, as the makeup of those at risk from infectious diseases evolves, it is essential to review the ethics of epidemiological research continually. Examining infections in Rivers State during the COVID-19 pandemic reveals significant differences in cases based on sex, age, and social and economic backgrounds. Being aware of these points clarifies why we should design health programs that cater to the specific needs of each group. It emphasises that all individuals should have equal access to healthcare and that public health initiatives must address these disparities. Ethical epidemiology must advocate for fairness in data collection, analysis, and response strategies to ensure that the most vulnerable populations receive appropriate care and resources, ultimately contributing to the effectiveness of public health initiatives in mitigating infectious diseases (Freeman, 2018; Soroye et al., 2024) (Figure 13.1).

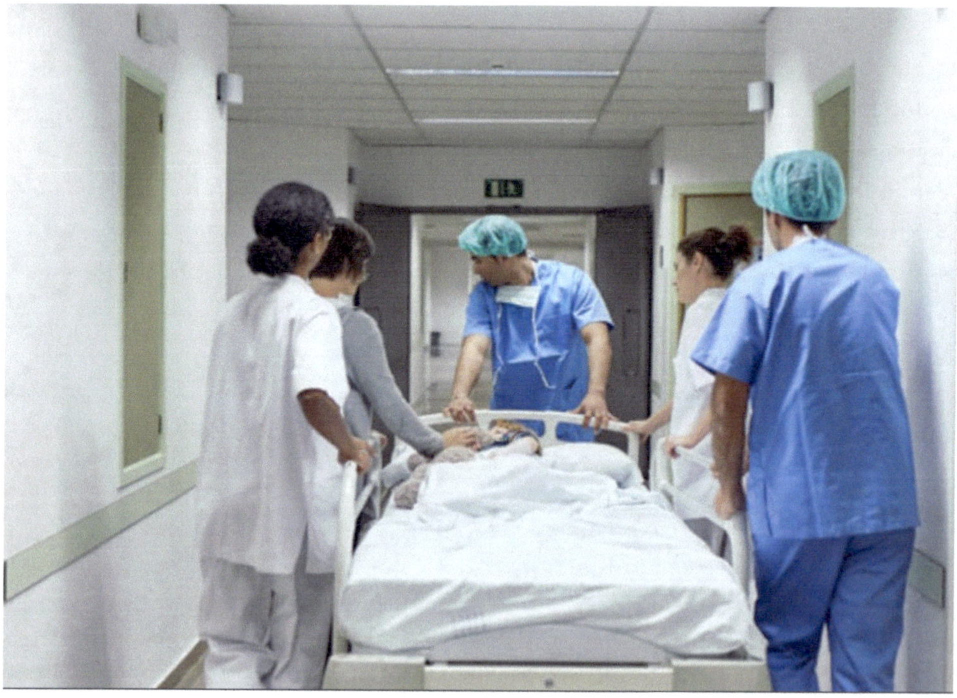

Figure 13.1. Public health, ethical considerations serve.

Source: https://www.sermo.com/wp-content/uploads/2022/03/ethical-issues-in-healthcare-img-2.jpeg.

Definition of Infectious Disease Epidemiology

The field of infectious disease epidemiology examines how infectious diseases affect populations, focusing on the various patterns, causes, and outcomes of health and disease. By merging several scientific approaches, this field can measure and study the prevalence of a disease. Epidemiology forms the basis for public health actions by identifying the causes of disease spread, establishing control methods, and informing health policy decisions. For this reason, the definition of infectious disease epidemiology is vital, as it helps design strategies that improve community health and reduce the incidence of diseases. This definition matters ethically because epidemiologists have to handle data in a way that respects individuals' rights and focuses on the health of the public, especially for vulnerable groups. There are many ethical issues in infectious disease epidemiology, since researchers must gather a lot of data while still respecting people's privacy and independence. Ethics require epidemiologists to obtain informed consent whenever possible and to be transparent about their research methods. Moreover, their findings often have broader implications, as epidemiological data can influence public opinions and health policies that impact the lives of many. For this reason, understanding social responsibilities is a key part of what infectious disease epidemiology is about. When performed ethically, infectious disease epidemiology fosters trust between the public and health authorities, which is crucial for the effective implementation of disease control strategies, particularly during outbreaks or pandemics that necessitate swift community responses (Beltrán-Aguilar et al., 2020). The field of infectious disease epidemiology needs to adapt as new infectious threats, such as emerging diseases or antibiotic resistance, emerge. Researchers are required to put the safety and welfare of people first when planning interventions. A good example is COVID-19, where rapid and flexible epidemiology was needed to help public health officials make informed decisions about actions and resources. Concern for ethical practices in infectious disease epidemiology stays vital from the beginning of data gathering and analysis all the way through disease management. When public health plans are developed using epidemiology, they should consider and address the unfair disparities among those affected. Ultimately, a robust definition of infectious disease epidemiology incorporates these ethical dimensions, affirming the critical role of this field in safeguarding public health and fostering social justice (Bhimraj et al., 2020).

Importance of Ethics in Public Health

Ethics in public health is paramount, particularly in the context of infectious disease epidemiology, where the consequences of decisions can profoundly impact entire populations. Ethics involves supporting the good of individuals while balancing societal expectations, which can sometimes be at odds. Public health may require people to follow rules like vaccinations or quarantine, which might limit their personal freedom. Therefore, ethical frameworks must guide these public health policies to prioritise equity, justice, and respect for all individuals. If these ethical issues are not addressed, communities may develop distrust, and public health efforts may be ineffective, potentially hindering disease prevention and health promotion. Also, using new technologies like genomic medicine and wastewater epidemiology in public health calls for a solid ethical base. Genomic medicine can significantly improve diagnostics and treatments, but it also raises issues about privacy, giving consent, and the risk of genetic discrimination. Therefore, creating guidelines that address these ethical issues is crucial for utilising these technologies safely in public health. Similarly, wastewater epidemiology offers powerful insights into disease prevalence and transmission patterns, but ethical considerations, including data collection, privacy protections, and equitable access, must also be addressed to foster public trust and maximise its effectiveness in disease surveillance (Liu, 2024). Community engagement is critical when discussing ethics in public health. When stakeholders take part, it leads to greater transparency and trust, which is very important for public health initiatives that might limit some personal freedoms. If public health authorities include communities in deciding on interventions, they can make sure the interventions are appropriate and ethical. If communities are involved, they are more likely to follow public health advice, which helps control infectious diseases. Hence, prioritizing ethics in public health not only aligns with moral imperatives but also improves overall health outcomes by creating policies that are more likely to be accepted and effective (Chauhan et al., 2025) (Figure 13.2).

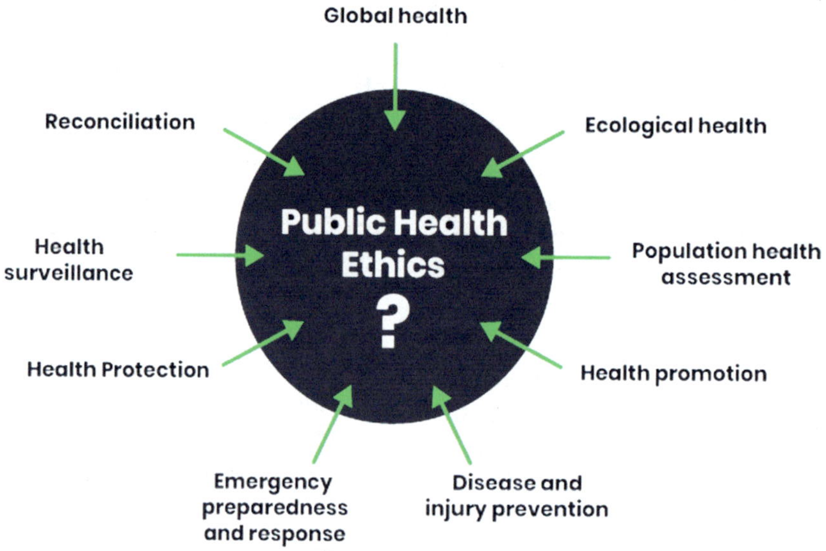

Figure 13.2. Ethics in public health.

Source: https://contensis.uwaterloo.ca/sites/courses/HLTH-602A%20[X]/media/images/ethical-issues.jpg.

Overview of Ethical Dilemmas in the Field

There are often ethical issues in infectious disease epidemiology, primarily related to data collection and patient confidentiality. It is a challenge for epidemiologists to collect detailed information for tracking diseases and, at the same time, respect people's privacy. The pressure increases even further when a public health emergency occurs, as a swift response is required. Because it is essential to trace contacts and learn about how the virus spreads, privacy can sometimes be put at risk, which might lead people in the community to become distrustful. Also, ethical questions about informed consent are fundamental when working with vulnerable groups. While managing outbreaks, researchers must consider the rights of individuals as well as the health of the public, which raises questions about how to utilise surveillance systems without compromising people's privacy. Another significant ethical dilemma arises from the deployment of technological innovations, such as artificial intelligence (AI), in the management of infectious diseases. AI could enhance epidemiology by improving diagnoses and treatments, but it also raises numerous ethical concerns. For example, relying on AI systems can lead to concerns about data and healthcare access disparities. If the data used to train AI does not cover a wide range of groups, there is a chance that marginalized communities will be disproportionately affected. Additionally, as decisions are made by algorithms rather than humans, issues of accountability become increasingly important. The integration of such technology into public health strategies necessitates a stringent ethical framework to ensure that AI serves the common good without perpetuating existing health disparities, highlighting the balance between innovation and ethical responsibility (Sarantopoulos et al., 2024). In addition, handling information systems in emergencies, especially during a pandemic, highlights the complexities of ethical issues in infectious disease epidemiology. The pandemic made it clear that contact tracing and surveillance systems had to deal with both technical issues and concerns about ethics and trust. When creating COVID Safe in Australia, it was necessary to consider issues such as data privacy, the need for swift public health action, and community confidence. The issue in these circumstances is to manage public health actions that are both timely and effective, while still considering privacy and community involvement. For strategies to be effective, people and groups involved should be engaged, and the information shared should be transparent and open. As infectious disease management increasingly navigates ambiguous ethical terrain, the need for robust theories and principles governing these systems becomes essential (Molla et al., 2024).

13.1. Historical Context

The historical context of infectious disease epidemiology is replete with ethical dilemmas that have shaped contemporary practices. There have been numerous moral issues surrounding the collection and study of patient data throughout history. The cholera outbreaks in the 19th century highlighted a conflict between the public's best interests and individual desires. While researchers like John Snow worked on mapping diseases, they had to contend with ethical issues regarding obtaining consent and the potential impact of their findings on individuals at risk. Because of these early examples, medical research and public health now prioritise obtaining informed consent and respecting individuals as they work to address the community's health. With the start of the 20th century, the emergence of more complex infectious diseases and the rise of global health initiatives made it increasingly challenging to address ethical issues in epidemiology. HIV/AIDS and similar epidemics made it clear that public health goals should always be balanced with human rights. Experiences of marginalized groups helped to influence the public's view of infectious diseases and led to a review of ethical guidelines. Various groups began to encourage the inclusion of people affected by health issues in decision-making, leading to more active participation in health interventions. This shift reflects a growing acknowledgment that ethical considerations must include the perspectives and rights of those directly impacted by infectious diseases (Bhimraj et al., 2020). Currently, epidemiologists and public health officials still rely on the lessons learned from previous ethical issues. Recognising the past reminds us that while data and statistics play a significant role in fighting infectious diseases, we must not forget to consider the ethical problems. As technology and data collection continue to advance rapidly, it is now more crucial than ever to discuss privacy, consent, and the fair use of data. In recent talks about the COVID-19 pandemic, it is clear that epidemiologists must pay close attention to how urgency in public health decisions interacts with ethics. All in all, being aware of these events enhances our understanding of today's ethical principles in infectious disease epidemiology and public health.

13.1.1. Notable Case Studies in Infectious Disease Outbreaks

Analysing significant cases of infectious disease outbreaks teaches us about the ethical issues that are part of epidemiology. A clear example is the Ebola virus outbreak in West Africa, which highlights the importance of public health efforts being transparent, involving informed consent, and engaging communities. The outbreak made it clear that there were insufficient plans for handling outbreaks, and this was most noticeable in how affected individuals were treated and how resources were allocated. Choosing who to treat and deciding on experimental therapies caused healthcare workers to apply their ethical frameworks. In current studies, ML techniques have demonstrated their ability to analyse large amounts of data, aiding in the prediction and control of outbreaks. This technological evolution not only improved understanding of disease dynamics but also raised questions regarding data privacy and the ethical implications of surveillance in predictive modelling (Senthil et al., 2023). The HIV/AIDS epidemic is another critical case, mainly because of its effects on sub-Saharan Africa. Ethical issues regarding getting treatment, educational resources, and health information have been very important and vital. It was clear that customized public health messages were needed because misconceptions and stigma often made it hard to help local communities. For instance, search data revealed significant gaps in the public's understanding of HIV-related content, highlighting the importance of addressing audience-specific health information needs (Abebe et al., 2019). This highlights the importance of providing equal access to accurate health information and resources. When trying to stop infectious diseases, it is important to involve the community and be sensitive to cultural differences during the design of health interventions. The 2015–2016 ZIKV outbreak contributed to the ethical challenges encountered in infectious disease epidemiology. Many ethical issues arose because of the quick spread of Zika, mainly about reproductive rights and how to handle public health responses for pregnant women. It was not easy to decide on urgent public health steps when personal freedom and knowledge of risks are involved. The use of genetic modification on mosquitoes to stop Zika led to concerns about what might happen to the environment and to people. As researchers utilise ML to enhance outbreak predictions, the need for ethical guidelines becomes increasingly apparent, ensuring that innovations in disease control are responsibly implemented without infringing on individual rights or autonomy (Senthil et al., 2023). All these case studies highlight the need to incorporate ethics into policy and epidemiology to prevent infectious disease outbreaks.

13.1.2. Evolution of Ethical Standards in Epidemiology

The ethical standards in epidemiology have undergone a significant evolution, particularly influenced by the historical context of public health crises. Initially, epidemiology primarily focused on collecting information rather than protecting the rights and well-being of individuals. Due to this approach, researchers sometimes compromised the dignity and autonomy of those involved. As people began to pay more attention to human rights and ethical research, the field started to follow principles of respect for persons, beneficence, and justice. The change is most noticeable in the creation of ethical rules for handling data, ensuring that studies are designed with the well-being of participants as the primary concern. As the scope of epidemiological research expands, these principles continue to evolve to address emerging ethical dilemmas, particularly in the age of big data and genetic research, where the potential for misuse of personal information has heightened privacy concerns and informed consent (Uffelmann et al., 2021). Furthermore, global events, such as pandemics, have a significant impact on the development of ethics in medicine. The COVID-19 pandemic has prompted people to reassess the balance between individual freedom and the greater good of the community. When a crisis occurs, it may become necessary to collect epidemiological data quickly, which can clash with the usual ethical standards on consent and privacy. The discussions around wastewater surveillance (WWS) during the pandemic exemplify this tension. While wastewater analysis has become a critical tool for tracking the spread of SARS-CoV-2, it raises complex ethical questions about surveillance and the potential stigmatisation of communities (Kitajima et al., 2020). The experience of this crisis will guide future ethics in epidemiology, encouraging practitioners to be transparent and ensure all people have fair access to health information. It is essential to see that collaboration between different fields helps improve the guidelines for ethical practice in epidemiology. Bringing bioethics, law, and social sciences into epidemiology has helped people see the ethical side of research more clearly. For example, considering the ethical issues associated with genomic research and the potential for genetic discrimination, the field now adopts a broader approach to managing risks and protecting participants. This way of working improves the quality of epidemiological research and helps create trust between researchers and the public. Additionally, as epidemiology continues to advance through technology, it is essential to continue discussing these issues with ethicists, public health officials, and the affected communities. This collaborative effort ensures that ethical standards remain responsive to the changing landscape of public health challenges and the evolving expectations of society (Uffelmann et al., 2021) (Figure 13.3).

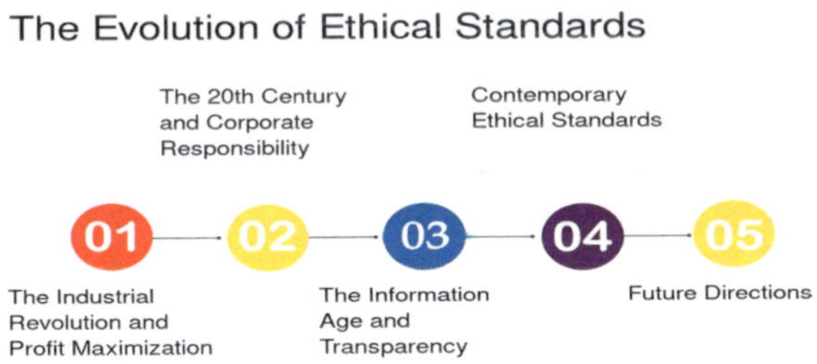

Figure 13.3. The ethical standards in epidemiology.

Source: https://fastercapital.co/i/Business-education-and-training--The-Role-of-Ethics-in-Business-Education--The-Evolution-of-Ethical-Standards.webp.

13.1.3. Impact of Historical Events on Current Practices

The ramifications of historical events significantly influence current practices in infectious disease epidemiology, particularly in the realm of ethical considerations. For example, dealing with past pandemics has shaped the way public health responds and the ethical standards it adheres to today. Because of the HIV/AIDS crisis in the 1980s, public health efforts put more emphasis on informed consent, privacy, and proper use of data to avoid further discrimination against marginalized groups. They point out that ethical guidelines should be updated to fit different cultures when dealing with EIDs. The ethical principles derived from past events ensure that current epidemiology prioritises fairness, justice, and respect for all individuals affected by infectious diseases. Due to events such as the Tuskegee Syphilis Study, the ethics of infectious disease epidemiology have undergone significant updates. To address these major violations, regulatory groups and ethics committees have been established to ensure that participants in clinical trials are appropriately treated. The establishment of Institutional Review Boards (IRBs) following the Tuskegee study reflects a growing commitment to safeguarding participant welfare and fostering trust between researchers and communities. This new way of thinking emphasises transparency and accountability, which enables modern practices to become more inclusive and ethical. By looking back at history, epidemiology now focuses on restoring trust and ensuring that research and practice are ethical. Furthermore, the COVID-19 pandemic demonstrates that our previous experiences influence how we approach EIDs and the ethical choices we make in epidemiology. The rapid update of treatment guidelines by the Infectious Diseases Society of America and others during the COVID-19 pandemic is based on lessons learned from past health crises. Evidence-based recommendations drawn from reviews of both peer-reviewed and gray literature reflect a dedication to honesty and fast decision-making.

The history of treatment reveals a persistent conflict between what is necessary for public health and what is required to ensure patient safety. Therefore, what we learn from history helps improve our current ethics, encouraging a more responsible and attentive approach to infectious disease epidemiology in the face of worldwide health issues.

13.2. Informed Consent

Informed consent remains a cornerstone of ethical medical practice, particularly in the realm of infectious disease epidemiology. It means that individuals are provided with all the necessary information about the risks, benefits, and consequences of participating in research or public health activities. It is essential to communicate clearly in epidemiology, particularly during outbreaks of disease. They should ensure that people without scientific training can understand how the disease spreads, what the interventions might cause, and how public health strategies are designed. If informed consent is not obtained, it can lead to ethical problems and erode trust between the public and health authorities, which is particularly crucial during public health crises such as COVID-19. Besides simply obtaining permission, informed consent has ethical implications that extend beyond it. In infectious disease research, especially studies utilising genetic data such as genome-wide association studies (GWAS), the potential for misuse of participants' data increases dramatically. Participants must be made aware not only of how their data will be utilised but also of the potential future applications that could arise from it (Uffelmann et al., 2021). Due to this complexity, a robust framework must address how researchers ensure confidentiality, the purpose of data collection, and how they will share the data. For these processes to be responsible, they must be based on clear rules, proper oversight, and openness. The of informed consent is even more complex due to cultural differences among people. If people have different levels of health literacy, it can significantly impact their ability to comprehend health information, raising concerns about equality in health research and care. For instance, a study conducted in Bangladesh during the early stages of the COVID-19 pandemic revealed notable variations in knowledge, attitudes, and practices among different demographic groups, which affected their responses to public health measures (Ferdous et al., 2020). This highlights the need to adapt our approach to seeking consent to accommodate varying educational and cultural levels. Ensuring that informed consent procedures are culturally competent and accessible is crucial for ethical compliance and to enhance participant engagement in research efforts aimed at controlling infectious diseases (Figure 13.4).

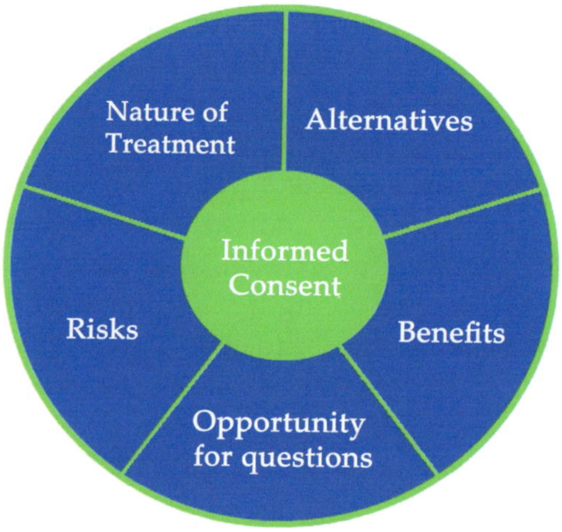

Figure 13.4. Informed consent remains a cornerstone of ethical medical practice.

Source: https://understandingmyositis.org/wp-content/uploads/2016/09/informed-consent-1.jpg.

13.2.1. Importance of Obtaining Informed Consent from Participants

In the realm of infectious disease epidemiology, obtaining informed consent from participants is not merely a regulatory requirement; it is a fundamental ethical obligation aimed at upholding the autonomy and dignity of individuals. To obtain informed consent, researchers must ensure that potential participants understand what the study is about, why it is being conducted, its potential risks and benefits, and make a voluntary decision about whether to participate. This approach fosters trust with participants, making them feel valued and respected throughout the research process. Also, the fact that women and pregnant people have been traditionally overlooked in research shows how essential it is to include everyone in research. As noted in King et al. (2024), the exclusion of these demographics has resulted in insufficient data regarding their health outcomes and treatment responses, emphasising that comprehensive informed consent processes are vital for equitable participant involvement and relevant research outcomes. Besides allowing someone to participate in a study, informed consent also reflects the ethical principle of respect for individuals, which is essential in research settings. Individuals participating in studies should be aware that their involvement could contribute to the production of crucial results that may influence public health policies and practices, particularly for infectious diseases. When people do not give informed consent, there is a danger of coercion or control which harms the research process. As highlighted in Mo et al. (2024), ethical nursing competence plays a moderating role in the intention to care for patients with infectious diseases, indicating that ethical frameworks must guide practitioners. Due to these frameworks, healthcare professionals are reminded to prioritise participants' knowledge and willingness to participate as key aspects of ethical research and practice. The process of informed consent must keep changing to address the new problems and challenges in current research on infectious diseases. They must educate participants about the short-term effects of their studies, as well as the broader societal implications. This is most important in EID studies, as the need to collect information quickly can sometimes make ethics less critical. Making communication clear and open, and consistently engaging with participants, can reduce worries and misunderstandings about joining the group. Further emphasizing the need for inclusivity, the importance of obtaining informed consent from historically marginalized populations cannot be overstated, as failure to do so has perpetuated gaps in knowledge and ultimately compromised public health outcomes, as indicated by King et al. (2024). As the science of infectious disease epidemiology progresses, we must also keep informed consent as a main ethical principle in our research.

13.2.2. Challenges in Obtaining Consent During Outbreaks

The process of obtaining informed consent during infectious disease outbreaks presents a significant ethical challenge for epidemiologists and healthcare professionals. When situations change quickly, such as during pandemics, it can be challenging to follow the usual consent process because action is required promptly. Due to stress and other factors, individuals may not be able to fully comprehend their decisions in a crisis, which could raise ethical concerns regarding autonomy and informed consent. Trying to achieve fast results can make researchers resort to forceful methods, which may prevent participants from choosing their own treatment options. This raises profound ethical questions about the balance between public health interests and individual rights, necessitating that health authorities are especially vigilant in adhering to ethical standards while navigating the complexities of consent amid outbreaks (Houri et al., 2023). Besides the sense of urgency in epidemics, the fact that some people have less health knowledge makes it harder to get consent. The extent to which people understand the possible risks, advantages, and unknowns of participating in research or using preventive measures depends on their education and past experiences with healthcare. Therefore, people from marginalised groups might have more challenges with informed consent, including differences in language or a lack of trust. If these disparities are not resolved, people may not get equal access to research and treatment, which could also violate ethical principles of justice and beneficence. Therefore, it becomes imperative to develop tailored communication strategies that can effectively address the diverse needs of different communities during outbreaks, ensuring that consent is not just a formality, but a genuine invitation to engage in informed participation (El-Hebsh, 2018). Also, when an outbreak happens, it is necessary to mobilise resources and people quickly, which can result in less attention to established rules for informed consent.

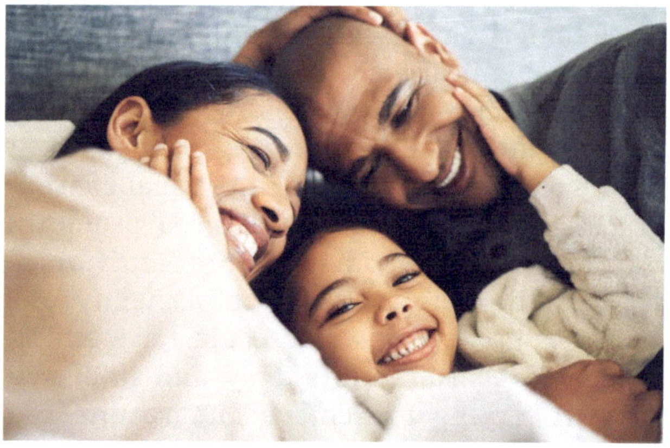

Figure 13.5. Challenges in obtaining consent during outbreaks.

Source: https://www.researchgate.net/profile/A-Preda/publication/267102112/figure/fig1/AS:295670394179584@1447504723015/Layout-of-the-analyzed-informed-consent-process-doi101371-journalpone0110139g001.png.

Because staff focus on immediate care, they may not have enough time to thoroughly discuss consent with the patient, making it hard for them to understand or ask questions. It is also a challenge to get consent from unconscious individuals, who cannot make decisions, or are too ill to give legal consent. Therefore, surrogate decision-makers may be necessary, which can complicate the process and lead to disagreements about the patient's true wishes. Thus, creating robust frameworks that can adapt to these urgent and unpredictable scenarios while safeguarding ethical integrity remains a critical challenge amidst the ongoing evolution of infectious disease epidemiology (Houri et al., 2023) (Figure 13.5).

13.2.3. Ethical Implications of Consent Violations

The ethical implications of consent violations in infectious disease epidemiology pose a profound challenge, raising significant moral concerns within the medical and research communities. People whose consent is not sought for study or treatment have their autonomy and rights seriously affected. It is most noticeable when people who are detained in compulsory treatment centers are part of the situation. Research has shown that these facilities often lack necessary ethical oversight, with many studies failing to adequately report on participant consent processes or the ethics approval required for research involving human subjects (Barhoush et al., 2025). When there is no consent, it weakens healthcare, and it can also lead to people being exploited and harmed, which adds to the moral duties of researchers and healthcare professionals. Besides, while trying to understand and control infectious disease outbreaks, it is essential always to follow ethical research guidelines. Informed consent helps protect the rights of individuals and ensures the accuracy of research results. As evidenced by recent investigations, a significant number of studies conducted in distressing environments, like drug detention centres, neglected to report on consent, raising alarms about the ethics of such research (Barhoush et al., 2025). When people are forced to participate, their answers may be inaccurate, and they might not disclose the truth about their health. As a result, research misconduct can lead to incorrect conclusions that exacerbate health problems instead of helping to solve them. It is also essential to strengthen ethical standards in the process of obtaining consent, especially for healthcare workers interacting with patients who have infectious diseases.

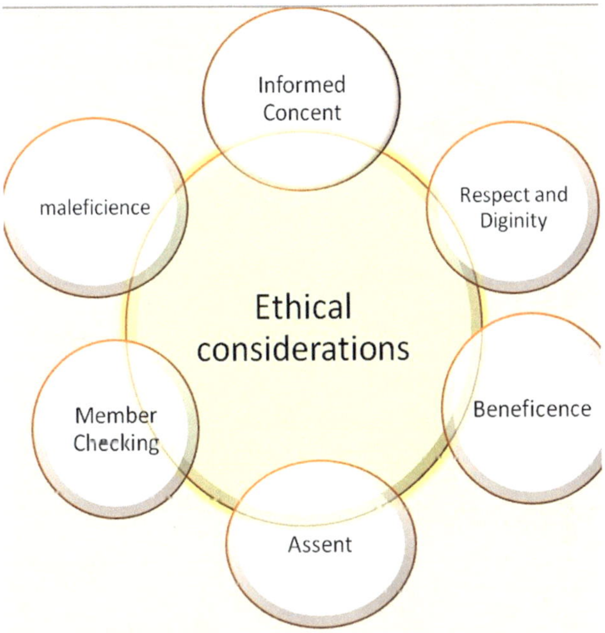

Figure 13.6. The ethical implications of consent violations in infectious disease epidemiology.

Source: https://www.researchgate.net/profile/Rose-Mugweni-2/publication/338435600/figure/fig1/AS:844821346394112@1578432513441/Ethical-considerations-Source-Designed-by-Authors_Q640.jpg.

The theory of planned behavior, which examines the intentions of nurses in treating patients with infectious diseases, points out that ethics play a key role in nursing. Being ethically competent helps nurses both understand the results of their actions and defend the rights of their patients. Encouraging ethical nursing education and training will help the healthcare system develop staff who value informed consent, which can result in better patient results and more trust among the community. This shift toward an ethics-centered approach in infectious disease epidemiology not only protects individual rights but also bolsters the overall efficacy of public health interventions (Figure 13.6).

13.3. Privacy and Confidentiality

In the realm of infectious disease epidemiology, the protection of privacy and confidentiality stands as a paramount ethical concern. Researchers and public health officials may need to collect sensitive information about people to monitor disease outbreaks and implement appropriate public health measures. This calls for finding a balance between getting the data and respecting the privacy of individuals. Improper handling of personal health records can result in stigma, discrimination, or legal consequences for people with infectious diseases. In this way, securing data and maintaining confidentiality is necessary both for legal reasons and to earn the trust of people needed for epidemiological surveillance to succeed. The integration of technology in epidemiological practices, particularly through artificial intelligence (AI) and data analytics, raises additional challenges regarding privacy and confidentiality. Researchers at the National Institute on Aging have found that more attention is being given to using technology ethically to safeguard older adults with long-term health problems. Anyone applying for a pilot grant in these programs had to explain how they would protect the privacy and confidentiality of participants' information, which reflected their knowledge of ethical issues in health research. It is essential to have these measures in place because people are more willing to participate in studies if they believe their personal data will be kept safe. By embedding privacy considerations into the research design, epidemiologists can enhance the integrity of their studies while also advancing broader health equity goals (Largent et al., 2025). Privacy concerns also have consequences for the whole public health system, not just for each participant. Modern public health management utilises data-driven technology to forecast outbreaks and make informed decisions about resource allocation. Yet, ensuring AI is used ethically involves addressing any privacy concerns or potential data breaches. Studies on AI in predicting infections emphasise that strong data governance should always incorporate ethical considerations, including consent, transparency, and accountability. Also, it is essential for systems to work together and for data to be standardized to protect privacy and respond well to health challenges. Thus, striking a balance between technological innovation and ethical responsibility remains a critical focus as public health organizations strive for improved response capabilities (Omale et al., 2025) (Figure 13.7).

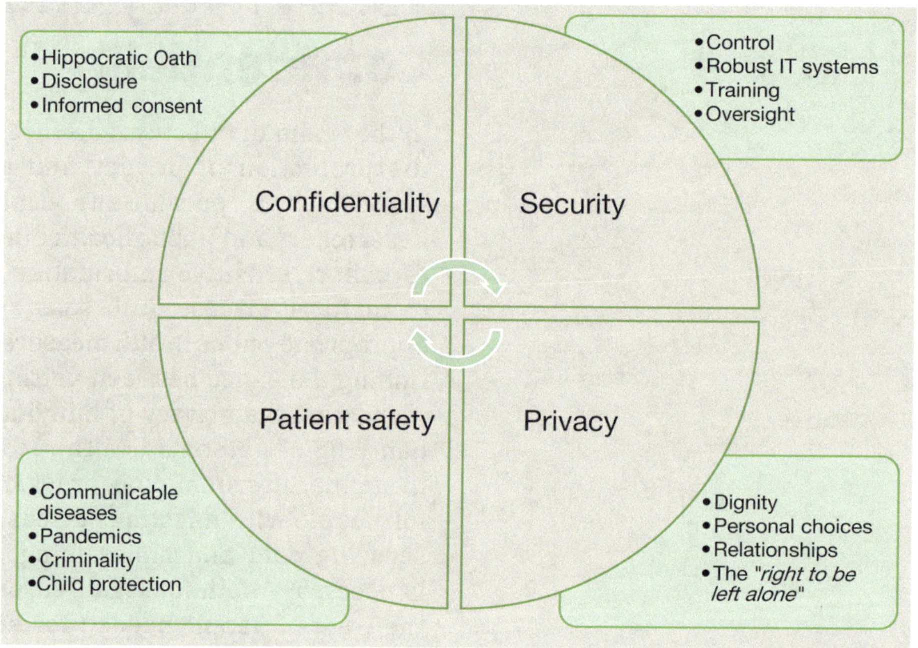

Figure 13.7. Privacy and confidentiality.

Source: https://www.anaesthesiajournal.co.uk/cms/attachment/beccf140-cd5e-4211-a416-30a7194aaf56/gr1_lrg.jpg.

13.3.1. Importance of Protecting Patient Data

In the realm of infectious disease epidemiology, protecting patient data is paramount, given the sensitivity and personal nature of health information. Because more health records are now digital, the possibility of unauthorised access and breaches has increased significantly. Ethics in public health requires officials and researchers to maintain patient confidentiality and ensure that research and public health activities are transparent and justified. Therefore, we must work with data to improve society while ensuring that individuals' rights and privacy are respected. If patient data is not protected, individuals can be harmed, and trust in health systems can be lost, which makes it harder to respond quickly and correctly to infectious disease outbreaks like COVID-19. Looking after patient data is not only about complying with the law; it also involves ensuring that patients are treated with respect and have control over their personal information. Public health officials must handle the balance between protecting people's health and their privacy sensitively. Ethics to hide or remove personal details from sensitive data whenever possible, thereby protecting individuals while ensuring confidentiality. However, the analysis and reporting can still take place. Also, obtaining informed consent for how data is collected and used increases ethical responsibility. Researchers and epidemiologists should be equipped with the knowledge and tools to communicate effectively with patients about their data, fostering a culture of transparency and trust that is essential for public health (Somekh et al., 2020). If data protection fails, it can cause serious problems, especially in the context of public health measures for infectious diseases. A lack of trust in data security may cause patients to conceal important health details, making it challenging to track and treat diseases effectively. Also, when people feel that health information is not shared openly, it can lead to more misinformation. For this reason, being responsible with patient data is crucial for earning the trust of the community, which is vital for public health to work well. Strong data protection helps protect both individuals and society as a whole by enabling informed decisions based on accurate disease data, which supports better management of infectious diseases.

13.3.2. Risks Associated with Data Breaches in Epidemiological Studies

Epidemiological studies are essential for understanding the dynamics of infectious diseases and informing public health interventions. At the same time, depending more on digital data increases the risk of data breaches for these studies. If private health details are exposed, it can erode the trust between researchers and participants, potentially deterring people from participating in research. Additionally, when data is stolen, it may lead to identity theft or discrimination for the affected individuals, which raises ethical questions about the importance of being informed and safeguarding personal information. Strictly protecting the privacy of people in epidemiological research is crucial, as any breach could compromise the quality of the data and reduce the effectiveness of public health actions against infectious diseases. Therefore, researchers must take strong measures to safeguard all data. Data breaches in epidemiological studies can pose problems for both the public and individuals. When data is leaked, it can lead to people sharing false information and feeling panicked, mainly during a disease outbreak. Resource allocation, vaccination plans, and public health messages are guided by the accurate data that epidemiologists and public health officials have. A mistake in data reporting can lead to incorrect policy decisions, potentially resulting in the spread of more infectious diseases and reduced trust in health advisories. As technology advances rapidly, researchers must remain cautious about cybersecurity, incorporate ethical considerations into their research, and balance scientific accuracy with public security. Due to the numerous dangers associated with data breaches in epidemiology, experts recommend employing robust data governance frameworks that prioritise ethics. Applying Differential Privacy and secure custody of data chains is necessary to protect health information and still allow research on the data. They work to reduce the risk of data misuse and re-identification, which helps make individuals feel secure about sharing their health information. In addition, having regulations ensures that those who handle sensitive data are held responsible by the authorities. When stakeholders promote openness and ethical ways of handling data, epidemiological studies can supply reliable information for public health without invading people's privacy. Ultimately, a proactive approach to data governance in the context of infectious disease epidemiology serves to enhance the ethical landscape of research while safeguarding public trust and participant welfare (Figure 13.8).

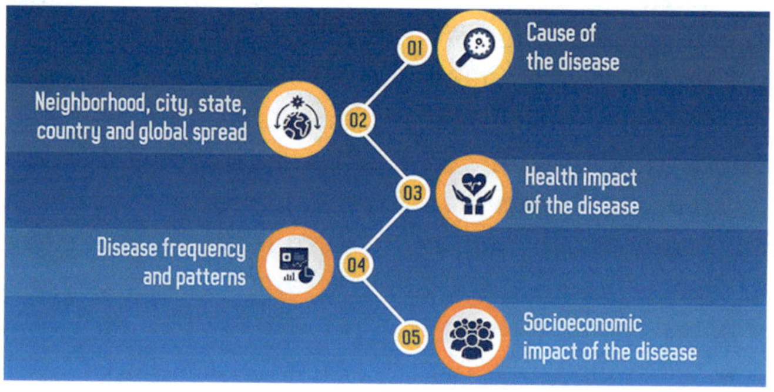

Figure 13.8. Risks associated with data breaches in epidemiological studies.

Source: https://s3.amazonaws.com/utep-uploads/wp-content/uploads/unr/2020/11/16165705/UNR-MPH-Q2-2020_Epidemiology-vs.-Biostatistics-IG01.jpg.

13.3.3. Balancing Public Health Needs with Individual Privacy Rights

The intersection of public health needs and individual privacy rights presents a complex ethical landscape in the context of infectious disease epidemiology. Public health officials employ data collection techniques that can sometimes compromise people's privacy as they attempt to control diseases. During public health emergencies, rapid data collection is crucial for managing the spread of diseases. However, when utilising these technologies, we must always consider how they may impact individuals' privacy. For instance, employing wastewater epidemiology enhances disease surveillance, revealing patterns of transmission while raising questions regarding the ethical handling of collected data (Liu, 2024). Therefore, it is essential to strike a balance between public health actions and respect for privacy to maintain public trust and ensure that health measures are followed. Additionally, AI and other emerging technologies are exacerbating the challenges of balancing public health and individual privacy rights. AI is data, which is beneficial for identifying infectious diseases early and improving health interventions. Even so, the use of government-held databases can lead to serious ethical concerns regarding the monitoring of people's information and the risk of its misuse. Studies suggest that while AI-powered phenotyping holds transformative potential for public health, it also necessitates stringent ethical and legal frameworks to safeguard individual privacy (Páč et al., 2024). If there are no strong safeguards, the government could gain more power and use this to increase its surveillance, which could threaten personal freedom. So, it is crucial to deal with these ethical issues by being transparent and accountable in managing data. Ultimately, ensuring that public health and privacy rights are balanced requires multiple strategies. Involving ethicists, public health officials, and the affected communities is necessary to ensure that both public welfare and personal privacy are considered in policies. There should be laws in place to outline how data can be used, ensuring that individual rights are still protected in times of crisis. Additionally, it is crucial to provide clear explanations of how data is collected, utilised, and safeguarded. This transparency helps build trust and encourages public participation in health initiatives. When ethics are prioritised in handling and using data, the public health system can improve its responses and still uphold the privacy of individuals. Following this method is necessary to ensure that ethical topics in infectious disease epidemiology are handled effectively.

13.4. Equity and Justice

The principles of equity and justice in the context of infectious disease epidemiology highlight the imperative to address systemic health disparities while ensuring fair treatment for all populations. As infectious diseases do not discriminate by socioeconomic status (SES) or demographic characteristics, the response to outbreaks must prioritise vulnerable groups who often bear a disproportionate burden of disease. Some of these groups are low-income communities, racial and ethnic minorities, and marginalised genders, who have additional difficulties getting good healthcare. It is essential to recognise these inequities to ensure that public health strategies address and overcome systemic disparities. Equity should be a key part of epidemiology from the beginning, not just added on later, to make a real difference and create an inclusive environment in health care. Additionally, the use of AI in public health may either exacerbate or mitigate the existing inequalities present in healthcare systems. Although AI aids in diagnosis and resource management, the ethical issue of fairness in algorithms should not be overlooked. Data quality and bias problems can significantly impact fair healthcare, as ML systems may inadvertently perpetuate biases against underrepresented groups. Responsible use of AI means we should focus on development that benefits people who are marginalised. The incorporation of diverse perspectives from affected communities, healthcare practitioners, and policymakers is crucial to ensure that AI solutions contribute to reducing health disparities rather than exacerbating them, especially in resource-limited settings where needs are greatest (Ibiam et al., 2025). In the realm of public health data, the use of claims-based algorithms to identify transgender and gender-diverse (TGD) populations presents both opportunities and ethical challenges. Since there is not much accurate health data about TGD individuals, it becomes necessary to use new methods in epidemiology, but using algorithms to assign gender identity to coded diseases can cause unfair treatment of TGD people. Such algorithms can perpetuate CIS beliefs and not recognise people's self-identification, which can silence TGD voices in health matters. It is essential to understand these aspects to design ethical research that values and supports TGD communities. To advance equity in research, stakeholders must engage TGD individuals directly and establish guidelines that minimise harms while maximising benefits, promoting a more just healthcare environment where all individuals receive the attention and care they deserve (Alpert et al., 2024).

13.4.1. Disparities in Disease Impact Among Different Populations

Disparities in disease impact among different populations can primarily be attributed to a confluence of socioeconomic factors, healthcare access, and systemic inequalities. People living in poverty are more likely to get infectious diseases since they do not have enough access to healthcare and preventive care. Because of this healthcare gap, communities that are already disadvantaged suffer more from disease outbreaks, since they lack the resources to fight illness. To address these differences, it is essential to understand how social factors influence the spread of diseases and impact people's health. It is essential to understand these factors to create interventions that handle urgent health issues and also help improve the system for these communities over time. Social determinants also encompass education, employment, and the living conditions in which people reside, not just access to healthcare. Those who live in poverty are more likely to face crowded homes and poor sanitation, which helps infections spread. Also, past injustices and discrimination can make it more difficult for certain groups to get prompt and suitable medical care. If social variables and the new findings in literature are not considered in epidemiological models, they may not accurately represent the situation faced by the communities. The capacity to integrate these dimensions into public health strategies can enhance our understanding of disease dynamics, contributing to more effective and ethical responses to health crises (Anderson et al., 2015). In addition, addressing health disparities highlights the need for equitable resource distribution across all populations. The COVID-19 pandemic clearly showed that marginalised groups were hit the hardest, so public health responses should focus on them to control the spread of the disease. According to ethical frameworks, public health policies should prioritise justice and equity, enabling vulnerable populations to access the necessary support to overcome health barriers. Involving these communities in health-related decision-making can strengthen them and help them handle future health emergencies. The importance placed on equity in healthcare is not merely a moral imperative but a practical necessity for effective epidemiological outcomes (Figure 13.9).

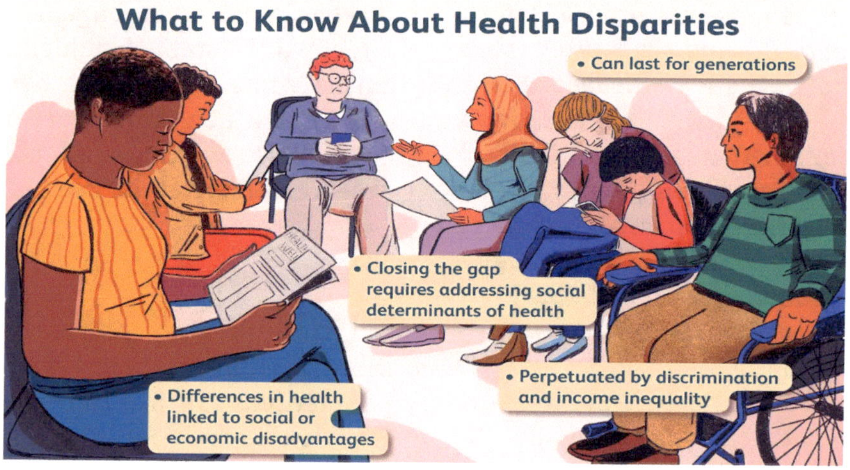

Figure 13.9. Disparities in disease impact among different populations.

Source: https://www.verywellhealth.com/thmb/28zhufSBRwb6RpQo2TPPie9tu8U=/750x0/filters:no_upscale():max_bytes(150000):strip_icc()/health-disparities-4173220_v1-e8914773af574e3d9f02b08d86835de5.jpg.

13.4.2. Ethical Considerations in Resource Allocation

Resource allocation in the context of infectious disease epidemiology presents significant ethical dilemmas that necessitate careful consideration and a balanced approach to multiple factors. Because EIDs need to be addressed quickly, decisions are often made fast, which may result in unequal distribution of resources. For instance, initiatives such as the Southern African Centre for Infectious Disease Surveillance (SACIDS) demonstrate the importance of a One Health approach, which integrates various sectors for effective disease management. Nonetheless, the fact that resources are not shared equally and data is not always available means that equity and justice are not always given importance. Dealing with these issues is essential, since they influence the success of public health efforts and the trust that communities have in health programs, which can change disease outcomes and the health of the population. The ethical allocation of resources is particularly critical when considering interventions such as antiretroviral therapy (ART) for HIV prevention. Although biological efficacy is significant, it is not enough to determine how resources are shared. The most effective way to allocate resources is to integrate epidemiology and economics to assess the overall impact on society. It is widely agreed upon in ART discussions that a multidisciplinary approach is necessary to help decide on resource allocation. When we review case studies, it is clear that ethical considerations, such as fair ART distribution, should prioritise those who are most likely to contract the infection. They can benefit people's health and help protect the community by lowering the number of diseases. Also, it is essential to be open and involve the community when deciding how to use resources in infectious disease epidemiology. Involving those affected in decision-making helps them feel responsible and more likely to follow the intervention, making it more effective. Ethical standards call for communities to be involved in the process of sharing resources, since they can point out what is needed locally and any ethical problems. Thus, policymakers should not make resource allocation decisions independently but should continue to consult stakeholders throughout the process. By establishing inclusive mechanisms that consider diverse viewpoints, public health strategies can align more closely with ethical principles, ultimately leading to more equitable and effective responses to infectious diseases (Figure 13.10).

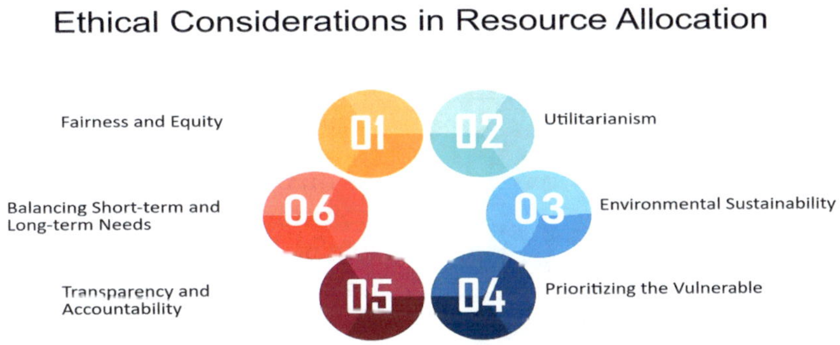

Figure 13.10. Resource allocation in the context of infectious disease epidemiology.

Source: https://fastercapital.co/i/Resource-distribution--Maximizing-Allocation-Rates-for-Optimal-Efficiency--Ethical-Considerations-in-Resource-Allocation.webp.

13.4.3. Strategies to Promote Health Equity in Epidemiology

Health equity in epidemiology is fundamentally about understanding and addressing the intricate interplay of social determinants that affect health outcomes, particularly in the context of infectious diseases. Health equity strategies should start by finding out who the vulnerable populations are, as they are more likely to face health problems due to their SES, location, and experience with discrimination. Examining epidemiological data closely can reveal that infectious diseases disproportionately affect certain groups more than others. Moreover, incorporating community-based participatory research methods can foster collaboration between epidemiologists and marginalised communities, ensuring that research reflects their specific health needs and perspectives (Elendu et al., 2024). This approach makes the research findings more useful, which helps achieve health equity by designing interventions for these groups. Promoting health equity in epidemiology also relies on the effective use of health communication strategies. When people lack sufficient health literacy, it can prevent marginalized groups from accessing essential health information and services. Using cultural messages in health communication helps bridge this gap and enables communities to make informed health choices. Utilising a mixed-methods approach that combines traditional media with innovative digital platforms can enhance outreach and engagement (Igwe et al., 2024). It is crucial to bring together health professionals, policymakers, and community leaders to ensure that communication strategies are effective for a wide range of people. Such partnerships facilitate a back-and-forth exchange, enabling the quick sharing of information and the gathering of community input for future health actions. Ethical issues related to resource allocation are significant for improving health equity in epidemiology.

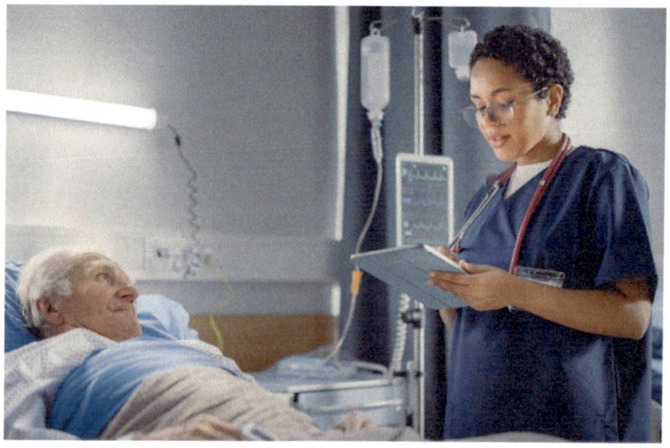

Figure 13.11. Health equity in epidemiology.

Source: https://med.nyu.edu/departments-institutes/population-health/divisions-sections-centers/health-behavior/sites/default/files/health-equity-integrative-framework-graphic.jpg.

Policies aimed at the equal distribution of resources must be created by public health officials when infectious diseases spread. Focusing on helping people in poorer regions and those who are at higher risk can reduce health inequalities. Being open about decisions on public health funding and resource allocation helps communities trust those in charge. Engaging stakeholders from diverse backgrounds in these discussions not only promotes accountability but also ensures that the voices of those most affected are heard (Elendu et al., 2024). Ultimately, promoting health equity in epidemiology requires an interdisciplinary approach that integrates effective communication, community engagement, and ethical resource management to create a more just health system for all (Figure 13.11).

13.5. Risk Communication

Effective risk communication is a critical component of infectious disease epidemiology, particularly in the context of public health crises. Authoritative advice and empathy are usually needed to help diverse groups trust the management of communicable diseases. Informing the public about disease risks helps them make informed decisions about vaccination and adopt healthy lifestyle choices. In Brazil, the Unified Health System has faced challenges from misinformation during the COVID-19 pandemic, which has led some groups to deny the seriousness of the disease. By addressing the infodemic and engaging in transparent dialogue, public health officials can help mitigate confusion and enhance public compliance with health advisories, thereby improving overall health outcomes (Júnior et al., 2024). Ethical questions about individual autonomy and rights add to the difficulties in risk communication. When an outbreak occurs, directives intended to keep everyone safe may sometimes conflict with what individuals want to do. For example, in vaccination campaigns, ethical risk communication involves presenting the science while also respecting cultural differences and individual views on risk. A failure to consider these factors can lead to public resistance and ultimately impede vaccination efforts (Freeman,

2018). For this reason, having inclusive and culturally aware approaches to communication encourages people to accept public health measures instead of opposing them. Emerging technologies are also critical in the field of risk communication. Information can be shared and the public can be reached more easily thanks to digital platforms, social media, and mobile applications. At the same time, they create issues because false information can travel faster than accurate news. As evidenced by the Brazilian experience during the COVID-19 pandemic, combating misinformation is essential for building trust and ensuring informed decision-making among the population (Júnior et al., 2024). Consequently, employing a multifaceted approach to risk communication—one that integrates traditional methods with modern technology—can bolster the public's understanding and responsiveness to infectious disease threats, contributing to overall health equity and better public health outcomes (Figure 13.12).

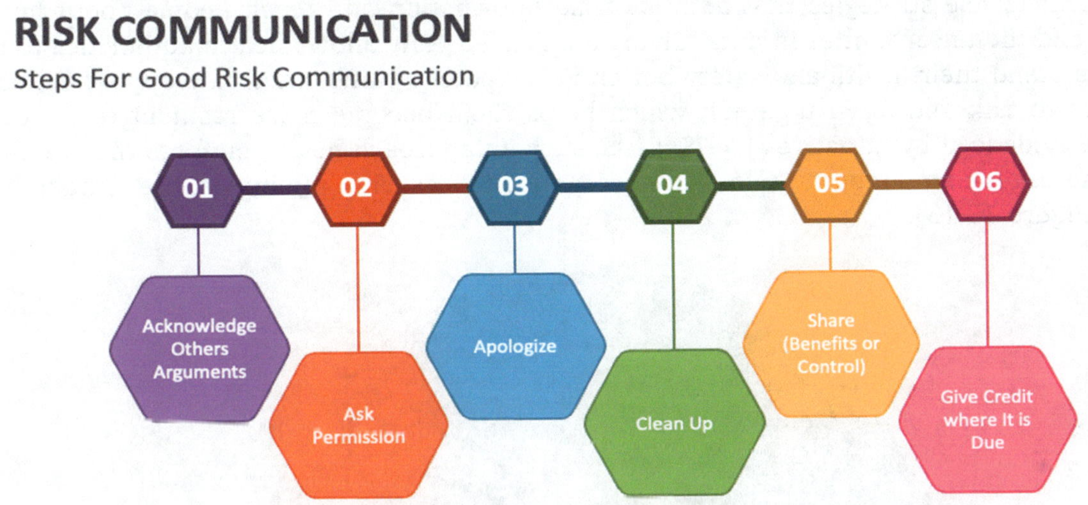

Figure 13.12. Effective risk communication is a critical component of infectious disease epidemiology.

Source: https://www.collidu.com/media/catalog/product/img/4/b/4bbc93af156af1253441023e4546221d156c808b007b3cf6eb894b4d4220f3ba/risk-communication-slide3.png.

13.5.1. Ethical Responsibilities in Communicating Risks to the Public

Effective communication of risks during infectious disease outbreaks is a fundamental ethical responsibility that public health authorities must prioritise. Because infectious diseases are complex, it is important to share information clearly and honestly. If public health officials fail to provide people with clear and complete information about risks, it can lead to reduced trust, increased fear, and the spread of misinformation. It is essential to ensure that all groups can understand information, taking into account literacy and cultural differences, so that vulnerable groups are not left out or left feeling worried. Initiatives like the SACIDS exemplify how integrated approaches can foster a better understanding of risks by engaging multiple sectors and promoting an informed citizenry (Anderson et al., 2018). In addition, maintaining public trust requires officials to share information that is always up to date with the latest scientific knowledge on infectious diseases.

In the framework of ethical communication, the principles outlined in the International Health Regulations (IHR) (2005) further underscore the importance of timely and accurate information dissemination. Such regulations require WHO Member States to undertake specific tasks, particularly during an international public health emergency. Therefore, health communication strategies should adhere to these legal rules to help communities and health systems manage risks effectively. This multifaceted approach, demonstrated at sites such as the Julius Nyerere International Airport, showcases how proper implementation of IHR can benefit from clear communication channels and best practices tailored to various contexts (Bakari et al., 2012). Ultimately, encouraging an ethical approach to risk communication fosters a public that understands the dangers, can protect themselves, and respond appropriately to health emergencies. Ethically, risk communicators should also deal with false information and help people understand when science is uncertain. Because misleading information spreads quickly on social media, health officials have to deal with it. Thus, it is important to use strategies that address false information and teach people about how to judge risks and the uncertainties in data. Giving a balanced view allows health authorities to help people understand their health and safety better. Participatory platforms create opportunities for communities to talk and learn together, which helps them become more resilient to infectious diseases. As evidenced by initiatives like SACIDS, such an approach helps reinforce the credibility of health messages and supports a collective response to ensuring public welfare (Anderson et al., 2018) (Figure 13.13).

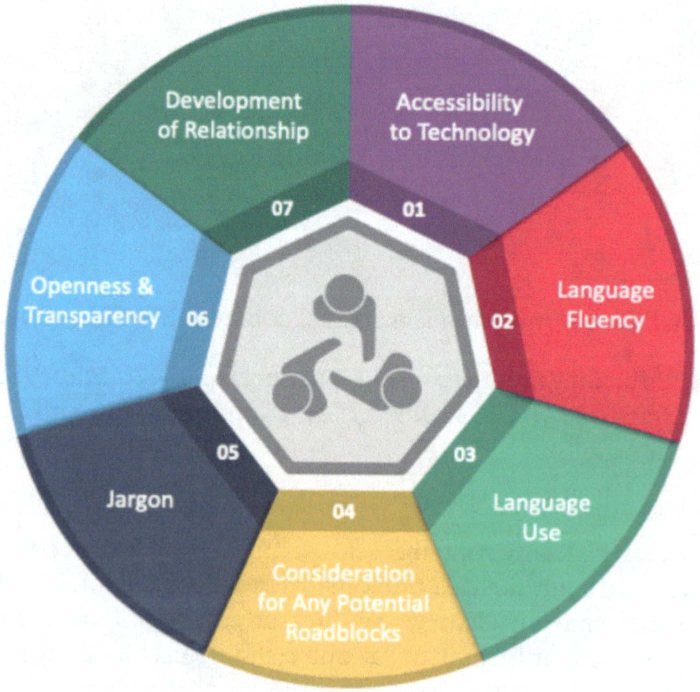

Figure 13.13. Effective communication of risks during infectious public health.

Source: https://cdn.sketchbubble.com/pub/media/catalog/product/optimized1/b/4/b41f067ed82b6b512d7b5527fff1b049b0fafc76a2b137446d26a885dd8ac976/ethical-communication-mc-slide1.png.

13.5.2. Challenges in Conveying Uncertainty and Complexity

Conveying uncertainty and complexity in infectious disease epidemiology presents significant ethical challenges, particularly when communicating risks to the public. The constant changes in contagious diseases often lead to fluctuations in data and knowledge, which can create confusion among health authorities. When people do not receive all the details about risks, they may misunderstand and fail to follow the rules provided by public health. Sometimes, when new variants of a virus emerge, explaining concepts such as how the virus spreads and how well vaccines work can be very challenging. Failing to address uncertainty can lead to people not trusting health officials and becoming confused, which can hinder the effective handling of health crises. In addition, the ethical aspect of public communication during outbreaks emphasises the importance of transparency and maintaining the public's trust. Epidemiologists and public health officials must ensure they do not cause unnecessary fear when providing information to the public. At times, the need to distribute data quickly can prompt people to explain complex concepts in simple terms. If health communication does not accurately represent the details of epidemiological findings, it may inadvertently lead people to doubt or fear the information. For this reason, it is essential to create ways of sharing uncertainty that are responsible. This issue is most severe in places where misinformation spreads quickly, which is why health communicators are crucial in reducing the problems caused by a lack of understanding about how diseases are spread and controlled. Additionally, using different types of data creates logistical and ethical challenges when sharing and interpreting epidemiological results. As highlighted in WWS programs during the COVID-19 pandemic, such as those discussed in Harris-Lovett et al. (2021), complexities arise from varying methodologies, local context, and the capabilities of surveillance systems, which can result in disparate interpretations of data. It is vital to communicate the findings to stakeholders and the public as well as to collect and analyse the data. People may start to doubt more if the reasons behind changing guidelines are not made clear. So, it is significant for researchers, healthcare professionals and communities to work together. When experts collaborate, information can be open, easy to understand and show the many aspects of uncertainty in infectious disease epidemiology.

13.5.3. The Role of Trust in Public Health Messaging

Trust serves as a cornerstone in the effective dissemination of public health messaging, particularly during infectious disease outbreaks, where accurate information is vital for community compliance and engagement. If public health officials and the public have a good relationship, the likelihood of people following health advice, including vaccinations, is significantly higher. If there is trust, individuals tend to listen to advice and follow the protocols meant to stop the spread of disease. If people do not trust, they may doubt the usefulness of health initiatives, which can reduce their success. Because of this, earn trust by being open, actively engaging with the public, and demonstrating accountability. When the community feels respected and informed, public health campaigns are more effective, encouraging everyone to respond to health crises and helping to reduce the impact of infectious diseases. Drawing on cultural and religious ideas, such as those from Islam, can help establish trust in public health messages. Concepts such as taharah (cleanliness) align well with public health objectives by promoting hygiene practices that are crucial in controlling infectious diseases. Using these culturally appropriate messages supports ethical behaviour in epidemiology, as respect for community values is crucial for health promotion. Moreover, involving community health workers (CHWs) and religious leaders can enhance the relatability and credibility of health messages, thus bridging gaps between health authorities and the population. By cooperating, they address false information and support the public's trust in public health actions, which allows for broader outreach. Acting ethically in this way pays attention to the context and helps the community feel involved, which is crucial for the success of public health actions. Because technology enables information to spread quickly, the use of AI-based chatbots for public health messaging raises new issues and challenges for trust. Having these tools means information is available immediately, but their success hinges on whether people trust the technology. A chatbot utilising AI should always prioritise data privacy and ensure accuracy, as a breach could severely damage the trust people have in the company. Therefore, it is crucial to maintain transparency, implement robust data security measures, and regularly evaluate the data utilised in AI applications. For public health messages to be effective today, these factors are very important. By addressing these ethical dilemmas, public health officials can utilize technology not only to enhance access to timely information but also to fortify the public's trust in health messaging efforts, ultimately contributing to better health outcomes during infectious disease outbreaks (Figure 13.14).

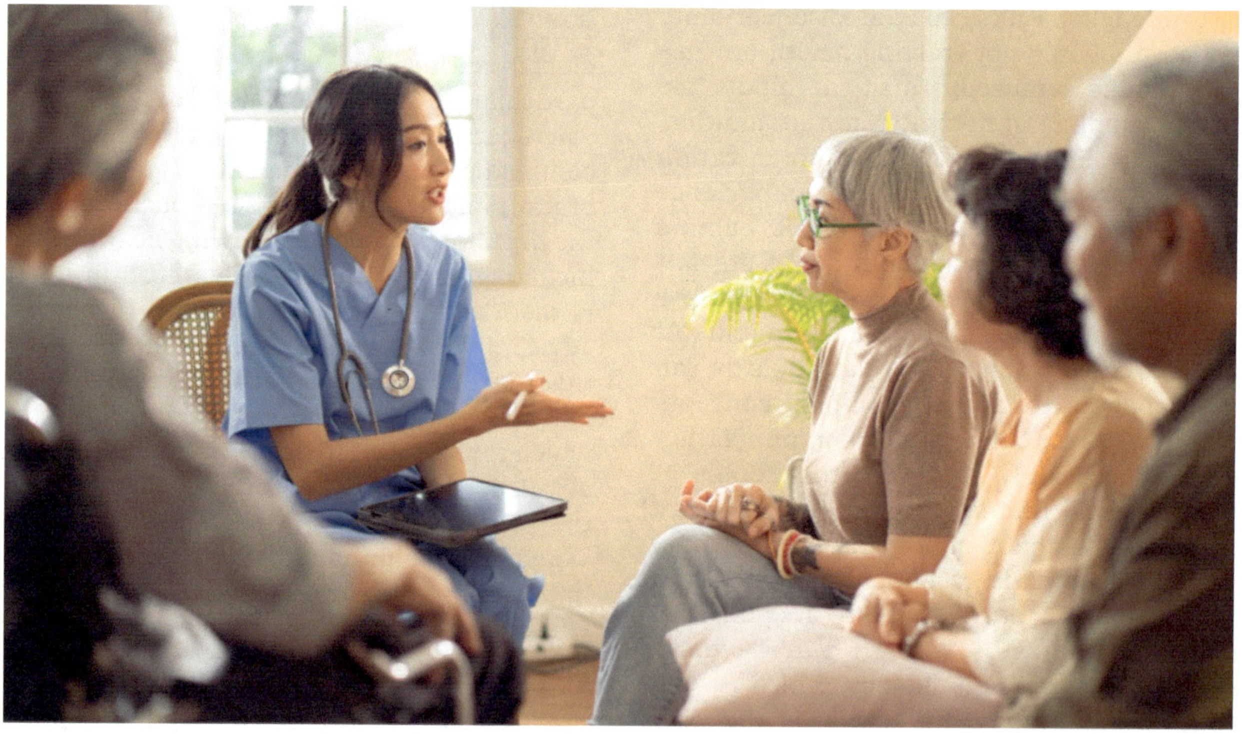

Figure 13.14. The role of trust in public health messaging.

Source: https://nightingale.edu/_resources/images/blog/public-health-rn.jpeg.

13.6. Global Health Considerations

The intersection of global health and infectious disease epidemiology underscores the necessity for a robust ethical framework to address disparities in healthcare access and outcomes. A notable example is Brazil, where the disparity between the rich and the poor has a substantial impact on public health. While the SUS works towards equal access to healthcare, it still faces problems because of an increasing number of elderly people and people with chronic diseases. Solving these problems is essential for the nation's health and also reflects global patterns of unfairness in healthcare. Effective vaccinations and public health strategies, as demonstrated by Brazil's National Immunisation Plan (PNI), underscore the importance of collaborative international efforts in combating infectious diseases and promoting overall health (Júnior et al., 2024). Due to globalisation, health issues are now more complex, demonstrating how closely connected the world is. Because infectious diseases can spread rapidly across the globe, it is clear that countries must cooperate and adhere to ethical principles in addressing them. While surveillance helps stop outbreaks, it also raises issues about privacy and personal freedom. The conflict between public health and individual rights raises significant concerns about how countries are governed and held accountable worldwide. Infectious disease prevention must, therefore, not only focus on scientific advancements but also on creating equitable systems that address the diverse needs of populations worldwide, promoting health as a fundamental human right (Freeman, 2018). Ultimately, encouraging informed decision-making motivates people to participate in and comply with health initiatives. Teaching people about infectious diseases is essential for controlling rumors and boosting community trust in public health measures. Informing people about the benefits of vaccinations and health interventions can lead to improved health outcomes for those who are most vulnerable. Ensuring ethical practices guide every part of health planning and execution, making sure various groups are included and heard. This inclusive approach to public health not only enhances community resilience but also reinforces the collective responsibility to safeguard global health (Freeman, 2018) (Figure 13.15).

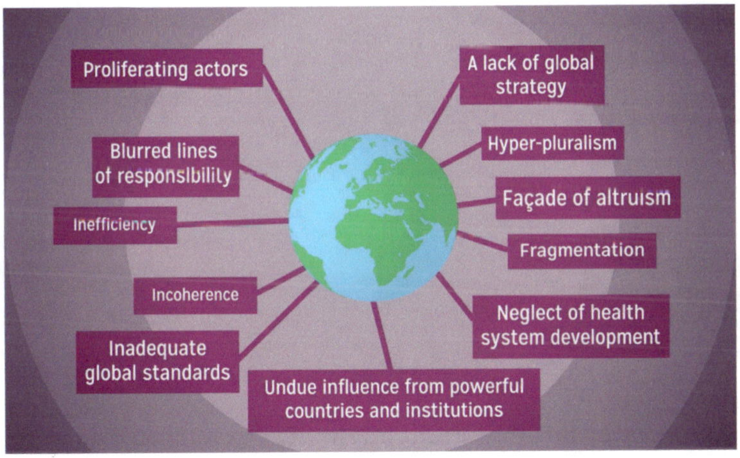

Figure 13.15. Global health considerations.

Source: https://penntoday.upenn.edu/sites/default/files/2021-05/global-health-governance-main.jpg.

13.6.1. Ethical Issues in International Epidemiological Research

The landscape of international epidemiological research is fraught with ethical challenges that require careful navigation to ensure the integrity and safety of both participants and researchers.

In many situations, researchers must address problems related to informed consent, particularly in groups that may not fully understand the implications of their participation. Ethical issues tend to arise when experiments are conducted on patients who have limited other treatment options. It can be challenging for scientists to balance learning new concepts with adhering to ethical guidelines. Furthermore, in instances of high-stakes research during outbreaks, such as EIDs, ethical oversight becomes even more critical, as rapid responses are often required, leading to potential ethical compromises that must be carefully assessed (Sharif et al., 2024). Additionally, being sensitive to cultural differences is crucial in international research ethics. Researchers should interact with local communities to learn about their traditions and values which helps build trust and teamwork. This means going beyond just following ethical rules; it requires companies to genuinely deal with what communities expect from them.

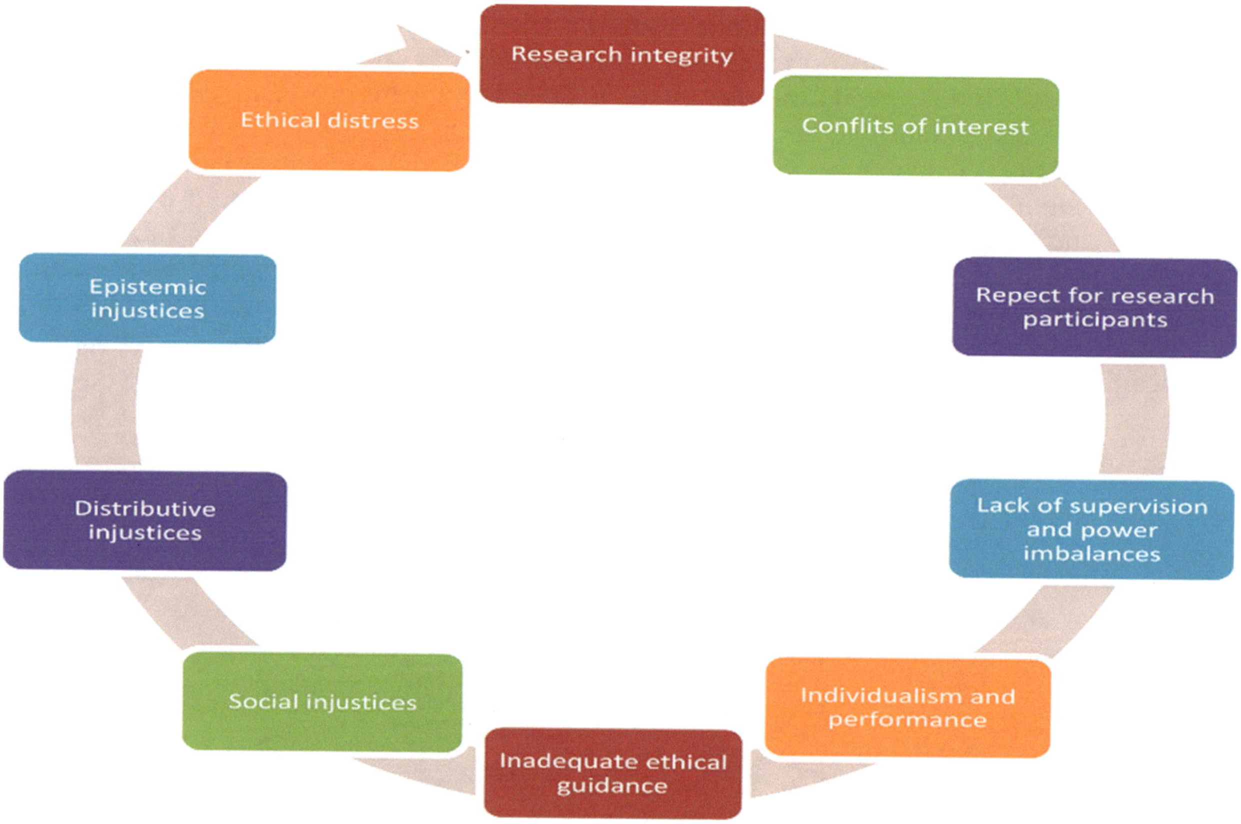

Figure 13.16. Ethical issue international epidemiological research.

Source: https://www.researchgate.net/profile/Bryn-Williams-Jones-2/publication/362663090/figure/fig1/AS:11431281360792825@1744093663492/Ethical-issues-in-research-according-to-the-participants.png.

There are times when the ethical rules from the West do not align with local customs, which can cause problems or confusion. Due to these differences, it is crucial to establish ethical guidelines that cater to the unique needs and values of each community. This necessity becomes increasingly evident during outbreaks when public suspicion may hinder participation, emphasizing the importance of ethical conduct that respects the community's historical and cultural context (Tajudeen et al., 2023). In addition, sharing biological samples and data introduces more ethical issues to international epidemiological research. Issues about ownership of samples and data become essential when they are taken from marginalised groups. Researchers must monitor these communities to ensure they do not relinquish their biological resources without fair compensation. It is vital to practice benefit-sharing, which means local people should have fair access to the benefits of research using their samples or data. Additionally, it is crucial to have rules governing data privacy and security, as data can be easily misused when shared across international borders. As the field of epidemiology continues to evolve, addressing these ethical issues effectively is crucial not only for maintaining the credibility of research but also for fostering goodwill and cooperation between researchers and the communities they serve (Sharif et al., 2024) (Figure 13.16).

13.6.2. Responsibilities Towards Vulnerable Populations

The responsibilities towards vulnerable populations in the context of infectious disease epidemiology are paramount, given the disproportionate burdens that such populations often face during health emergencies. Groups that are at risk, such as people with health problems, low-income or marginalised communities, are commonly not considered in public health interventions that lack equity. Based on recent research, incorporating health equity into epidemic responses can significantly mitigate the adverse effects on these groups. It is not enough to provide medical resources; active involvement, open communication, and teamwork with local leaders are also necessary to create and implement community-specific interventions. Overall, prioritising equity in health response efforts not only addresses immediate health concerns but also strengthens the resilience of affected communities against future public health crises (Cummings et al., 2025). At the same time, the use of advanced technologies such as AI requires us to carefully consider how they may impact vulnerable groups. Since data-based approaches are now used more often in fighting infectious diseases, there is a possibility that AI could unintentionally support discrimination against marginalized groups.

As an illustration, if AI is used, it could strengthen existing inequalities and repeat biases against sexual and gender minorities, which would lead to decisions that miss essential viewpoints. It is critical to monitor AI technologies to avoid contributing to the stigmatisation or discrimination of these populations. By actively engaging with diverse voices during the development of these systems, public health officials can foster an inclusive approach that addresses potential disparities and cultivates algorithmic justice (Racine, 2025). In essence, addressing the needs of vulnerable groups in infectious disease epidemiology requires employing multiple strategies that prioritise inclusion and equitable treatment for all. Working together with those who are affected is essential for creating responses that meet their needs. Given technology's significant role in public health, it is crucial to continually review the use of AI and other data tools in light of their ethical considerations. The link between community engagement and new technologies creates an opportunity to rewrite public health stories, prioritizing those who have been marginalized in the past. Collectively, these efforts represent a commitment to fostering healthier, more resilient populations that are better equipped to navigate the challenges posed by infectious diseases (Cummings et al., 2025; Racine, 2025) (Figure 13.17).

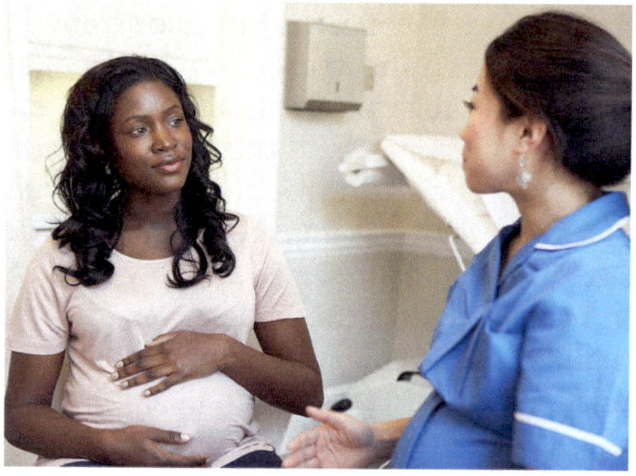

Figure 13.17. Responsibilities towards vulnerable populations.

Source: https://www.eatrightpro.org/-/media/images/eatrightpro-articles/eatrightpro-article-image-804x602/researchvulnerablepopulrations-804x602.jpg?h=602&w=804&hash=1D88CB45064DE4B98373697CDBE3ABDC.

13.6.3. Collaboration Between Countries and Ethical Implications

Working together on infectious disease epidemiology enables countries to employ different strategies that can significantly enhance public health. When countries share resources and experiences, they can establish robust surveillance systems to handle EIDs. As an illustration, the SACIDS is a transnational group that works to unite different health areas and reduce the risk of diseases in its member countries. By working together, these countries demonstrate the importance of nations being responsible and sharing resources and data equally, as unequal access can compromise the effectiveness of their efforts to protect global health. Additionally, fostering open communication and involving all countries in decision-making helps ensure that everyone feels included, thereby addressing potential ethical concerns about unequal participation and contributions in health projects. At the same time, there are ethical problems that need to be considered when countries collaborate globally. Factors such as unequal budgets, differing national priorities, and variations in regulations can hinder countries' ability to cooperate in managing infectious diseases. The evaluation framework developed by the Network for Evaluation of One Health (NEOH) highlights the importance of assessing One Healthiness, which encompasses the interconnectedness of various health disciplines. In many cases, unequal sharing and collaboration exacerbate ethical issues, particularly when richer nations dominate decision-making and resources. When a country has poor infrastructure, it is at a disadvantage in working together to fight diseases. Therefore, crucial for ethical frameworks to prioritize fairness and equity, ensuring that partnerships lead to sustainable and inclusive health improvements in all participating nations, thereby addressing global health inequalities. Besides operations, ethics in collaboration also covers public health policy and community involvement. An example is the effort made by health advocates in Alaska to add meningitis vaccination to school schedules, demonstrating the importance of changing policies through teamwork. The project employed community awareness campaigns to educate the public and promote informed choices about vaccination. While the campaign reached many people, it also highlighted the need for more organized legislation to support health interventions. Any such work should focus on ethical values that support both personal and community health. It is necessary to address ethical issues when collaborating internationally on public health, so that partnerships can last and all countries can gain from the efforts.

SUMMARY

In conclusion, the landscape of infectious disease epidemiology is fraught with ethical challenges that necessitate careful consideration and action. The unequal access to healthcare in Brazil highlights the need to develop public health policies that consider individuals' economic circumstances. How the public views government decisions affects both health behaviours and health policies. In Brazil, misinformation can damage the scientific consensus and create health problems, mainly for marginalised populations. Strategies to counteract these issues must emphasise community engagement and transparent communication to ensure that ethical standards are upheld in the dissemination of health information and intervention strategies (Júnior et al., 2024). Also, since congenital anomalies are more common in low and middle-income countries like Iran, it shows the urgent need for strong preventive steps and ethical healthcare practices. Epidemiologists and public health officials should employ a method that not only collects data but also considers the ethical implications of their findings.

Ensuring that participants' rights are respected and their privacy is protected is part of this. By enhancing prenatal care and developing effective screening procedures, stakeholders can work to rectify the growing prevalence of congenital anomalies while adhering to ethical standards in health promotion and disease prevention (Tarighat et al., 2021). Additionally, ethical issues in infectious disease epidemiology extend beyond health and impact the broader community. It is crucial for different fields to collaborate, as integrating ethics with science can lead to more effective public health strategies. People responsible for healthcare should ensure fairness and justice, and also pay attention to what individuals and communities require. As new public health problems emerge, regularly considering ethical issues will inform decisions and contribute to a fairer and healthier society. Advocating for such principles will be essential in maintaining the integrity of public health initiatives and ensuring their effectiveness in improving health outcomes for all populations (Júnior et al., 2024).

Ethical considerations in infectious disease epidemiology are multifaceted, encompassing issues related to consent, privacy, and equity in the distribution of health resources. An essential part of these discussions is the principle of informed consent, which requires individuals to understand the study and agree to participate voluntarily. This can be very challenging when it comes to vulnerable people who are not able to give consent. Besides, it is critical to respect privacy; researchers should weigh the need to collect a lot of data against the need to protect personal information from being misused or exposed. Because these challenges are complex, the rules for research ethics must be updated to ensure everyone is protected and respected during the research. Another crucial ethical point is making sure that different groups of people share the benefits and burdens fairly. It is common for epidemiologists to need to decide which groups should receive priority, which can lead to differences in the distribution of healthcare and resources. For example, the SACIDS highlights the importance of using a One Health approach which sees how human, animal and environmental health are connected.

Although SACIDS successfully combines different sectors to combat infectious diseases, it also highlights that member countries have unequal funding and resources, which raises ethical concerns. Ensuring that all participating nations receive equitable support fosters an environment of mutual benefit rather than a hierarchical system that privileges certain regions over others (Anderson et al.,

2018). In addition, it is essential for ethical practices in infectious disease epidemiology to evolve and reflect on new problems continually. Since new pathogens and changing environments appear, the methods used in epidemiology should be able to adapt. It means encouraging researchers to share openly with communities, so that local and traditional knowledge can be included in health programs. Moreover, ethical frameworks should encourage different disciplines to cooperate, which improves the trustworthiness of research and helps participants feel more comfortable. By actively engaging with communities and emphasizing equitable partnerships, public health initiatives can promote a more just approach to infectious disease management (Pearson et al., 2001). It is vital in epidemiology and public health ethics to balance scientific accuracy with ethical duties.

CLOSER LOOK

GENOME-WIDE ASSOCIATION STUDIES (GWAS):

Genome-wide association studies (GWAS) are a powerful tool in modern genetics, designed to uncover the genetic factors underlying complex traits and diseases. Unlike traditional genetic studies that focus on a few candidate genes, GWAS scan the entire genome for small variations called single nucleotide polymorphisms (SNPs) to identify associations with specific traits or health conditions. This approach has revolutionized our understanding of the genetic basis of diseases, providing insights into risk factors, biological pathways, and potential therapeutic targets.

The process of a GWAS begins with the collection of genetic data from a large group of individuals, often thousands or even hundreds of thousands. These participants are typically categorized based on the trait or disease being studied—for example, individuals with type 2 diabetes versus those without. Researchers then analyze millions of SNPs across the genome to determine whether any genetic variants occur more frequently in one group compared to the other. Statistical methods are used to identify significant associations, while controlling for confounding factors such as population structure and environmental influences.

GWAS have successfully identified genetic variants linked to a wide range of complex diseases, including cardiovascular disease, diabetes, autoimmune disorders, and psychiatric conditions. For example, studies have pinpointed loci associated with increased risk of Alzheimer's disease, shedding light on potential biological mechanisms and paving the way for new drug development. Beyond disease risk, GWAS also help explain variations in traits like height, body mass index, and response to medications, enabling personalized medicine approaches.

Despite their power, GWAS have limitations. They often detect variants with small effects, meaning that individual SNPs may contribute only modestly to disease risk. Moreover, most studies have focused on populations of European ancestry, limiting the generalizability of findings to other populations. Researchers are now working to increase diversity in GWAS and to integrate these findings with other types of data, such as gene expression and epigenetic profiles, to better understand the complex interactions between genes and the environment.

Technological advancements, including high-throughput genotyping, whole-genome sequencing, and advanced computational tools, continue to enhance the accuracy and scope of GWAS. As datasets grow larger and more diverse, GWAS are expected to play an increasingly central role in precision medicine, public health, and our understanding of human biology.

In conclusion, genome-wide association studies provide a comprehensive approach to uncovering the genetic underpinnings of complex traits and diseases. By linking genetic variation to health outcomes, GWAS not only advance scientific knowledge but also open new avenues for personalized medicine, early disease detection, and targeted therapeutic strategies.

REFERENCES

1. Abebe, R., Hill, S., Schwartz, H. A., Small, D., et al. (2019). *Using Search Queries to Understand Health Information Needs in Africa.* https://arxiv.org/abs/1806.05740 (accessed on 30th May 2025).
2. *Registries for Evaluating Patient Outcomes: A user's guide.* (2020b). https://doi.org/10.23970/ahrqepcregistries4Al Houri, A. N., Alhouri, A. N., Zahrawi, H., Al Houri, H. A., Abu-Hussein, B., Arrouk, D. M. N., Jarrar, Y., et al. (2023). The prevalence and risk factors of COVID-stress syndrome. *Cureus, 15.* https://www.semanticscholar.org/paper/72e02521a053daba6e161d61fa91edd72d8c4fea (accessed on 30th May 2025).
3. Al Sharif, N. A., Kabi, K. M. H., Alshayeb, H. A. A., Asiri, A. O. H., Asiri, J. A. H., Alzaid, E. D. I., Muqarbish, M. A. H., et al. (2024). Healthcare workplace hazards: A multilingual assessment of nursing, pharmacy, optics, social sciences, and epidemiology. *Journal of Ecohumanism.* https://www.semanticscholar.org/paper/a76366ae6740f2bdddb92dbc7852952230b46c36 (accessed on 30th May 2025).
4. Alpert, A., Babbs, G., Sanaeikia, R., Ellison, J., Hughes, L. D., Herington, J., Dembroff, R. (2024). Doing justice: Ethical considerations identifying and researching transgender and gender diverse people in insurance claims data. *Journal of Medical Systems, 48.* https://www.semanticscholar.org/paper/e65a8650dba4caf8d3030466757be898a711b186 (accessed on 30th May 2025).
5. Anderson, R. M., Aunger, R., Banaji, M., Barnett, T., Denton, D., et al. (2015). Some considerations concerning the challenge of incorporating social variables into epidemiological models of infectious disease transmission. *Global Public Health.* https://core.ac.uk/download/36778292.pdf (accessed on 30th May 2025).
6. Anderson, R., Aragrande, M., Argyris, G., Chomel, B., Coker, R., Epstein, J., Gibbs, E., et al. (2018). *A One Health Evaluation of the Southern African Centre for Infectious Disease Surveillance.* https://core.ac.uk/download/159106431.pdf (accessed on 30th May 2025).
7. Bakari, E. (2012). Assessment of implementation of International Health Regulations (2005) on preventing infectious diseases: A case study of Julius Nyerere International Airport, Dar es Salaam. https://core.ac.uk/download/pdf/11307882.pdf (accessed on 30th May 2025).
8. Barhoush, Y., & Amon, J. (2025). Research in compulsory drug detention centers in China: Characteristics and ethical considerations. *Global Public Health, 20*(1), 2447795. https://www.semanticscholar.org/paper/ac9d9cab7cb58b1abcb126cc976d815807ceed12 (accessed on 30th May 2025).
9. Beltrán-Aguilar, E. D., Benzian, H., & Niederman, R. (2020). Rational perspectives on risk and certainty for dentistry during the COVID-19 pandemic. *American Journal of Infection Control, 49,* 131–133. https://doi.org/10.1016/j.ajic.2020.06.007.
10. Bhimraj, A., Morgan, R. L., Shumaker, A. H., Lavergne, V., Baden, L. R., Cheng, V. C. C., Edwards, K. M., et al. (2020). Infectious Diseases Society of America guidelines on the treatment and management of patients with COVID-19. *Clinical Infectious Diseases, 78,* e83–e102. https://doi.org/10.1093/cid/ciaa478.
11. Branda, F., Stella, M., Ceccarelli, C., Cabitza, F., Ceccarelli, G., Maruotti, A., Ciccozzi, M., et al. (2025). The role of AI-based chatbots in public health emergencies: A narrative review.

Future Internet. https://www.semanticscholar.org/paper/7278104e56e9214a42bdde6e0706dbe096a2e806 (accessed on 30th May 2025).

12. Cenedesi, Jr. M. A., Rodrigues, D. P. V., Merege, M. C., Schwarz, F. S., Gomes, G. S. B. F., Vasconcelos, J. L. A., Melo, J. L. N., et al. (2024). The challenges in rebuilding a quality public health in Brazil. *Observatório de la Economía Latinoamericana*. https://www.semanticscholar.org/paper/89310a27393328d4d308eb85ab914cc69115a6df (accessed on 30th May 2025).

13. Chauhan, C., Khunger, A., Lachyan, A., Choudhary, K., & Aloona, S. (2025). Integrating genomic medicine into public health: A comprehensive review of advancements, challenges, and ethical considerations. *Majmaah Journal of Health Sciences*. https://www.semanticscholar.org/paper/c1d410fe1a1e059af2b38a5cc028c37dc8998038 (accessed on 30th May 2025).

14. Cummings, P. J. D. W., Baker, K. K., Appell, L., Del Rios, M., Diekema, D. J., Kitzmann, T., Marroquin, N., et al. (2025). Equity in epidemic response: An action-oriented framework for guiding public health in equitable responses to major infectious disease emergencies. *International Journal for Equity in Health, 24*. https://www.semanticscholar.org/paper/47699e6bc69459afb9650c9e3ecba1a477db3040 (accessed on 30th May 2025).

15. Delva, W., & HIV Modeling Consortium Treatment as Prevention Editorial Writing Group, The. (2012). HIV treatment as prevention: Models, data, and questions—Towards evidence-based decision-making. *PLoS Medicine*. https://core.ac.uk/download/55802467.pdf (accessed on 30th May 2025).

16. Ebron, J. G. A., Endaya, J. K. L., Lat, N. O. S., Levardo, F. A. N., Libaton, M. L. A., Rivera, J. R. M., Solar, J. J. J. B., et al. (2024). Modeling and simulation of infectious disease dynamics utilizing SEIR model. *2024 ASU International Conference in Emerging Technologies for Sustainability and Intelligent Systems (ICETSIS)*. https://www.semanticscholar.org/paper/4d110c1b5393c443275b86d26851a8c8ef57550c (accessed on 30th May 2025).

17. Elendu, C., Osamuyi, E. I., Afolayan, I. A., Opara, N., Chinedu-Anunaso, N. A., Okoro, C. B., Nwankwo, A. U., et al. (2024). Clinical presentation and symptomatology of Guillain-Barré syndrome: A literature review. *Medicine, 103*. https://www.semanticscholar.org/paper/15f20b046385ffe333e3bd0106b720b193c88549 (accessed on 30th May 2025).

18. El-Hebsh, H. S. (2018). Nurses' knowledge and practice about infection control in outpatient clinics of governmental hospitals at Al-Mukalla City – Yemen. *Assiut Scientific Nursing Journal*. https://www.semanticscholar.org/paper/3227940b680e42d6da7d9889596c7b793212ffb9 (accessed on 30th May 2025).

19. Ferdous, M. Z., Islam, M. S., Sikder, M. T., Mosaddek, A. S. M., Zegarra-Valdivia, J., & Gozal, D. (2020). Knowledge, attitude, and practice regarding COVID-19 outbreak in Bangladesh: An online-based cross-sectional study. *PLOS ONE, 15*, e0239254–e0239254. https://doi.org/10.1371/journal.pone.0239254.

20. Freeman, M. (2018). *The Ethics of Public Health*. https://www.semanticscholar.org/paper/6b0b1d251404e6bfb9b4fa4d4e082ffe8f8b081f (accessed on 30th May 2025).

21. Giuffrè, M., & Shung, D. (2023). Harnessing the power of synthetic data in healthcare: Innovation, application, and privacy. *NPJ Digital Medicine, 6*. https://doi.org/10.1038/s41746-023-00927-3.

22. Harris-Lovett, S., Nelson, K. L., Beamer, P. I., Bischel, H. N., Bivins, A., Bruder, A., Butler, C. S., et al. (2021). Wastewater surveillance for SARS-CoV-2 on college campuses: Initial efforts,

lessons learned, and research needs. *International Journal of Environmental Research and Public Health, 18*, 4455. https://doi.org/10.3390/ijerph18094455.

23. Hulstine, A. (2017). *Vaccine Implementation: Alaska 2017.* https://core.ac.uk/download/286607590.pdf (accessed on 30th May 2025).
24. Ibiam, V. A., Omale, L. E., & Taiwo, O. (2025). The role of artificial intelligence models in clinical decision support for infectious disease diagnosis and personalized treatment planning. *International Journal of Science and Research Archive.* https://www.semanticscholar.org/paper/2eb92ff69739febe03ab53228c14952fb2b7333f (accessed on 30th May 2025).
25. Igwe, M. C., & Obeagu, E. (2024). The scopes and implications of health communication in public health practices in Nigeria. *Journal of Bacteriology and Mycology.* https://www.semanticscholar.org/paper/a7bb77f81e9031b112dd463796095bc517bf6757 (accessed on 30th May 2025).
26. Irfan, B., Khleif, A., Badarneh, J., Abutaqa, J., Allam, A., Kweis, S., Tarab, B., et al. (2025). Considering Islamic frameworks to infectious disease prevention. *Open Forum Infectious Diseases.* https://www.semanticscholar.org/paper/c841c4594c7b5d36f4580ddcce61aebb579bf37f (accessed on 30th May 2025).
27. King, L. P., & Pincus, J. B. (2024). ACOG Committee Statement No. 9: Ethical considerations for increasing inclusivity in research participants. *Obstetrics & Gynecology, 143*, e155–e163. https://www.semanticscholar.org/paper/ab2fd5ad43176da8a69fc60e98f44df32997d024 (accessed on 30th May 2025).
28. Kitajima, M., Abe, H., Honda, R., Kobayashi, H., Kuroita, T., Nemoto, A., Shirakashi, R., et al. (2025). Biobanking: Possibilities for wastewater-based epidemiology. *Biopreservation and Biobanking.* https://www.semanticscholar.org/paper/623793280a82ba1bae0a8d59aaa911e7c3780e8b (accessed on 30th May 2025).
29. Kitajima, M., Ahmed, W., Bibby, K., Carducci, A., Gerba, C. P., Hamilton, K. A., Haramoto, E., et al. (2020). SARS-CoV-2 in wastewater: State of the knowledge and research needs. *The Science of The Total Environment, 739*, 139076. https://doi.org/10.1016/j.scitotenv.2020.139076.
30. Kováč, P., Jackuliak, P., Bražinová, A., Varga, I., Aláč, M., Smatana, M., Lovich, D., et al. (2024). Artificial intelligence-driven facial image analysis for the early detection of rare diseases: Legal, ethical, forensic, and cybersecurity considerations. *AI.* https://www.semanticscholar.org/paper/48b479a78ec64873f6078910115f3812c2a5ebf3 (accessed on 30th May 2025).
31. Largent, E., Kim, Y., Karlawish, J., & Wexler, A. (2025). Ethics from the outset: Incorporating ethical considerations into the AI Tech Collaboratories' pilot projects. *The Journals of Gerontology. Series A, Biological Sciences and Medical Sciences.* https://www.semanticscholar.org/paper/b2561fdc2755b9d13a8246fa39a86d057c145153 (accessed on 30th May 2025).
32. Liu, X. (2024). Application and development of wastewater epidemiology in public health: Current status and future trends. *Theoretical and Natural Science.* https://www.semanticscholar.org/paper/b7fd8d729fe3121f8d3d19c302cec967f7c07805 (accessed on 30th May 2025).
33. Mo, M., Moon, S., & Song, E. (2024). Nurses' intention to care of COVID-19 patients in hospitals dedicated to infectious disease in South Korea: Application of the theory of planned behavior and verification of the moderating effect of ethical nursing competence. *BMC Nursing, 23.* https://www.semanticscholar.org/paper/8f8da366eb3e9d1b4be3e2997b0cf5518a682737 (accessed on 30th May 2025).

34. Molla, A., Kruse, L. C., Karanasios, S., Cheong, C., & Hoang, G. (2024). Designing information systems for infectious disease management in VUCA situations: Insights from a design archaeology analysis of COVIDSafe. *Journal of the Association for Information Systems, 25*(2). https://www.semanticscholar.org/paper/ece7b0f4310d81a17f1b827d1a34c4f999603bda (accessed on 30th May 2025).

35. Muteeb, G., Rehman, M. T., Shahwan, M., & Aatif, M. (2023). Origin of antibiotics and antibiotic resistance, and their impacts on drug development: A narrative review. *Pharmaceuticals, 16*, 1615. https://doi.org/10.3390/ph16111615.

36. N/A. (2025). *Advisory Committee on Immunization Practices (ACIP) Summary Report: September 22, 2020, Atlanta, Georgia*. https://core.ac.uk/download/363141593.pdf (accessed on 30th May 2025).

37. Omale, L. E., Ibiam, V. A., Sidikat, L. W., & Taiwo, O. (2025). Transformative applications of artificial intelligence in infectious disease forecasting and public health decision support systems. *World Journal of Advanced Research and Reviews*. https://www.semanticscholar.org/paper/bbdb6f7ea15878fbb8dbba8d8d9c682aa1c36813 (accessed on 30th May 2025).

38. Pearson, G. S. (2001). *New Scientific and Technological Developments of Relevance to the Fifth Review Conference*. https://core.ac.uk/download/6242.pdf (accessed on 30th May 2025).

39. Racine, E. E. (2025). Que(e)rying artificial intelligence use for infectious disease surveillance: The need for a reparative algorithmic praxis. *Big Data & Society*. https://www.semanticscholar.org/paper/4998a4b4e83d3c6d448502d4f8cf673ad91d5a80 (accessed on 30th May 2025).

40. Sarantopoulos, A., Kourmpani, C. M., Yokarasa, A. L., Makamanzi, C., Antoniou, P., Spernovasilis, N., & Tsioutis, C. (2024). Artificial intelligence in infectious disease clinical practice: An overview of gaps, opportunities, and limitations. *Tropical Medicine and Infectious Disease, 9*. https://www.semanticscholar.org/paper/f028c84a668fae5b4b6648bcdaf9b90bc3e1f7e6 (accessed on 30th May 2025).

41. Senthil, R., Gopal, R., Rahman, S. Z., & Ramalingam, V. (2023). *Predicting Infectious Disease Outbreaks with Machine Learning and Epidemiological Data*. https://core.ac.uk/download/591404868.pdf (accessed on 30th May 2025).

42. Somekh, I., Somech, R., Pettoello-Mantovani, M., & Somekh, E. (2020). Changes in routine pediatric practice in light of Coronavirus 2019 (COVID-19). *The Journal of Pediatrics, 224*, 190–193. https://doi.org/10.1016/j.jpeds.2020.05.053.

43. Soroye, M., Owhonda, G., Nwadiuto, I., Livingstone, T., Ameh, S., Ordinioha, B., Akeredolu, P. A. (2024). An analysis of COVID-19 statistics in Rivers State, Nigeria: A study of demographic patterns, geographic distribution, and prevalent symptoms from April 2020 to March 2021. *Asian Journal of Research in Infectious Diseases*. https://www.semanticscholar.org/paper/93cd694a6809fb01aa3f8019936f83b56f9505ca (accessed on 30th May 2025).

44. Tajudeen, R., Silaigwana, B., Yavlinsky, A., & Edwards, S. (2023). Research ethics during infectious disease outbreaks: A survey of African research stakeholders using the Ebola virus disease outbreak as a case. *Journal of Public Health in Africa, 14*. https://www.semanticscholar.org/paper/6ba95dd47ffb1792bf8e5a2fda5d58b3e94b02e1 (accessed on 30th May 2025).

45. Tarighat, F., Golshan, E., & Dastgiri, S. (2021). Prevalence of congenital anomalies in the Northwest of Iran. *Depiction of Health*. https://www.semanticscholar.org/paper/a223fd217a7dba6a8036260a1e4991698b95f984 (accessed on 30th May 2025).

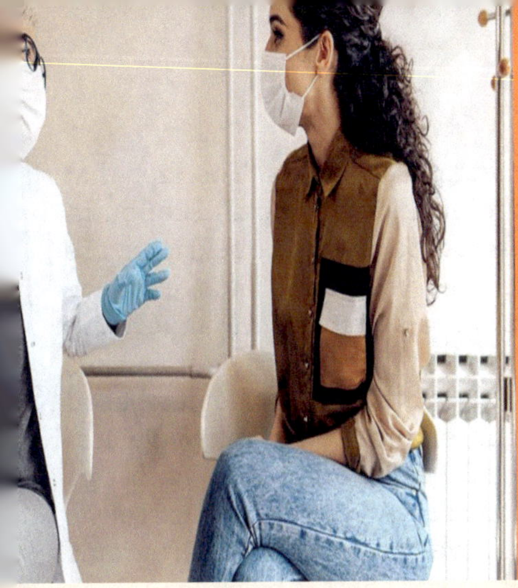

Chapter 14

SOCIAL AND BEHAVIOURAL FACTORS IN INFECTIOUS DISEASE EPIDEMIOLOGY

Contents

Introduction

The exploration of social and behavioral factors in infectious disease epidemiology is crucial for understanding how these elements influence disease spread and control. Infectious diseases are linked to people's behaviours, societal norms, and the state of the economy. Risky habits like smoking or drinking can make people in low-resource areas more likely to get diseases during an outbreak. It becomes clear that special health interventions are necessary when we see the data showing how common these behaviours are. Research in Bushbuckridge, South Africa, indicates that 51.3% of the participants smoked, and 76.2% did not consume enough fruits and vegetables in their diets. Such statistics underscore the urgent need for tailored strategies aimed at mitigating these behaviours to improve public health outcomes (Pilusa et al., 2025). Social determinants, including poverty, unemployment, and the ease of access to healthcare, are also crucial in the study of infectious diseases. In many rural areas, these factors contribute to unhealthy lifestyle choices that exacerbate the risk of non-communicable diseases (NCDs) and, indirectly, infectious diseases. The fact that these determinants are related means public health strategies should include social, economic, and cultural aspects. It is clear from the data that unemployed people in Bushbuckridge are more likely to drink alcohol, which is connected to social and economic problems. Thus, effective interventions must not only address immediate health behaviours but also target the underlying social determinants that create an environment conducive to unhealthy practices (Pilusa et al., 2025). To help change behaviours in vulnerable groups, using health promotion strategies based on established behavioural theories is very effective. Evidence from intervention mapping suggests that addressing specific community challenges can lead to improved health outcomes. With this methodology, stakeholders work together to identify what stops adolescents from choosing healthy living, such as a lack of motivation and resources. Using social cognitive theory in these programs helps them use the influence of peers and community leaders to encourage better behavior, which supports the overall health of the public. Such targeted efforts are pivotal in cultivating environments that not only prevent infectious diseases but also promote long-term wellness (Figure 14.1).

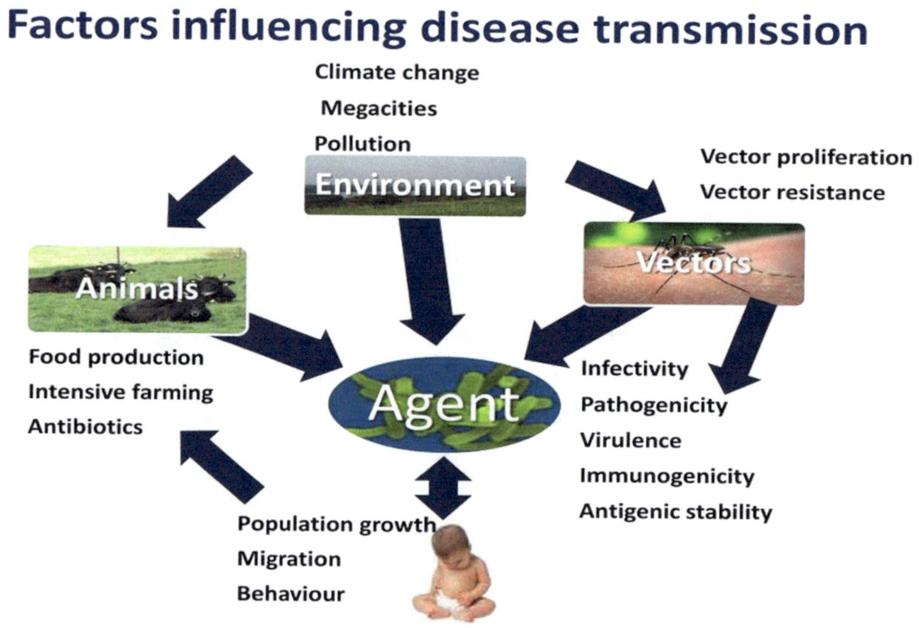

Figure 14.1. The exploration of social and behavioral factors in infectious disease epidemiology.

Source: https://image.slideserve.com/661052/factors-influencing-disease-transmission-l.jpg.

Definition of infectious disease epidemiology

Infectious disease epidemiology is a crucial subfield of public health that focuses on the distribution, patterns, and determinants of infectious diseases in populations. The primary tasks are to determine the prevalence of specific diseases, identify their causes, and understand how they are transmitted. It is essential to look at social and behavioural factors when trying to understand how diseases are spread. Factors such as cultural practices, socioeconomic status (SES), and individual health behaviours can significantly affect infection rates and overall public health outcomes. As a result, infectious disease epidemiology considers both the biology of diseases and the social factors that influence health behaviours, which shows the value of using a wide range of measures to prevent and control diseases. Additionally, the complex relationship between infectious diseases and social factors in health makes epidemiological studies more challenging. An example is HIV/AIDS, which has shown that simply looking at how people behave cannot explain the differences between groups, especially where multiple infectious diseases are found, like in sub-Saharan Africa. Prof. Stillwagon's work illustrates this complexity, showcasing how examining social and behavioural dimensions can lead to more effective interventions and policies tailored to specific communities (Sawers et al., 2018). Thanks to this approach, epidemiologists can design strategies that address both the pathogens and the environmental and societal factors that facilitate their spread, thereby enhancing the success of public health actions. Finally, the role of psychosocial factors in infectious disease epidemiology cannot be understated, especially concerning diseases like tuberculosis (TB). Recent studies have demonstrated that psychosocial stressors can significantly modulate immune function, impacting susceptibility to infections and responsiveness to vaccines, such as the BCG vaccine for tuberculosis (Boccia et al., 2019). Researchers have begun to investigate how social factors influence the immune system and health outcomes through a review of the available literature. It demonstrates that human actions, societal factors, and the body's response to infections are closely linked, so a more integrated approach is needed in infectious disease epidemiology.

Importance of Social and Behavioural Factors

Understanding the significance of social and behavioral factors in infectious disease epidemiology is essential for comprehending how diseases spread and are managed within populations. Economic status, education, and cultural habits are social determinants that significantly influence a person's health and the likelihood of contracting or spreading infectious diseases. Places where healthcare is not readily available usually have more cases of tuberculosis and HIV/AIDS. This highlights that traditional epidemiology often overlooks the social and economic factors that significantly influence people's health choices. As researchers recognise these complexities, the integration of social and behavioural factors becomes vital for crafting public health interventions that are both effective and equitable, ensuring that strategies resonate with the populations at risk (Hoye et al., 2018). Additionally, the willingness of people to get vaccinated, their understanding of health, and their compliance with public health rules are significant factors in controlling outbreaks. People's choices about vaccinations and adherence to health advice are often influenced by their trust in healthcare and assessment of the risks, which can significantly impact the number of people following health guidelines during epidemics. For example, during the COVID-19 pandemic, differences in vaccination rates revealed that both personal choices and social factors, including misinformation and unequal access to healthcare, played a role. Super spreaders are individuals who transmit the disease at a rate much higher than others, illustrating how personal actions can significantly impact epidemics. Therefore, understanding these behavioural patterns is critical for effective epidemiological modelling and response strategies (Hoye et al., 2018). Taking social and behavioural aspects into account in epidemiology supports a complete approach to preventing and controlling diseases. Public health strategies that consider social factors are more effective in addressing the primary reasons for vulnerability and distress within communities. Programs that support education and economic security can help individuals strengthen their defences against infectious diseases by providing them with helpful information and tools. In addition, when sociology, anthropology, and psychology work together, it can help explain how social factors shape health behaviors. This integrative approach can yield more comprehensive strategies, ultimately leading to improved health outcomes across populations and a more robust response to infectious disease threats (Herval et al., 2018) (Figure 14.2).

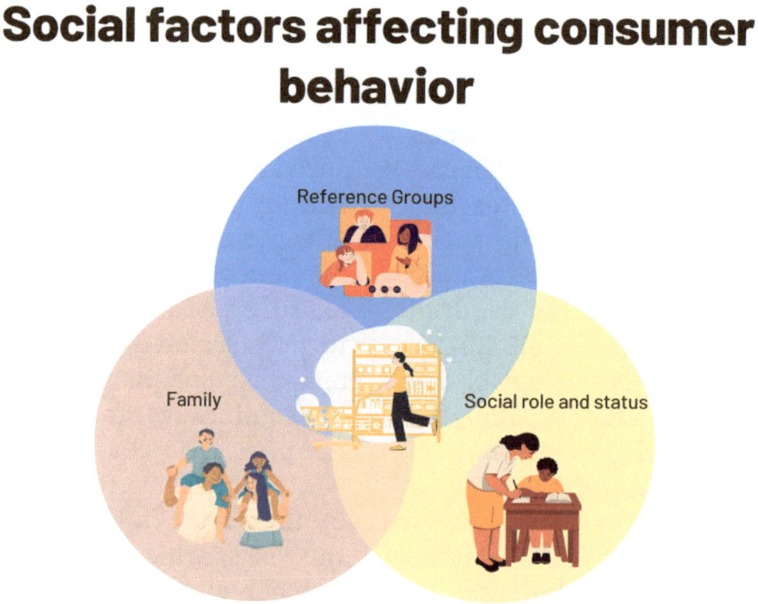

Figure 14.2. The significance of social and behavioral factors in infectious disease epidemiology.

Source: https://www.superheuristics.com/wp-content/uploads/2023/02/Sage-Green-Abstract-Floral-Social-Networking-Venn-Diagram-Graph-1.png.

14.1. Historical Context of Infectious Diseases

The historical context of infectious diseases reveals a complex interplay between social determinants and disease propagation, demonstrating that societal structures significantly shape health outcomes. In the past, pandemics such as the Black Death in the 14th century and the 1918 influenza pandemic made it clear that people from certain SES and geographic groups were more affected by infectious diseases. Especially, people from marginalised groups faced the worst of these crises because they had less access to healthcare, faced existing health differences, and lived in areas with more environmental problems. These patterns persist in contemporary pandemics, such as COVID-19, wherein racial and ethnic minorities in the United States face elevated risks of exposure and mortality, echoing historical inequities (Domingo, 2020). Therefore, understanding these historical factors is crucial for identifying solutions to today's health inequalities and developing interventions for at-risk populations. Additionally, the behaviour of societies and the response of public health have played a significant role in shaping the course of infectious disease management. For example, in the 19th century, the response to cholera outbreaks in cities led to changes in public health policies, demonstrating that water use and sanitation played a crucial role in spreading the disease. Governments and health officials began implementing changes, such as repairing buildings and educating people about health, to prevent the spread of more diseases. Because of this, modern epidemiology developed, emphasising the importance of social involvement in fighting infectious diseases. It is crucial today, as we saw during the COVID-19 pandemic, because following public health guidelines has been necessary. However, as evident from writings on gender and health disparities, the varied experiences of different demographics toward these guidelines illustrate the influence of social factors on health behaviours (Gausman et al., 2020). Additionally, the history of infectious diseases underscores the importance of addressing stigma and discrimination during outbreaks. Stigmatizing marginalized groups usually worsens their problems and makes it harder for public health to respond. Communities dealing with HIV/AIDS in the late 20th century were often stigmatized, which made many people hesitant to get help. Because of this misunderstanding, there are still differences in the way diverse populations are treated and supported. During the COVID-19 pandemic, some racial and ethnic groups have been mistreated or marginalized, which has made them less likely to seek medical help. Acknowledging these historical injustices is crucial for future public health strategies, as they guide us in fostering more inclusive and equitable approaches to disease prevention and control that actively involve affected communities (Domingo, 2020). It points out that strong epidemiology depends on understanding the social and cultural aspects of health behaviors, so that infectious disease threats can be dealt with effectively.

14.1.1. Major Pandemics and Their Social Impacts

Pandemics have historically triggered substantial shifts in societal structures, presenting both challenges and transformations across various dimensions. This is clearly evident in the current COVID-19 pandemic, which has significantly impacted public health, economies, and social life in numerous ways. When the virus spread around the world, it revealed that some healthcare systems were not strong enough, exacerbating existing disparities among people. Those with pre-existing health problems were much more at risk, which prompted researchers to study how social factors affect health. For instance, emerging data indicate a correlation between obesity and severe COVID-19 outcomes, further highlighting the relationship between social behaviours, lifestyle factors, and susceptibility to illness (Kitajima et al., 2020). Thus, the pandemic showed that we need to address both social and behavioural aspects when dealing with infectious diseases. Besides affecting health, major pandemics have traditionally changed the way people interact and behave in society. COVID-19 required people to stay apart and isolate, which brought changes to how communities interacted. As a result of remote work and virtual meetings, the traditional way people communicate face-to-face has been significantly changed. The change caused people to worry about mental health and social well-being, mainly for those who are elderly or live by themselves. Additionally, cultural practices were impacted, as gatherings and rituals were either restricted or had to be conducted differently. Research indicates that such disruptions can lead to increased anxiety and depression, underscoring the intricate interplay between infectious disease spread and psychosocial outcomes (Kitajima et al., 2020). It is clear from the way social connectivity changed during the pandemic that community-focused changes are essential in public health planning. Pandemics have a profound impact on the economy and give rise to long-lasting social problems. The pandemic resulted in many people losing their jobs, businesses closing, and an unexpected economic crisis, which mainly hurt marginalised communities. For example, industries that rely on in-person meetings, such as hospitality and retail, suffered significantly, which exacerbated socioeconomic disparities. The government's next measures, such as unemployment support and stimulus packages, were designed to reduce financial hardship, yet they led to arguments about fairness and access. It also became clear during the pandemic that gig economy jobs are not secure, and essential workers are at risk. The economic fallout not only highlighted existing systemic inequities but also necessitated a reevaluation of labour policies and worker protections to foster resilience against future public health challenges (Sattar et al., 2020). It is essential to understand the social and economic factors that influence how people and communities respond to pandemics.

14.1.2. Evolution of Public Health Responses

The interplay of social and behavioral factors has significantly influenced the evolution of public health responses to infectious diseases. Before, public health measures mainly involved improving sanitation and vaccinations to handle the epidemics caused by industrialisation and urbanisation. In the 19th century, people started to focus on enhancing sewers and getting clean water after realising how diseases were spread. Focusing on community interventions rather than just changing individual habits was a significant shift in public health. It is clear from the HIV/AIDS situation in sub-Saharan Africa that health differences are not only caused by individual choices but also by the influence of structures and health inequities. Thus, the evolution of public health responses now requires a multifaceted approach that recognizes these social determinants (Sawers et al., 2018). Currently, how people react to infectious disease risk is considered an essential aspect of epidemiology. Now, public health policy covers both medical treatments and methods that address how people in communities behave and what risks they face. When diseases such as avian influenza occur, policymakers have noted that livestock producers adjust their methods in response to the risks, which in turn affects the spread of the disease. Because community actions, trade, and the environment are interconnected, public health authorities should collaborate more closely. Research indicates that fostering specific farmer behaviours—like vaccination and depopulation—can either mitigate or exacerbate disease transmission, highlighting the need for targeted public health strategies that encompass behavioural economics and risk perception (Boni et al., 2019). The primary challenge in public health evolution is to integrate scientific information with human behaviour. Progress in vaccines and treatments should go hand in hand with actions to inform and involve people in healthy behaviours. The COVID-19 pandemic made it clear that trusting public health advice and following the rules is essential and that social norms and community participation help make public health efforts more effective. Collaboration among different fields should be a primary goal for future public health frameworks so that they can address both the biological and social sides of infectious disease transmission. By recognizing the importance of behavioral factors, public health responses can evolve to be more adaptive, equitable, and impactful in tackling the complexities of infectious disease epidemiology (Figure 14.3).

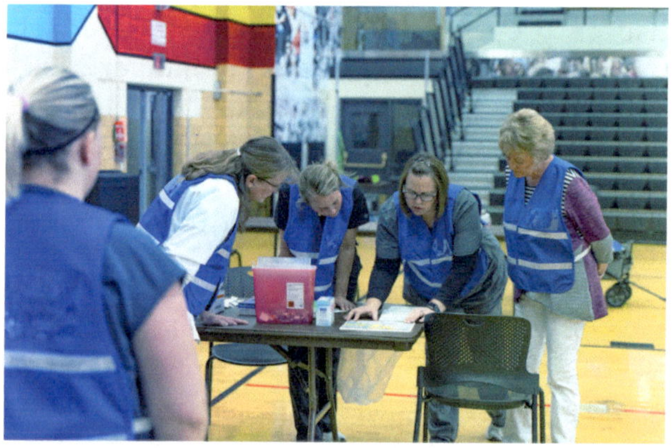

Figure 14.3. The evolution of public health responses to infectious diseases.

Source: https://clcpublichealth.org/wp-content/uploads/2022/06/CLCPH-PublicHealthResponse-Photo.jpg.

14.1.3. Lessons Learned from Past Outbreaks

The experience of past infectious disease outbreaks has revealed critical lessons related to social and behavioural factors that significantly influence public health responses. Events such as the HIV and SARS epidemics show that stigma and discrimination make health crises worse. Because of stigma, some people avoid being diagnosed and treated, which causes the disease to spread more widely in the community. When public health officials understand the socio-ecological model of stigma, they can develop strategies to mitigate its effects. Education is a strong way to inform groups and enable individuals to address stigmatising behaviours. Given this context, comprehensive communication strategies are crucial for enhancing public understanding of infectious diseases and dispelling prevalent myths during outbreaks (Sharma et al., 2023). Past outbreaks have shown that including epidemiology in clinical care is very important. The pandemic made it clear that existing health systems had issues, and it showed that health professionals should be well-versed in epidemiology. Public health training in educational reforms prepares healthcare providers to handle new health risks. This training enables doctors to utilise clinical skills and comprehend the social factors that influence patient care and community health. Through the incorporation of epidemiological knowledge, clinicians can better navigate public health challenges, ultimately leading to improved health outcomes for society as a whole (Sharma et al., 2023). It has become clear that both individual behavior and societal influence play a significant role in infectious disease outbreaks. The pandemic made it clear that how people behaved, such as wearing masks and getting vaccinated, depended significantly on their trust in health officials and the actions of others in society. If community leaders and healthcare workers encourage health interventions, it can significantly increase public involvement. Also, helping people cope with the mental effects of illness can greatly ease their fears and help reduce stigma. Helping those who are affected and encouraging togetherness among people can help communities work as one. If health authorities use behavioral insights, they can be more prepared for future outbreaks and improve their public health responses.

14.2. Social Determinants of Health

Understanding the social determinants of health is essential for addressing disparities in health outcomes, particularly within the context of infectious disease epidemiology. Among the social determinants are SES, education, features of the neighbourhood, and the ease of getting healthcare. Such elements may increase people's risk of infection and impair their ability to manage their health effectively. People living in poor neighbourhoods might not be able to get proper healthcare, which could prevent them from finding out about and treating infections quickly. In addition, when people have a hard time getting nutritious food, their immune systems may not work properly and they are more likely to get infectious diseases. Addressing these social factors is crucial for designing effective public health measures that prevent the spread of diseases and enhance community health. In addition, the COVID-19 pandemic has made it clear that social factors are very important in shaping health. Due to the pandemic, existing inequalities have become more pronounced, and vulnerable individuals now face even greater challenges. Living in under-resourced communities, children and adolescents have faced significant health problems because of school closures and losing their everyday routines, resulting in less healthy food and fewer opportunities to be physically active. The pandemic has shown that when parents are very stressed, combined with job losses and isolation, it can harm children's health, especially affecting their weight and mental health. Such vulnerabilities necessitate a comprehensive approach to public health that not only addresses medical treatment but also integrates support for the social contexts in which individuals live and grow (Browne et al., 2020). Chronic diseases, which are on the rise, often make people more likely to suffer from severe infections. Obesity, which became a significant issue during the pandemic, is a good example of this. Those who are obese as children have a higher risk of overall health problems and also face worse outcomes if they get infectious diseases such as COVID-19. The biopsychosocial dangers associated with obesity exacerbate inflammatory responses and undermine immune functionality, leading to worse health trajectories in such populations (Roth et al., 2020). For this reason, addressing social factors such as inequalities and environments that promote obesity is crucial for developing plans that improve health equity and mitigate the risks of infectious diseases. Ultimately, understanding and addressing these determinants within an epidemiological framework can enhance public health responses to current and future disease threats (Figure 14.4).

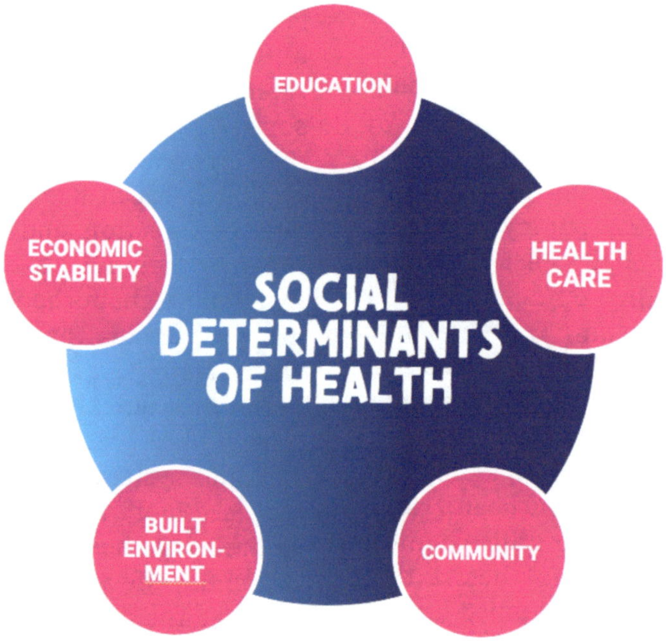

Figure 14.4. The social determinants of health.

Source: https://www.edpost.com/hubfs/Imported_Blog_Media/lDkde7sgrCY3YaBOSAQ3zWvvTMrJiXFIdLbXYIdXlpu8EK_9CNzeSCME0ZSGOdI1wCoYpPM_f6_uZpMoQZ_ts501HNrFuC1j51hqCJ58la4BUgDdw5oGLLmbdfwStn6P4LsFrvJ6-1.png -.

14.2.1. Socioeconomic Status and Disease Susceptibility

Understanding the relationship between SES and disease susceptibility is vital for informing public health policy and intervention strategies. Those from lower SES groups are more likely to suffer from infectious diseases because they have less access to healthcare, housing, and healthy food. All these factors increase the likelihood of health problems, making it more challenging for these communities to take effective measures to prevent diseases. Additionally, the anxiety caused by economic issues can weaken the immune system, making people more susceptible to illness. Studies have found that those living in poverty-stricken areas usually have more chronic diseases, which can make infectious diseases worse. Overall, the intersection of socioeconomic factors and health outcomes emphasises the necessity of integrating social determinants into epidemiological studies to address systemic inequalities that hamper effective disease control and prevention strategies (Sattar et al., 2020). Socioeconomic differences play a significant role in shaping the overall spread of disease and the likelihood of outbreaks. Areas with a lower SES are often crowded, which makes it more likely for diseases to spread. In addition, the social connections found in these communities can lead people to live in congested areas, making it easier for diseases to spread. If it is difficult for people to get vaccinated or learn about health, these problems are made worse, and more people suffer from diseases. Recent pandemics showed that places with less healthcare access had higher cases of infection and worse outcomes. This underscores the critical need for interventions tailored to address these socioeconomic barriers, fostering resilience within vulnerable populations and thereby curtailing the spread of infectious diseases (Gausman et al., 2020). The COVID-19 pandemic has made it evident that there is a strong connection between SES and the likelihood of getting sick. It has been shown by the data that those with lower SES are more likely to suffer from severe illness and death due to the pandemic. Because many in these communities lack healthcare and deal with other social issues, they have suffered more infections and higher death rates. Noticing these inequalities in real time prompts public health officials to make health equity a priority in their actions. By investing in social programs that enhance health literacy and improve access to care, policymakers can mitigate the impact of socioeconomic disparities on infectious disease susceptibility and foster a healthier, more equitable society in the face of future health crises (Sattar et al., 2020).

14.2.2. Access to Healthcare and Preventive Measures

Access to healthcare is a critical factor in managing infectious diseases, as it directly influences both the initiation of treatment and the implementation of preventive measures within communities. Lack of access to healthcare is often related to a person's economic situation, where they live, and their cultural background, which makes underprivileged people more at risk. It is concerning because quick medical care and regular preventive services, such as vaccinations and screenings, help reduce the spread of infectious diseases. In areas where healthcare is not readily available, people may not be vaccinated, which can lead to increased outbreaks. Lack of equal access weakens the health of individuals and prevents communities from responding effectively to disease threats, which is why comprehensive strategies are needed to help all groups access healthcare. Actions such as providing education, administering vaccines, and promoting public health initiatives help control infectious diseases. Sometimes, social factors significantly impact the effectiveness of these measures. SES, education, and cultural practices influence how people in communities perceive health issues and adopt preventive measures. For example, programs that explain why vaccination is essential can encourage more people in the community to follow the rules. Still, unless these social factors are addressed, such efforts might not be successful. Therefore, it is essential to integrate education with broader socioeconomic activities to ensure that preventive measures are both accessible and culturally suitable for all communities, thereby improving public health. The link between healthcare access and preventive actions highlights the importance of addressing infectious diseases, taking into account their social and cultural contexts. Many studies, including those conducted in Zambia, have demonstrated that understanding the local context is crucial. The lack of resources and reliable data makes it challenging to use epidemiological methods to tackle infectious diseases in Zambia. Additionally, planning that incorporates healthcare access, along with other health-related factors, is crucial for achieving long-term healthcare success. For example, the Go To 2040 regional master plan explains that a mix of strategies targeting population, economy, and education is essential for enhancing the community's health. Thus, making sure all people can access healthcare is a key approach to fighting infectious diseases and promoting better health for the population.

14.2.3. Education and Health Literacy

Effective education and health literacy are undeniably critical in the context of infectious disease epidemiology, as they significantly influence an individual's ability to engage in preventive behaviours. A study in Korea found that foreign students' COVID-19 preventive behaviours were strongly linked to their health literacy, which included knowing about the virus and having access to eHealth resources. Participants with higher eHealth literacy not only understood the risks associated with the disease but also demonstrated more effective preventive behaviours, such as mask-wearing and social distancing (Lee et al., 2023).

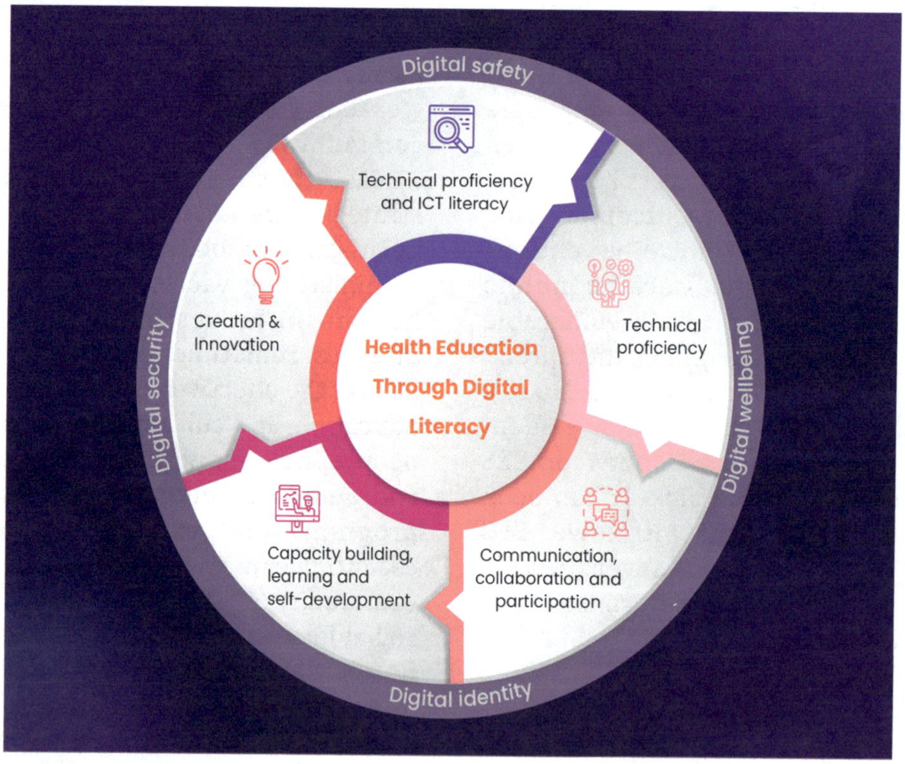

Figure 14.5. Education and health literacy.

Source: http://mypulse360.com/wp-content/uploads/2022/09/information.png.

This suggests that individuals with better health literacy can effectively manage health information and make informed decisions during outbreaks, potentially reducing infection rates and supporting community health initiatives. Additionally, discussions about health literacy extend beyond individual actions and focus on social factors that influence the way communities address health threats. Health literacy and education are closely related, as gaps in knowledge can exacerbate health inequities in infectious disease epidemiology. As articulated in the examination of various infectious diseases, such as HIV and tuberculosis, it has become clear that individual risk behaviours are embedded within larger socio-economic frameworks that either facilitate or hinder effective health communication (Dean et al., 2010).

Communities that lack educational resources often struggle to share health information, which increases their vulnerability during health emergencies. Therefore, addressing these larger issues is crucial for developing health literacy that leads to informed public health actions. It is crucial to incorporate education and health literacy into public health initiatives to enhance communities' resilience against infectious diseases. A holistic strategy requires people to change their habits and also for systems to be improved so that education and resources become more accessible. Using creative ways to connect education with the community can inspire people in marginalized areas to make better health choices. By promoting comprehensive educational programs that encompass basic health literacy as well as specific disease-related information, public health practitioners can cultivate a more informed populace that actively participates in preventive measures against infectious diseases (Lee et al., 2023). Ultimately, the cultivation of health literacy serves as a foundational element in developing effective strategies to combat infectious diseases and reduce health disparities across diverse populations (Figure 14.5).

14.3. Behavioural Factors Influencing Disease Spread

Understanding the behavioural factors influencing disease spread is essential in the realm of infectious disease epidemiology. The spread of pathogens depends on the actions people take and their interactions, which can affect the way outbreaks unfold. For example, during the COVID-19 pandemic, Twitter and Instagram were used to share information, which showed that user engagement can help spread accurate news as well as false rumours. These platforms enable people to discuss health, and the prevalence of misinformation on each platform illustrates the relationship between behaviour, messaging, and disease spread. The realisation that behavioural patterns can mirror epidemic models, such as those quantifying the basic reproduction number R_0, highlights the necessity of considering social media interactions as integral components of disease spread frameworks (Cinelli et al., 2020). Besides using the internet, how people travel, practice culture, and follow health instructions also have a significant impact on the progress of infectious diseases. Tuite et al. highlight this with their research on international travellers from Iran during the COVID-19 pandemic, showing how nations are easily linked and can spread the disease. Research has shown that an increase in travellers visiting different places leads to more cases of imported infections, highlighting the importance of travel decisions in disease spread. These findings suggest that understanding the cultural context and practices of specific populations is crucial for predicting and controlling disease transmission, thus highlighting the interplay between societal norms and epidemiological outcomes (Tuite et al., 2020). Additionally, the community's response to health interventions and messages plays a significant role in managing diseases.

People tend to follow public health rules, such as getting vaccinated and maintaining social distancing, when they trust the healthcare system and believe the disease is a significant risk. The differences in adherence to COVID-19 restrictions across various regions demonstrate that public health campaigns should be tailored to each area's unique beliefs and attitudes. Behavioural theories, such as the Health Belief Model, help explain these differences and create strategies that are effective for specific groups of people. Analysing past outbreaks through this lens can yield insights into effective communication and engagement strategies that enhance overall public health responses, ultimately leading to more effective containment of infectious diseases (Cinelli et al., 2020).

14.3.1. Personal Hygiene Practices

Personal hygiene practices are foundational to preventing the transmission of infectious diseases, particularly in the context of social and behavioural factors that influence epidemiological outcomes. Personal hygiene encompasses regularly washing your hands, bathing properly, and maintaining a clean living space. Research indicates that effective hand hygiene significantly reduces the burden of respiratory and gastrointestinal infections, making it a vital public health strategy (Aprillia et al., 2024). Even though these practices are effective, how much people follow them can depend on their culture, income, and available resources, which illustrates the connection between individual actions and social structures. It is essential to know these factors to develop public health measures that encourage everyone to care about personal hygiene. The pandemic has demonstrated that maintaining personal hygiene is crucial in preventing infections and that collective actions can significantly impact the spread of diseases. The pandemic's emergence has led to widespread public health campaigns promoting handwashing, mask-wearing, and sanitising practices as universal preventive measures (Qin et al., 2021). It is argued that the negative attitude toward those who do not follow hygiene guidelines might isolate people, mainly in communities where clean water and sanitation are not readily available. Making personal hygiene easier also requires reducing stigma, involving the community, and ensuring that resources are equally accessible to all. When public health authorities build an inclusive environment that promotes hygiene, communities become stronger against infectious diseases. Interventions that educate people about hygiene can encourage them to adopt better practices, which can help prevent the spread of infectious diseases. Such initiatives should encompass tailored messaging that resonates with specific populations, emphasising not only the benefits of hygiene but also the role of individual agency within a collective health framework (Aprillia et al., 2024). Self-efficacy programs about hygiene may encourage people, especially those with unique health crisis challenges, to change their habits. Additionally, applying the socio-ecological model in education promotes the maintenance of good hygiene habits at all levels, thereby supporting public health. When personal hygiene, social habits, and health are viewed as interconnected, stakeholders can develop strategies to prevent the spread of infectious diseases in various communities.

14.3.2. Vaccination Attitudes and Compliance

The attitudes surrounding vaccination play a crucial role in public health, particularly in the management and prevention of infectious diseases. The perceived effectiveness, safety, and necessity of vaccines significantly influence people's decision to get vaccinated. Sadly, doubts about medical advice and false rumours can cause people to avoid getting vaccinated, which makes it harder to reach herd immunity. Talking about concerns and presenting clear, scientific evidence helps people accept vaccines. For example, if people are frequently informed about the safety and effectiveness of vaccines, it can help them overcome their fears based on stories or exaggerated news. Moreover, fostering a strong sense of community and collective responsibility may encourage compliance among individuals who prioritise social norms and public health over personal apprehensions, illustrating the importance of social and behavioural factors in vaccination uptake (Belton et al., 2020). To understand how vaccination attitudes develop, we must examine the social and behavioural factors that influence health decisions. Behavioural science shows that how a person identifies with a group and the group's norms can strongly influence their decision to get vaccinated. If people believe their peers are being vaccinated, they are more likely to follow suit, as social networks create an environment where it is expected. Also, if society is strongly in favour of vaccination and if people disapprove of not getting vaccinated, individuals might feel pressured to get the shot. Therefore, it suggests that social approaches, such as involving peers or community leaders, may encourage more people to get vaccinated. A concerted effort to create a collective identity focused on health can encourage compliance while addressing the underlying behavioural factors affecting vaccination attitudes (Hayashi et al., 2016). Additionally, mathematical models can help explain the relationship between individuals' views on vaccination and their decision to comply. Adding variables for social norms, risks, and individual behaviour can help researchers build models that predict the number of people who choose to get vaccinated. For example, game theory and evolutionary dynamics can help us understand the relationship between perceived risk and willingness to follow public health instructions in an outbreak scenario. Models that link changes in community actions to disease spread, such as cleaning up after an outbreak, can help explain how vaccination compliance works. As demonstrated during the Ebola outbreak, shifts in societal practices significantly corresponded with improvements in public health outcomes, reinforcing the importance of addressing behavioural factors in the epidemiological landscape (Hayashi et al., 2016; Belton et al., 2020) (Figure 14.6).

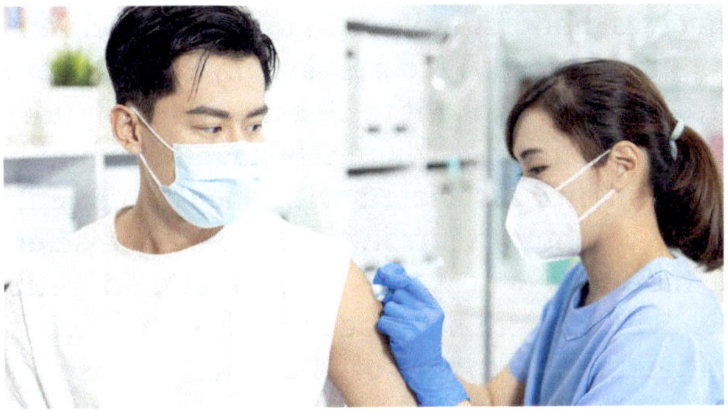

Figure 14.6. The attitudes surrounding vaccination play a crucial role in public health.

Source: https://www.rafflesmedicalgroup.com/wp-content/uploads/2023/04/importance-of-vaccination-singapore.jpg.

14.3.3. Risk-Taking Behaviours in Populations

Risk-taking behaviours within populations significantly influence the spread of infectious diseases, particularly through patterns of health-related decision-making. How much someone vaccinates, follows public health instructions, and engages in risky activities all say something about their risk-taking tendencies. One example is vaccine hesitancy, which happens when people believe vaccines are dangerous and less important than the benefits of immunising many people. As more people are allowed to opt out of vaccination for philosophical reasons, it is clear that some groups prioritise their own ideas over the health of everyone, which increases the risk of outbreaks. Therefore, it is crucial to employ health communication strategies that shape public perceptions and promote the adoption of preventive health measures, thereby reducing the incidence of infectious diseases and fostering a more resilient community. In addition, social expectations and group behaviour play a significant role in influencing people to misuse antibiotics. Many people follow the lead of others, which can result in the overuse of antibiotics for uncomplicated infections. Because antibiotics are often seen as safe and effective by many, people keep using them, which results in more drug-resistant infections. It adds to the difficulties in controlling and managing infectious diseases. When we study the reasons behind these behaviours, public health teams can develop programs to change how society views medicine use, which can improve the health of the entire population. In addition, recognising risk-taking behaviours in infectious disease epidemiology involves understanding that health interventions are not universally perceived. Although many people question vaccines, usually because of false information and fear of side effects, antibiotics are generally thought to be extremely helpful. It highlights the need to address the mental shortcuts that influence how people behave in public health. It is challenging to clearly articulate the risks and benefits associated with each treatment option. Reducing dangerous health habits requires using community involvement, teaching science, and building trust in medical services. As noted in the context of vaccine hesitancy and antibiotic misuse, it is imperative to contextualise these behaviours within broader social frameworks to craft effective public health policies aimed at mitigating the spread of infectious diseases (Wagner et al., 2020; Ruden, 2024).

14.4. Cultural Influences on Health Practices

The relationship between culture and health practices is multifaceted, significantly influencing healthcare behaviours among various populations. The beliefs and actions of communities influence their understanding of health and illness, leading to varied approaches to seeking healthcare. For example, the Phu Thai ethnic group in Thailand bases its interactions with healthcare and the environment on its cultural traditions and rituals. The COVID-19 pandemic demonstrated that traditional habits can meet new health risks, which means public health strategies should be sensitive to local cultures and encourage safer habits. The adoption of health interventions must consider these cultural contexts to ensure efficacy and community buy-in, as behaviour change is more readily accepted in alignment with established cultural beliefs, thereby addressing both health risks and community values (Bubpa et al., 2025). The way someone identifies with their culture also influences the health decisions they make, particularly in marginalised communities. Within Native Hawaiian and Pacific Islander (NHPI) populations, significant disparities in health outcomes persist, often rooted in sociocultural and historical contexts. Studies show that not having access to culturally appropriate health care and facing language difficulties prevent many people of colour from getting preventive screenings, which leads to worse health results than those seen in white people. For instance, individuals from these communities who struggle to communicate with healthcare providers are less likely to receive cancer screenings, highlighting the importance of cultural and linguistic compatibility in achieving good healthcare. Therefore, enhancing provider training on cultural competence and integrating traditional health beliefs into public health campaigns could improve screening rates and broader health outcomes among NHPI populations (Willingham et al., 2024). The relationship between culture and health behaviours shows that public health should respect and include cultural aspects of communities. Participating in local practices helps health programs function more effectively and fosters trust between the community and the healthcare system. Studies have shown that public health messages that fit a community's culture encourage people to follow the recommendations. It becomes especially significant for infectious disease epidemiology, since considering culture can lower the risks of zoonotic diseases and help communities cope better with outbreaks. Emphasising culturally relevant strategies can significantly reduce barriers to healthcare access while promoting the adoption of safer health practices, ultimately contributing to improved health outcomes for diverse populations (Willingham et al., 2024; Bubpa et al., 2025) (Figure 14.7).

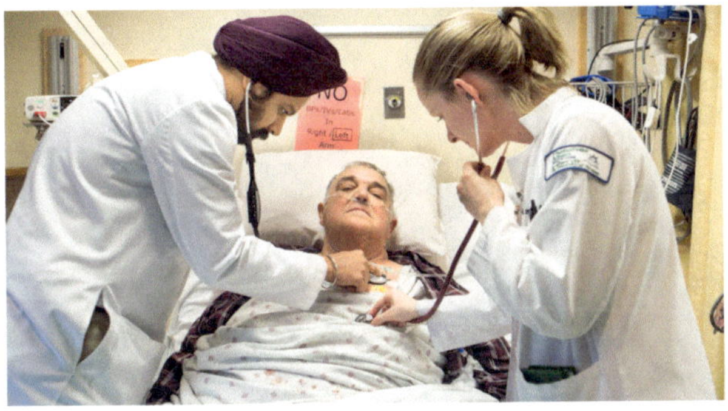

Figure 14.7. The relationship between culture and health practices.

Source: https://www.uvm.edu/publichealth/wp-content/uploads/2014/09/Diversity.jpg.

14.4.1. Cultural Beliefs and Their Impact on Health Behaviours

Cultural beliefs serve as powerful determinants of health behaviours, shaping how individuals perceive and respond to health-related issues. Such beliefs influence how a person perceives diseases, the available treatments, and methods for prevention, which can be crucial for infectious disease epidemiology. For some people, traditional ideas about illness cause them to choose alternative therapies over those supported by science. Health policymakers and public health officials need to be aware of these cultural frameworks to develop effective health education programs. Using cultural knowledge, interventions can be tailored to suit particular communities, which improves their response. In short, recognising and handling cultural ideas about health can greatly encourage people to take protective measures to stop infectious diseases, as shown in many epidemiological studies on following health recommendations. The success of health measures often depends on their acceptance within the culture, as evidenced by the behaviour of the entire population. During the recent Mpox pandemic, self-care behaviours among men who have sex with men in Brazil varied a lot because of different cultural beliefs. It was found in qualitative studies that people's beliefs about hygiene, partners and following health advice were influenced by both their own and others' beliefs. Men's efforts to lower their number of sexual partners and use protection are tied to their cultural ideas about being a man and having sex. Based on what participants shared, dealing with misinformation and relying on trust among people were key to promoting good health habits. Thus, understanding these cultural dynamics is essential for developing interventions that resonate and elicit positive behavioural change within targeted populations (Bulcão et al., 2024). Additionally, combating the stigma surrounding disease can significantly enhance health practices. In infectious disease cases, cultural views tend to influence the extent to which people practice self-care and risk avoidance. Because of the stigma around sexually transmitted infections, individuals may be reluctant to get treatment or follow prevention advice. Using Dorothea Orem's Self-Care Theory in public health enables healthcare providers to support patients by teaching them in a manner that respects their cultural background and addresses their personal concerns. This approach will enable individuals to prioritise their health and contribute to creating an environment that accepts and addresses stigma. Consequently, understanding and integrating cultural beliefs into public health strategies can create a more robust framework for enhancing health behaviors and reducing the impact of infectious diseases across diverse populations (Rodriguez-Cartes et al., 2024).

14.4.2. Stigma Associated with Certain Diseases

Stigma surrounding certain diseases significantly influences public perceptions and responses to infectious disease outbreaks. Because HIV and monkeypox are associated with particular groups, people with these diseases have often faced discrimination and isolation. Talks about the monkeypox outbreak highlighted that linking the disease to MSM led to stigmatising the disease and those who got it. Due to this stigma, it is more challenging to accurately describe disease outbreaks and prevent them. As history shows, misnaming or categorising diseases based on prevalent social beliefs can perpetuate discrimination while undermining trust in public health messaging, making it imperative for health authorities to present epidemiological data transparently and to address these societal perceptions to combat stigma (Daskalakis et al., 2022).

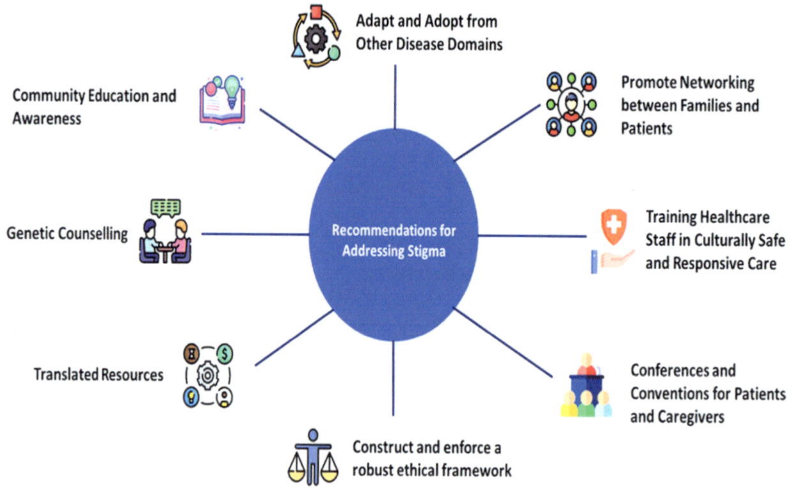

Figure 14.8. Stigma surrounding certain diseases significantly influences public perceptions and responses to infectious disease outbreaks.

Source: https://www.frontiersin.org/files/Articles/1335768/fgene-15-1335768-HTML/image_m/fgene-15-1335768-g002.jpg.

The way social, economic, and behavioural factors interact greatly influences the stigma associated with certain diseases. As an example, the COVID-19 pandemic showed that marginalised groups faced more stigma because of their links to the virus. Those who were affected by HIV/AIDS were at risk for their health and also struggled to get the treatment and help they needed because of social discrimination and fear. This problem is more noticeable in places where people already face health problems, and the way society views obesity has added to their stress and health issues. Evidence suggests that stigma exacerbates the psychosocial implications of diseases by fostering environments that discourage individuals from seeking help, thereby perpetuating cycles of illness and neglect in necessary care (Browne et al., 2020). Addressing the stigma around infectious diseases involves teaching people, encouraging advocacy, and engaging communities. Public health campaigns should be developed to address misunderstandings and clarify that everyone is at risk, not just certain groups. For example, learning from past epidemics like HIV, it becomes evident that messages should focus on bringing people together and encouraging empathy. Involving community leaders and using appropriate cultural ways to talk about stigma can encourage people to seek medical care without fearing discrimination. A collective effort toward dismantling stigma will not only enhance individuals' health outcomes but also strengthen the resilience of communities against future health crises (Browne et al., 2020; Daskalakis et al., 2022) (Figure 14.8).

14.4.3. Community Engagement and Health Promotion

Community engagement plays a pivotal role in health promotion by fostering collaboration between public health officials and community members, ultimately leading to the development of tailored interventions that address local needs. When community members are involved, they tend to trust health plans and take preventive actions. It helps make health messages more effective and also allows communities to be involved in decision-making. Additionally, community involvement helps identify factors that influence health outcomes, including the availability of healthcare services and socioeconomic issues. Talking with communities in the context of infectious disease epidemiology helps them become more aware of health risks and take steps to prevent diseases. Due to the growing issue of antimicrobial resistance, it is now more crucial than ever to engage the community in health education and promotion.

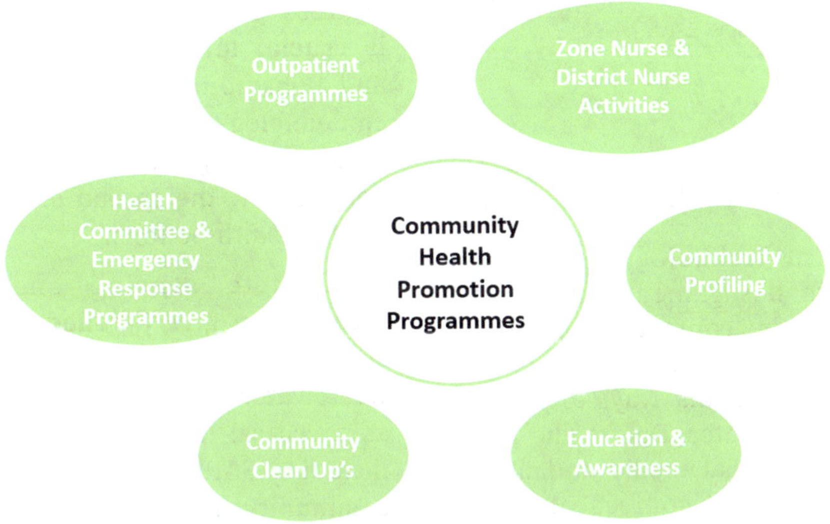

Figure 14.9. Community engagement plays a pivotal role in health promotion.

Source: https://thinkpacific.com/app/uploads/2020/06/Community-health-promotion.png.

As antimicrobial resistance (AMR) remains a pressing global health threat, understanding how community behaviours directly contribute to its propagation is essential. If people are better informed about using antibiotics appropriately, it can significantly lower the spread of resistant microbes. Salam et al. (2023) highlight the alarming rise in antimicrobial-resistant bacteria, which often originates from the inappropriate use of antibiotics in both healthcare and agricultural settings. So, programs that encourage communities to use antibiotics wisely can help address the threats from AMR. Consulting with the community can lead to educational campaigns that are more effective for the target group, ultimately improving health outcomes. Biodiversity and health also demonstrate another area where community involvement is essential. Studies show that biodiversity is vital for human health, as it supplies essential resources for medicine and enhances mental well-being. Marselle et al. (2021) elaborate on the beneficial impacts of biodiversity, such as reducing exposure to environmental pollutants and enhancing physical activity through accessible green spaces. As a result, community actions for preserving local biodiversity help the environment and also support public health by creating areas that support well-being. Involving the community in conservation allows public health organizations to use these ties to help ensure health equity and inform people about the relationship between the environment and infectious diseases. Overall, understanding these interconnected factors through community engagement is essential for effectively promoting health and preventing infectious diseases (Figure 14.9).

14.5. Role of Technology and Media

The intersection of technology and media with public health has gained prominence, particularly within the context of infectious disease epidemiology. Digital tools help to spread news about outbreaks, ways to prevent them, and the latest updates. Due to the rapid spread of COVID-19, social media and health apps have become crucial sources of timely information for many people. With these new technologies, advice on disease prevention can be shared more widely, leading people to take actions that help stop the spread of diseases. Even so, misinformation can be a significant problem, as incorrect information may cause people to panic and harm their health, which is not what public health aims to achieve. Finding ways to utilise technology for health communication that avoids misinformation remains a significant concern when attempting to achieve public health goals during outbreaks. Media platforms play a role in moulding how people perceive infectious diseases, which can change how people act and spread the disease. The presentation of health-related news on the internet or in the media may influence the community's reactions to health advisories and efforts.

Because of sensational news about COVID-19, many people may be less likely to seek care or report their symptoms. With the help of technology, especially during emergencies, public health officials can launch proactive initiatives to reduce the stigma associated with illnesses and encourage people to prioritise their health. Moreover, technology enables health authorities to quickly gauge public sentiment, which helps them tailor their messaging to address people's concerns. Being adaptable is crucial for navigating the diverse social and behavioural factors that impact disease epidemiology. In addition, technology is used for data gathering and modelling diseases, which helps follow the spread of illnesses and direct public health actions.

Remote sensing and digital health records can give detailed information on the spread and number of diseases. For instance, wastewater surveillance (WWS) has emerged as a critical method for detecting viral RNA, including SARS-CoV-2, providing insights into community infection rates beyond traditional testing boundaries (Kitajima et al., 2020). They help you understand epidemiological trends and support the planning of resources and actions. In addition, using behavioral data and technology can help public health officials see how different groups follow health warnings. As the global community navigates persistent infectious disease challenges, embracing the multifaceted capabilities of technology and media will be crucial in shaping effective public health strategies to mitigate future outbreaks (Hossain et al., 2020) (Figure 14.10).

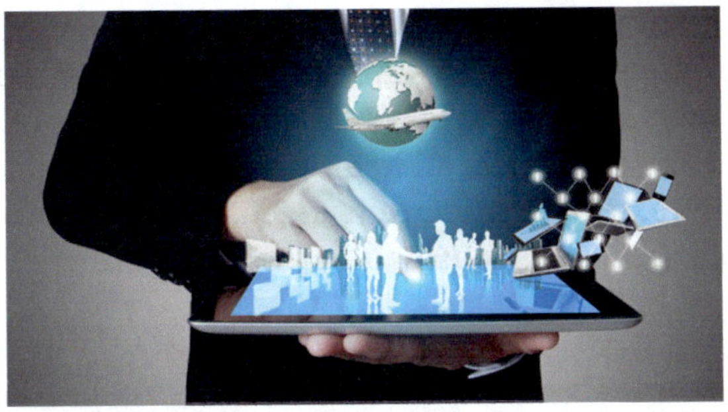

Figure 14.10. The role of technology and media with public health.

Source: https://www.alphonsolabs.com/wp-content/uploads/2017/03/Roles-Of-Technology.jpg.

14.5.1. Influence of Social Media on Public Perception

The profound impact of social media on public perception, particularly during health crises such as the COVID-19 pandemic, underscores its pivotal role in shaping collective understanding. The rapid spread of information on Twitter and Instagram has altered traditional methods of public health communication. At the onset of the COVID-19 outbreak, social media played a pivotal role in disseminating crucial health messages, facilitating discussions about the virus, and reflecting public opinion. Because misinformation is prevalent on these platforms, it has made it difficult for health authorities to disseminate accurate information. This phenomenon highlights the dual-edged nature of social media. At the same time, it can enhance awareness and mobilise communities, but it simultaneously risks perpetuating false narratives that can mislead public perception and health behaviours, as demonstrated by the findings in studies analysing social media's role during COVID-19 (Shu-Tsao et al., 2021). Additionally, data from social media platforms indicates that the process of sharing information and how the public perceives it is not straightforward. Discussing politics on Reddit and YouTube has helped spread both accurate and incorrect information, making it difficult for people to find reliable news. It appears that misinformation, originating from any source, tends to spread in a manner similar to genuine health information. It shows that likes, shares, and comments do not always help people distinguish between real and false health information, which makes it harder for them to understand and respond to health crises. As a result, the potentially harmful effects of misinformation can exacerbate public fear and anxiety, necessitating further examination of how social media shapes societal responses to infectious diseases (Cinelli et al., 2020). Additionally, social media influences public opinion by showcasing the social habits and trends prevalent in society. Online discussions and debates about health interventions, such as vaccination, often reflect the same fears, beliefs, and attitudes prevalent in society. Social media platforms not only reflect existing societal biases but also influence how people respond to health policies and advice. This interplay poses significant implications for public health strategies. It is essential to utilise these platforms in a manner that curbs the dissemination of false news and fosters the dissemination of accurate information. Achieving this balance is essential for enhancing public perception and fostering trust in health authorities during future public health emergencies, ultimately influencing the success of health interventions (Shu-Tsao et al., 2021).

14.5.2. Telehealth and Its Impact on Disease Management

The advent of telehealth has significantly transformed the landscape of disease management, particularly in the context of infectious diseases. Telehealth enables patients to consult healthcare professionals remotely, thereby overcoming common challenges associated with attending appointments, including the lack of transportation or insufficient time. It is vital for marginalised groups, since they often encounter systemic challenges in getting healthcare; the COVID-19 pandemic made these disparities clear for Latinx and Black people. Telehealth has enabled these groups to safely access healthcare providers during outbreaks, thereby improving the control of diseases. As a result, there has been a notable increase in health literacy and engagement among patients who utilise these digital platforms, paving the way for more proactive health management and preventive measures as communities adapt to evolving public health challenges (Zuluaga et al., 2023). With the development of telehealth, we must recognise its ability to help with mental health management, mainly for people who are at a higher risk of severe infectious diseases. When mental health screenings and social health factors are integrated into care models, there is a good chance that patients will experience less stress from their illness. It has been found that those with chronic conditions or increased chances of getting an infection, such as COVID-19, may have more severe mental health issues. Telehealth services offer individuals access to mental health resources, support groups, and patient navigator programs, which support both mental wellness and adherence to treatment plans. This dual approach of addressing physical and psychological health through telehealth not only enhances patient outcomes but also encourages a holistic view of health necessary for effective disease management during public health crises (N/A, 2021). In addition, telehealth raises essential topics about health equity and access issues that could persist or worsen due to digital solutions. Although telehealth is very convenient and easily accessible, it also runs the risk of leaving behind individuals who cannot use the internet or are unfamiliar with digital tools. Because health gaps in minority communities existed before the pandemic, it is vital to find ways to close the digital divide. Policies and studies in the future should focus on making telehealth resources available to all people to ensure everyone can use these new tools for managing diseases. By addressing these challenges, we can establish more resilient and inclusive healthcare systems that hold promise for improving overall health outcomes amid the complexities of infectious disease epidemiology (N/A, 2021; Zuluaga et al., 2023) (Figure 14.11).

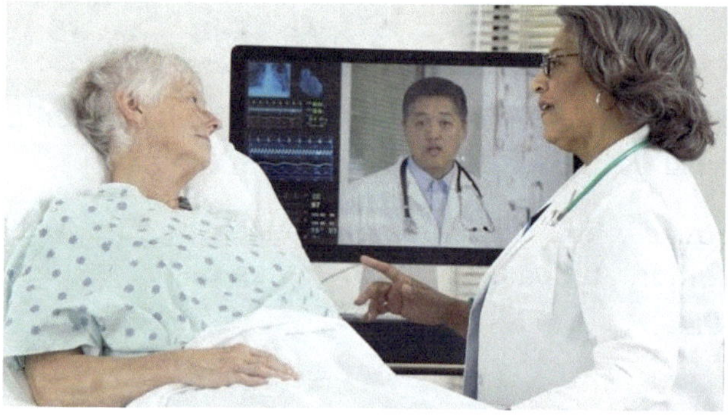

Figure 14.11. The telehealth has significantly transformed the landscape of disease management.

Source: https://www.hhmglobal.com/wp-content/uploads/news/23433/Telemedicine-696x398.jpg.

14.5.3. Misinformation and Its Consequences

In contemporary society, misinformation has become a significant factor influencing public health outcomes, particularly during infectious disease outbreaks. In Italy, during the measles outbreak, not many people chose to get vaccinated because of both doubts about vaccines and false information spread on social media. The rise in this phenomenon is attributed to people losing trust in vaccines due to the widespread dissemination of false scientific information. Due to this misinformation, communicating about health and implementing effective public health strategies becomes more challenging, highlighting the need for further education on vaccines. The intersection of misinformation with socioeconomic factors underscores the importance of addressing these issues through a holistic approach, enabling health authorities to formulate targeted strategies that promote vaccine uptake and mitigate the consequences of misinformation (Scire, 2021). It is also worrying how misinformation can affect other infectious disease outbreaks, as was the case with COVID-19. People became confused about the virus, its spread, and how to stay safe due to misinformation, leading to health disparities among various groups. Public health experts stress that inequalities should be addressed by making settings that encourage people to change their behaviours, which requires challenging false information. It is essential to engage diverse groups, including government agencies and community organisations, when creating public health messages that resonate with various audiences.

The ongoing struggle against misinformation necessitates a coordinated response that draws upon multidisciplinary perspectives, ensuring that communication strategies are tailored to the specific needs and beliefs of targeted communities (Auerbach et al., 2022). The problems caused by misinformation are not confined to individual health actions, as they can seriously affect the progress of public health. Policymakers need to realise that social factors play a significant role in how diseases like measles progress, as shown by their periodic outbreaks. Building models that relate social behaviors, actions by institutions, and misinformation helps health authorities identify the reasons for infectious disease outbreaks. Also, dealing with misinformation as a complex matter requires different experts to work together, which makes health policies more effective in stopping outbreaks. Investment in research exploring the relationship between misinformation and public health measures will be pivotal in informing future strategies designed to protect population health and support behavioral change in the face of infectious diseases (Scire, 2021) (Figure 14.12).

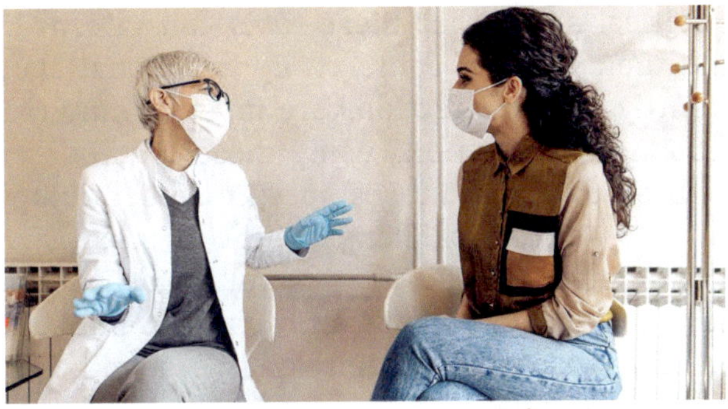

Figure 14.12. Misinformation has emerged as a critical factor influencing public health.

Source: https://www.aamc.org/sites/default/files/styles/scale_and_crop_1200_x_666/public/dear-pandemic-1200.jpg?itok=5szq6QfD.

14.6. Policy Implications and Public Health Strategies

The intricate relationship between social and behavioural factors and infectious disease epidemiology significantly shapes public health policy and strategic responses. As indicated by recent studies, psychosocial stressors, including social isolation or trauma, can adversely affect immune responses, potentially increasing susceptibility to diseases such as tuberculosis (TB). Because of this, public health policies should focus on bringing mental health and social support systems together as a means of prevention. These strategies may enhance the body's resistance to infections by promoting psychological well-being, in addition to receiving medical care. Implementing these policies can result not only in a reduction of disease incidence but also in improved health outcomes, emphasising the necessity of a comprehensive, interdisciplinary approach to infectious disease prevention (Boccia et al., 2019). Additionally, epidemiological tools are crucial in developing effective public health plans. It is clear from a critical study that these tools can inform health interventions tailored to specific populations and their cultural contexts. By using spatial analysis and serological tests, it becomes possible to identify where infections are most common and what causes them, allowing for a better focus in responses. In Zambia, using these methods enables officials to plan resources and interventions tailored to the country's specific epidemiology. It highlights the need to continually update these tools to address challenges such as insufficient resources and unreliable data. Thus, refining the methodologies used in infectious disease epidemiology plays a pivotal role in informing policy decisions that can significantly enhance public health initiatives (Arthur et al., 2023). Besides affecting health, psychosocial factors and epidemiological strategies can impact the structure of society and existing inequalities. For public health strategies to be effective, everyone should have access to healthcare, the community should be involved, and social capital should be enhanced. Policies that consider social factors are expected to be more effective in combating infectious diseases among those who are most at risk. Understanding that social context affects health means that health professionals, policymakers, and community leaders should team up. Tackling both biological and social aspects of health through initiatives helps societies create strong public health systems that can handle the challenges caused by infectious diseases. Ultimately, integrating these multifaceted approaches is essential for achieving long-term health equity and sustainability in public health policy (Boccia et al., 2019) (Figure 14.13).

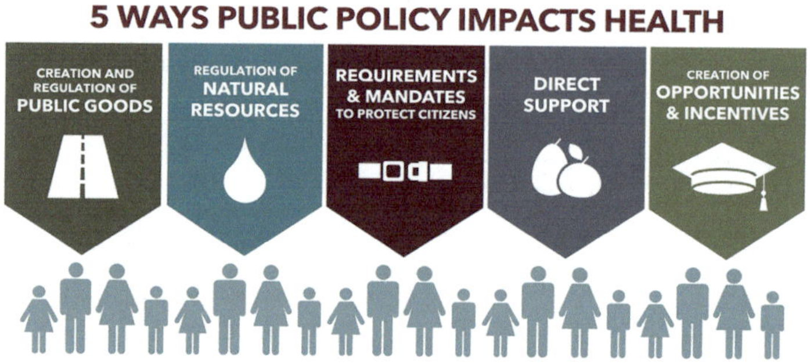

Figure 14.13. The public health policy.

Source: https://sycamoretn.org/wp-content/uploads/2017/05/5-ways-policy-impacts-health-e1532716467411.png.

14.6.1. Importance of Community-Based Interventions

Addressing the social and behavioural causes of infectious diseases is greatly helped by community-based interventions. These interventions utilise local communities' strengths to design health projects that meet the needs and culture of the people living there. This approach increases the likelihood that community members will be involved and trust the health professionals. For example, community stakeholders involved in the opioid overdose crisis found that utilising data dashboards could facilitate informed decision-making, demonstrating the importance of local input in public health strategies (Fareed et al., 2024). Getting community members involved in health discussions helps them feel responsible for their own health, which leads to better health habits and a reduced spread of infectious diseases. Additionally, community-based efforts have been shown to enhance awareness and knowledge about infectious diseases among residents in the area. A pertinent example can be seen in the efforts to combat Taeniasis/cysticercosis (TC/CC) in Bali. Community-based epidemiological surveys demonstrated that targeted interventions elevated public knowledge and behavioural changes regarding TC/CC, leading to a measurable decline in disease risk factors (Agung et al., 2024). It proves that when communities are included in the design of interventions and involved in decision-making, their health can improve significantly. Using local knowledge supports communities in making positive changes, which leads them to adopt healthier behaviours that match public health goals. This demonstrates that projects that consider community life are more likely to be successful. Such strategies also help in regularly reviewing and boosting public health initiatives. Employing frameworks such as the System Usability Scale and Technology Adoption Model, as illustrated by the Community that HEAL (CTH) initiative, enables stakeholders to assess the usability of health interventions and address gaps in their design and implementation (Fareed et al., 2024).

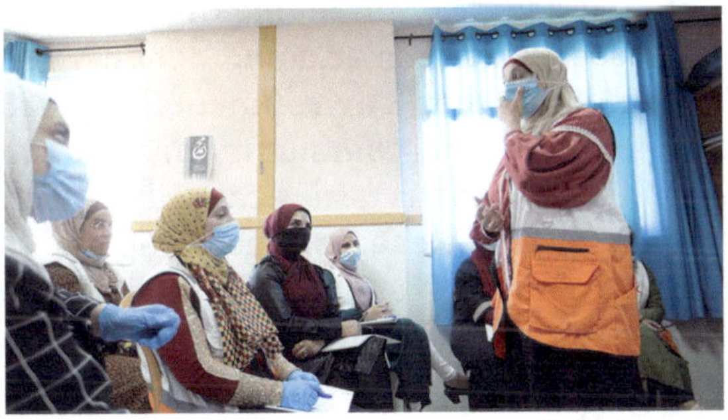

Figure 14.14. Importance of community-based interventions.

Source: https://www.palestinercs.org/public/files/image/2023/cw/Community-Based-Interventions-Program.jpg.

By repeating this process, health resources become easier to use and understand, and they also meet the changing needs of the community. When communities encourage constant feedback and adaptation, their interventions will remain up-to-date as public health evolves. Therefore, the integration of local perspectives in designing health interventions not only strengthens their impact but also embodies a proactive approach to infectious disease epidemiology, ultimately leading to healthier, more resilient communities (Figure 14.14).

14.6.2. Role of Government in Disease Prevention

The role of government in disease prevention is pivotal, particularly in the context of infectious diseases that are highly influenced by social and behavioural factors. Strong governance supports the effective use of policies that manage public health issues by utilising resources efficiently, establishing clear rules, and educating the public. crucial for this role to develop a robust public health system that provides essential services, including immunisation and disease monitoring. For example, by passing laws, the government can provide clean water, sanitary surroundings, and vaccines, all of which are crucial for preventing infectious diseases. Government programs also focus on helping groups that are at risk, such as those facing health problems caused by social factors, including income and access to healthcare. It is also clear from history that government actions significantly influence how public health responds to new health issues. As chronic diseases became more common in the United States, health officials shifted their attention to more than infectious diseases and started involving communities and promoting changes in people's behaviour. Health education has shifted to emphasise the importance of changing habits and considering the impact of one's surroundings and society. For example, the HIV epidemic caused people to reconsider public health priorities, and it showed that teaching and informing people can work better than just providing medical treatments for complex health behaviours. Efforts to combat smoking-related illnesses through legislation, taxation, and public awareness campaigns exemplify how governments can successfully influence health outcomes through collective action (Speers, 1996). Additionally, a strong government response is now considered essential for controlling and preventing the spread of infectious diseases in our global society. Due to urbanisation and increased migration across borders, diseases can now spread rapidly from one community to another and from one country to another. Therefore, creating and maintaining international partnerships and agreements is necessary to prevent diseases. Working together, governments can enhance their disease prevention efforts by following best practices and sharing their knowledge and resources. Recognizing the connection between globalization and disease trends highlights the importance of addressing social, behavioral, and environmental factors in tandem. This holistic approach aligns with recent findings indicating that addressing root causes linked to social determinants can significantly reduce vulnerability and enhance the overall health of populations (Caiaffa et al., 2011) (Figure 14.15).

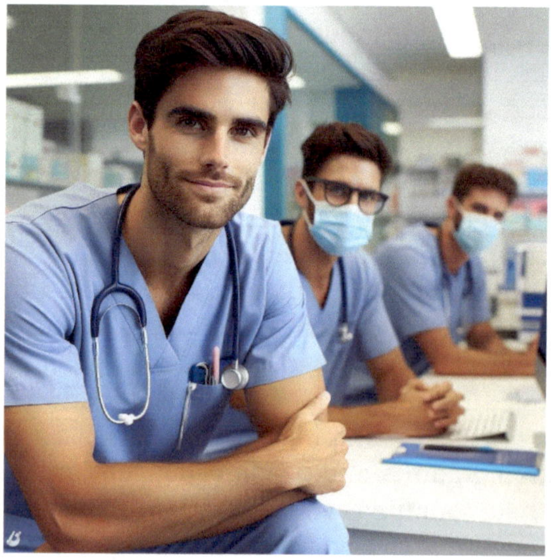

Figure 14.15. The role of government in disease prevention is pivotal.

Source: https://aussiecareerinsights.com/wp-content/uploads/2024/01/Disease-Prevention-Roles-in-Australia1.jpeg.

14.6.3. Collaboration Between Sectors for Effective Responses

Effective responses to infectious diseases necessitate collaboration between multiple sectors, recognising that the determinants of health extend beyond the traditional boundaries of healthcare. Public health agencies, government structures, non-profit groups, and private businesses should collaborate to develop a comprehensive response that considers multiple social and behavioural factors. In the field of sexual health, using a rights-based approach is now essential to deal with the spread of STIs. When human rights are included in public health and the social factors affecting health are recognised, it becomes easier to reduce stigma and discrimination, which improves access to care for groups at risk. Such collaboration ensures that interventions are not only evidence-based but also socially and culturally relevant, thus maximising their effectiveness in reducing disease prevalence (Tucker et al., 2019). Infectious disease epidemiology also benefits from intersectoral collaborations (ISCs), particularly in managing mosquito-borne diseases like malaria and dengue. These ISCs bring together environmental agencies, urban planners, and community organisations to address the various issues caused by vector-borne diseases. Research has shown that managing diseases sustainably depends on understanding the environmental, economic, and social factors that contribute to their spread. Involving the community can help ensure that insecticide-treated nets and local sanitation are implemented correctly. Initiatives such as the Kilusan Ligtas Malaria program in the Philippines serve as exemplary models of how a network of diverse sectors can synergise efforts to achieve impressive declines in malaria cases, showcasing the effectiveness of integrated strategies (Rivera et al., 2019). Because infectious diseases are complex, it is essential to address them in ways that fit each community, which makes collaboration necessary. When communities are involved in health interventions, there is more trust and easier sharing of knowledge, which helps the outcomes last longer. By leveraging the strengths of healthcare, education, and social services, it becomes possible to address both urgent health problems and the social factors behind them. This way of working helps prevent and control diseases, and it also improves health equity. Understanding how social behaviors, such as mobility and socio-economic conditions, interact with disease spread further underscores the importance of collaboration among sectors to create effective public health strategies (Rivera et al., 2019) (Figure 14.16).

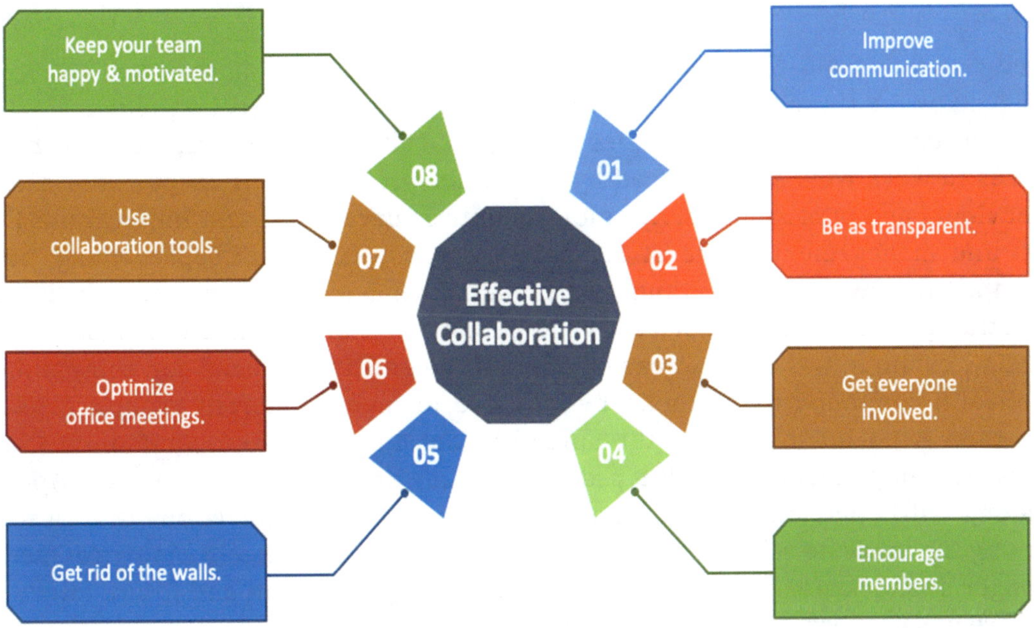

Figure 14.16. Effective responses to infectious diseases necessitate collaboration between multiple sectors.

Source: https://www.collidu.com/media/catalog/product/img/a/2/a2b441f4a674766739809c95fced97cb3b6c4d64fe2a8215872a573921952013/effective-collaboration-slide1.png.

SUMMARY

In conclusion, the role of social and behavioural factors in the epidemiology of infectious diseases is profound and multifaceted. They play a role in how diseases are spread and also how people respond to health actions. The way populations perceive risks and follow health advice is significantly influenced by social networks, culture, and behaviours. For instance, the GBD Study highlights the increasing prevalence of cardiovascular diseases, indicating a potential public health crisis that may be exacerbated by social determinants of health, such as socio-economic status, access to healthcare, and lifestyle choices related to diet and exercise (Roth et al., 2020).

Therefore, addressing these factors is essential for reducing disease and improving public health. Also, knowing these social and behavioral aspects helps in creating effective interventions. It is essential for public health strategies to respect cultural differences and the behaviours of communities to work well. As evidenced by recent analyses of COVID-19 patterns, the nuances of travel behaviours and interconnectivity among countries have significant implications for outbreak prediction and management (Tuite et al., 2020). Because diseases keep evolving, public health needs to adjust to new social situations and changing behaviours. When public health authorities use these strategies, they can better reach the public and manage infectious diseases. Ultimately, strengthening communities and increasing their involvement is crucial for combating infectious diseases. Health communication should be adjusted to match different groups, assisting people to change their behavior to prevent the spread of the disease. When communities are involved in planning and implementing health programs, trust and outcomes improve. Applying social science, along with epidemiology, will make it easier to manage infectious diseases as a whole. By leveraging the intricate relationship between social, behavioural, and biological factors, we can build stronger public health systems capable of responding to current and future infectious disease threats, thereby safeguarding global health (Roth et al., 2020).

Social and behavioural aspects have a substantial impact on the pattern of infectious diseases. The pandemic showed that individuals from low-income families and marginalised communities are more likely to suffer from health problems because they do not have enough resources and live in poor conditions. The evidence from studies shows that disaggregated data is key to designing fair health programs that address the needs of groups often overlooked in healthcare. By utilising health monitoring data, as discussed in Finnish health system case studies, one can gain a deeper understanding of and address the inequities faced by vulnerable groups, thereby improving overall health outcomes during crises such as pandemics (Tynkkynen et al., 2023). The health problems that refugees and migrants experience during migration show how critical social systems are. Many people who move to Switzerland are from parts of the world where both health conditions and medical care are unstable.

If there are no regular checks for common infectious diseases upon arrival, this can pose a threat to the health of individuals and also concern public health officials in the host nation. As evident in the health conditions reported among Eritrean refugees, many present with untreated infectious and non-communicable diseases, making early intervention crucial to protect both individual and community health (Chernet, 2018). Also, mental health and other behavioural issues are essential in determining the impact of infectious diseases on migrants. Stressful situations during migration can cause post-traumatic stress disorder, which underlines the importance of providing mental health care together with physical care. It is crucial to address these social challenges and adopt whole-person health approaches to ensure refugees and migrants have full access to healthcare. Collaborative efforts among policymakers, NGOs, and health professionals are essential to foster an equitable healthcare system, thereby minimising public health disparities and enhancing the overall well-being of immigrant communities (Chernet, 2018).

CLOSER LOOK:

LONG-LASTING SOCIAL PROBLEMS:

Long-lasting social problems are persistent issues that affect communities and societies over extended periods, often resisting simple solutions. These problems—such as poverty, inequality, discrimination, and inadequate access to education or healthcare—have deep-rooted causes and wide-ranging consequences. Understanding their complexity is essential for designing effective policies and interventions that can bring about meaningful and sustainable change. Poverty is one of the most pervasive social problems worldwide. It limits access to basic necessities like food, clean water, shelter, and healthcare, creating cycles of hardship that can span generations. Closely related is economic inequality, where wealth and resources are concentrated in the hands of a few, leaving large segments of the population marginalized. Both poverty and inequality contribute to social instability, poor health outcomes, and limited opportunities for upward mobility.

Discrimination based on race, gender, religion, or other characteristics is another long-lasting social issue. Systemic discrimination not only denies individuals equal opportunities but also perpetuates social divisions and fosters exclusion. For example, marginalized communities often face barriers to education, employment, and political participation, which reinforce cycles of disadvantage and limit social cohesion.

Access to quality education and healthcare is also a persistent challenge in many regions. Unequal educational opportunities can prevent individuals from developing skills needed to participate fully in society, while inadequate healthcare systems lead to preventable diseases and reduced life expectancy. These disparities often intersect with poverty and discrimination, compounding the impact on vulnerable populations. Addressing long-lasting social problems requires a multifaceted approach. Policy interventions must tackle both immediate needs—such as food security or healthcare access—and the underlying structural causes, like unequal distribution of resources or discriminatory practices. Community engagement, public awareness campaigns, and social programs can empower individuals and promote social inclusion. Additionally, international cooperation and sustainable development strategies are vital for addressing global challenges such as poverty, migration, and environmental injustice.

Technological advancements and data-driven approaches are increasingly being used to identify and target social problems more effectively. For instance, social surveys, geographic mapping, and predictive analytics can help policymakers understand where interventions are most needed and assess their impact over time.

In conclusion, long-lasting social problems are complex and deeply embedded in society. Successfully addressing them requires comprehensive, sustained efforts that combine policy reform, community engagement, and innovative solutions. By tackling both the symptoms and root causes, societies can create more equitable, resilient, and inclusive communities for future generations.

REFERENCES

1. Sudewi, A. a. R., Swastika, K., Sudarmaja, I. M., Wulanyani, N. M. S., Dharmawan, N. S., Wirawan, I. M. A., Kumbara, A. a. N. A., Pramitasuri, T. I., Karang, A. a. a. S. I., & Susilawathi, N. N. M. (2024). One health approach for taeniasis/cysticercosis control measure in Bali, Indonesia: updated situations, implementations, and challenges. *Bali Medical Journal, 13*(1), 709–714. https://doi.org/10.15562/bmj.v13i1.4982Aprillia, Y. T., Adawiyah, A. R., Ambarwati, K., & Tenrilemba, F. (2024). Factors associated with breastfeeding self-efficacy and COVID-19 pandemic anxiety in postpartum mothers. *Jurnal Kesehatan Masyarakat*. https://www.semanticscholar.org/paper/485f425f53595c6aef0af183b65940b8645b1e25 (accessed on 30th May 2025).
2. Arthur, C., Banda, H., Chazya, R., Chijoka, et al. (2023). Epidemiological tools in focus: A comprehensive assessment of their role in addressing infectious disease challenges in Zambia. Journal for Research in Applied Sciences and Biotechnology. https://core.ac.uk/download/597862448.pdf (accessed on 30th May 2025).
3. Auerbach, J. D., Davey, C., Forsyth, A. D., Hargreaves, et al. (2022). Living with COVID-19 and preparing for future pandemics: Revisiting lessons from the HIV pandemic. *Lancet HIV*. https://core.ac.uk/download/552461338.pdf (accessed on 30th May 2025).
4. Belton, C., Lavin, C., Lunn, P., McGowan, et al. (2020). *Using Behavioral Science to Help Fight the Coronavirus (ESRI Working Paper No. 656, March 2020)*. https://core.ac.uk/download/288435971.pdf (accessed on 30th May 2025).
5. Bibbins-Domingo, K. (2020). This time must be different: Disparities during the COVID-19 pandemic. *Annals of Internal Medicine, 173*, 233–234. https://doi.org/10.7326/m20-2247.
6. Boccia, D., Dowd, J. B., Fletcher, H., Hayward, et al. (2019). A systematic review of the impact of psychosocial factors on immunity: Implications for enhancing BCG response against tuberculosis. SSM – Population Health. https://core.ac.uk/download/286270876.pdf (accessed on 30th May 2025).
7. Boni, M. F., & Delabouglise, A. (2019). Game theory of vaccination and depopulation for managing livestock diseases and zoonoses on small-scale farms. *Epidemics*. https://core.ac.uk/download/268904901.pdf (accessed on 30th May 2025).
8. Browne, N. T., Snethen, J., Greenberg, C. S., Frenn, M., Kilanowski, J. F., Gance-Cleveland, B., Burke, P. J., et al. (2020). When pandemics collide: The impact of COVID-19 on childhood obesity. *Journal of Pediatric Nursing, 56*, 90–98. https://doi.org/10.1016/j.pedn.2020.11.004.
9. Bubpa, N., Suwannarong, K., Thammasutti, K., Ponlap, T., Thongkan, W., Boonyakawee, P., Kanthawee, P., et al. (2025). Cultural practices, healthcare-seeking behaviors, and wildlife interface: Zoonotic disease risks among the Phu Thai ethnic group in Thailand. *Veterinary World*. https://www.semanticscholar.org/paper/93cea2f53117a21218a11c9eae5fda89d16c1ece (accessed on 30th May 2025).
10. Bulcão, C. Da. S., Prates, P. E. G., Pedrosa, I., De Santana, S. G. R., De Oliveira, L. B., De Souza, J. J., De Almeida, L. C. G., et al. (2024). Exploring self-care practices and health beliefs among men in the context of emerging infectious diseases: Lessons from the Mpox pandemic in Brazil. *Nursing Inquiry*. https://www.semanticscholar.org/paper/15b6c5cd8425a350fa64e3ecefedc94b08cab388 (accessed on 30th May 2025).

11. Caiaffa, W., & Rossi, D. (2011). Viral hepatitis and vulnerability among cocaine users in South America. *Cadernos de Saude Publica, 27*(9), 1664, 1665. https://www.semanticscholar.org/paper/5225031f470ace635b9e6b69b67732a1954d08a0 (accessed on 30th May 2025).

12. Chernet, A. (2018). Infectious and non-communicable health conditions among newly arrived Eritrean migrants and refugees at arrival and post integration in Switzerland. https://www.semanticscholar.org/paper/c0d0a5c4c19e9eaf1a0c38fc470a799d53c3c9c4 (accessed on 30th May 2025).

13. Cinelli, M., Quattrociocchi, W., Galeazzi, A., Valensise, C. M., Brugnoli, E., Schmidt, A. L., Zola, P., et al. (2020). The COVID-19 social media infodemic. *Scientific Reports, 10*. https://doi.org/10.1038/s41598-020-73510-5.

14. Cluj-Napoca, challenge of., Société Française, Robert, 23 EB Van 1, Keskimäki, L. K., Tynkkynen, et al. (2023). Power and politics of health system data: How data shape responses and equity during pandemics. *The European Journal of Public Health, 33*. https://www.semanticscholar.org/paper/d6dd3f2ceeb49d92b596991dd84ceac0398d38d9 (accessed on 30th May 2025).

15. Darukaradhya, T. B., & Jayanna, K. (2024). Development of a health promotion intervention in managing behavioral risk factors for non-communicable diseases in adolescents: An intervention mapping approach. *Journal of the Epidemiology Foundation of India*. https://www.semanticscholar.org/paper/0e89774d5fcd77ad976ca40567b68010b166190b (accessed on 30th May 2025).

16. Daskalakis, D., McClung, R. P., Mena, L., Mermin, J., McQuiston, J. H., Damon, I. K., Monroe, B., et al. (2022). Monkeypox: Avoiding the mistakes of past infectious disease epidemics. *Annals of Internal Medicine, 175*, 1177, 1178. https://doi.org/10.7326/m22-1748.

17. Dean, H., & Fenton, K. (2010). Addressing social determinants of health in the prevention and control of HIV/AIDS, viral hepatitis, sexually transmitted infections, and tuberculosis. *Public Health Reports, 125*, 1–5. https://www.semanticscholar.org/paper/a98036d476ced2936f862a97f0f5bb394eedf17d (accessed on 30th May 2025).

18. Fareed, N., Olvera, R. G., Wang, Y., Hayes, M., Larimore, E., Balvanz, P., Langley, R., et al. (2024). Lessons learned from developing dashboards to support decision-making for community opioid response by community stakeholders: Mixed methods and multisite study. *JMIR Human Factors, 11*. https://www.semanticscholar.org/paper/a30f96296d2526fbda0668e81ed4b7153505166f (accessed on 30th May 2025).

19. Gausman, J., & Langer, A. (2020). Sex and gender disparities in the COVID-19 pandemic. *Journal of Women's Health, 29*, 465, 466. https://doi.org/10.1089/jwh.2020.8472.

20. Hayashi, M. A. L. (2016). Integrating mathematical models of behavior and infectious disease: Applications to outbreak dynamics and control. http://deepblue.lib.umich.edu/bitstream/2027.42/133434/1/mhayash_1.pdf (accessed on 30th May 2025).

21. Herval, Á. M., & de Mello Rode, S. (2018). Advances required for epidemiological studies. *Journal of Oral Research, 7*, 166, 167. https://www.semanticscholar.org/paper/b27212660f7060861bc88510c3f708fd8b3f5085 (accessed on 30th May 2025).

22. Hossain, M. M., Tasnim, S., Sultana, A., Faizah, F., Mazumder, H., Zou, L., McKyer, E. L. J., et al. (2020). Epidemiology of mental health problems in COVID-19: A review. *F1000Research, 9*, 636. https://doi.org/10.12688/f1000research.24457.1.

23. Hoye, B., & Fenton, A. (2018). Animal host–microbe interactions. *The Journal of Animal Ecology, 87*(2), 315–319. https://www.semanticscholar.org/paper/f611f6990ab09370893b9f03a35dc54cf35c223e (accessed on 30th May 2025).

24. Imamura, T., Saito, T., & Oshitani, H. (2020). Roles of public health centers and cluster-based approach for COVID-19 response in Japan. *Health Security, 19*, 229–231. https://doi.org/10.1089/hs.2020.0159.

25. Kerr, C. C., Stuart, R. M., Mistry, D., Abeysuriya, R., Rosenfeld, K., Hart, G. R., Núñez, R. C., et al. (2021). Covasim: An agent-based model of COVID-19 dynamics and interventions. *PLoS Computational Biology, 17*, e1009149. https://doi.org/10.1371/journal.pcbi.1009149.

26. Kitajima, M., Ahmed, W., Bibby, K., Carducci, A., Gerba, C. P., Hamilton, K. A., Haramoto, E., et al. (2020). SARS-CoV-2 in wastewater: State of the knowledge and research needs. *The Science of The Total Environment, 739*, 139076. https://doi.org/10.1016/j.scitotenv.2020.139076.

27. LeBreche, A., Lenihan, D. P., & Sewell, R. (2009). *Health Report*. https://core.ac.uk/download/71346006.pdf (accessed on 30th May 2025).

28. Lee, E., & Kang, J. H. (2023). Influences of COVID-19 knowledge, eHealth literacy, COVID-19 literacy, and social support on COVID-19 preventive behaviors among foreign students in Korea. *Journal of Korean Academy of Fundamentals of Nursing*. https://www.semanticscholar.org/paper/9346145c169cfeeec90fafa1a22352e37ddf345b (accessed on 30th May 2025).

29. Marselle, M., Hartig, T., Cox, D. T. C., De Bell, S., Knapp, S., Lindley, S., Triguero-Mas, M., et al. (2021). Pathways linking biodiversity to human health: A conceptual framework. *Environment International, 150*, 106420. https://doi.org/10.1016/j.envint.2021.106420.

30. N/A. (2021). Interventions to support mental health among those with health conditions that present risk for severe infection from coronavirus disease 2019 (COVID-19): A scoping review of English and Chinese-language literature. *Int. J. Environ. Res. Public Health*. https://core.ac.uk/download/479112532.pdf (accessed on 30th May 2025).

31. Pilusa, T. D., Ntimana, C., & Maimela, E. (2025). The prevalence and behavioral risk factors contributing to non-communicable diseases in Bushbuckridge, Mpumalanga Province, South Africa. *Frontiers in Epidemiology, 5*. https://www.semanticscholar.org/paper/3cdd0cff07161a252f94b0b882b74dda5a4c8460 (accessed on 30th May 2025).

32. Qin, X., & Song, L. (2021). Addressing stigma in the context of the coronavirus disease 2019 (COVID-19) outbreak: A socio-ecological approach. *Infection Control and Hospital Epidemiology*. https://www.semanticscholar.org/paper/9d7855c3c1437edb2c3159f9a8d46afb9e4cb920 (accessed on 30th May 2025).

33. Rivera, P. T. (2019). Editorial. *Acta Medica Philippina*. https://www.semanticscholar.org/paper/1298c02e8e9d93394e234b86530a064ecfd54ffd (accessed on 30th May 2025).

34. Rodriguez-Cartes, S. A., Mayorga, M. E., Özaltin, O. Y., & Swann, J. L. (2024). Incorporating face mask usage in agent-based models using personal beliefs and perceptions: An application of the Health Belief Model. *2024 Winter Simulation Conference (WSC)*. https://www.semanticscholar.org/paper/22670921cdd2966e1ded37bc764eea83350dc4bc (accessed on 30th May 2025).

35. Roth, G. A., Mensah, G. A., Johnson, C. O., Addolorato, G., Ammirati, E., Baddour, L. M., Barengo, N. C., et al. (2020). Global burden of cardiovascular diseases and risk factors, 1990–2019. *Journal of the American College of Cardiology, 76*, 2982–3021. https://doi.org/10.1016/j.jacc.2020.11.010.

36. Ruden, V. (2024). Level of awareness managers of medical institutions and health care bodies of Lviv Oblast regarding the theoretical foundations of non-infectious diseases (according to the results of a sociological study). *Lviv Clinical Bulletin*. https://www.semanticscholar.org/paper/4c0c86c4e2d2244c017f92bb83fd16bde457e42c (accessed on 30th May 2025).

37. Salam, M. A., Al-Amin, M. Y., Salam, M. T., Pawar, J. S., Akhter, N., Rabaan, A. A., Alqumber, M. A. A. (2023). Antimicrobial resistance: A growing serious threat for global public health. *Healthcare, 11*, 1946. https://doi.org/10.3390/healthcare11131946.

38. Sattar, N., McInnes, I. B., & McMurray, J. J. V. (2020). Obesity is a risk factor for severe COVID-19 infection. *Circulation, 142*, 4–6. https://doi.org/10.1161/circulationaha.120.047659.

39. Sawers, L., & Stillwaggon, E. (2018). *Understanding HIV/AIDS in the African Context*. https://cupola.gettysburg.edu/cgi/viewcontent.cgi?article=1030&context=econfac (accessed on 30th May 2025).

40. Scirè, G. (2021). *Modeling and Assessing Public Health Policies to Counteract Italian Measles Outbreaks*. https://core.ac.uk/download/479995892.pdf (accessed on 30th May 2025).

41. Sharma, D., & Kumar, S. (2023). A call for greater participation of academia in public health. *The Indian Journal of Surgery*. https://www.semanticscholar.org/paper/53f3452f15b29ef2eba9f5f972d97943cd107105 (accessed on 30th May 2025).

42. Somekh, I., Somech, R., Pettoello-Mantovani, M., & Somekh, E. (2020). Changes in routine pediatric practice in light of coronavirus 2019 (COVID-19). *The Journal of Pediatrics, 224*, 190–193. https://doi.org/10.1016/j.jpeds.2020.05.053.

43. Speers, M. (1996). Encouraging trends in health promotion in the United States. *Health Promotion International, 11*, 69–72. https://www.semanticscholar.org/paper/fa10a1cc2631f427a6051741b2f68bd48e6b3273 (accessed on 30th May 2025).

44. Tsao, S. F., Chen, H., Tisseverasinghe, T., Yang, Y., Li, L., & Butt, Z. A. (2021). What social media told us in the time of COVID-19: A scoping review. *The Lancet Digital Health, 3*, e175–e194. https://doi.org/10.1016/s2589-7500(20)30315-0.

45. Tucker, J., Meier, B., Devoto, C., Szunyogová, E., & Baral, S. (2019). Sexual health and human rights: Protecting rights to promote health. *BMC Infectious Diseases, 19*. https://www.semanticscholar.org/paper/726f9df022e74ce2aaf52ca066453e61fd581d8b (accessed on 30th May 2025).

46. Tuite, A. R., Bogoch, I. I., Sherbo, R., Watts, A., Fisman, D. N., & Khan, K. (2020). Estimation of coronavirus disease 2019 (COVID-19) burden and potential for international dissemination of infection from Iran. *Annals of Internal Medicine, 172*, 699–701. https://doi.org/10.7326/m20-0696.

47. Wagner, C., Prentice, J. A., Saad-Roy, C., Yang, L., Grenfell, B., Levin, S., & Laxminarayan, R. (2020). Economic and behavioral influencers of vaccination and antimicrobial use. *Frontiers in Public Health, 8*. https://www.semanticscholar.org/paper/f0db9d81e18bfa175969a27c67476b0c92be0e8e (accessed on 30th May 2025).

48. Willingham, M., Cassel, K. D., Zhang, W., Diaz, T., Sy, A., Pagano, I., Ta'afaki, M. R., et al. (2024). Abstract PR012: Social and structural influences of preventive cancer screenings for Native Hawaiian and Pacific Islander adults in Hawai'i. *Cancer Epidemiology, Biomarkers & Prevention*. https://www.semanticscholar.org/paper/9653fd4f25ec31fc3301ccc14928aee9a

Chapter 15

HEALTHCARE SYSTEMS AND INFECTIOUS DISEASE CONTROL

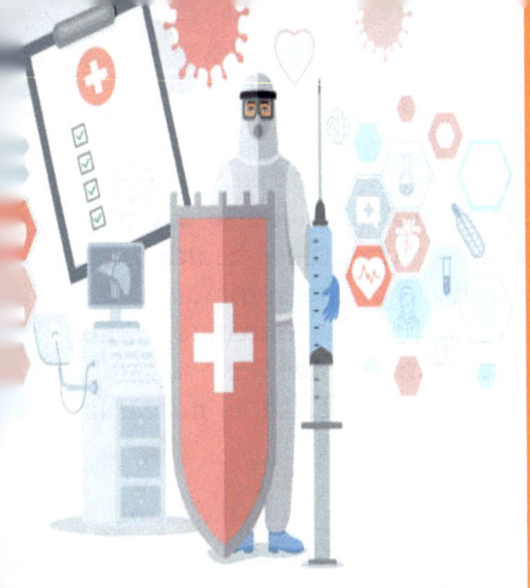

Contents

Introduction

The complexities of healthcare systems play a pivotal role in the management and control of infectious diseases. Understanding these systems helps you see how they affect public health. Healthcare systems are effective when they utilise policies, monitoring, and treatment plans in conjunction. All of these elements are crucial for achieving the goal of preventing the spread of infections, such as tuberculosis and other emerging health risks. Research suggests that clear policy recommendations, particularly in LMICs, are crucial for enhancing healthcare delivery and preventing disease outbreaks (Aarestrup et al., 2015). As antimicrobial resistance becomes increasingly severe worldwide, it is now more important than ever to have complete healthcare systems. Infectious diseases, particularly those caused by drug-resistant pathogens like multidrug-resistant tuberculosis (MDR-TB), pose significant public health challenges worldwide. The rise of such diseases can be attributed to various factors, including inadequate healthcare infrastructure, insufficient funding, and lack of public awareness

(Gamon et al., 2013). India demonstrates how healthcare systems ought to be strengthened quickly to address the problems of chronic and infectious diseases. Countries need to establish robust monitoring systems and promote early detection to manage and control these health crises effectively. In addition, using treatment programs that match the culture of the community can help people adhere to treatment and understand their health, resulting in better outcomes. Since healthcare policies and infectious disease control are so linked, different sectors need to cooperate. A One Health approach, which considers human, animal, and environmental health, is necessary for creating strategies that address the many aspects of infectious diseases.

Enhanced collaboration among healthcare providers, government agencies, and communities can support initiatives for improved public health programs, particularly in countries with under-resourced healthcare systems (Aarestrup et al., 2015). Given the challenges of managing disease, using standard assessments to evaluate the effectiveness of policies becomes vital. The ongoing development of responsive healthcare frameworks not only addresses existing health threats but also prepares systems for future challenges by fostering resilience and adaptability in the face of evolving pathogens (Figure 15.1).

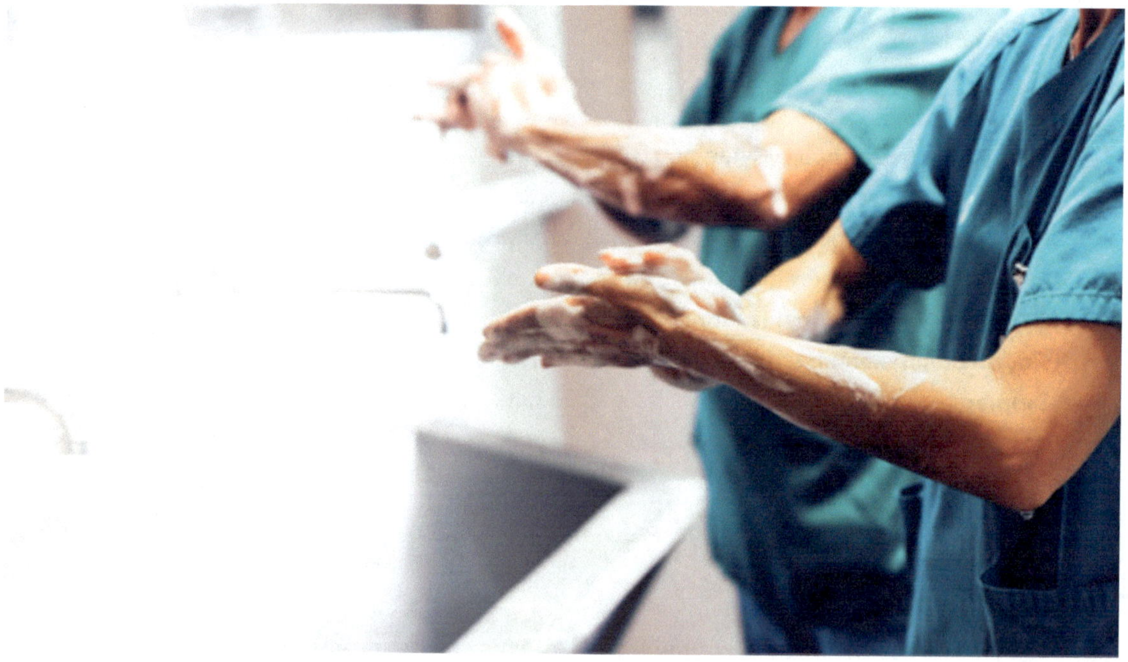

Figure 15.1. The complexities of healthcare systems.

Source: https://o.quizlet.com/GfY64But60JakB3eLpW-nQ_b.png.

Definition of Healthcare Systems

Healthcare systems encompass a complex network of organisations, institutions, and resources that deliver health care services to populations. It comprises hospitals, clinics, preventive health services, primary care, and public health initiatives. A healthcare system aims to improve health for everyone, ensuring that care is accessible, of high quality, and equitable for all. Because infectious diseases continue to be a problem, healthcare systems are more critical than ever in carrying out effective surveillance and response. For instance, the integration of technology, such as Artificial Neural Networks (ANNs), into healthcare management demonstrates how modern systems can adapt rapidly to the fluctuating demands of infectious disease control, significantly improving resource allocation and patient outcomes (Mothilal et al., 2023). The ability of healthcare systems to identify and address new health issues is crucial to their effectiveness. This includes the adoption of standardised classifications such as the International Classification of Diseases (ICD), which facilitates systematic tracking of diseases, including novel infectious ones. The introduction of codes like U09.9 for post-acute sequelae of COVID-19 (PASC) illustrates how healthcare systems can evolve to meet new clinical realities. It aids in epidemiology and also guides doctors in treating and managing patients with COVID-19 symptoms, thereby improving care and optimising resource utilisation.

As evidence from various healthcare systems indicates, the variable positive predictive value (PPV) of the U09.9 code highlights the necessity for precise operational definitions, ensuring accurate identification and treatment of patients (Zhang et al., 2023). Besides treating infections, healthcare systems focus on preventing them and teaching the public about prevention. Utilising vaccination and education for health is crucial for a comprehensive healthcare system aimed at reducing the incidence of infectious diseases. The ability of systems to adjust to new health problems encourages action ahead of outbreaks and allows them to respond and limit the damage quickly. Working together with governments, healthcare providers, and community organisations, healthcare systems can become more resistant to infectious diseases. It is critical to understand and define these systems because they provide care and also help guide public health policies and strategies as infectious diseases change.

Importance of Infectious Disease Control

The control of infectious diseases is crucial in ensuring public health and safety, particularly within healthcare systems. Communities can be severely affected by infectious diseases, which often result in more cases of sickness and death. Besides, they consume a significant amount of healthcare resources, which can cause the system to become overloaded during epidemics. The emergence of the novel coronavirus SARS-CoV-2 has underscored the need for robust measures to control diseases. The world's response to COVID-19 demonstrates that a well-structured approach to observing, reporting, and acting early on diseases is necessary to prevent infections from spreading. This not only saves lives but also maintains the functionality of healthcare systems by preventing surges in patient volume that can lead to system breakdowns and reduced care quality (Colavita et al., 2020). Infectious disease control is closely tied to the idea of being ready for public health emergencies. Strong health systems employ methods that prioritise prevention, education, and making resources accessible to respond to outbreaks promptly. The pandemic made it clear that global health systems depend on and support local community health efforts. Vaccination programs, travel restrictions, and public health information are essential for combating infectious diseases. When communities are involved in learning about health, they understand why hygiene and vaccination matter, and the number of contagious diseases can decrease a lot. Hence, developing and implementing robust public health policies is essential for nurturing a culture of health awareness and resilience in the face of infectious threats (Dewey et al., 2020). Additionally, it is essential for different experts to collaborate to fight infectious diseases. Working together, healthcare providers, government agencies, and community organizations are key to facing outbreaks successfully. Sharing information and resources helps healthcare systems react quickly to new infectious diseases. As an example, during the COVID-19 pandemic, sharing information among different countries allowed for the fast creation of diagnostic tests and vaccines. Additionally, teaching healthcare workers to recognise and treat infectious diseases enables prompt and informed responses. Incorporating the **one health approach**, which recognizes the link between human, animal, and environmental health, further emphasizes the need for comprehensive strategies. Consequently, investing in disease control not only protects public health but also fortifies the entire healthcare infrastructure against future outbreaks (Colavita et al., 2020) (Figure 15.2).

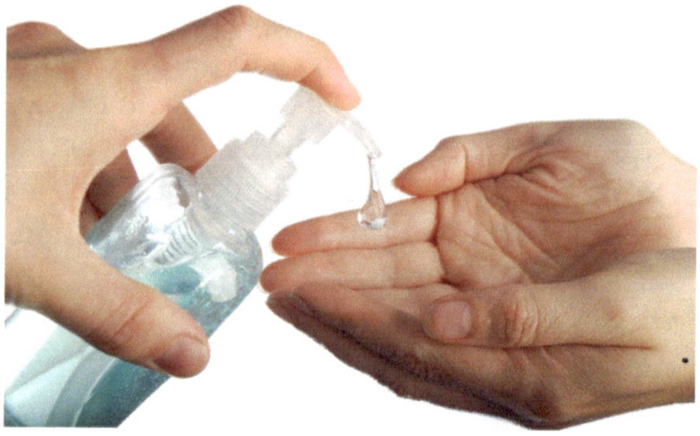

Figure 15.2. Importance of infectious disease control.

Source: https://www.firstaidforfree.com/wp-content/uploads/2015/02/Infection-Control-First-Aid.jpg.

Overview of the Relationship Between Healthcare Systems and Disease Management

The intricate connection between healthcare systems and disease management is underscored by the necessity of having robust infrastructure and protocols in place to combat infectious diseases. Surveillance, prevention, and treatment of disease are made possible by the strong healthcare systems in place. For example, the emergence of COVID-19 in 2020 demonstrated that healthcare services struggle when faced with unexpected diseases. In South Korea, for instance, managers and practitioners involved in the response to COVID-19 experienced considerable confusion due to insufficient preparation and a lack of clear guidelines, which further intensified during this health crisis (Pyo et al., 2025). Because of these inefficiencies, it was clear that healthcare systems should focus on regular training and set up clear ways to communicate, which would help them deal with infectious disease outbreaks more effectively. Additionally, research in African countries has demonstrated that the connection between healthcare systems and disease management is crucial in areas with limited resources. The research introduced an econometric model that analyzes what affects malaria mortality, proving that healthcare resources and disease outcomes are linked. Notably, the number of healthcare professionals, hospital beds, and confirmed disease cases plays a crucial role in managing infectious diseases such as malaria and tuberculosis (Kostyrin et al., 2025). The study reveals that inadequate healthcare infrastructure contributes to challenges in disease control and increased mortality, underscoring the importance of ongoing support for healthcare systems. Addressing these structural issues is crucial in managing diseases and promoting public health. In short, understanding the relationship between healthcare systems and disease management enables more effective responses to infectious diseases. It is essential for government bodies, healthcare workers, and public health organisations to work together to support existing systems and put in place new strategies to be ready for epidemics. What healthcare has learned from previous infectious disease outbreaks can be applied to future policies and practices to strengthen the system. As evidenced by the personnel's reflections in Ulsan, South Korea, the pressing need for comprehensive training, adequate resource allocation, and proactive policy development must be prioritised to mitigate the adverse effects of infectious diseases and improve health outcomes for populations at risk (Pyo et al., 2025). As global health evolves, improving the interaction between healthcare systems and disease management is crucial.

15.1. Types of Healthcare Systems

The structure of healthcare systems globally is diverse, significantly impacting their efficacy in managing infectious diseases. In general, healthcare systems are organized into public, private and mixed types. The government primarily finances and operates public healthcare, providing services to everyone, typically with little to no fee. The goal of this model is to focus on universal healthcare and fairness, which is essential for containing infectious diseases, as evidenced by effective vaccination and health programs. For example, countries with sound public health systems tend to respond more quickly to outbreaks because their systems are organized centrally. Private healthcare systems can enhance care and utilise modern technologies, but they often make it more challenging for vulnerable individuals to access care during infectious disease outbreaks. Many countries are now using mixed healthcare systems, which try to provide both access and good quality care. In such systems, people can use public services for basic needs and look for private care when they need something specific or quicker. Working together in this way enables healthcare to address public health crises more effectively, as was seen during the COVID-19 pandemic. A mixed system could speed up vaccine distribution by using private healthcare providers and have public health agencies oversee outbreak management. Still, difficulties exist, mainly in ensuring that private providers adhere to national public health standards, which is crucial for the effective control of infectious diseases. Besides these parts, the way healthcare is regulated and how it is funded also play a significant role in how effective the system is. Countries that focus on healthcare infrastructure and regulations are usually better prepared for infectious disease outbreaks. Research has shown that strong healthcare systems, supported by adequate funding and effective management, can effectively allocate resources during health emergencies. If there is not enough money for surveillance, it can lead to a failure to respond to outbreaks, which allows infectious diseases to spread rapidly. Moreover, studies show that regions with substantial health data collection and reporting systems can identify and respond to infectious disease threats more swiftly, minimizing their societal impact (Murray et al., 2022). As nations continue to adapt to emerging health challenges, understanding the interplay between healthcare system types and infectious disease control remains paramount (Harrison et al., 2020) (Figure 15.3).

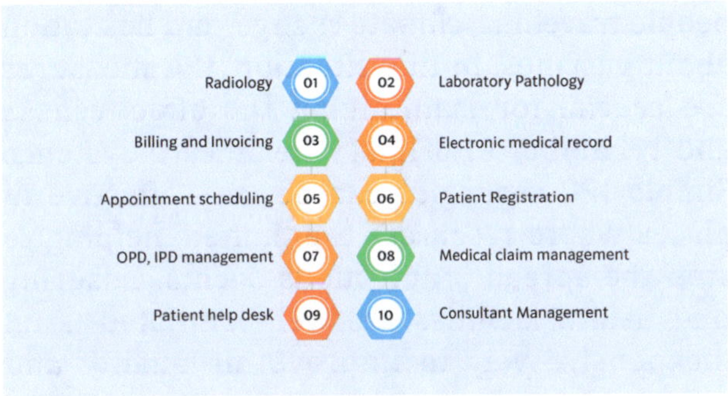

Figure 15.3. Types of healthcare systems.

Source: https://blogimages.softwaresuggest.com/blog/wp-content/uploads/2020/03/23115716/Types-of-Health-Information-Technology-Healthcare-Software-System_02-777x420.png.

15.1.1. Public Healthcare Systems

Public healthcare systems play a crucial role in managing infectious diseases, particularly in resource-constrained settings. Public health systems can utilise their services to monitor, identify, and control outbreaks before they spread widely. These systems improve when different types of data are combined, as mentioned by the need to focus on monitoring risks linked to exposure, disease, or death. It is important in cases where testing and diagnosis are limited, which may delay a response. Utilising electronic medical records and surveillance systems enables public health authorities to gather additional intelligence that supports facility-based surveillance. This integration not only enhances the ability to predict potential outbreaks but also aids in the targeted allocation of resources to high-risk populations, which is crucial for effective epidemic preparedness and response (Ingelbeen et al., 2025). Additionally, the situation with infectious diseases can be influenced by the constant changes in healthcare challenges, such as environmental shifts and changes in human behaviour. Public healthcare systems need to respond to dangers caused by more people travelling, climate change, and hesitation about vaccines. In this situation, IPC measures are crucial for maintaining the effectiveness and reliability of primary healthcare systems. Simple IPC strategies can be very effective in places where resources are limited, helping to stop the spread of infectious agents. Ensuring that health facilities are well-ventilated is an inexpensive way to improve air quality and reduce the risk of airborne infections. These adaptations not only protect patients and healthcare workers but also build resilience within the healthcare system to better handle future epidemics and health crises (Crews et al., 2024). In addition, the fact that infectious diseases affect marginalized communities more strongly shows the importance of equal access to public healthcare. In many cases, inadequate healthcare and poverty together increase the adverse effects of epidemics on vulnerable people. Inclusivity should be the primary goal in public healthcare strategies for disease prevention and control so that all people can access the proper care when needed. Concentrating on community-based health efforts enables public health authorities to support the most vulnerable individuals. Additionally, investing in infrastructure and training for healthcare workers can enhance the effectiveness of these systems and foster a proactive approach to managing infectious diseases. This holistic focus on equity not only maximizes the positive impact of public healthcare systems but also strengthens the public health response necessary for maintaining the health of populations at large (Crews et al., 2024; Ingelbeen et al., 2025) (Figure 15.4).

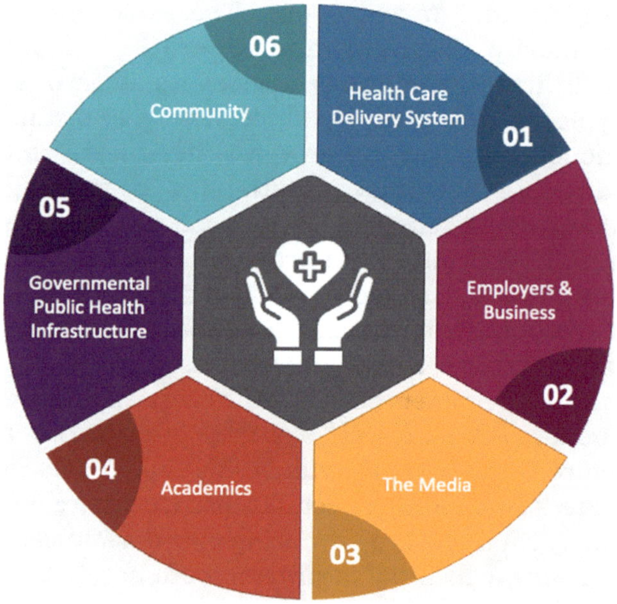

Figure 15.4. The Public healthcare systems.

Source: https://www.collidu.com/media/catalog/product/img/d/7/d7a8b2ed3478aa38ab3a823ac7 eed1ace4854 00ede4cf65d201191e72d7a42c6/public-health-systems-slide1.png.

15.1.2. Private Healthcare Systems

Private healthcare systems play a crucial role in managing infectious disease control, particularly in countries where public health infrastructure is limited. These systems typically enable individuals to access medical care more quickly, as they can afford to invest in advanced technology and facilities for early detection and treatment. For example, private companies can soon implement new rules in response to infectious diseases, as was the case with COVID-19. During this time, private healthcare entities adapted rapidly by adopting telehealth services and enhancing infection control measures to safeguard patients and staff (Ballif et al., 2025). Still, even though these systems provide fast care, their primary goal is profit, which may result in unfair access to healthcare for those who are less well-off. When profits drive healthcare, it can lead to differences in how infectious diseases are managed. This is particularly evident in settings where there is inadequate investment in Water, Sanitation, and Hygiene (WASH) facilities, which are vital in preventing the spread of infectious diseases. A study highlighted that in various healthcare facilities, particularly in lower-income regions, the lack of comprehensive WASH infrastructure directly impacts the control of infections, often exacerbating outbreaks if not addressed (Ogbonna et al., 2024). So, while private healthcare works efficiently and utilises the latest technology, its primary goal of generating a profit can hinder its support for key preventive measures, which is detrimental to public health efforts against infectious diseases. It seems that combining the strengths of private healthcare with the goals of public health could lead to better health results. In this way, private institutions might be encouraged to offer community health services, therefore including prevention in their services. For example, lessons gleaned from the COVID-19 pandemic should encourage private healthcare providers to maintain robust infection control practices and further invest in preventive health measures that facilitate early diagnosis and treatment of diseases like tuberculosis (Ballif et al., 2025). Encouraging private companies to collaborate with public health systems could improve the sharing of resources and the condition of WASH facilities, which could result in improved health for the population. Consequently, re-evaluating the role of private healthcare in infectious disease management is essential for improving access and efficacy in health service delivery (Figure 15.5).

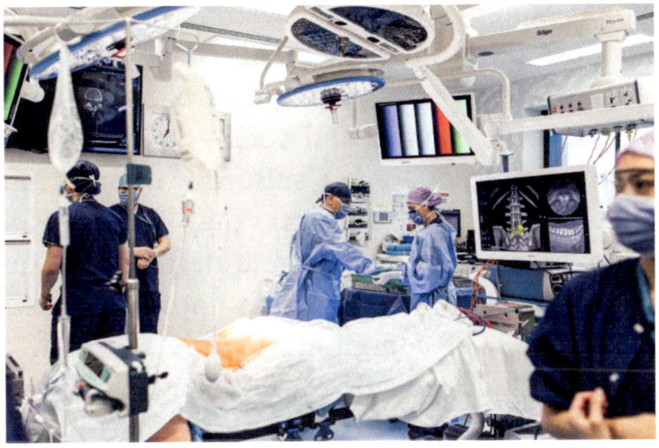

Figure 15.5. Private healthcare systems.

Source: https://cdn.vox-cdn.com/thumbor/dgJUrnkCwzi05AihjKAr83KR8QI=/0x0:2924x1950/1520x0/filters:focal(0x0:2924x1950):no_upscale()/cdn.vox-cdn.com/uploads/chorus_asset/file/19573141/0Q1A4017.jpg.

15.1.3. Mixed Healthcare Systems

In exploring mixed healthcare systems, one must consider their complex interplay with infectious disease control. When a country has both public and private healthcare providers, it can offer various ways to finance and provide health services, which helps more people in LMICs access them. They may address infectious diseases by employing community-based strategies that help reduce the number of people who are sick and dying. For this reason, the use of oral amoxicillin to treat pneumonia at home suggests that treatment guidelines should be flexible in mixed healthcare systems. Implementing such evidence-based practices can significantly reduce hospitalisations and improve health outcomes by shifting care to outpatient settings, thus addressing the challenges faced by healthcare systems in high-mortality regions such as sub-Saharan Africa, as indicated by Qazi et al. (2014). Additionally, mixed healthcare systems can effectively address the unique needs of diverse populations, particularly during challenging situations like the COVID-19 pandemic. F

or example, Native Hawaiians and Pacific Islanders have shown adaptable care approaches because their health problems are made worse by historical trauma and social factors. When healthcare providers use culturally appropriate practices in mixed systems, they can provide better mental health care and help reduce the stigma of seeking care, which improves health for marginalised communities. This intersection between infectious disease management and mental health is critical, as highlighted by the disproportionate mental health risks faced by these populations during the pandemic Enomoto et al. (1971). By studying these dynamics, we can gain a better understanding of how mixed healthcare systems respond to infectious disease threats. In addition, by leveraging technology and community involvement, mixed healthcare systems can do an even better job of controlling contagious diseases. Telehealth services, which gained popularity during the pandemic, demonstrate how technology enables people in rural and underserved areas to access the care they need. Telemedicine enables health workers to connect with patients who might not receive treatment due to their location or financial situation. Early intervention and regular surveillance of infectious diseases help mixed healthcare systems build a strong system for disease control and prevention. When these strategies are employed, patients are healthier and emergency services are less stressed, which enhances the ability of mixed healthcare systems to manage infectious diseases.

15.2. Role of Government in Healthcare

The role of government in healthcare is pivotal, especially in the context of infectious disease control. It is the government's role to develop policies that manage how people get care, how much it costs, and its quality. Intensive surveillance and swift action against outbreaks are essential components of public health plans that governments should implement. When the ZIKV outbreak happened in India, the government took steps to strengthen healthcare and start vector control programs. They are based on the idea that working together is essential to limit the spread of disease, as governments can utilise their resources and issue effective public health orders. By prioritising health education and accessible healthcare services, governments strengthen the resilience of their populations against infectious diseases, demonstrating their critical role in maintaining public health safety and effectively managing health crises, as underscored in the comprehensive analysis of the Zika outbreak (Chandra et al., 2024). It is also essential for governments to make sure healthcare professionals, especially infectious disease specialists, are well-educated and trained. Due to the COVID-19 pandemic, it is evident that healthcare systems in many areas are underfunded and require a robust team of ID specialists to tackle emerging health challenges. To address these shortages, governments could provide grants for training, promote the establishment of specialised infectious disease departments in medical schools, and enforce certifications to ensure adherence to common standards. Additionally, by supporting young doctors in underserved regions, we can enhance healthcare and improve the country's preparedness for pandemics. By developing a workforce capable of responding effectively to infectious diseases, the government plays a fundamental role in safeguarding public health (Hagiya, 2024). It is also essential for healthcare management, especially in the context of infectious diseases, that government agencies and international organisations cooperate closely. During health crises, governments should encourage cooperation that facilitates communication, research, and resource sharing. For example, when there was a Zika outbreak, governments worked together to reduce the virus's impact by using broad public health measures such as controlling mosquitoes and involving the community. Because health systems are linked globally, these efforts help protect global health security and highlight the need for combined efforts to address infectious diseases. Ultimately, it is the government's responsibility to establish the framework for such cooperation, facilitating comprehensive responses to health challenges that transcend national boundaries while promoting long-term preparedness against future outbreaks (Chandra et al., 2024; Hagiya, 2024) (Figure 15.6).

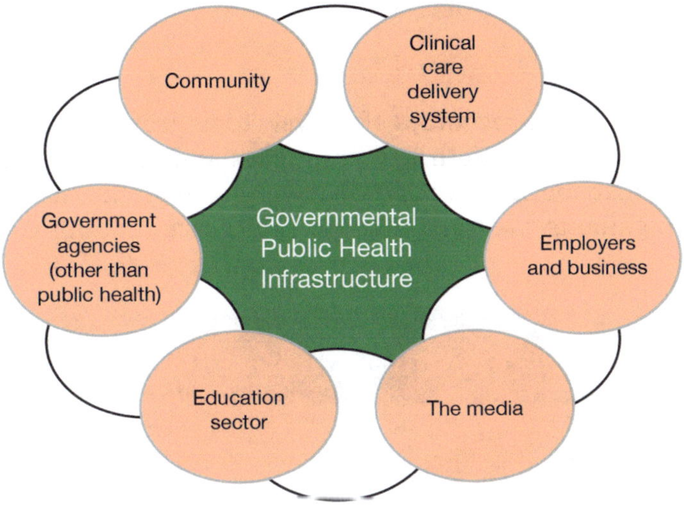

Figure 15.6. The role of government in healthcare.

Source: https://nap.nationalacademies.org/openbook/13093/xhtml/images/p17-01.jpg.

15.2.1. Policy-Making and Regulation

Policy-making and regulation play critical roles in shaping healthcare systems, particularly in the context of infectious disease control. An organised policy framework establishes rules for good healthcare and encourages measures to prevent the spread of communicable diseases. As the threat of antimicrobial resistance (AMR) escalates globally, regulatory bodies must implement stringent protocols to monitor antibiotic usage and promote stewardship programs. It is essential since AMR can stop common treatments from working, which causes more sickness and deaths. The development of comprehensive policies that integrate surveillance, research, and public education is essential for addressing the multifaceted challenges posed by AMR, facilitating a more resilient healthcare system capable of protecting public health from emerging infectious threats (Sultana et al., 2024). Because contagious diseases spread globally, healthcare regulations are now shaped by increased international cooperation. Public health problems are often seen to cross borders, so countries are taking steps to cooperate and adhere to global health standards. For instance, the recent reorganisation of public health infrastructure in Georgia reflects an effort to build a system capable of dealing with contemporary public health challenges through a decentralised approach (Verulava et al., 2022). By adopting European principles in public health reform, Georgia has shown that policy changes can effectively control epidemics and promote preventive healthcare. This highlights the importance of establishing robust governance systems that enable regional and municipal bodies to succeed in implementing major public health plans. Policies and regulations should be made by considering the opinions of healthcare professionals, patients, and communities. Involving different stakeholders in decision-making provides a more comprehensive understanding of healthcare issues and leads to policies grounded in real experiences. When policies are developed collaboratively, the strategies may be more suitable for various communities, which can enhance the control of infectious diseases. Additionally, it is essential to regularly review and update these policies to keep pace with changes in healthcare, ensuring they continue to protect the public effectively. If healthcare systems involve stakeholders and respond well, they can become stronger and manage the complications of infectious diseases in a global setting.

15.2.2. Funding and Resource Allocation

It is essential to manage funding and resources effectively to improve healthcare systems, particularly when addressing infectious diseases. Both fast responses and strategic plans for the future, such as vaccine production and distribution, depend on having enough financial resources. For example, the problem of malaria highlights the need to align healthcare funding with the specific needs of each region.

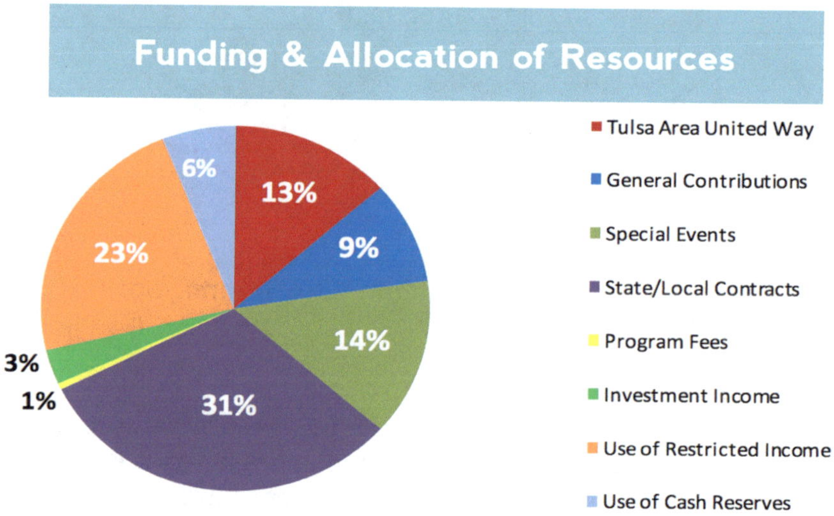

Figure 15.7. The effective management of funding and resource allocation of infectious disease control.

Source: https://www.parentchildcenter.org/wp-content/uploads/2017/04/Funding-Allocation-of-Resources.png.

The WHO's decision to promote the RTS,S malaria vaccine demonstrates how targeted investments can have a substantial impact on health. Nevertheless, the problem of unequal resource distribution complicates healthcare systems in sub-Saharan Africa, which must contend with both infectious diseases and the broader effects of economic disparities. Sustainable funding mechanisms, therefore, must prioritise these areas to ensure adequate disease prevention and treatment strategies

(Seitzinger et al., 2024). Additionally, the use of advanced technologies, such as AI, in public health planning underscores how funding needs can evolve over time. The ability of AI to identify health trends and predict outbreaks underscores the importance of investing in technology. AI being used for syndromic surveillance in current health advancements indicates that funding should cover both usual healthcare and new methods for infectious disease control. Healthcare systems can make better use of resources and act quickly to save lives by using AI's data-analysis abilities. Thus, a dual approach that combines traditional funding with investments in technology is crucial for building resilient healthcare infrastructures capable of addressing EIDs efficiently (Seitzinger et al., 2024). Ultimately, the impact of the COVID-19 pandemic has led many countries to reallocate their budgets, often resulting in reduced funding for other health initiatives. Therefore, it is evident that funding strategies should be adaptable and capable of handling unexpected situations. For malaria to be effectively managed, there needs to be continuous and coordinated funding for prevention and for the introduction of vaccines. This money should also cover the challenges of both pandemics and the diseases that continue to exist in the background. By establishing resilient funding frameworks that prioritize both current infectious disease threats and long-term healthcare infrastructure improvements, public health authorities can cultivate an environment prepared to mitigate the impacts of various health crises (Narain et al., 2022) (Figure 15.7).

15.2.3. Public Health Initiatives

Public health initiatives are foundational to the effective management and control of infectious diseases within healthcare systems. These initiatives often incorporate a multifaceted approach that includes surveillance, vaccination programs, and health education. Having well-developed surveillance systems enables public health departments to monitor diseases and identify outbreaks promptly, which is crucial for preventing the spread of infections. Vaccines are also used to avoid many communicable diseases from happening in the first place. Teaching people about health and diseases encourages them to manage their health effectively and helps build a culture where individuals are proactive about their well-being. They work to limit the spread of diseases and also make healthcare systems more prepared for new infectious threats. The use of advanced technologies in public health has significantly improved the management of infectious diseases. As an example, predictive modelling is now vital for predicting and controlling outbreaks. By employing machine learning (ML) algorithms that analyse extensive datasets—from patient records to environmental conditions—public health officials can identify high-risk areas and optimise resource allocation accordingly. Because of this technology, it is possible to prevent infections from developing into widespread outbreaks. Additionally, having IoT-based surveillance systems enables immediate monitoring, allowing threats to be addressed promptly. By embracing these technological innovations, healthcare systems can enhance their ability to manage infectious diseases and protect public health more effectively (Palla et al., 2025). Testing in laboratories has become very important for public health, especially during the COVID-19 pandemic. Efficient and precise identification of infectious agents supports effective patient care and also aids in broader public health initiatives. Therefore, diagnostic tests are now crucial for predicting and managing outbreaks, as they can help identify trends that may signal more infections. Additionally, by monitoring wastewater, scientists can determine the prevalence of pathogens in a community and estimate the severity of an impending outbreak. These diagnostic and monitoring strategies underscore the necessity of a well-coordinated public health initiative, allowing healthcare systems to allocate resources more effectively and prepare for future infectious disease threats, establishing a framework for managing potential outbreaks of Disease X (Lippi et al., 2025) (Figure 15.8).

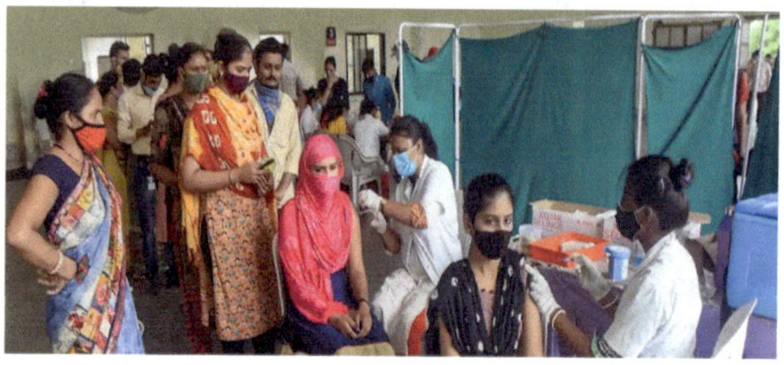

Figure 15.8. Public health initiatives.

Source: https://miro.medium.com/v2/resize:fit:1200/1*URV-OpMg5BQdkBLHat2EMA.jpeg.

15.3. Infectious Disease Surveillance

Infectious disease surveillance is a critical component of healthcare systems, serving as the foundation for monitoring, controlling, and preventing outbreaks of infectious diseases. Proper surveillance systems gather, analyse, and share information about diseases, allowing for prompt responses to new health risks. They typically employ several methods, combining information from clinical examinations, laboratory results, and disease tracking. In India, the Zika outbreak was effectively managed due to the government's strong surveillance efforts, which included disseminating health information and upgrading healthcare facilities. This example underscores the importance of having comprehensive infectious disease surveillance networks to ensure swift action during health crises. It highlights the need for continuous improvement in data collection methodologies and inter-agency collaboration in future responses (Chandra et al., 2024). Moreover, the rapid evolution of pathogens and the increasing prevalence of antimicrobial resistance (AMR) add complexity to the practice of infectious disease surveillance. AMR is a significant problem for public health, reducing the effectiveness of common infection treatments and making healthcare more difficult. Antibiotic resistance patterns should be a focus of surveillance systems, which requires professionals from microbiology, epidemiology, and clinical practice to work together. How well infectious diseases and AMR are controlled in healthcare is closely connected to the effectiveness of surveillance. Regularly following resistance trends enables healthcare providers to refine their treatment plans and take appropriate actions. This proactive stance not only aids in managing existing diseases but also fortifies the healthcare framework against future outbreaks, making it essential for policymakers to prioritise the integration of AMR monitoring into established surveillance systems (Sultana et al., 2024). Because people are connected worldwide, it is necessary to use a single method to watch for infectious diseases across borders. As shown by many global outbreaks, EIDs can spread fast, which highlights the importance of countries teaming up for surveillance. For international health security to improve, countries must develop standard procedures and share data in real time so that infectious diseases can be handled quickly. These initiatives rely on securing sufficient funding, providing training, and disseminating valuable information in public health. If countries create a cooperative and honest environment, they can improve their ability to handle both pandemics and endemic diseases. Ultimately, the comprehensive integration of infectious disease surveillance into healthcare systems will empower nations to safeguard public health more effectively, ensuring that they are equipped to face the ever-evolving landscape of infectious threats (Chandra et al., 2024; Sultana et al., 2024) (Figure 15.9).

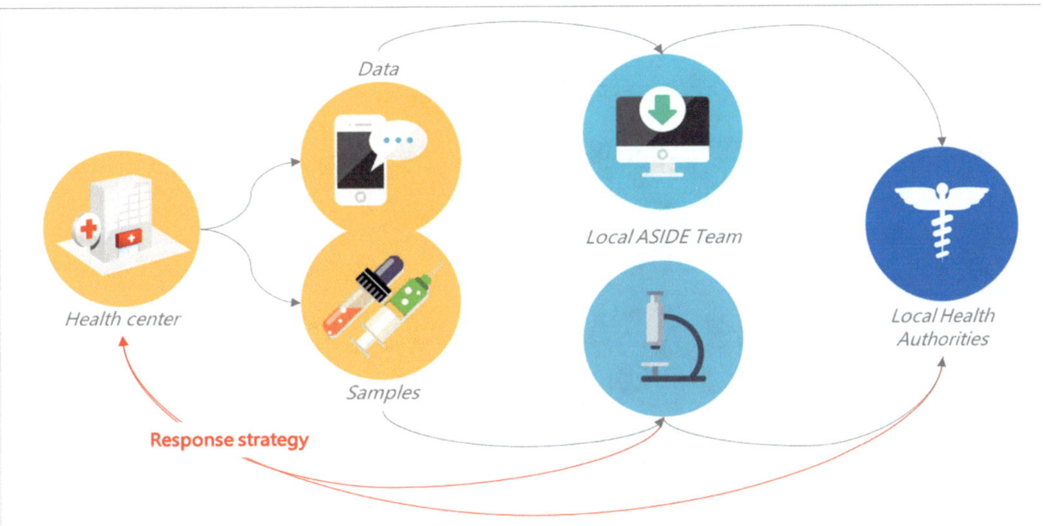

Figure 15.9. Infectious disease surveillance is a critical component of healthcare systems.

Source: https://research.pasteur.fr/wp-content/uploads/2015/05/research_pasteur-alerting-and-surveillance-for-infectious-disease-epidemics-warning-system.png.

15.3.1. Importance of Data Collection

The significance of data collection in healthcare systems, particularly in the context of infectious disease control, cannot be overstated. Effective data collection enables health authorities to track the progression of diseases, assess the effectiveness of control efforts, and allocate resources accordingly. The pandemic clearly demonstrated what can happen when there is insufficient data. Those nations that used organised data collection were able to act quickly and find areas with the most cases. In Indonesia, early in the pandemic, reviews revealed significant gaps in both knowledge and the number of healthcare workers. This highlights that robust data collection informs strategic planning and policy decision-making within healthcare systems, enabling targeted interventions that can enhance public health resilience and response capabilities (Ibrahim et al., 2025). In addition to providing immediate responses, collecting data systematically enables healthcare systems to be prepared for any future infectious disease outbreaks. The knowledge gained from previous health crises, such as the COVID-19 pandemic, typically leads to improved data infrastructure. For example, research in various countries has shown that individuals who monitor epidemiological patterns, such as those in Rwanda, can make more informed decisions about their healthcare systems. By analysing correlations between public mobility and infection rates, authorities can institute timely measures to mitigate risks associated with increased contact (Umutoni et al., 2024). Therefore, data collection is essential in public health because it allows decision-makers to anticipate emerging health issues and improve healthcare during emergencies. The effectiveness of a healthcare response often depends on the quality and thoroughness of the collected data. When data management is used in health systems, it becomes easier to prevent and manage infectious diseases. Moreover, when healthcare professionals, government agencies, and community members collaborate in collecting data, the quantity and accuracy of the information improve. As evidenced in several studies, including an examination of Indonesia's healthcare readiness during the pandemic, effective data collection promotes collaboration and shared responsibility across various sectors (Ibrahim et al., 2025). In conclusion, prioritizing data collection within healthcare systems not only addresses current challenges but also fortifies preparedness against future infectious disease threats (Figure 15.10).

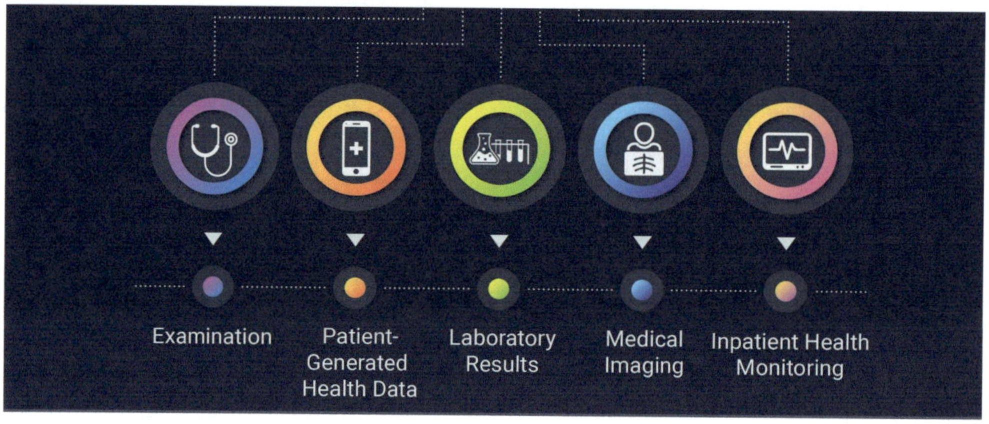

Figure 15.10. The significance of data collection in healthcare systems.

Source: https://www.infocleanse.com/wp-content/uploads/2022/05/why-is-healthcare-data-collection-essential.jpg.

15.3.2. Role of Technology in Surveillance

The integration of technology in surveillance plays a crucial role in enhancing healthcare systems and managing infectious disease control. In recent times, digital tools have greatly improved how health authorities monitor, record, and manage disease outbreaks. The use of geographic information systems and mobile health applications enables real-time data collection and analysis, facilitating the early detection of potential outbreaks. This new technology is most noticeable in cross-border health efforts, since sharing information and communicating well among countries is vital for a combined approach. For instance, in the context of Mpox management across the Kenya-Uganda border, the deployment of robust surveillance systems significantly enhances situational awareness and resource allocation in health interventions, ultimately contributing to more effective control measures for infectious diseases (Peter, 2025). ML and AI help health surveillance systems predict outbreaks, enabling timely action before diseases spread. The use of a wide range of data about patients, the environment, and past outbreaks enables these technologies to provide healthcare professionals with useful information about areas with high risk and potential outbreaks. By using predictive modelling, it becomes easier to quickly use resources and respond effectively, which helps control the spread of infectious diseases.

Moreover, the integration of Internet of Things (IoT) devices further enhances real-time monitoring and data collection, enabling health authorities to track infection dynamics and identify hotspots for targeted intervention. As seen in various healthcare settings, robust data-driven approaches, supported by predictive analytics, are instrumental in fostering resilience against emerging health threats (Pallaet al., 2025). Although technology can be instrumental in surveillance, it is sometimes limited by a lack of infrastructure and resources. In many countries, a lack of healthcare facilities, trained workers, and financial resources makes it challenging to implement technological solutions. For instance, in the case of Kenya and Uganda, healthcare workers recognise that border health posts are crucial for monitoring infections like Mpox; however, there are still difficulties with training staff and teamwork between the two countries. To address these problems, funds should be invested in technology and staff training to enhance the effectiveness of surveillance systems. By aligning technological advancements with comprehensive training programs and enhanced infrastructure, healthcare systems can better leverage surveillance technologies to improve outcomes in infectious disease control (Palla et al., 2025; Peter, 2025).

15.3.3. Case Studies of Successful Surveillance Programs

Effective surveillance programs play a crucial role in controlling infectious diseases, as demonstrated by numerous successful case studies worldwide. Cooperative healthcare work between Kenya and Uganda in the battle against Mpox is a good example. According to research, the fact that Mpox cases have appeared in both countries has encouraged both nations to cooperate more, making it easier to monitor and respond to the outbreak. A survey found that 55.6% of healthcare workers thought their countries were good at sharing resources, which reflects success in cross-country collaboration. However, difficulties such as insufficient trained staff and inadequate facilities hinder the achievement of optimal health outcomes. This situation highlights the need to strengthen healthcare systems and improve surveillance frameworks to address the persistent challenges in controlling infectious diseases across borders (Peter, 2025). A further case study demonstrating the effectiveness of surveillance programs involves the use of advanced technologies, such as AI and genomic surveillance. Because of these tools, managing outbreaks has become more accurate and faster. Recently, the use of ML algorithms to analyse large datasets has helped quickly identify infection hotspots related to COVID-19 and the Zika virus, allowing interventions to be targeted accordingly. In addition, these technologies have enabled public health authorities to exchange data instantly, which is crucial for a unified response. The lessons learned from these outbreaks emphasize the potential of technological integration in surveillance systems, highlighting that with adequate international support and investment in digital infrastructure, healthcare systems can enhance their preparedness and resilience against future infectious disease challenges (Ugwu et al., 2025). Additionally, community involvement is crucial, along with the implementation of new surveillance tools, to effectively manage infectious diseases. It is essential for successful surveillance programs to cooperate with the local population to make sure people are aware of and follow health rules. Mpox cases in Kenya and Uganda have demonstrated that local communities respond differently, highlighting the need to incorporate their knowledge and practices into official health plans. The study shows that border health posts are crucial for detecting diseases, but they face challenges in contact tracing and mobilizing the community. Informing communities through health education campaigns might lead to better reporting and better management of diseases. Overall, the efficacy of surveillance programs hinges not only on technological advancements and intergovernmental cooperation but also on the systematic involvement of communities in the fight against infectious diseases (Peter, 2025; Ugwu et al., 2025).

15.4. Vaccination Programs

Vaccination programs represent a crucial component of healthcare systems focused on combating infectious diseases. These initiatives are designed to immunise populations against specific pathogens, thus reducing disease incidence and prevalence. Vaccination programs often struggle to ensure that many people are vaccinated, as this is influenced by disparities in wealth, misinformation, and vaccine scepticism. Ensuring that everyone can get vaccinated enhances community immunity and reduces the likelihood of outbreaks. For instance, during the monkeypox virus outbreak, effective vaccination strategies were deployed, which underscored the importance of timely and coordinated public health responses (Rashid et al., 2025). Including vaccination in the overall health system is necessary to keep diseases under control and help the system deal with new infectious diseases. Recent studies have highlighted that the effectiveness of vaccination programs depends on the population's connectivity and the vaccination rate of the area. Even in places where most people are vaccinated, studies have shown that differences in vaccination can result in outbreaks. For example, a study in the Serengeti district, Tanzania, showed that increased spatial heterogeneity in dog vaccination contributed to persistent rabies transmission, emphasising how localised outbreak risks can emerge despite ongoing vaccination campaigns (Ferguson et al., 2024). This analysis of vaccination strategy effectiveness points out that we should use approaches that consider both demographic and geographic factors. If health authorities use detailed monitoring and adjust vaccination strategies, they can make vaccination programs more effective and able to prevent disease transmission among people. In addition, constantly reviewing and updating vaccination strategies helps keep them effective against infectious diseases. Lessons from vaccination efforts during rabies and monkeypox outbreaks demonstrate the importance of utilising real-time data and making prompt decisions in health policy. Such frameworks help understand the spread of diseases and the areas where vaccination rates are low so that actions can be taken promptly. For example, leveraging data from rabies contact tracing has shown that localized vaccination efforts yield better outcomes than generalized approaches (Ferguson et al., 2024). Such findings advocate for a systems thinking perspective in healthcare, where vaccination programs are continuously assessed and adjusted based on emerging epidemiological data, ultimately ensuring sustained protection for the population against infectious diseases (Figure 5.11).

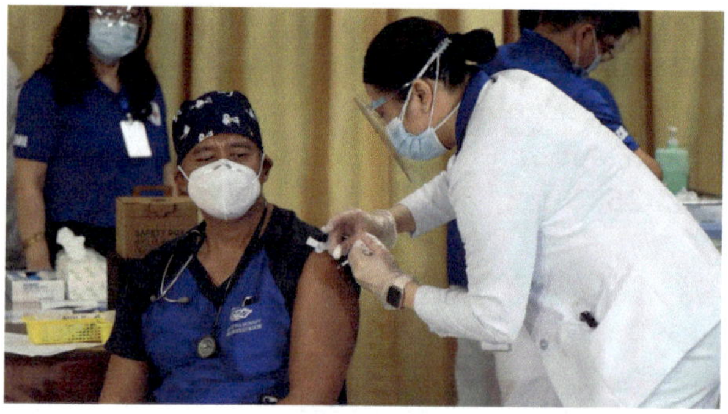

Figure 15.11. Vaccination programs.

Source: https://www.frontiersin.org/files/Articles/550510/fmicb-11-01526-HTML/image_m/fmicb-11-01526-g001.jpg.

15.4.1. Historical Context of Vaccination

Throughout history, the development of vaccination has emerged as a pivotal advancement in public health, dramatically reshaping healthcare systems and infectious disease control. Edward Jenner developed the smallpox vaccine from cowpox in the late 18th century, which marked the beginning of vaccination. As a result, people could now prevent a disease that had been a problem for many generations, and it also formed the basis for immunology. As vaccination programs were implemented and put into practice, infectious diseases were controlled, significantly reducing the number of people affected and dying from these diseases. Efforts by various international health organisations further catalysed the introduction of vaccines as an essential component of global health policy, reflecting an increasing recognition of their role in infectious disease management (Forman et al., 2021). As more people were vaccinated, the story of how vaccination was adopted suggests that there are many challenges in public health and respecting personal freedoms. Different countries had laws requiring vaccination, deciding how much to protect health and how much to respect individual freedom. In Australia, discussions are underway about whether healthcare workers should be required to get vaccinated, highlighting the legal and ethical issues involved. Such discussions often raise issues of public health ethics, social responsibilities, and individual rights, which underscore the challenges healthcare systems face in implementing mandatory vaccination policies.

Consequently, countries have had to navigate these philosophical and legal debates while developing effective and equitable vaccination strategies that can withstand scrutiny and societal resistance (Kevat et al., 2021). There has been a significant increase in vaccination programs in the 20th and 21st centuries, mainly to fight diseases such as polio, measles, and recently, COVID-19. With global health organizations like GAVI and the Global Fund, it has become much easier for LMICs to get and use vaccines quickly. Outbreaks are effectively controlled, and herd immunity is achieved when vaccination campaigns are implemented. Yet, modern problems persist, including a decline in vaccination rates due to misinformation and doubts about health services. Examining the history of vaccination, it is evident that effective public health communication and community engagement are essential to achieving widespread vaccination acceptance. As healthcare systems evolve, lessons learned from the past will be pivotal in combating infectious diseases and securing population health for future generations (Forman et al., 2021).

15.4.2. Impact on Infectious Disease Control

In evaluating the impact of healthcare systems on infectious disease control, it becomes imperative to understand the operational challenges posed during outbreaks. The Centres for Disease Control and Prevention (CDC) plays a pivotal role in managing these health crises, particularly in identifying infected individuals and their geographical locations. This task often involves tackling a Target-to-Area (TTA) problem, where the effectiveness of resource allocation can determine the outcome of an epidemic response. Recent advancements, such as the integration of Point-In-Polygon (PIP) techniques and K-Nearest Neighbours (KNN) algorithms, hold promise for enhancing classification accuracy in tracking disease spread. However, if there is insufficient sample data, it can be more challenging to respond quickly to problems. Therefore, the adoption of innovative technological frameworks is essential to optimise resource distribution and bolster the healthcare system's capacity for infectious disease control and responsiveness to emerging threats (Chen et al., 2025). Because of their close-contact nature, long-term care facilities make infectious diseases much more likely. The pandemic clearly showed that nursing homes are vulnerable, as people living there, visiting, and working interact often and can spread the disease quickly. Simulating these environments reveals how different methods of transmitting the disease interact with one another when interventions are implemented. For example, studies found that super-spreader healthcare workers caused a greater increase in the number of infections than other sources in these facilities. Using up-to-date data, healthcare systems can plan their actions more efficiently, choosing the most affordable measures that benefit the public the most. This nuanced understanding of transmission dynamics allows for more tailored healthcare responses that can effectively curb outbreaks while considering the complexities of human interaction (Ghosh et al., 2024). The ability to manage infectious disease outbreaks better depends on the combination of technology and strong strategies in healthcare. The intersection of rigorous data analysis, such as the adaptation of KNN against TTA challenges, and the implementation of targeted non-pharmaceutical interventions (NPIs) demonstrates a sophisticated approach to public health management. Strategies such as surface cleaning and wearing masks should be changed according to the phase of the outbreak to keep up with the latest epidemiological situation. When costs are modeled as these interventions are carried out, healthcare providers can decide how to manage the disease and its prevention costs. Consequently, strengthening healthcare systems through comprehensive planning and innovative solutions becomes crucial to mitigating the impacts of infectious diseases in our interconnected society (Ghosh et al., 2024) (Figure 15.12).

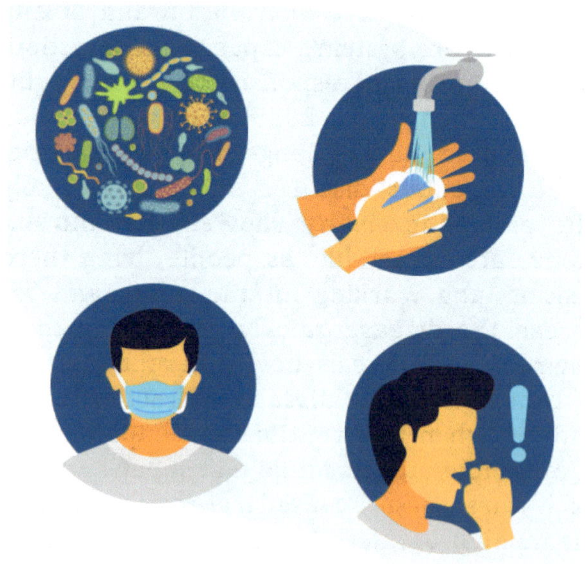

Figure 15.12. The impact of healthcare systems on infectious disease control.

Source: https://pdihc.com/wp-content/uploads/2021/01/InfectionPreventionTrendBlog_2021.png.

15.4.3. Challenges in Vaccination Implementation

The implementation of vaccination programs is fraught with multifaceted challenges that undermine their effectiveness in controlling infectious diseases. Many people are reluctant to get vaccines because they fear they are not safe or effective, and this is often made worse by false claims on the internet. Such doubt can lead to fewer people getting vaccinated, allowing diseases that could be avoided to return to communities. In addition, some people in marginalised groups do not have easy access to healthcare, which leads to uneven vaccination rates. Different geographical locations, financial constraints, and cultural barriers can hinder patients' access to vaccination, highlighting the need to address these inequalities to improve control of infectious diseases. It is also challenging to store, move, and give vaccines because the process involves a lot of logistics. Many vaccines require storage at very low temperatures, which is not always feasible in places with limited resources. Disruptions from events such as natural disasters or pandemics, for example, the recent COVID-19 crisis, often make it more challenging to manage logistics, resulting in waste and hindering the prompt delivery to the intended groups. Also, making sure healthcare staff are trained to manage vaccines and run effective vaccination campaigns is essential, but is not always given enough attention when planning resources. Collaboration among health agencies, governments, and global organisations helps manage logistics effectively, increasing the chances of successful vaccination programs. Finally, the way governments handle politics can influence vaccination programs by causing policies to change frequently, which can hinder the development of effective strategies. Governments can sometimes focus more on quick results than on long-term health benefits, which results in uneven support for vaccination programs. Additionally, neglecting infectious disease prevention can make people less likely to get vaccinated. Case studies of countries like Kazakhstan prove that strong political support, proper resource planning, and educating the public greatly affect the success of vaccination programs. Addressing these political challenges requires a committed approach that not only informs the public about the importance of vaccinations but also fosters collaboration among various stakeholders to create a cohesive strategy that prioritizes health equity and disease control (Kokebayeva et al., 2024; Vecchia et al., 2025) (Figure 15.13).

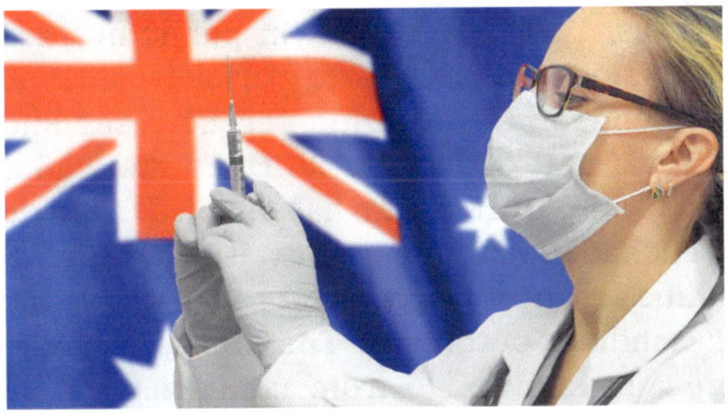

Figure 15.13. Challenges in vaccination implementation.

Source: https://content.api.news/v3/images/bin/a6953f4a9636ac1b9a2c6f7325d8f022.

15.5. Global Health Organizations

Global health organisations are vital for handling infectious diseases around the world. These entities, such as the WHO and the Centres for Disease Control and Prevention (CDC), are designed to facilitate collaborative efforts among nations to combat public health challenges. They work to establish systems for tracking diseases, help distribute vaccines, and encourage research that enhances global health security. The emergence of antimicrobial resistance (AMR), as noted in recent literature, underscores the critical need for international cooperation and robust healthcare systems to manage threats that transcend national boundaries effectively (Sultana et al., 2024). Their skill in mobilising resources and responding to emergencies during outbreaks is crucial, highlighting why they are essential for managing global health infrastructures facing increases in infectious diseases. International health organisations are primarily responsible for educating people about communicable diseases and methods to prevent them. They do this by organising campaigns to inform people and healthcare workers about the newest information on controlling, preventing, and treating diseases. For example, the WHO provides guidance on vaccinations and encourages the prudent use of antimicrobials to prevent the growth of resistant pathogens. They not only alleviate current health issues but also establish sustainable methods for managing diseases in healthcare. The interplay between education, policy formulation, and active participation by global health organisations is vital in driving practical actions against infectious diseases, ensuring that communities around the world are adequately prepared and responsive to emerging health threats (Omotayo et al., 2024). Besides, the combined actions of international health organizations support the creation of policies that tackle both communicable and non-communicable diseases. By sharing their experiences and data from various locations, these organisations identify weaknesses in healthcare systems and work to improve them. Recognising the interconnectedness of infectious and non-communicable diseases, it is crucial to employ an integrated strategy in public health. As highlighted in discussions surrounding NCDs, the challenges posed by preventable diseases require a concerted response, utilizing a variety of interventions, including lifestyle modification and public health education (Omotayo et al., 2024). The role of global health organizations in this context is crucial, as they advocate for cross-sectoral collaborations that promote sustainable health initiatives and drive home the importance of public health policies that encompass a wider array of health challenges (Figure 15.14).

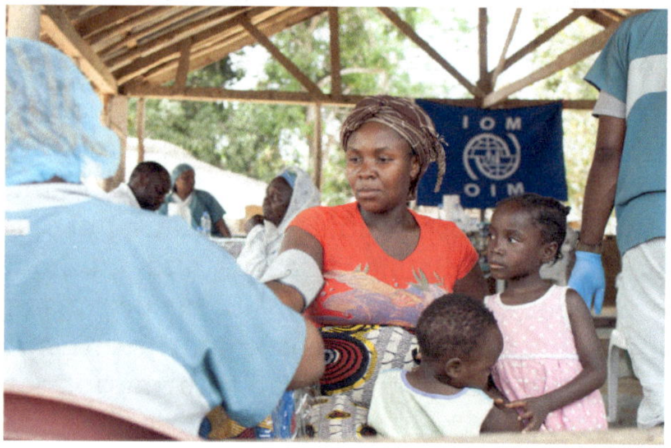

Figure 15.14. Global health organizations.

Source: https://borgenproject.org/wp-content/uploads/16369812974_83ba830af2_k.jpg.

15.5.1. Role of the World Health Organisation (WHO)

The WHO plays a pivotal role in strengthening global healthcare systems, particularly in the context of infectious disease control. Being the central health authority in the United Nations system, the WHO develops standards and guidelines to handle health emergencies, organise responses to outbreaks, and ensure that essential healthcare is available to all. A primary focus of its mission is to strengthen the health systems of LMICs, which regularly face both common and outbreak diseases. In this context, WHO's guidelines and frameworks enhance the resilience of healthcare systems, enabling nations to manage better and prevent infectious disease outbreaks, thus reducing mortality and morbidity associated with such diseases (Murray et al., 2022). Additionally, by sharing knowledge and resources, the WHO helps enhance the effectiveness of public health programs worldwide. In the face of rising antimicrobial resistance (AMR), the WHO's role becomes even more critical. AMR seriously affects global health, and it is thought that millions of people die from it each year. It has been key in organizing actions for AMR surveillance, awareness and research. The Global Action Plan on AMR from WHO aims to unite countries in combating AMR by integrating approaches across human, animal, and environmental health. This multifaceted approach is crucial as resistant pathogens do not recognize borders and can spread quickly through international travel and trade (Nkengasong et al., 2020). WHO is leading this effort because it is committed to addressing existing health issues and preventing future problems caused by AMR and other infectious diseases. The WHO's work in public health is evident in its response to various epidemics and pandemics, including recent cases such as Ebola and COVID-19. WHO, as the leading agency for global health, has enabled countries to exchange critical information, provided technical support, and established guidelines for handling outbreaks. The ability to gather help and knowledge from many nations has been key to handling outbreaks and limiting their effects on public health. It also highlights that improved public health infrastructure and training for healthcare workers will enable the country to handle future health emergencies better. The lessons learned from managing these crises underscore the necessity of international collaboration and the integration of global health agendas into national policies, reinforcing WHO's integral role in evolving healthcare systems that are responsive to infectious disease threats (Murray et al., 2022; Nkengasong et al., 2020).

15.5.2. Contributions of Non-Governmental Organizations (NGOs)

Non-governmental organisations (NGOs) play a crucial role in enhancing healthcare systems, particularly in the realm of infectious disease control. These entities often bridge gaps in funding, infrastructure, and expertise, especially in underserved regions where government resources may be insufficient. NGOs help local communities by providing medical care and sharing information about disease prevention. They are crucial for managing outbreaks, as they enable the quick implementation of effective emergency response plans. Because global health problems are so complex, NGOs rely on teaming up with governments and agencies to develop healthcare solutions that fit the community's needs. NGOs are also crucial in supporting global efforts to detect and monitor infectious diseases. Because they work with communities, they to collect epidemiological data quickly, which helps with understanding and handling disease outbreaks. Partnerships with local health authorities enable NGOs to identify patterns and issue early warnings to prevent further cases. Additionally, many NGOs are conducting research and advocacy, promoting greater openness and accountability in health systems to address issues such as corruption that can hinder disease control. As highlighted in discussions about health-related corruption, the integrity of such systems is vital; NGOs often lead the charge toward reform by raising awareness and proposing solutions around governance in healthcare (Clare et al., 2016). NGOs have also played a significant role in mitigating the environmental impacts of healthcare services. They advocate for sustainable healthcare, considering both the immediate health of individuals and the long-term environmental impacts of healthcare activities. According to research on the service sector's environmental impact, NGOs stress the need to address hazardous waste and prevent pollution in hospitals. NGOs are making sure that efforts to stop infectious diseases do not damage the environment. This interconnected approach underscores the multifaceted role of NGOs in building resilient healthcare systems that can effectively control diseases while promoting sustainable development (Davies et al., 2025) (Figure 15.15).

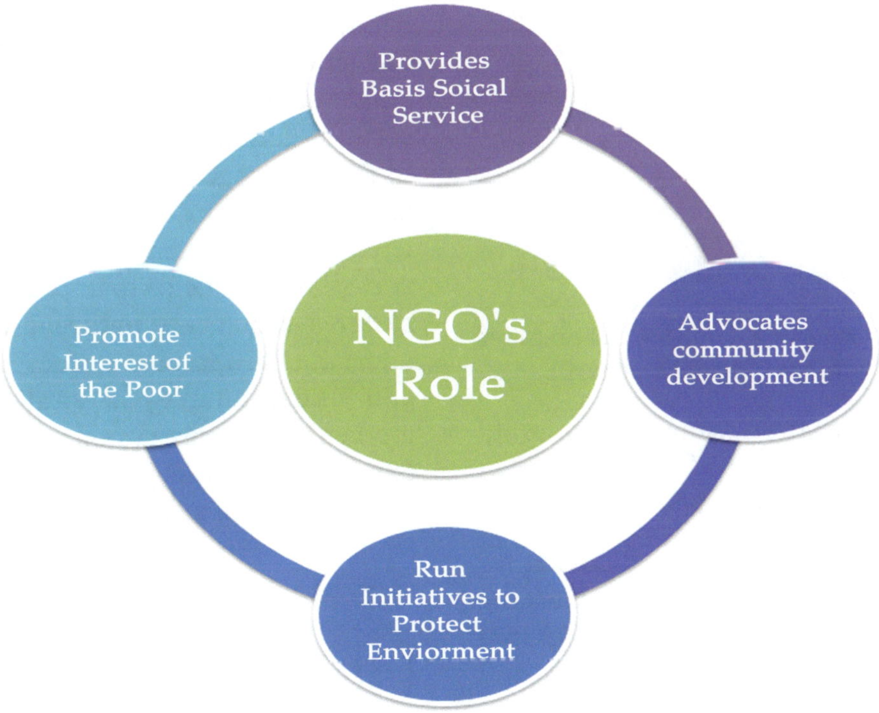

Figure 15.15. Non-governmental organizations (NGOs) healthcare systems.

Source: https://corpbiz.io/learning/wp-content/uploads/2020/08/image-99.png.

15.5.3. International Collaboration in Disease Control

International collaboration plays a pivotal role in effective disease control, particularly in the face of increasingly resilient infectious agents. Global health efforts depend on sharing knowledge and resources to improve the detection and management of diseases. Groups like the WHO help nations form partnerships that enable them to track health threats and prevent outbreaks by sharing information and joining forces. For instance, the National Centre for Preparedness, Detection, and Control of Infectious Diseases (NCPDCID) exemplifies such collaboration by working closely with international and domestic partners to conduct research, enhance public health capacities, and implement surveillance systems.

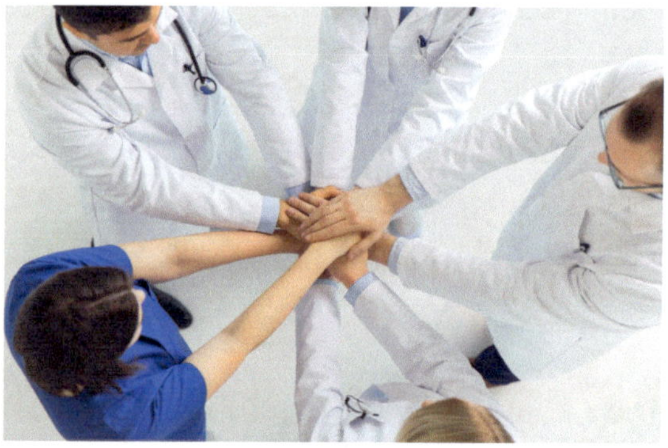

Figure 15.16. International collaboration plays a pivotal role in effective disease control.

Source: https://prognocis.com/wp-content/uploads/2022/01/group-of-doctors-with-hands-together-at-hospital-scaled.jpg.

This network of cooperation is crucial for early detection and responses to emerging diseases, ultimately safeguarding global populations from widespread outbreaks and associated morbidity and mortality (N/A). Moreover, the challenge of antimicrobial resistance (AMR) highlights the necessity for coordinated international policies in disease management. Because healthcare systems and resources vary among countries, it is challenging to apply the same strategies to combat AMR globally. Those who create policies must be mindful of the factors that can impact the effectiveness of interventions across different income groups and sectors. Analysing all these areas—the responsible use of antibiotics, improved surveillance, and effective prevention of infections—can make a significant difference in the health of people in a region or country. Recommendations from experts call for standardised policy assessments to determine the cost-effectiveness and applicability of measures tailored to the unique needs of different countries and their healthcare systems (Aarestrup et al., 2015). In the end, One Health unites efforts in human, animal, and environmental health, allowing for teamwork in controlling diseases that normally stay separate. This approach recognises that health is linked across various environments and encourages cooperation among multiple stakeholders. Working together with other sectors, nations can more effectively respond to the challenges posed by infectious diseases, including zoonotic ones that often originate from environmental changes. Working together on such platforms helps to improve the way health systems can tackle outbreaks. Ultimately, an international approach anchored in cooperation and understanding is vital for developing resilient healthcare systems formidable enough to mitigate the risks posed by infectious diseases on a global scale (Figure 15.16).

15.6. Challenges in Infectious Disease Control

The complexities and challenges inherent in infectious disease control are multifaceted, particularly in regions characterised by limited healthcare resources and infrastructural deficiencies. Recent cases of Mpox (Monkeypox) in Kenya highlight the pressing need for effective cross-border collaboration in managing infectious diseases. It is shown that although border health posts help detect diseases, they are frequently hindered by a shortage of trained staff, as 30% of healthcare workers in Kenya have identified this as a significant issue. Also, improving healthcare infrastructure and funding plays a key role in reducing these gaps. The effectiveness of infectious disease surveillance is further compromised by limited communication and data exchange between neighbouring countries, illustrating how systemic weaknesses can exacerbate the spread of contagion and stymie containment efforts (Peter, 2025). In addition, the pandemic has shown that global healthcare systems were not as ready for infectious diseases as many people thought. It is now clear that many countries were not prepared to handle a pathogen of such danger. The lessons learned from fighting COVID-19 confirm that we should utilise knowledge from previous epidemics to address current problems. For example, the experience gained from past health restrictions, especially during significant epidemics in Kazakhstan, highlights the need for thorough preparedness. To control diseases such as smallpox and cholera, which had been significant dangers before, these strategies introduced vaccination and improved sanitation. Such historical precedents can inform current policies and enhance the overall efficacy of public health initiatives (Kokebayeva et al., 2024). Also, the influence of social factors and public attitudes makes it more challenging to control infectious diseases. False information erodes trust in health interventions, making them less effective. During the Mpox outbreak, wrong beliefs stopped people from taking enough precautions and from joining community efforts which are necessary for controlling the disease. This highlights the importance of effective strategies that offer medical help, involve the community, and provide education to increase people's trust and willingness to follow the plan. Also, making sure there are no gender disparities in healthcare roles is crucial for any control strategy, since they can influence how resources are distributed and how responses are carried out. By paying attention to both the system and society, healthcare systems can handle infectious diseases more efficiently.

15.6.1. Emerging Infectious Diseases

EIDs pose significant challenges to global healthcare systems, particularly in the wake of the COVID-19 pandemic. After NPIs were relaxed, many infectious diseases resurfaced, illustrating how easily healthcare systems can be overwhelmed during an outbreak. The pandemic made it clear that using NPIs, such as wearing masks, maintaining social distancing, and washing hands, helps control the spread of diseases. acute infections increased in number post-COVID-19, which highlights the importance of having strong management plans in place. Furthermore, the disruption of established health protocols, combined with the absence of international collaboration, has introduced a heightened risk of infectious diseases re-emerging and spreading uncontrollably, underscoring the urgent need for a concerted global response to maintain public health stability and readiness for future outbreaks (Abiri et al., 2025). The ability of healthcare systems to function effectively and withstand challenges is vital, crucial for addressing EIDs efficiently. Since hospitals are the leading institutions in the fight against these health crises, better management and utilisation of resources are necessary. The challenges brought by disease outbreaks require preparing and building strong systems to resist worldwide health problems. Recent studies have proposed comprehensive evaluation systems designed to assess hospital resilience, focusing on factors such as medical response capacity, risk communication, and command coordination (Cheng et al., 2025).

Using these leading indicators, healthcare institutions can identify their weaknesses, which helps them become more flexible and respond more quickly to EIDs. Increasing the resilience of hospitals is crucial for both operational stability and the protection of public health in future health emergencies and pandemics. Because of the link between EIDs and healthcare, it is clear that controlling diseases needs a worldwide and multi-layered strategy. Paying more attention to NPIs and developing effective ways to assess hospital resilience are key components of this effort. Better international cooperation and communication between health organisations allows them to share applicable practices and resources, which is key to managing outbreaks and diseases. Additionally, investing in research and education will help communities become more aware and prepared for disasters. Establishing these foundational elements will not only mitigate the impact of current and EIDs but also fortify healthcare systems for future challenges, ensuring a more resilient response to global health threats (Abiri et al., 2025; Cheng et al., 2025) (Figure 15.17).

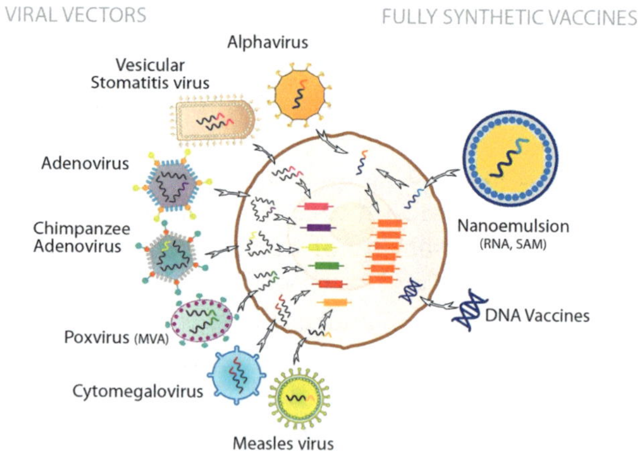

Figure 15.17. Emerging infectious diseases.

Source: https://www.pnas.org/cms/10.1073/pnas.1701410114/asset/172136ba-73bc-48c6-bd36-e59d56019720/assets/graphic/pnas.1701410114fig02.jpeg.

15.6.2. Antimicrobial Resistance

Antimicrobial resistance (AMR) represents one of the most pressing challenges to global health systems, complicating the management of infectious diseases. AMR is increasing because of factors such as giving antibiotics too often, poor infection control, and wrong use of antimicrobials in both healthcare and veterinary medicine. To respond effectively to AMR, healthcare systems must adopt comprehensive strategies such as Antimicrobial Stewardship (AMS) programs that optimise the use of antibiotics. They aim to help patients by choosing the right antibiotic, administering the correct dose, and selecting the appropriate duration, all to prevent the growth of antibiotic resistance. The urgent need for such measures is underscored by the increasing prevalence of resistant pathogens, such as *Helicobacter pylori,* which, as emerging evidence suggests, significantly undermines standard eradication therapies (Hsu et al., 2025). To fight AMR, healthcare practices must use advanced diagnostic equipment. Policymakers and healthcare staff need to utilise technologies such as polymerase chain reaction and next-generation sequencing to inform the selection of the right antibiotics for each local situation. Because of these advances, doctors can select more effective treatment methods and concentrate on the specifics of each infection. It is also essential to use a One Health approach, which means seeing the connections among human, animal, and environmental health, to fight the emergence and spread of resistant organisms. As globalised trade and travel continue to facilitate the transmission of infectious diseases, coordinated efforts across sectors can significantly mitigate AMR's impact on public health authorities (Onyebuchi et al., 2025). In addition, efforts to tackle AMR should include raising awareness and educating people, both in healthcare and the broader public, about the risks associated with misusing antimicrobials. Improving knowledge about proper antibiotic use can lead clinicians to prescribe better and motivate patients to stick to their treatment plans. In addition, such campaigns can highlight that vaccination and good hygiene practices help to reduce infections, thus lowering the need for antibiotics. If we encourage different experts to team up and make sure everyone has access to healthcare resources, our healthcare systems will be better prepared for diseases caused by AMR. Ultimately, a collective effort is required to implement sustainable solutions that safeguard against the looming threat of antimicrobial resistance into the future (Onyebuchi et al., 2025) (Figure 15.18).

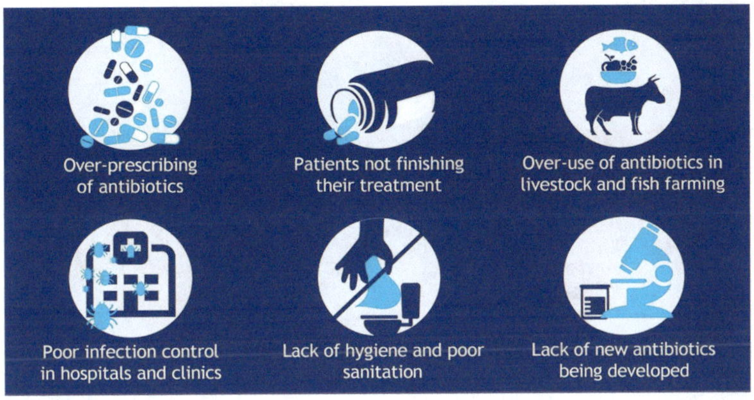

Figure 15.18. Antimicrobial resistance represent challenges to global health.

Source: https://www.afro.who.int/sites/default/files/infographics/Antimicrobial_Resistance_causes.jpg.

15.6.3. Socioeconomic Factors Affecting Healthcare Access

The interplay between socioeconomic status (SES) and healthcare access is a crucial consideration in the realm of infectious disease control. It is often challenging for individuals from lower socioeconomic backgrounds to access quality healthcare services. Some of these barriers are financial, while others involve insufficient insurance or limited access to healthcare facilities. As a result, when infectious diseases emerge, those who are most at risk may not receive a timely diagnosis or treatment, which can exacerbate the outbreak and heighten public health concerns. In addition, individuals with limited resources and education may be unaware of crucial preventive measures, such as vaccines and screenings, which can hinder the effectiveness of public health initiatives. So, improving socioeconomic conditions is crucial for better healthcare access and stronger infection control. Furthermore, environmental and societal conditions play a significant role in determining how different groups access healthcare, making it more challenging to manage infectious diseases. If there is not enough healthcare infrastructure, communities may find it difficult to offer basic services which leads many residents to either skip medical care or travel far for treatment. Such geographic issues are often exacerbated by social-environmental problems, including poor housing and increased exposure to harmful germs. Health literacy is also important, critical; those with lower SES may not know enough about preventing diseases, which can lead to more infections among them. Public health actions should consider socioeconomic factors to ensure that the right messages and services are provided to those most likely to spread disease due to their social and environmental circumstances. Stunting, which is caused by a lack of healthcare and economic challenges, highlights the broader effects on public health, mainly in children. Stunting is found in many regions, which indicates that there are systemic problems preventing access to healthcare, including malnutrition and unequal health services. Notably, studies indicate significant associations between stunting prevalence and factors like acute respiratory infections and poverty levels (Rinjani et al., 2024). The results highlight how healthcare access is related to long-term health outcomes, mainly for those who are vulnerable. Giving importance to health care and social factors helps public health systems make communities stronger against infectious diseases. Integrating socioeconomic considerations into healthcare delivery and public health strategies is crucial in mitigating future outbreaks and improving population health outcomes (Figure 15.19).

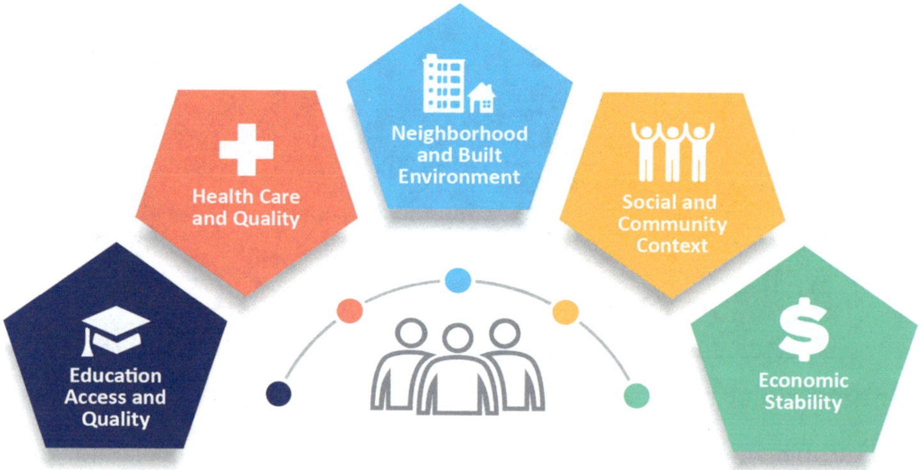

Figure 15.19. Socioeconomic and healthcare access of infectious disease control.

Source: https://www.cdc.gov/public-health-gateway/media/images/images/sdoh/SDOH-icons.png.

SUMMARY

In conclusion, the interplay between healthcare systems and infectious disease control is increasingly critical in a world marked by globalisation and interconnectivity. The fact that infectious diseases are increasing in Kenya and Uganda, which are neighbouring countries, highlights the importance of international cooperation in addressing these issues. The latest Mpox cases have shown that healthcare systems still have significant shortfalls in training, infrastructure, and communication. As mentioned, a study found that 75% of those surveyed agreed on the need to strengthen healthcare monitoring at border points to address new health issues. This collaboration not only fosters a more unified response to outbreaks but also enhances the overall resilience of healthcare systems facing infectious disease challenges (Peter, 2025).

Moreover, the successful application of innovative healthcare frameworks, such as Failure Mode and Effects Analysis (FMEA), presents promising avenues for improving infectious disease control strategies. FMEA helps identify where healthcare systems could fail, which helps spot weaknesses in IPC. By using this method, emergency readiness can be enhanced, processes can be streamlined, and patient safety can be improved in healthcare settings. It appears that FMEA is now being used more frequently to study healthcare processes related to infectious diseases, suggesting that people are turning to systematic risk assessment tools to enhance public health strategies. The literature reviewed highlights the need for ongoing research and the integration of such methods, ensuring that healthcare systems can adapt and evolve in response to emerging threats (Vecchia et al., 2025). Surveillance, teamwork among healthcare professionals, and innovative approaches are the key elements of a robust response to infectious diseases in healthcare systems. The issues identified in various healthcare settings suggest that for systems to function effectively, they must both operate independently and collaborate with others across borders. Stronger infrastructure, data sharing, and more training for healthcare staff play key roles in reducing the risks of infectious diseases. It is clear from this study that making healthcare systems stronger helps control diseases, improves community health, and prepares for future health disasters. A concerted effort towards these objectives will ensure that healthcare systems evolve in ways that prioritize safety and efficiency in the face of infectious disease challenges (Peter, 2025; Vecchia et al., 2025).

It is essential to understand how healthcare systems relate to infectious disease control in order to create effective ways to mitigate their impact. An issue is that HAIs are common, which may result in more cases of illness and death, and also put more pressure on healthcare finances. Regularly monitoring microbes in healthcare environments enables more effective and precise actions to control infections. The study detailed in Ackers et al. (2024) highlights the presence of *Staphylococcus* spp. on high-touch surfaces in a newly constructed hospital ward, emphasising the importance of rigorous cleaning protocols and ongoing environmental surveillance to combat HAIs and safeguard patient health. Additionally, it is crucial to understand how infectious diseases spread in order to take the right, timely, and effective public health actions. Accurate modelling of disease spread, as presented in the Generalised Compartmental Transmission Model (GCTM) discussed in Santosh et al. (2024), allows healthcare professionals to assess critical dependencies that influence infection rates, such as population density and demographic factors. The GCTM explains the different stages of disease transmission by using logistic growth equations. Thanks to such models, health officials can identify where outbreaks are likely to occur and develop plans to manage them by focusing on prevention and control. These studies suggest that a combination of methods is necessary in healthcare systems to effectively manage infectious diseases. Combining rigorous environmental monitoring, as illustrated in Ackers et al. (2024), with sophisticated modelling techniques discussed in Santosh et al. (2024) effectively enhances our capability to predict, prevent, and manage infectious outbreaks. The combined actions of healthcare workers, policymakers, and researchers are vital for better public health, which helps healthcare systems face infectious disease challenges. Addressing environmental issues and disease transmission helps create a setting that supports all aspects of healthcare.

CLOSER LOOK

K-NEAREST NEIGHBOURS (KNN)

K-Nearest Neighbours (KNN) is one of the simplest yet widely used algorithms in machine learning, particularly for classification and regression tasks. It is a type of instance-based or "lazy" learning method, meaning that it does not build an explicit model during the training phase. Instead, KNN stores the training data and makes predictions only when a new query point needs to be classified or estimated. Despite its simplicity, KNN is highly effective in scenarios where patterns in the data are locally consistent. The core idea of KNN is intuitive. To classify a new data point, the algorithm identifies the 'k' closest points in the training dataset based on a distance metric, commonly Euclidean distance for numerical data. The class most frequently represented among these neighbors is then assigned to the new point. For regression tasks, the prediction is typically the average or weighted average of the neighbors' values. Choosing an appropriate value for 'k' is critical: a small k may lead to overfitting and sensitivity to noise, while a large k may oversimplify the model and overlook local patterns.

Distance metrics play a central role in KNN performance. While Euclidean distance is standard for continuous features, other metrics such as Manhattan distance, Minkowski distance, or cosine similarity can be used depending on the data type and domain. Feature scaling is also essential because KNN is sensitive to differences in feature magnitude; unscaled features can dominate the distance calculation and distort predictions.

KNN offers several advantages. It is simple to understand and implement, requires no assumptions about data distribution, and can adapt naturally to multi-class problems. Additionally, it can handle non-linear decision boundaries because predictions are based on local neighborhoods rather than global models. However, KNN has limitations. It can be computationally expensive with large datasets, as distances must be calculated for all training points. It also struggles with high-dimensional data due to the "curse of dimensionality," where distance metrics become less meaningful. KNN is widely applied in various domains, including medical diagnosis, recommendation systems, image recognition, and anomaly detection. Its interpretability and straightforward mechanism make it an excellent choice for exploratory data analysis and baseline models.

In conclusion, K-Nearest Neighbours is a fundamental machine learning algorithm that relies on local similarity to make predictions. By carefully selecting parameters like 'k', choosing appropriate distance metrics, and preprocessing data correctly, KNN can provide reliable and intuitive results in both classification and regression problems, making it a valuable tool in the data scientist's toolkit.

REFERENCES

1. Dar, O. A., Hasan, R., Schlundt, J., Harbarth, S., Caleo, G., Dar, F. K., Littmann, J., Rweyemamu, M., Buckley, E. J., Shahid, M., Kock, R., Li, H. L., Giha, H., Khan, M., So, A. D., Bindayna, K. M., Kessel, A., Pedersen, H. B., Permanand, G., . . . Heymann, D. L. (2015d). Exploring the evidence base for national and regional policy interventions to combat resistance. *The Lancet, 387*(10015), 285–295. https://doi.org/10.1016/s0140-6736(15)00520-6Abiri, E., Raesi, R., & Kashani, M. H. Q. (2025). The role and position of non-pharmacological interventions (NPI) in the management and control of emerging and re-emerging infectious diseases in the post-COVID-19 era: A systematic review. *The Open Public Health Journal.* https://www.semanticscholar.org/paper/f04c687b0d79bfa2602875d90bcd1fbec60657fd (accessed on 30th May 2025).
2. Ackers, G., McLaughlin, D., Doyle, A., Lewis, J. M., Neal, T., Todd, S., Roberts, A. P., et al. (2024). Investigating the changing taxonomy and antimicrobial resistance of bacteria isolated from door handles in a new infectious disease ward pre- and post-patient admittance. *Microbiol. Spectr.* https://www.semanticscholar.org/paper/a4b99118f9c08b245c122ce385b1d3b9f1c0c6bc (accessed on 30th May 2025).
3. Ballif, M., Banholzer, N., Perrig, L., Avihingsanon, A., Nsonde, D. M., Obatsa, S., Muula, G., et al. (2025). The long-term impact of the COVID-19 pandemic on tuberculosis care and infection control measures in anti-retroviral therapy (ART) clinics in low- and middle-income countries: A multiregional site survey in Asia and Africa. *BMJ Global Health, 10.* https://www.semanticscholar.org/paper/616a75269aad85e7c5ba46d27e16b198028ac6b6 (accessed on 30th May 2025).
4. Chandra, V., Gaidhane, A., & Choudhari, S. G. (2024). Public health strategies in the face of crisis: A comprehensive review of the Zika outbreak in India. *Cureus, 16.* https://www.semanticscholar.org/paper/46371d00ded47b5d1497227c5d2d2285e0d62771 (accessed on 30th May 2025).
5. Chen, J. S., Hung, R. W., & Yang, C. Y. (2025). An efficient target-to-area classification strategy with a PIP-based KNN algorithm for epidemic management. *Mathematics.* https://www.semanticscholar.org/paper/e0989dd3928e847fcca1416e93a9385c6c34652d (accessed on 30th May 2025).
6. Cheng, K., Xu, Z., Zhang, Y., Chen, R., & Gui, L. (2025). Construction of an evaluation index system for hospital resilience to emerging infectious diseases: A Delphi study from China. *BMC Public Health, 25.* https://www.semanticscholar.org/paper/eef9f1d32ef8a668272c957213aaed43a52c7299 (accessed on 30th May 2025).
7. Clare, J., Lewis, M., Mackey, T., et al. (2016). The disease of corruption: Views on how to fight corruption to advance 21st century global health goals. BMC Medicine https://open.bu.edu/bitstream/2144/31130/1/mackey_disease.pdf (accessed on 30th May 2025).
8. Colavita, F., Lapa, D., Carletti, F., Lalle, E., Bordi, L., Marsella, P., Nicastri, E., et al. (2020). SARS-CoV-2 isolation from ocular secretions of a patient with COVID-19 in Italy with prolonged viral RNA detection. *Annals of Internal Medicine, 173,* 242, 243. https://doi.org/10.7326/m20-1176.
9. Crews, C., Angwaawie, P., Abdul-Mumin, A., Yabasin, I., Attivor, E., Dibato, J., & Coffee, M. (2024). Assessing ventilation through ambient carbon dioxide concentrations across multiple healthcare levels in Ghana. *PLOS Global Public Health, 4.* https://www.semanticscholar.org/paper/de949f72400b32a6e785920394df25ebeaf8171c (accessed on 30th May 2025).

10. Davies, J. C., & Lowe, A. (2025). *Environmental Implications of the Health Care Service Sector*. https://core.ac.uk/download/pdf/9307987.pdf (accessed on 30th May 2025).

11. Dewey, C. M., Hingle, S., Goelz, E., & Linzer, M. (2020). Supporting clinicians during the COVID-19 pandemic. *Annals of Internal Medicine, 172*, 752, 753. https://doi.org/10.7326/m20-1033.

12. Dopelt, K. (2025). Sustainable public health policies: Understanding influenza vaccination uptake among college students in a changing society. *World*. https://www.semanticscholar.org/paper/e29da93ce2f868ae43d0ddb04765fbd3b427a016 (accessed on 30th May 2025).

13. Enomoto, M., Iwata, H., & Iida, M. (1971). Past. *PS: Political Science & Politics, 4*, 89–92. https://www.semanticscholar.org/paper/bbc5d2d0cd3a49c8f6219050cd4ea6567585a25e (accessed on 30th May 2025).

14. Ferguson, E., Lugelo, A., Czupryna, A. M., Anderson, D., Lankester, F., Sikana, L., Dushoff, J., et al. (2024). Reducing spatial heterogeneity in coverage improves the effectiveness of dog vaccination campaigns against rabies. *bioRxiv*. https://www.semanticscholar.org/paper/d2204da32f70839070ea07fda8d1be237c72918d (accessed on 30th May 2025).

15. Forman, R., & Mossialos, E. (2021). The EU response to COVID-19: From reactive policies to strategic decision-making. *JCMS: Journal of Common Market Studies, 59*, 56–68. https://doi.org/10.1111/jcms.13259.

16. Gamon, M. (2013). *Multidrug-Resistant Tuberculosis in India: Solving a Problem by Reconstructing the Public Health Infrastructure*. https://core.ac.uk/download/67755957.pdf (accessed on 30th May 2025).

17. Ghosh, A., Castillo, Y., Garzon, A. D. N., Arriola, L., & Mubayi, A. (2024). COVID-19 transmission dynamics in close-contacts facilities: Optimizing control strategies. *Computational and Mathematical Biophysics*. https://www.semanticscholar.org/paper/97b7b49eddf01423db87563a80c4028bf4dfe961 (accessed on 30th May 2025).

18. Hagiya, H. (2024). Thoughts on and proposal for the education, training, and recruitment of infectious disease specialists. *Acta Medica Okayama, 78*(3), 205–213. https://www.semanticscholar.org/paper/ef0d4c8db4893a39fd26be62cdec059278d1a62d (accessed on 30th May 2025).

19. Harrison, A. G., Tao, L., & Wang, P. (2020). Mechanisms of SARS-CoV-2 transmission and pathogenesis. *Trends in Immunology, 41*, 1100–1115. https://doi.org/10.1016/j.it.2020.10.004.

20. Hsu, J. Y., Wu, U. I., Wang, J. T., Sheng, W. H., Chen, Y. C., & Chang, S. C. (2025). Managing *Helicobacter pylori* as an infectious disease: Implementation of antimicrobial stewardship. *Helicobacter, 30*(1), e70013. https://www.semanticscholar.org/paper/a6a8475303d838cdda86b1793dd997e2d16257a6 (accessed on 30th May 2025).

21. Ibrahim, N. A., Samosir, F. A. H. H., Putri, D. T., Sekarfitri, A. S., Reezal, A. I., & Putri, M. D. (2025). Fish bone analisis respon kesiapan sistem kesehatan di Indonesia terhadap penyakit pandemi: Sumber daya manusia, keuangan, pemerintah, dan informasi. *SCRIPTA SCORE Scientific Medical Journal*. https://www.semanticscholar.org/paper/931d8f7a084dc1880dd460d0be39a0a2820cb78a (accessed on 30th May 2025).

22. Ingelbeen, B., van Kleef, E., Mbala, P., Danis, K., Macicame, I., Hens, N., Cleynen, E., et al. (2025). Embedding risk monitoring in infectious disease surveillance for timely and effective outbreak prevention and control. *BMJ Global Health, 10*. https://www.semanticscholar.org/

paper/8bff2b8437c9dc2376609397095c4132b4071965 (accessed on 30th May 2025).

23. Kevat, D., Panaccio, D., Pang, S. C., Dean, J., Farmer, C. C., & Mahar, P. (2021). Medico-legal considerations of mandatory COVID-19 vaccination for high risk workers. *The Medical Journal of Australia, 215*, 22. https://doi.org/10.5694/mja2.51128.

24. Kokebayeva, G., Shildebai, S., & Smanova, A. (2024). Infectious disease epidemics in Kazakhstan in the 1900–1930s and their impact on healthcare development. *Pertanika Journal of Social Sciences and Humanities*. https://www.semanticscholar.org/paper/b05ec9b3f4cc0b438143308eca7d952b7755a35a (accessed on 30th May 2025).

25. Kostyrin, E., & Loua, M. P. (2025). Econometric model of infectious disease management in Africa. *Ekonomika i Upravlenie: Problemy, Resheniya*. https://www.semanticscholar.org/paper/c37a358ec48ef9cd214ab6347ad28e6bd1efce63 (accessed on 30th May 2025).

26. Lippi, G., Henry, B., & Mattiuzzi, C. (2025). The crucial role of laboratory medicine in addressing future public health infectious threats: Insights gained from the COVID-19 pandemic. *Diagnostics, 15*. https://www.semanticscholar.org/paper/d00e97f9e8624cc05b84972fa7477095cff4f3d4 (accessed on 30th May 2025).

27. Mothilal, T., Aluvala, S., Paranthaman, V., & Socrates, S. (2023). Artificial neural network-driven healthcare resource management for improved outcomes in infectious disease control. *2023 IEEE International Conference on ICT in Business Industry & Government (ICTBIG)*. https://www.semanticscholar.org/paper/67c335fcd9ae3111f222236a447e3997f3936306 (accessed on 30th May 2025).

28. Murray, C. J. L., Ikuta, K. S., Sharara, F., Swetschinski, L. R., Robles, A. G., Gray, A. P., Han, C., et al. (2022). Global burden of bacterial antimicrobial resistance in 2019: A systematic analysis. *The Lancet, 399*, 629–655. https://doi.org/10.1016/s0140-6736(21)02724-0.

29. N/A. (2025). *National Center for Preparedness, Detection, and Control of Infectious Diseases (CVK)*. https://core.ac.uk/download/144193641.pdf (accessed on 30th May 2025).

30. Narain, K., Rackimuthu, S., Nawaz, F., Okonji, O. C., Ashworth, H., Du Plessis, S. D., Shah, J. (2022). Strategies for malaria vaccination during the COVID-19 pandemic in African countries. *Bulletin of the World Health Organization, 100*, 582–582A. https://www.semanticscholar.org/paper/74f9db384b2b2a0951d4fb384a85c3a6003f3b59 (accessed on 30th May 2025).

31. Nkengasong, J. N., & Tessema, S. K. (2020). Africa needs a new public health order to tackle infectious disease threats. *Cell, 183*, 296–300. https://doi.org/10.1016/j.cell.2020.09.041.

32. Ogbonna, P. C., Oparaocha, E., & Anyanwu, E. C. (2024). Water, sanitation and hygiene services in healthcare facilities in Bayelsa State Nigeria: A primordial prevention strategy for infectious disease control. *Med Discoveries*. https://www.semanticscholar.org/paper/ef3116f89999f0a089bb89e21f104320bac26d34 (accessed on 30th May 2025).

33. Omotayo, O., Maduka, C. P., Muonde, M., Olorunsogo, T. O., & Ogugua, J. O. (2024). The rise of non-communicable diseases: A global health review of challenges and prevention strategies. *International Medical Science Research Journal*. https://www.semanticscholar.org/paper/026b8695b8e5552cf2704c4921324c8b801095ac (accessed on 30th May 2025).

34. Onyebuchi, C., Okeke, H. N., Uzochukwu, O. H., Racheal, A. O., Kolade, E., Onyebuchi, A. O., Odekhe, E., et al. (2025). Emerging infectious diseases and global response strategies: A systematic review and meta-analysis. *International Journal of Research and Scientific Innovation*.

https://www.semanticscholar.org/paper/278b7b6b2a3f4bbe997310e0677c4c9cbf456442 (accessed on 30th May 2025).

35. Palla, U., & Iwunwa, M. G. (2025). Leveraging predictive models to enhance infection control and reduce cross-contamination in public health settings. *International Journal of Research Publication and Reviews*. https://www.semanticscholar.org/paper/471be7429ec568067fea0cc7a399c7db7d75d031 (accessed on 30th May 2025).

36. Peter, W. W. (2025). Cross-border healthcare collaboration and surveillance systems for MPOX control between Kenya and Uganda: A case study of Busia County. *International Journal of Innovative Science and Research Technology*. https://www.semanticscholar.org/paper/227862fe1aaac787cc2903f8a1af3f2b8cea5de3 (accessed on 30th May 2025).

37. Prajapati, R. N., Bhushan, B., Singh, K., Chopra, H., Kumar, S., Agrawal, M., Pathak, D., et al. (2024). Recent advances in pharmaceutical design: Unleashing the potential of novel therapeutics. *Current Pharmaceutical Biotechnology*. https://www.semanticscholar.org/paper/1b52ec250292988718ad39438dc8f92e26af0c62 (accessed on 30th May 2025).

38. Pyo, J., Jeong, J., Jeong, H., & Ock, M. (2025). Exploring the experiences of managers and practitioners in infectious disease management organizations during the COVID-19 response: A qualitative study. *Journal of Korean Medical Science, 40*(16), e58. https://www.semanticscholar.org/paper/5a4eec043b6295700b3253fae7961fec3505481c (accessed on 30th May 2025).

39. Qazi, S., Fox, M. P., & Thea, D. (2014). Editorial commentary: Ambulatory management of chest-indrawing pneumonia. *Clinical Infectious Diseases: An Official Publication of the Infectious Diseases Society of America, 60*, 1225–1227. https://www.semanticscholar.org/paper/37b0ae70f0d392011288dd87604e037717f43653 (accessed on 30th May 2025).

40. Rashid, S., Bariq, A., Ali, I., Sultana, S., Siddiqa, A., & Elagan, S. K. (2025). Dynamic analysis and optimal control of a hybrid fractional monkeypox disease model in terms of external factors. *Scientific Reports, 15*. https://www.semanticscholar.org/paper/400c7281a49d87da223015dc8d5043344818dcac (accessed on 30th May 2025).

41. Rinjani, E. Z. V., Briawan, D., & Kustiyah, L. (2024). Ecological analysis of infectious diseases, healthcare access, and socioeconomic factors on stunting prevalence in West Sumatra, Indonesia. *AcTion: Aceh Nutrition Journal*. https://www.semanticscholar.org/paper/500185747e107b3f8b85784fe277ab2ea1e616e9 (accessed on 30th May 2025).

42. Santosh, C. J., & Shakya, A. (2024). Understanding infectious disease transmission: A generalized compartmental transmission model (GCTM) approach. *ShodhKosh: Journal of Visual and Performing Arts*. https://www.semanticscholar.org/paper/c14cf740dea59e86d429af9b454218cf4f369dc3 (accessed on 30th May 2025).

43. Seitzinger, P., Rafid-Hamed, Z., & Kalra, J. (2024). Artificial intelligence for cluster detection and targeted intervention in healthcare: An interdisciplinary system approach. *Artificial Intelligence and Social Computing*. https://www.semanticscholar.org/paper/f09d32a7fba1e82b229c7ce0983c821d96ee79f2 (accessed on 30th May 2025).

44. Sultana, M., Perves, N., Uddin, N., Chowdhury, M. E. E., & Amin, N. (2024). The vicious impact of antimicrobial resistance on global public health security and the role of healthcare systems and policy in combating AMR. *World Journal of Public Health*. https://www.semanticscholar.org/paper/67a094fc5755c7be7d117f710d5c385bf9f890d4 (accessed on 30th May 2025).

45. Ugwu, D., Amofah, A. D., & Kaiser, F. (2025). Enhancing the detection and response to infectious disease outbreaks. *International Medical Science Research Journal*. https://www.semanticscholar.org/paper/9ed5c7395e56eb4df0cc1b1ef0a37546c5a116fc (accessed on 30th May 2025).
46. Umutoni, B., Tumushime, J. C., Hewins, B., Udahemuka, J. C., Ndishimye, P., Kelvin, D. J., Martinez, G. S., et al. (2024). The impact of public transportation on the transmission of COVID-19 in Rwanda. *Frontiers in Public Health, 12*. https://www.semanticscholar.org/paper/6df5dfced7f9420421d4c6d1cfa873227adee720 (accessed on 30th May 2025).
47. Vecchia, M., Sacchi, P., Marvulli, L. N., Ragazzoni, L., Muzzi, A., Polo, L., Bruno, R., et al. (2025). Healthcare application of failure mode and effect analysis (FMEA): Is there room in the infectious disease setting? A scoping review. *Healthcare, 13*. https://www.semanticscholar.org/paper/1ea112a3e1448879654b74c91202a000f96d718c (accessed on 30th May 2025).
48. Verulava, T., & Jorbenadze, A. (2022). Development of public health in independent Georgia. *Economics and Business*. https://www.semanticscholar.org/paper/0db7a1f9c631b23a07e7820bea02ba27bd80f317 (accessed on 30th May 2025).
49. Zhang, H., Honerlaw, J., Maripuri, M., Samayamuthu, M., Beaulieu-Jones, B., Baig, H., L'Yi, S., et al. (2023). *Characterizing the Use of the ICD-10 Code for Long COVID in 3 US Healthcare Systems*. https://www.semanticscholar.org/paper/6251d6a429c23cdbb64a10c34a73f1c16d3bbc7b (accessed on 30th May 2025).

INDEX

E

F

G

H

I

L

M

N

O

P